WORLD HEALTH ORGANIZATION

INTERNATIONAL AGENCY FOR RESEARCH ON CANCER

NASOPHARYNGEAL CARCINOMA: ETIOLOGY AND CONTROL

Proceedings of an International Symposium jointly supported by IARC, the National Cancer Institute (USA) and the Japan Society for the Promotion of Science and help in Kyoto, Japan, 4-6 April 1977

EDITORS

G. de-THÉ

Y. ITO

TECHNICAL EDITOR FOR IARC

W. DAVIS

IARC Scientific Publications No. 20

INTERNATIONAL AGENCY FOR RESEARCH ON CANCER

LYON

1978

The International Agency for Research on Cancer (IARC) was established in 1965 by the World Health Assembly as an independently financed organization within the framework of the World Health Organization. The headquarters of the Agency are at Lyon, France, and it has Research Centres in Iran, Kenya and Singapore.

The Agency conducts a programme of research concentrating particularly on the epidemiology of cancer and the study of potential carcinogens in the human environment. Its field studies are supplemented by biological and chemical research carried out in the Agency's laboratories in Lyon and through collaborative research agreements, in national research institutions in many countries. The Agency also conducts a programme for the education and training of personnel for cancer research.

The publications of the Agency are intended to contribute to the dissemination of authoritative information on different aspects of cancer research.

ISBN 92 832 11200

The authors alone are responsible for the views expressed in the signed articles in this publication.

PRINTED IN SWITZERLAND

CONTENTS

Foreword ix

Introduction xi

Participants xiii

PATHOLOGY OF NASOPHARYNGEAL CARCINOMA

Histological typing of nasopharyngeal carcinoma
K. Shanmugaratnam 3

Histological types of nasopharyngeal carcinoma in an intermediate risk area
M. Cammoun, R. Ellouz, J. Behi & R. Ben Attia 13

Histopathological types of nasopharyngeal carcinoma in a low-risk area: Japan
H. Sugano, S. Sawaki, G. Sakamoto & T. Hirayama 27

The histopathological spectrum of nasopharyngeal carcinoma
L.H. Weiland 41

Diagnosis and differential diagnosis of lymphoepithelial carcinoma in lymph nodes: histological, cytological and electron-microscopic findings
K. Lennert, E. Kaiserling & T. Mazzanti 51

A histopathological study of lymphoid tissue reaction to metastatic nasopharyngeal carcinoma in nude mice
H.-C. Chen, A. Kawamura, Jr, M. Murata, K. Hamajima & M. Osono 65

Animal models for nasopharyngeal carcinoma
D.V. Ablashi, J.M. Easton & R. Glaser 85

Discussion Summary - M. CAMMOUN 95

CLINICAL ASPECTS OF NASOPHARYNGEAL CARCINOMA

Stage classification of nasopharyngeal carcinoma: A review
J.H.C. Ho 99

Nasopharyngeal carcinoma in children and adolescents in Tunisia: Clinical aspects and the paraneoplastic syndrome
R. Ellouz, M. Cammoun, R. Ben Attia & J. Bahi 115

Clinical aspects and natural history of nasopharyngeal carcinoma in Western Europe
Y. Cachin, H. Sancho-Garnier, G. Schwaab, P. Marandas . . 131

Analytical aspects of symptoms of nasopharyngeal malignancies
S. Sawaki, H. Sugano & T. Hirayama 147

EPIDEMIOLOGY OF NASOPHARYNGEAL CARCINOMA

Descriptive and analytical epidemiology of nasopharyngeal cancer
T. Hirayama 167

Variations in nasopharyngeal cancer incidence among specific Chinese communities (dialect groups) in Singapore
K. Shanmugaratnam 191

Etiological factors in nasopharyngeal carcinoma: A hospital-based, retrospective, case-control, questionnaire study
K. Shanmugaratnam, C.Y. Tye, E.H. Goh & K.B. Chia 199

Environmental factors in the etiology of nasopharyngeal carcinoma: Report on a case-control study in Hong Kong
A. Geser, N. Charnay, N.E. Day, H.C. Ho & G. de-Thé . . . 213

Environmental backgrounds of young Chinese nasopharyngeal carcinoma patients
E.N. Anderson, Jr, M.L. Anderson & H.C. Ho 231

Epidemiology of malignant tumours of the nasopharynx in France: Retrospective and prospective studies
J. Brugère, H. Sancho-Garnier, D. Point & G. Schwaab . . 241

Discussion of risk factors for nasopharyngeal carcinoma
B.E. Henderson & E. Louie 251

ETIOLOGY OF NASOPHARYNGEAL CARCINOMA - GENETIC AND CHEMICAL FACTORS

HLA frequencies in cancer: A third study
S.T. Perdue, P.I. Terasaki & M.R. Mickey 263

Nasopharyngeal carcinoma and histocompatibility antigens
M.J. Simons, S.H. Chan, G.B. Wee, K. Shanmugaratnam, E.H. Goh, J.H.C. Ho, J.C.W. Chau, S. Darmalingam, U. Prasad, H. Betuel, N.E. Day & G. de-Thé 271

Genetic components in susceptibility to nasopharyngeal carcinoma
R.L. Kirk, N.M. Blake, S. Serjeantson, M.J. Simons & S.H. Chan 283

Cytogenetic observations on the malignant epithelial cells and infiltrating lymphocytes of nasopharyngeal carcinoma
J.E. Jarvis, S. Finerty, M.A. Epstein, P.A. Trumper, G. Ball & B.C. Giovanella 299

Analysis for volatile nitrosamines in salt-preserved foodstuffs traditionally consumed by Southern Chinese
D.P. Huang, T.A. Gough & J.H.C. Ho 309

Carcinoma of the nasal and paranasal regions in rats fed Cantonese salted marine fish
D.P. Huang, D. Saw, T.B. Teoh, J.H.C. Ho 315

Discussion Summary - N.E. DAY 329

ETIOLOGY OF NASOPHARYNGEAL CARCINOMA - VIROLOGICAL FACTORS

Epstein-Barr virus - Discovery, properties and relationship to nasopharyngeal carcinoma
M.A. Epstein 333

The association between undifferentiated nasopharyngeal carcinoma and Epstein-Barr virus shown by correlated nucleic acid hybridization and histopathological studies
M. Andersson-Anvret, N. Forsby, G. Klein & W. Henle 347

Morphological transformation of nasopharyngeal epithelial cells *in vitro* by Epstein-Barr virus from B95-8 cells
D.P. Huang, J.H.C. Ho & M.H. Ng 359

Epstein-Barr virus-regulation studies on somatic-cell hybrids derived from the fusion of Burkitt's lymphoma and nasopharyngeal carcinoma cells with human or mouse partners
G. Klein 369

Epstein-Barr virus epithelial cell interaction and its implication in the etiology of nasopharyngeal carcinoma
G. Lenoir & G. de-Thé 377

Early and late components of Epstein-Barr virus-associated membrane antigen in superinfected Daudi cells and their reactivity with sera from nasopharyngeal carcinoma patients
Y. Hinuma, T. Sairenji & M. Maeda 385

Heterogeneity of Epstein-Barr virus derived from P3HR-1 cells
H. zur Hausen & K.-O. Fresen 391

Expression of latent Epstein-Barr virus genomes in human epithelial/Burkitt's lymphoblastoid hybrid cells
M. Nonoyama, A. Tanaka & R. Glaser 397

Detection and quantitation of adenovirus type 12 transforming DNA segments and their application in etiological studies of human neoplasia
K. Fujinaga, S. Yano, S. Ojima & Y. Sawada 403

Interaction between Epstein-Barr virus and type-C virus in human cells
T. Osato, K. Yamamoto, T. Matsuo, T. Aya, F. Mizuno & M. Nonoyama 413

Discussion Summaries - W. HENLE 421

ETIOLOGY OF NASOPHARYNGEAL CARCINOMA - IMMUNOLOGICAL FACTORS

Epstein-Barr virus-related serology in nasopharyngeal carcinoma and controls
W. Henle, G. Henle & J.H.C. Ho 427

Clinical evaluation of EBV serology in American patients with nasopharyngeal carcinoma
G.R. Pearson, H.L. Coates, H.B. Neel III, P. Levine, D. Ablashi & J. Easton 439

The genetic and antigenic basis for the IgA antibody response to Epstein-Barr viral capsid antigen
M.H. Ng, H.C. Ho & H.C. Kwan 449

Presence of Epstein-Barr virus specific IgA in saliva of nasopharyngeal carcinoma patients: their activity, origin and possible clinical value
C. Desgranges & G. de-Thé 459

Differences in EBV-antibody titres of patients with nasopharyngeal carcinoma originating from high, intermediate and low incidence areas
G. de-Thé, M.F. Lavoué & L. Muenz 471

Cell-mediated immunity, Epstein-Barr virus and nasopharyngeal carcinoma
P.H. Levine, J.-P. Lamelin & D.A. Stevens 483

General immunological status of nasopharyngeal carcinoma patients in Singapore
S.H. Chan, E.H. Goh, T.H. Khor & T.S. Chew 495

Effect of levamisole on cell-mediated immune responses in patients with nasopharyngeal carcinoma
E.H. Goh, S.H. Chan & M.J. Simons 503

Changes in T-cell subsets and their clinical significance in cancer patients
J. Yata, T. Shimbo & S. Sawaki 511

Autoantibodies (cold lymphocytotoxins, antiactin antibodies and antinuclear factors) in nasopharyngeal carcinoma patients
J.-P. Lamelin, J.P. Revillard, G. Gabbiani & G. de-Thé . . 523

Discussion Summary - T. TACHIBANA 537

PRESENT CONCEPTS ON TREATMENT AND CURRENT CLINICAL RESEARCH

In vivo cell-mediated immunity in Chinese patients with nasopharyngeal carcinoma
J.H.C. Ho, J.C.W. Chau, K.C. Tse, M.H. Ng & P.H. Levine . 545

Clinical evaluation of cytological diagnosis of nasopharyngeal malignancies
R. Molinari, S. Pilotti & F. Rilke 553

European Organization for Research on Treatment of Cancer (E.O.R.T.C.) controlled trials of chemotherapy as an adjuvant or palliative treatment of nasopharyngeal carcinoma
R. Molinari 565

Use of immunological studies in evaluating the clinical course of nasopharyngeal carcinoma
S. Sawaki, A. Kawamura, Jr & T. Tachibana 575

Discussion Summary - R.A. MANAKER 587

RECOMMENDATIONS

Histopathological classification 593

Clinical staging 594

Epidemiology 597

Genetics 599

Virology 601

Immunology 603

Histological classification of tumours of the nasopharynx recommended by World Health Organization 605

INDEX OF AUTHORS 609

FOREWORD

I am frequently asked about the progress being made in cancer research. In this volume we have an opportunity to review the information available today and to compare it with that presented at the first symposium on nasopharyngeal carcinoma held in 1964 in Singapore[1]*, and organized by Professor K. Shanmugaratnam and Dr C.S. Muir, under the auspices of the International Union Against Cancer.*

At that time, emphasis was laid on the possibility that inhaled chemicals were the potential causes. Although the role of viruses and especially adenoviruses was considered, the results were negative, and no mention was made of Epstein-Barr virus. The 1964 meeting agreed that racial susceptibility was an important factor, but no objective criteria were identified, and the risk attributable to such susceptibility remained uncertain. There was no discussion about the role of immunological factors in the disease.

The present volume shows that scientists now accept the need to utilize a multidisciplinary approach in investigating human cancer. It is further obvious that laboratory scientists are learning from epidemiologists and vice versa.

A series of papers are included that further implicate the Epstein-Barr virus as a cause of nasopharyngeal cancer. Several papers emphasize the importance of the role that immunological factors may play in the course of this disease. It appears to me that the exact role of the Epstein-Barr virus in nasopharyngeal cancer remains to be clarified, and I still feel that the Scottish verdict of 'non-proven' is apt. It is thus very important that during the next few years we answer definitively the question posed by Professor Shanmugaratnam whether or not cancers of the nasopharynx which do not contain the viral genome are true nasopharyngeal carcinomas but unrelated to the Epstein-Barr virus. It is possible that not all nasopharyngeal carcinomas are related to Epstein-Barr virus but that other etiological factors are involved in some of them. The role of racial susceptibility now seems to be more widely accepted, and important new data expressing such susceptibility in objective immunological terms have been presented. Lastly, although no satisfactory animal model has

---

[1] Muir, C.S. & Shanmugaratnam, K., ed. (1967) *Cancer of the Nasopharynx, UICC Monograph Series*, Vol. 1, Copenhagen, Munksgaard

yet been developed to simulate nasopharyngeal carcinoma there have been real advances in the study of Epstein-Barr virus in different primates.

To sum up, considerable progress has been made since the last meeting; new problems and hypotheses have been identified. It is essential that these be examined and that more sophisticated techniques for the epidemiological study of viruses be developed. Large-scale human studies are expensive and should be based on clearcut hypotheses; this has been the case in the excellent studies already carried out to date. Close collaboration between viral oncologists and epidemiologists would appear to offer considerable possibilities for future research, and it is my hope that the Agency will continue to play a major role in these developments.

In conclusion, I want to express my thanks on behalf of the Agency to all those who contributed scientifically and financially to the realization of the Symposium from which this volume has resulted, and in particular to thank the Japan Society for the Promotion of Science and the National Cancer Institute (USA) Virus Cancer Program for their support.

John HIGGINSON, M.D.

Director

International Agency
for Research on Cancer,
Lyon, France

INTRODUCTION

Few human tumours have yielded so much new and unexpected data in studies over the last ten years as nasopharyngeal carcinoma. This epithelial tumour of the upper respiratory tract, displays very large differences in incidence rate around the world - up to one hundred fold - and was assumed to be caused by an exogenous agent that, for example, affected the Chinese population in Singapore but spared the Indians and Pakistanis there. To date, however, no chemical carcinogen has been clearly associated with nasopharyngeal carcinoma but genetic factors and the Epstein-Barr virus are suspected of playing a role in its development. Proof that this role is etiological are still being sought, and the purpose of this book is to review and evaluate the available data on the pathological, clinical, and epidemiological characterization of nasopharyngeal carcinoma and to consider the possible etiological factors - genetic, viral and chemical - and the strength of their association with nasopharyngeal carcinoma.

Clinicians, pathologists, epidemiologists, immunologists, virologists, and molecular virologists have contributed to the present volume based on the proceedings of a symposium held in Kyoto, Japan. Specific agreements were reached on clinical staging, on pathological classification, and on their systematic use in joint clinico-experimental studies.

Recommendations that should help to conduct future studies aimed at controlling nasopharyngeal carcinoma were prepared by sub-groups. It is clear that the control of cancer may come before its etiology is known, and Epstein-Barr virus serology could help the management of nasopharyngeal carcinoma, whether or not the virus is an etiological factor. However, prevention, the ultimate goal of cancer research, will depend on knowledge of etiological factors, and multidisciplinary studies directed to this goal must remain the most important task of those involved in research on nasopharyngeal carcinoma.

G. de-Thé

Y. Ito

PARTICIPANTS

D.V. ABLASHI	National Cancer Institute, National Institutes of Health, Bethesda, Maryland 20014, USA
J. BRUGERE	Fondation Curie, 26 rue d'Ulm, 75231 Paris, Cédex 5, France
Y. CACHIN	Institut Gustave-Roussy, 16bis Avenue P. Vaillant-Couturier, 94800 Villejuif, France
M. CAMMOUN	Institut Salah Azaiz, Bab Saadoun, Tunis Tunisia
B. CERCEK	Paterson Laboratories, Christie Hospital & Holt Radium Institute, Manchester M20 9BX, UK
L. CERCEK	Paterson Laboratories, Christie Hospital & Holt Radium Institute, Manchester M20 9BX, UK
S.H. CHAN	WHO Immunology Research and Training Centre, Faculty of Medicine, University of Singapore, McAlister Road, Singapore 3
C.W. CHAU	Medical and Health Department Institute of Radiology, Queen Elizabeth Hospital, Kowloon, Hong Kong
N.E. DAY	International Agency for Research on Cancer, 150 cours Albert Thomas, 69372 Lyon, Cédex 2, France
G. DE-THE	International Agency for Research on Cancer, 150 cours Albert Thomas, 69372 Lyon, Cédex 2, France
R. ELLOUZ	Institut Salah Azaiz, Bab Saadoun, Tunis, Tunisia

M.A. EPSTEIN	Department of Pathology, University of Bristol, Medical School, Bristol BS8 1TD, UK
K. FUJINAGA	Department of Molecular Biology, Sapporo Medical College, Cancer Research Institute, S1 W17 Chuo-ku, Sapporo 060, Japan
N. FUKUZUMI	Institute of Medical Science, University of Tokyo, Minato-ku, Tokyo 108, Japan
A. GESER	International Agency for Research on Cancer, 150 cours Albert Thomas, 69372 Lyon, Cédex 2, France
E.H. GOH	Singapore General Hospital, Singapore
B.E. HENDERSON	University of Southern California, 2025 Zonal Avenue, Los Angeles, California 90033, USA
G. HENLE	University of Pennsylvania, Children's Hospital of Philadelphia, 34th Street, Civic Centre Bd, Philadelphia, Pennsylvania 19104, USA
W. HENLE	University of Pennsylvania, Children's Hospital of Philadelphia, 34th Street, Civic Centre Bd, Philadelphia, Pennsylvania 19104, USA
J. HIGGINSON	International Agency for Research on Cancer, 150 cours Albert Thomas, 69372 Lyon, Cédex 2, France
Y. HINUMA	Kumamoto University, Medical School, Kumamoto 860, Japan
T. HIRAYAMA	National Cancer Centre, Research Institute, Tsukiji 5, Chuo-ku, Tokyo, Japan
J.H.C. HO	Medical and Health Department Institute of Radiology and Oncology, Queen Elizabeth Hospital, Kowloon, Hong Kong
M.M. HSU	National Taiwan University Hospital, 1 Chang-Te Street, T'aipei, Taiwan
D.P. HUANG	Medical and Health Department Institute of Radiology and Oncology, Queen Elizabeth Hospital, Kowloon, Hong Kong

Y. IKAWA	Cancer Institute, 1-37-1 kami-ikebukuro, Toshima-ku, Tokyo 170, Japan
Y. ITO	Department of Microbiology, Faculty of Medicine, University of Kyoto, Kyoto, Japan
A. KAWAMURA	Institute of Medical Science, University of Tokyo, Minato-ku, Tokyo 108, Japan
G. KLEIN	Karolinska Institute, Department of Tumor Biology, S-104 01 Stockholm 60, Sweden
J.-P. LAMELIN	International Agency for Research on Cancer, 150 cours Albert Thomas, 69372 Lyon, Cédex 2, France
K. LENNERT	Institut für Pathology, Hospitalstrasse 42, 23 Kiel, Federal Republic of Germany
G. LENOIR	International Agency for Research on Cancer, 150 cours Albert-Thomas, 69372 Lyon, Cédex 2, France
T.M. LIN	National Taiwan University, College of Medicine, T'aipei, Taiwan
R.A. MANAKER	National Cancer Institute, Laboratory of DNA Tumor Viruses, Bethesda, Maryland 20014, USA
C. MICHEAU	Institut Gustave-Roussy, Département d'Anatomie Pathologique, 16bis Avenue P. Vaillant-Couturier, 94800 Villejuif, France
J.F. MILLER	Walter & Elisa Hall Institute, Royal Melbourne Hospital, Melbourne 3050, Australia
H. MITSUI	Tokyo Metropolitan Institute of Medical Science, Honkomagome 3-18-22, Bunkyoku, Tokyo, Japan
R. MOLINARI	National Cancer Institute, Head and Neck Department, Via Venezian 1, 20133 Milano, Italy
J.B. MOLONEY	National Cancer Institute, National Institutes of Health, Bethesda, Maryland 20014, USA

M.H. NG	Department of Microbiology, Faculty of Medicine, University of Hong Kong, Pathology Building, Queen Mary Hospital Compound, Hong Kong
K. NISHIOKA	Tokyo Metropolitan Institute of Medical Science, Honkomagome 3-18-22, Bunkyoku, Tokyo, Japan
M. NONOYAMA	Life Sciences Inc., Department of Molecular Virology, 2900 72nd Street North, St Petersburg, Florida 33710, USA
T. OSATO	Hokkaido University, Cancer Institute, Department of Virology, Sapporo N15 W7, Japan
G. PEARSON	Mayo Clinic, Rochester, Minnesota 55910, USA
Y.F. POON	Medical and Health Department Institute of Radiology and Oncology, Queen Elizabeth Hospital, Kowloon, Hong Kong
U. PRASAD	Medical Faculty, University of Malaysia, Kuala-Lumpur, Malaysia
D. SAW	Medical and Health Department Institute of Radiology and Oncology, Clinical Pathology Unit, Queen Elizabeth Hospital, Kowloon, Hong Kong
S. SAWAKI	Yokohama City University, School of Medicine, 3-46 Urafune, Minami-ku, Yokohama, Japan
K. SHANMUGARATNAM	University of Singapore, Department of Pathology, Outram Road, Singapore 3
M.J. SIMONS	Immuno-Diagnostic Centre, P.O. Box 4558, Melbourne 3001, Australia
N.F. STANLEY	Perth Medical Centre, University of Western Australia, Department of Microbiology, Perth, Western Australia 6000
D.A. STEVENS	Stanford University, Santa Clara Valley Medical Centre, 751 South Bascom Avenue, San Jose, California 95128, USA
H. SUGANO	Cancer Institute, 1-37-1 Kami-Ikebukuro, Toshima-ku, Tokyo 170, Japan

T. TACHIBANA — Research Institute for T.B. Leprosy and Cancer, Tohoku University, Department of Immunology, 4-12 Hirose-machi, Sendai, Japan

P. TERASAKI — University of California, Department of Surgery and Biomathematics, School of Medicine, Los Angeles, California 90024, USA

L.H. WEILAND — Mayo Clinic, Rochester, Minnesota 55901, USA

T. YAMAMOTO — Institute of Medical Science, University of Tokyo, Minato-ku, Tokyo 108, Japan

J. YATA — Toho University, Department of Pediatrics, 6-11-1, Omorinishi, Otaku, Tokyo, Japan

T.O. YOSHIDA — Hamamatsu University, Department of Microbiology, School of Medicine, 3600 Handa, Hamamatsu, Japan

H. ZUR HAUSEN — Institut für Virologie, Zentrum für Hygiene, Universität Freiburg, 78 Freiburg, Federal Republic of Germany

PATHOLOGY OF NASOPHARYNGEAL CARCINOMA

HISTOLOGICAL TYPING OF NASOPHARYNGEAL CARCINOMA

K. SHANMUGARATNAM

Department of Pathology,
University of Singapore,
Outram Road,
Singapore 3, Singapore

Nasopharyngeal carcinoma (NPC) has several distinctive epidemiological and biological features, but its classification, like that of other forms of cancer, is based only on its topography and histopathology. Like other tumours, its histological appearance varies. It is one of the objectives of this conference to examine whether correlations can be made between such variations and those observed in its epidemiological and biological behaviour.

TYPES OF NASOPHARYNGEAL CANCER AND THEIR RELATIVE FREQUENCIES

Many different types of cancer may arise in the nasopharynx, which correspond to the variety of normal tissue elements that exists in this area. Although the relative proportions of tumour types have been found to vary in different countries, it is evident that the most common form of nasopharyngeal cancer in man, regardless of geography or race, is NPC: the ratio of NPC to other forms of nasopharyngeal cancer is highest in countries with a high incidence of these cancers; it is this tumour that is essentially responsible for variations in the incidence of nasopharyngeal cancer. The report of a high incidence of nasopharyngeal lymphoma in Japan, 15.8% of nasopharyngeal malignancies (Sawaki et al., 1976), should be investigated further. An exceptionally high frequency of lymphomas (67 of 312 histologically confirmed cases) was reported in London by Lederman (1967), but this was almost certainly due to the author's method of classifying tumours: many of the tumours in his series appear to have been classified as lymphomas on the basis of their response to radiotherapy rather than on the basis of their histological appearance.

Histological examination of nasopharyngeal biopsies generally allows a clear separation of NPC from other types of malignancies. Difficulties may arise in the identification of a small proportion of highly undifferentiated NPCs that have lost their epithelioid features or of those whose appearances are complicated by artefactual traumatic distortion; these can be mistaken for lymphomas or sarcomas by persons with no particular experience with this neoplasm. Differences in pathological diagnoses are sometimes due to sampling variations; when multiple biopsies are taken, only some may contain tumour tissue. Furthermore, tissue specimens taken for other purposes, and alternatively frozen and thawed before fixation, are seldom suitable for histopathological evaluation in difficult cases.

HISTOGENESIS OF NASOPHARYNGEAL CARCINOMA

NPC arises from the squamous or respiratory epithelium lining the surface and crypts of the nasopharynx. The histological features are unquestionably those of a malignant epithelial tumour: the continuity of the tumour with the epithelium lining the surfaces and crypts of the nasopharynx, the structural pattern of fairly well-defined masses of tumour cells and the presence of varying degrees of keratinization in a proportion of cases. The epithelial nature of the tumour has been further demonstrated by the electron microscopic finding of desmosomes and cytoplasmic fibrils in most tumours. The clinical features and mode of spread are those of a carcinoma. There have, indeed, been virtually no accounts in the medical literature during the last 30 years, with the solitary exception of that of Lederman (1967), in which the epithelial nature of the tumour has been questioned.

Recognition of the tumour as a carcinoma does not, however, deny the existence of distinctive histological features, which are related to the characteristics of the epithelium from which the tumour arises. The nasopharyngeal epithelium is endodermal and branchiogenic in derivation. It is, for the most part, a respiratory-type, non-keratinizing epithelium without intercellular bridges, although foci of squamous metaplasia may occur. It is intimately related to lymphocytes, which occur in abundance in this region. Consequently, although some NPCs may be indistinguishable from squamous-cell carcinomas arising at other sites, many tumours and their metastases display cytological and structural features which allow a presumptive diagnosis of NPC.

HISTOLOGICAL CLASSIFICATION OF NASOPHARYNGEAL CARCINOMA

Disagreement among pathologists over the classification of NPC into histological sub-types is long-standing and has been acrimonious. Some have used two broad categories - squamous or undifferentiated and keratinizing or non-keratinizing; others have divided them into a variety of sub-types. There have been variations in diagnostic criteria - some have classified tumours as 'squamous' only when they are obviously keratinizing; others have used this term for tumours with no more than a doubtful suggestion of squamous differentiation. There have been variations in terminology - the terms 'undifferentiated carcinoma', 'undifferentiated carcinoma of nasopharyngeal type', 'non-keratinizing carcinoma', 'transitional-cell carcinoma' and 'anaplastic carcinoma' have all been used for the poorly differentiated carcinomas that occur commonly in this region (Shanmugaratnam & Muir, 1967). Some have restricted use of the term 'lymphoepithelioma' to undifferentiated carcinomas with lymphocytic admixture; others have applied it to all types of NPC with lymphocytic admixture. Consequently, comparisons of the relative frequencies of various histological types of NPC in different countries on the basis of published reports are of doubtful value. However, while the relative proportions of the various histological types may vary in different populations, it is evident that the incidence levels of both differentiated and undifferentiated carcinomas are generally higher in populations with high risks for nasopharynx cancer.

According to the classification proposed by WHO (1978), three histological types of NPC can be recognized on the basis of their predominant pattern as seen by light microscopy:

(1) *Squamous-cell carcinoma (keratinizing squamous-cell carcinoma):* a tumour showing definite evidence of squamous differentiation with the presence of intercellular bridges and/or keratinization over most of its extent (Fig. 1).

(2) *Non-keratinizing carcinoma:* a tumour showing evidence of differentiation, with a maturation sequence resulting in cells in which squamous differentiation is not seen by light microscopy (Fig. 2). The cells have fairly well-defined cell margins and show an arrangement that is stratified or pavemented and not syncytial. A plexiform pattern is present in many tumours. Some may exhibit a clear-cell structure, due to the presence of cytoplasmic glycogen.

(3) *Undifferentiated carcinoma (undifferentiated carcinoma of the nasopharyngeal type):* The cells in this type of tumour generally have vesicular nuclei and prominent nucleoli (Fig. 3). The cell margins are indistinct, and the tumour exhibits a syncytial rather than a pavemented appearance. Spindle-shaped tumour cells, some with hyperchromatic nuclei, may be present. The tumour cells are arranged in irregular and moderately well-defined masses and/or in strands of loosely connected cells in a lymphoid stroma (Fig. 4). These cytological and histological features are fairly characteristic and may enable a presumptive diagnosis of NPC even when identified in metastatic tumours.

The term 'lymphoepithelial carcinoma' (lymphoepithelioma) is used to describe non-keratinizing and undifferentiated NPCs in which numerous lymphocytes are found among the tumour cells. The lymphoid elements in such tumours are not neoplastic.

The histological distinctions among these three types are by no means sharp. The prototypes are distinguished easily enough, but many lesions show intermediate features, and some are histological

FIG. 1. NASOPHARYNGEAL CARCINOMA

Squamous-cell carcinoma with intercellular bridges and keratinization. x 190

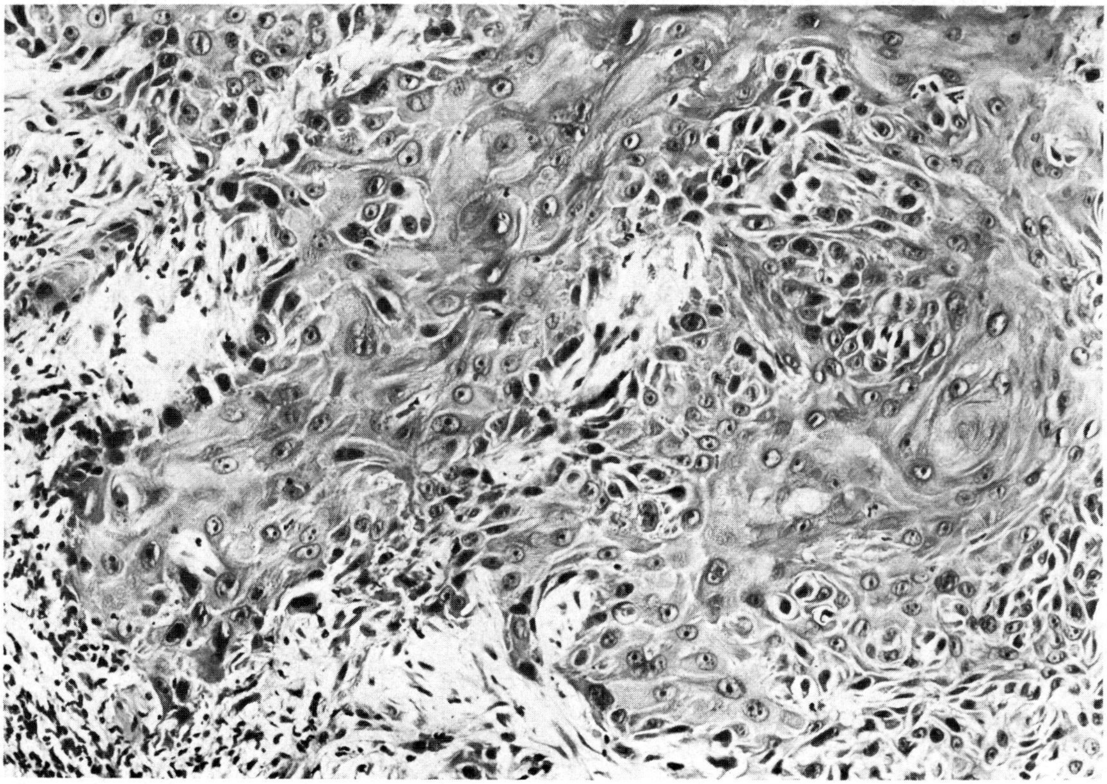

hybrids (Shanmugaratnam, 1972). There has been a strong personal equation in the separation of such tumours, as indicated by the reviewing of histological specimens by panels of experienced pathologists. I have often felt that their separation is more an exercise in histological grading than one in typing.

My own experience, based on the histological examination of more than 2 000 cases diagnosed in Singapore since 1950, leads me to believe that the types of NPC outlined above are to a large extent histological variants of a homogeneous group of tumours. This view is supported by the observation that all types are found with high frequencies in high-risk populations and is not discounted by observed correlations between histological type and other biological variables. Correlations between degree of differentiation, age of patient, response to radiotherapy and survival after treatment are known to occur with tumours of homogeneous

FIG. 2. NASOPHARYNGEAL CARCINOMA

Non-keratinizing carcinoma with pavemented tumour cells and plexiform arrangement. x 190

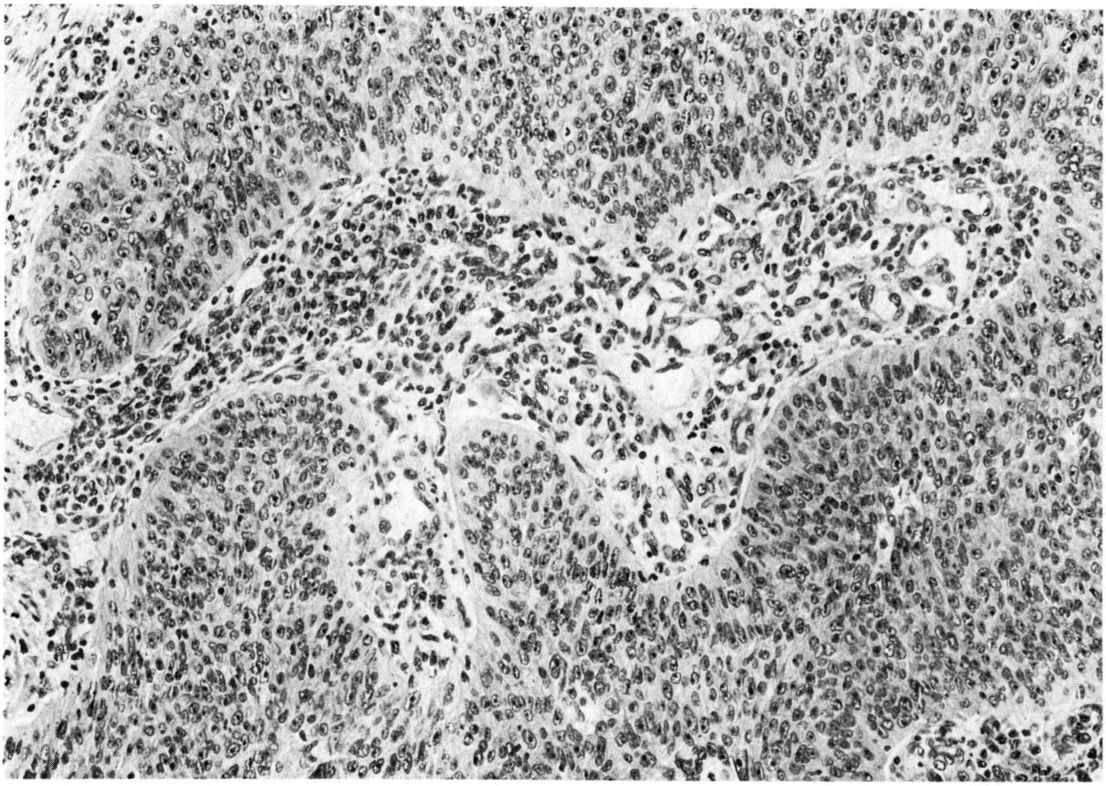

groups in other situations. It is also known that host immune responses are often reflected by the degree of lymphocytic infiltration into the tumour. Such phenomena must be taken into account in the interpretation of correlations between histological type and variations in the epidemiological and biological characteristics of NPC.

CORRELATIONS BETWEEN HISTOLOGICAL TYPES OF NASOPHARYNGEAL CARCINOMA AND OTHER BIOLOGICAL CHARACTERISTICS

Clinical features, mode of spread and response to radiotherapy

It is generally accepted that undifferentiated carcinomas of the nasopharynx, especially those referred to as 'lymphoepithelioma', are

FIG. 3. NASOPHARYNGEAL CARCINOMA

Undifferentiated carcinoma showing syncytial arrangement of tumour cells with vesicular nuclei and prominent nucleoli x 480

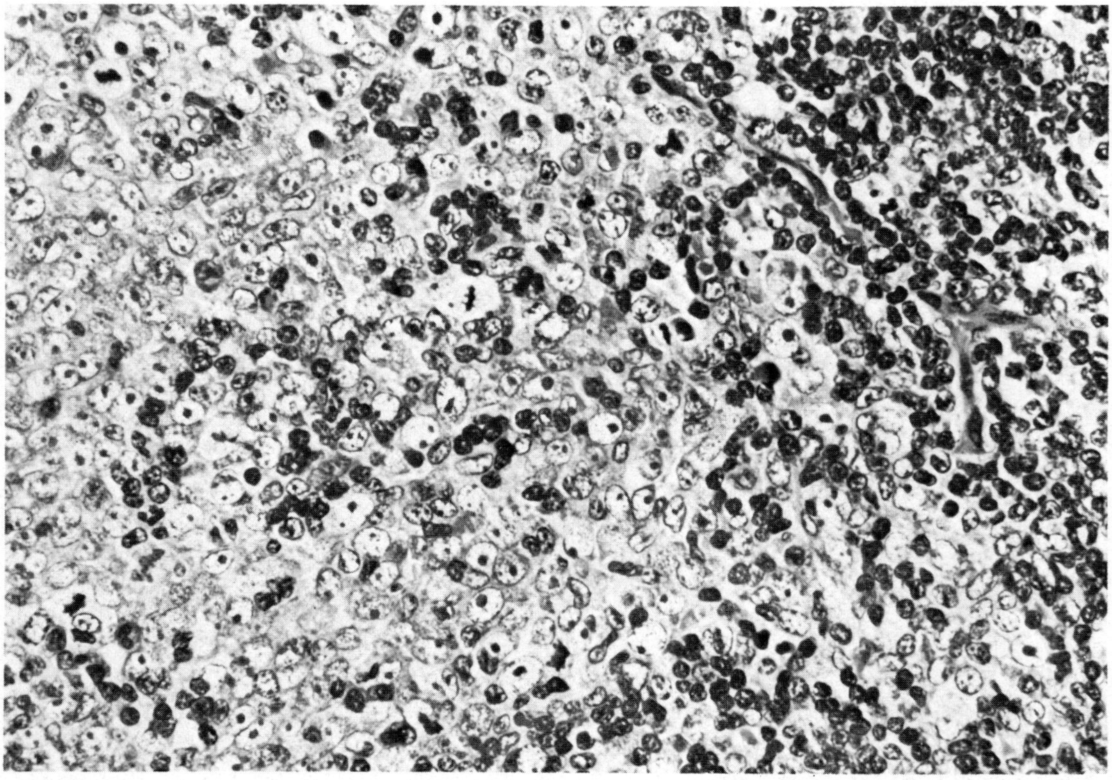

particularly radiosensitive and that five-year survival rates for patients with this tumour are better than for those with squamous-cell carcinomas (Bloom, 1961; Frank et al., 1941; Lenz, 1942; Scanlon et al., 1967). Our findings in Singapore would support this view. Wang et al. (1962) reported that the survival rate for patients with transitional-cell carcinoma was even better than that for patients with lymphoepithelioma. Other authors, however, have failed to find any correlation between histopathological type and five-year survival (Snelling, 1954; Vaeth, 1960; Yeh, 1962).

Geography and race

It is probable that all histological types occur with higher frequencies in high-risk populations. It is interesting to note, however, that not a single case of squamous-cell carcinoma with keratinization or prickles was reported in a series from Uganda (Schmauz & Templeton, 1972);

FIG. 4. NASOPHARYNGEAL CARCINOMA

Undifferentiated carcinoma showing loosely connected tumour cells in a lymphoid stroma. x 350

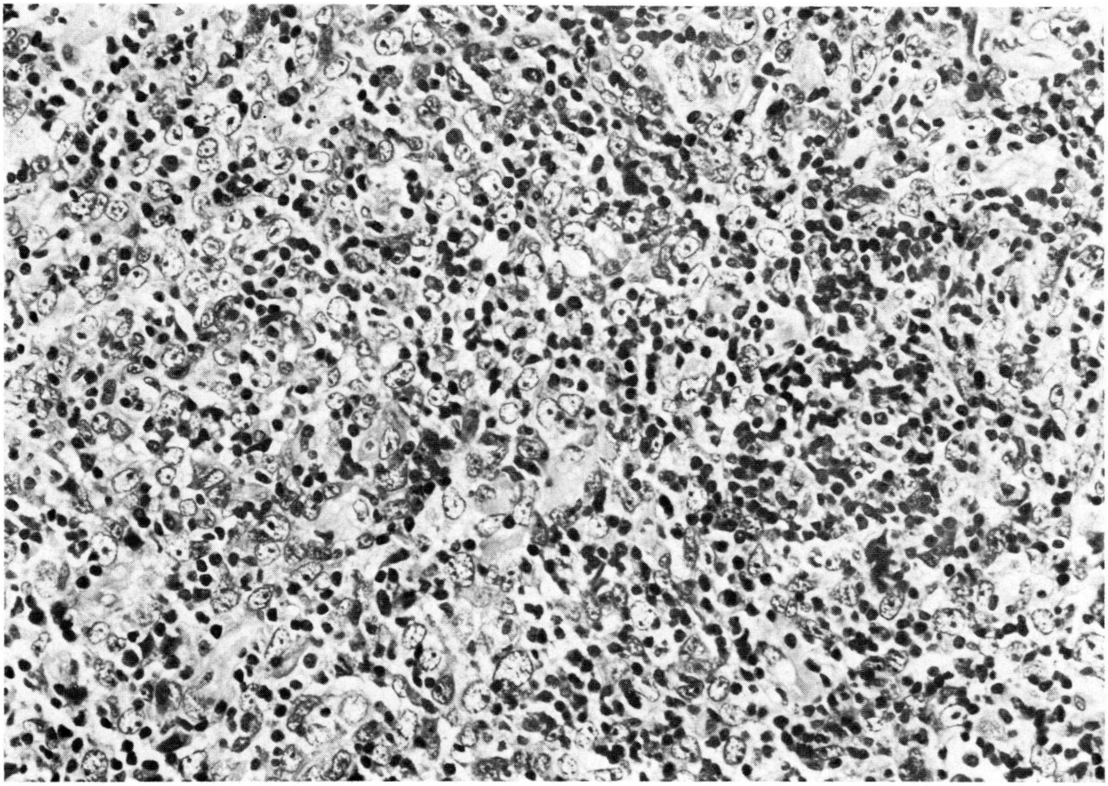

all of the cases in this series were poorly differentiated or anaplastic carcinomas.

Age and sex

It has been suggested that the frequency of well-differentiated squamous-cell carcinoma increases with age and that the frequencies of 'transitional' carcinoma and lymphoepithelioma decrease with age (Sawaki et al., 1976). We have not been able to demonstrate significant correlations between age, sex and histological type in the cases occurring in Singapore. It would be interesting to examine the data from Tunisia, where a substantial proportion (14.6%) of NPCs occur in persons under the age of 16 (Cammoun et al., 1974), and that from Uganda, where some 18% (15/83) of NPCs occur in patients under the age of 19 (Schmauz & Templeton, 1972).

Epstein-Barr virus

It has been reported that patients with the lymphoepithelial type of NPC have higher mean titres of serum antibodies to Epstein-Barr virus than do patients with other types of NPC (Miller et al., 1971; Sawaki et al., 1976). We have found that the mean titres of antibodies against Epstein-Barr virus nuclear antigen are higher in persons with non-keratinizing carcinomas and undifferentiated carcinomas than in those with squamous-cell carcinomas. There were no significant differences with respect to antibodies against Epstein-Barr viral capsid antigen or early antigen. The biological significance of this finding should be investigated. It has also been reported that the presence of Epstein-Barr viral genome in tumour cells is restricted to those of poorly differentiated or anaplastic NPCs (Klein, 1975). This finding requires confirmation.

Other variables

Patients with NPC have been reported to have depressed cell-mediated immunity (Chan et al., 1976) and to differ from controls in their HLA antigen profiles (Simons et al., 1974, 1976). We have found no significant correlations between histological types and HLA profiles.

The histopathological spectrum of NPC in countries where the risk is high, intermediate or low is discussed elsewhere[1], with particular reference to the biological characteristics of the neoplasm. The use of uniform terminology and diagnostic criteria, as proposed by WHO, would facilitate and improve such international comparisons.

SUMMARY

There is little agreement about correlations between histological type and the epidemiological and biological characteristics of NPC. This is largely due to variations in terminology and diagnostic criteria. The use of the terminology and definitions proposed by WHO would facilitate and improve international comparisons.

---

[1] See pp. 13, 27, 41

REFERENCES

Bloom, S.M. (1961) Cancer of the nasopharynx, with special reference to the significance of histopathology. *Laryngoscope*, *71*, 1207-1260

Cammoun, M., Hoerner, G.V. & Mourali, N. (1974) Tumors of the nasopharynx in Tunisia. *Cancer*, *33*, 184-192

Chan, S.H., Chew, T.S., Goh, E.H., Simons, M.J. & Shanmugaratnam, K. (1976) Impaired general cell-mediated immune functions *in vivo* and *in vitro* in patients with nasopharyngeal carcinoma. *Int. J. Cancer*, *18*, 139-144

Frank, I., Lev, M. & Blahd, M. (1941) Transitional cell carcinoma of the upper respiratory tract. *Ann. Otolaryngol.*, *50*, 393-420

Klein, G. (1975) The Epstein-Barr virus and neoplasm. *New Engl. J. Med.*, *293*, 1353-1357

Lederman, M. (1967) Cancer of the pharynx; a study based on 2417 cases with special reference to radiation treatment. *J. Laryngol. Otolaryngol.*, *81*, 151-172

Lenz, M. (1942) Roentgen therapy of primary cancer of nasopharynx. *Amer. J. Roentgenol.*, *48*, 816-832

Miller, D., Goldman, J.M. & Goodman, M.L. (1971) Etiologic study of nasopharyngeal cancer. *Arch. Otolaryngol.*, *94*, 104-108

Sawaki, S., Sugano, H. & Hirayama, T. (1976) *Nasopharyngeal malignancies in Japan*. In: Shanmugaratnam, K., Nambiar, R., Tan, K.K. & Chan, L.K.C., eds, *Proceedings of the 2nd Asian Cancer Conference*, Singapore, Singapore Cancer Society, pp. 263-267

Scanlon, P.W., Rhodes, R.E., Woolner, L.B., Devine, K.D. & McBean, J.B. (1967) Cancer of the nasopharynx: 142 patients treated in the 11 year period 1950-1960. *Amer. J. Roentgenol.*, *99*, 313-325

Schmauz, R. & Templeton, A.C. (1972) Nasopharyngeal carcinoma in Uganda. *Cancer*, *29*, 610-621

Shanmugaratnam, K. (1972) *The pathology of nasopharyngeal carcinoma*. In: Biggs, P.M., de-Thé, G. & Payne, L.N., eds, *Oncogenesis and Herpesviruses (IARC Scientific Publications No. 2)*, Lyon, pp. 239-242

Shanmugaratnam, K. & Muir, C.S. (1967) *Nasopharyngeal carcinoma - origin and structure*. In: Muir, C.S. & Shanmugaratnam, K., eds, *Cancer of the Nasopharynx (UICC Monograph Series No. 1)*, Copenhagen, Munksgaard, pp. 153-162

Simons, M.J., Wee, G.B., Day, N.E., Morris, P.J., Shanmugaratnam, K. & de-Thé, G.B. (1974) Immunogenetic aspects of nasopharyngeal carcinoma. I. Differences in HL-A antigen profiles between patients and control groups. *Int. J. Cancer, 13*, 122-134

Simons, M.J., Wee, G.B., Goh, E.H., Chan, S.H., Shanmugaratnam, K., Day, N.E. & de-Thé, G. (1976) Immunogenetic aspects of nasopharyngeal carcinoma. IV. Increased risk in Chinese of nasopharyngeal carcinoma associated with a Chinese-related HLA profile (A_2 Singapore 2). *J. nat. Cancer Inst., 57*, 977-980

Snelling, M.D. (1954) In: Discussion on treatment of carcinoma of nasopharynx. *Proc. roy. Soc. Med., 47*, 547-560, 549-554

Vaeth, J.M. (1960) Nasopharyngeal malignant tumors; 82 consecutive patients treated in period of 22 years. *Radiology, 74*, 364-372

Wang, C.C., Little, J.B. & Schulz, M.D. (1962) Cancer of the nasopharynx: its clinical and radiotherapeutic considerations. *Cancer, 15*, 921-926

WHO (1978) *Histological Typing of Tumours of the Upper Respiratory Tract*, Geneva (in press)

Yeh, S. (1962) A histological classification of carcinomas of the nasopharynx with a critical review as to the existence of lymphoepitheliomas. *Cancer, 15*, 895-920

HISTOLOGICAL TYPES OF NASOPHARYNGEAL CARCINOMA IN AN INTERMEDIATE RISK AREA

M. CAMMOUN, R. ELLOUZ, J. BEHI & R. BEN ATTIA

Department of Pathology and Cytology,
Salah Azaïz Institute,
Bab-Saadoun,
Tunis, Tunisia

INTRODUCTION

Histological classifications of nasopharyngeal carcinomas (NPC) are difficult to establish: biopsies are often small and distorted and may give only a partial picture of the tumour. Although classifications have been proposed by many authors, none has yet been accepted universally by pathologists.

Perez et al. (1969) demonstrated the epidermoid nature of undifferentiated NPC by electron microscopy. However, classification by light microscopy is still valuable when the histological types correspond to the clinical and biological findings.

In 1974, we established a histological classification of NPC. In this paper, after a brief presentation of the different histological types, we examine the relationship between these types and clinical/ anatomical findings and results of treatment.

MATERIALS AND METHODS

Between April 1969 and December 1974, 485 cases of NPC were seen at the Salah Azaïz Institute in Tunis. Only carcinomas were considered for study, and 39 cases were excluded due to insufficient data. All of the remaining 446 cases were examined histologically. Of these, 76 patients were less than 20 years of age, and 370 were adults (over 20 years of age). Among the younger patients, 58 had had curative treatment, and among the adults, 220. All patients, treated or not, were classified clinically according to the TNM classification (UICC, 1974).

RESULTS

Our study has led us to define three principal histological types:

(1) *Well-differentiated squamous-cell carcinoma* (Fig. 1). This carcinoma is the least common but the easiest to define. It consists of squamous-cell proliferation and various degrees of keratinization, with or without the presence of intercellular bridges.

FIG. 1. WELL-DIFFERENTIATED SQUAMOUS-CELL CARCINOMA, WITH KERATINIZATION AND INTERCELLULAR BRIDGES x 90

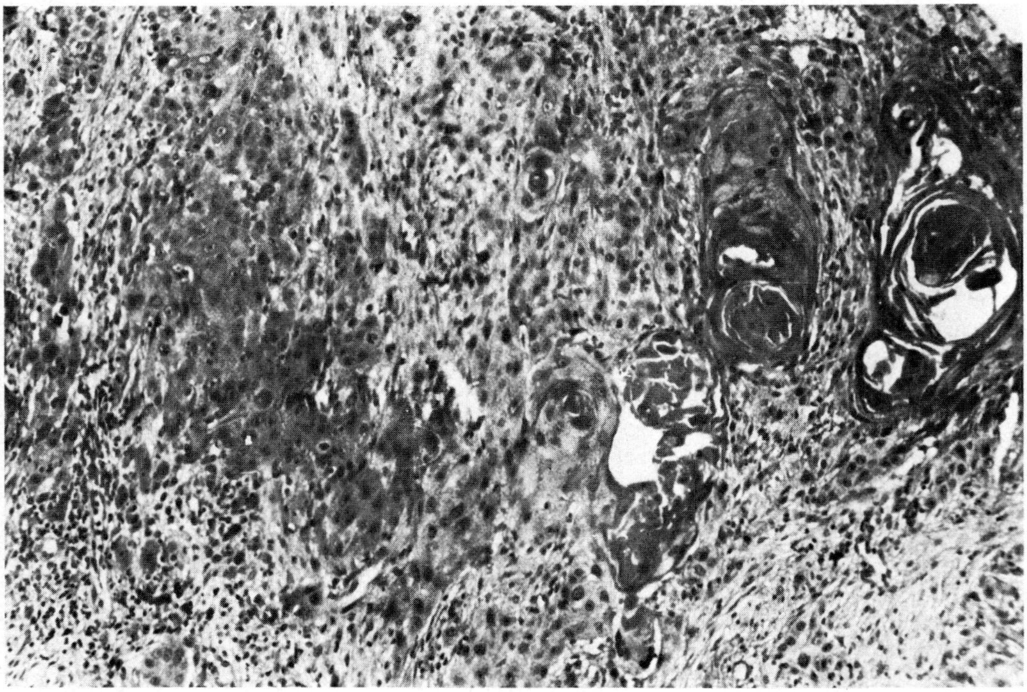

Only 29 cases of this type were found among the adult patients (7.8%) and none among the children.

(2) *Poorly-differentiated squamous-cell carcinoma*. Generally, this carcinoma consists of trabecular and lobular patterns, sometimes with a basement-like membrane (Fig. 2), but with no keratinization; the cells, rather than always being polyhedral, may be spindle-shaped (Fig. 3), round (Fig. 4) or oval. They demonstrate a definite

FIG. 2. POORLY-DIFFERENTIATED SQUAMOUS-CELL CARCINOMA, WITH BASEMENT-LIKE MEMBRANE x 90

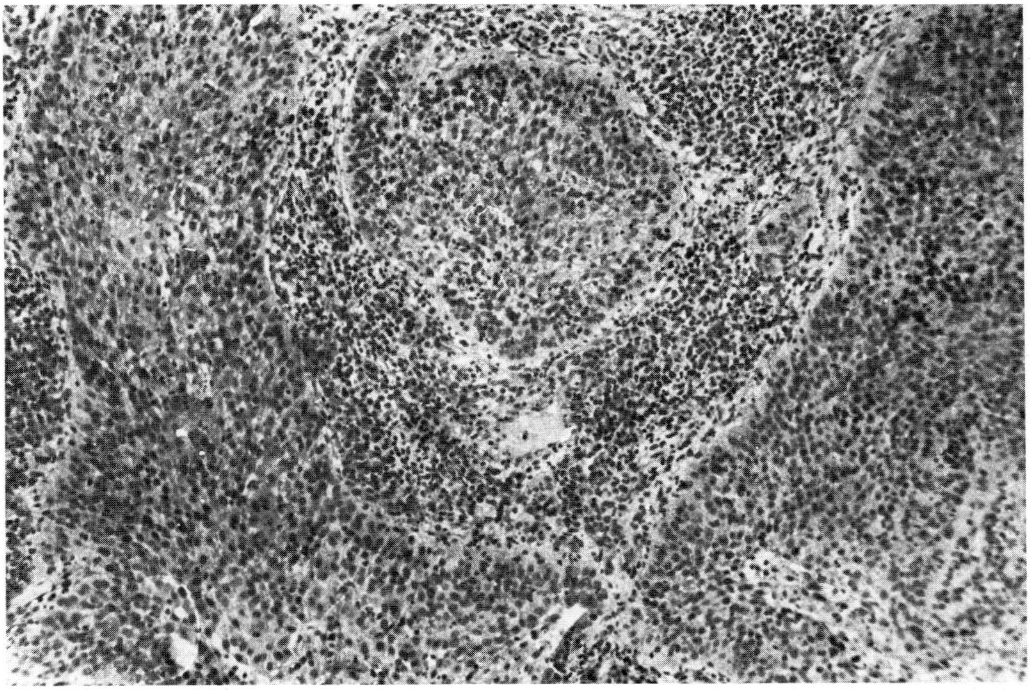

FIG. 3. POORLY-DIFFERENTIATED SQUAMOUS-CELL CARCINOMA, WITH SPINDLE-SHAPED CELLS x 225

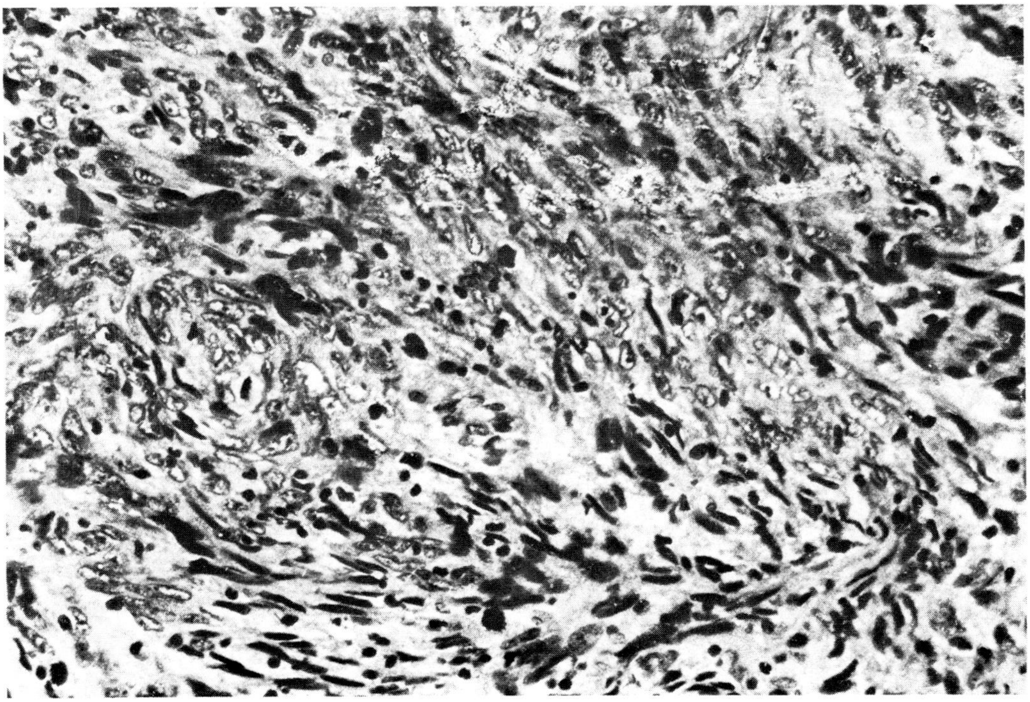

FIG. 4. POORLY-DIFFERENTIATED SQUAMOUS-CELL CARCINOMA, SHOWING A LOBULAR PATTERN, WITH ROUNDED CELLS x 90

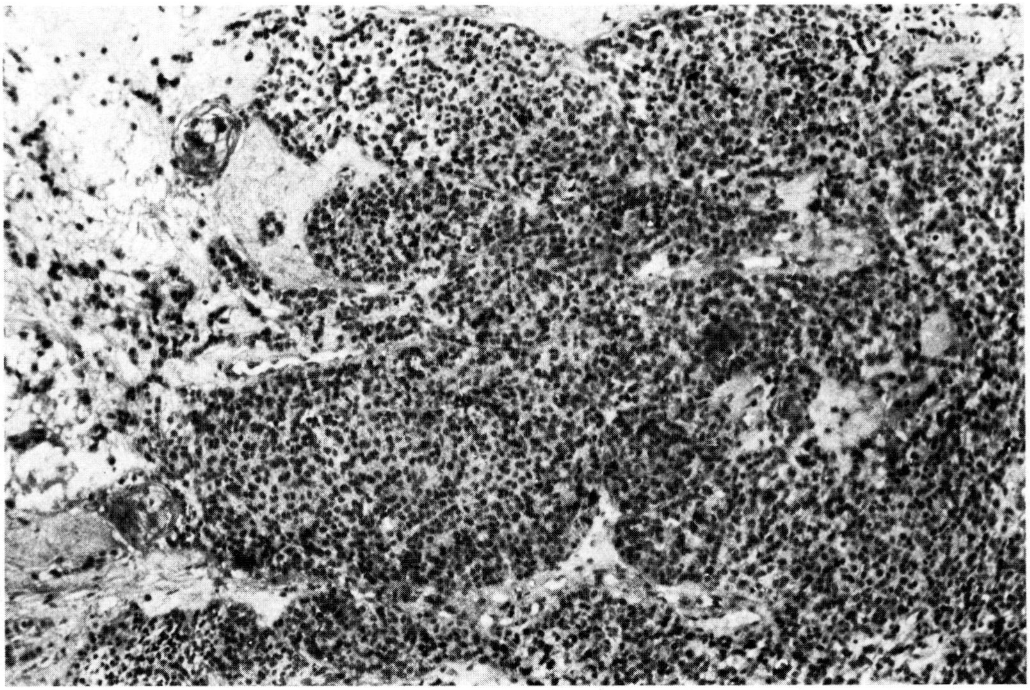

cellular border, and the nucleus and cytoplasm are highly stained (Figs 5-7). The margin of the epithelial component is clearly delineated from the stroma. This kind of tumour can be seen at any level of the Malpighian or para-Malpighian mucosa, especially in the cervix, the oesophagus and the oral cavity.

There was a higher incidence of this type among adults (281 cases, 76%) than among children (37 cases, 48.6%).

(3) *'Nasopharyngeal' carcinoma*. This type is more easily defined, corresponding directly to the form described by Regaud (1921) and Schminke (1921); the classification also includes some of the so-called 'transitional carcinomas'. This type of tumour consists of bulky, alveolar, syncytial masses (Fig. 8). The tumour-cell borders are not definite, and chromatin is scarce; the nuclei are clear and appear to be 'holed' (Fig. 9); they often exhibit two or three distinct nucleoli. The margins of the alveolar masses are often blurred by lymphoid infiltrations from the stroma. Table 1 presents a comparison of poorly-differentiated squamous-cell carcinomas and 'nasopharyngeal' carcinomas with regard to certain histological parameters.

FIG. 5. POORLY-DIFFERENTIATED SQUAMOUS-CELL CARCINOMA, SHOWING DEFINITE CELLULAR BORDER, HIGHLY-STAINED NUCLEI AND BASEMENT-LIKE-MEMBRANE x 225

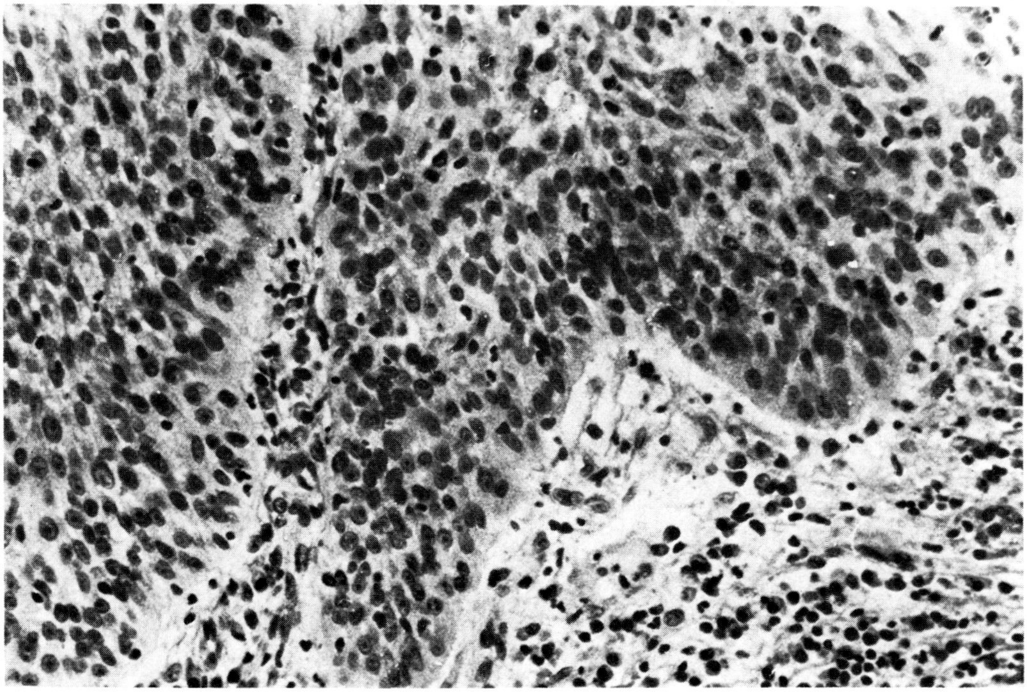

FIG. 6. POORLY-DIFFERENTIATED SQUAMOUS-CELL CARCINOMA, SHOWING MULTISTRATIFICATION AND HIGHLY-STAINED CELLS x 90

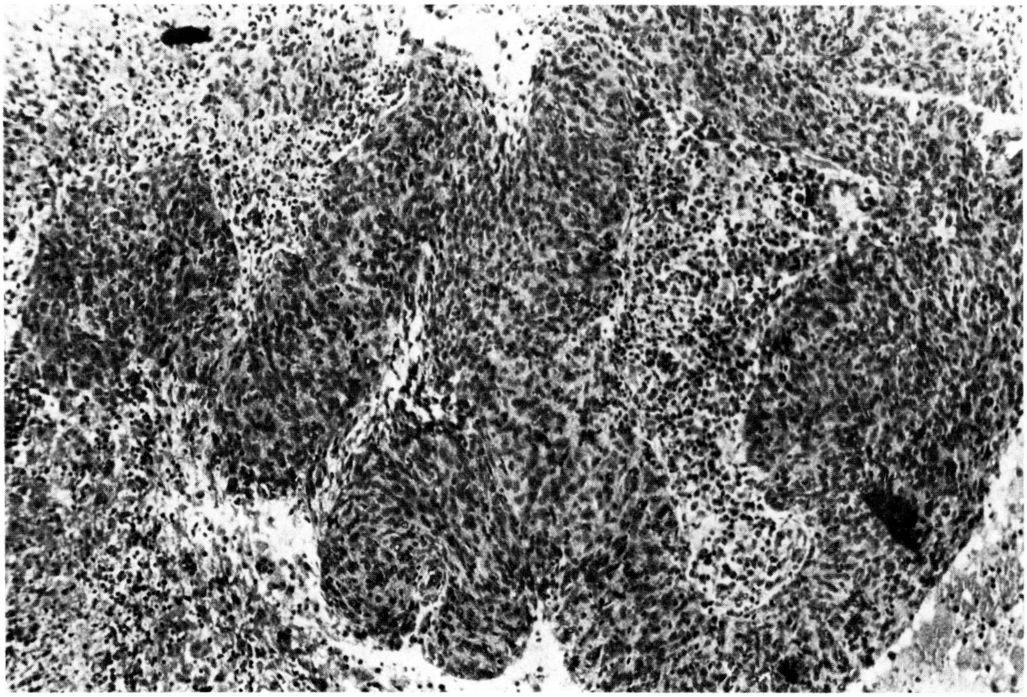

FIG. 7. HIGHER MAGNIFICATIONS OF CELLS SHOWN IN FIG. 6
x 225

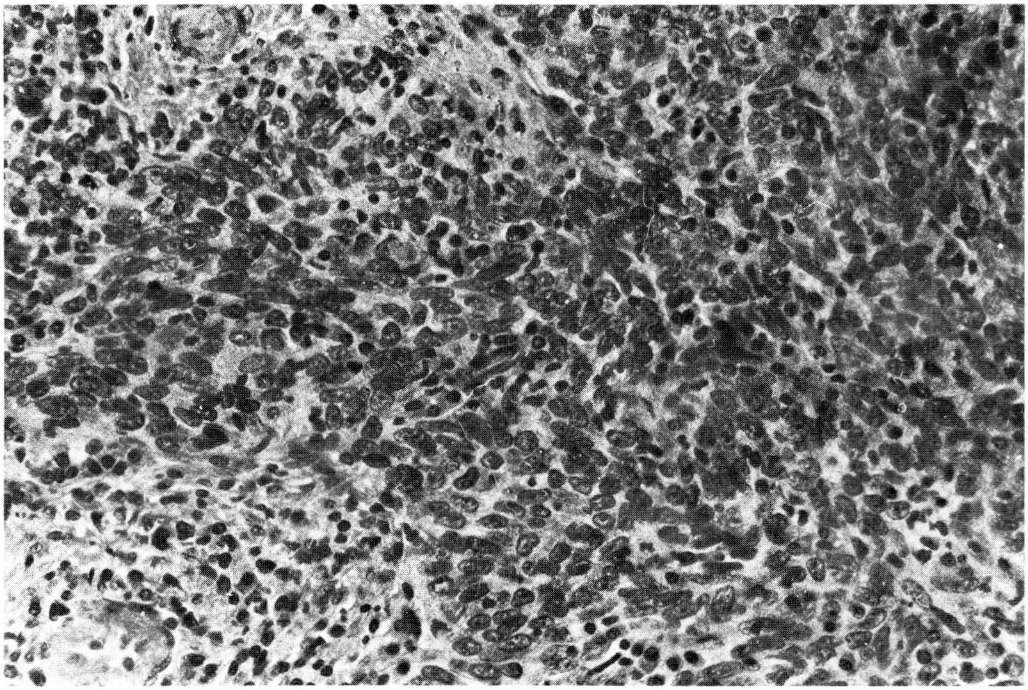

FIG. 8. 'NASOPHARYNGEAL' CARCINOMA
SHOWING BULKY, ALVEOLAR, SYNCYTIAL MASSES x 90

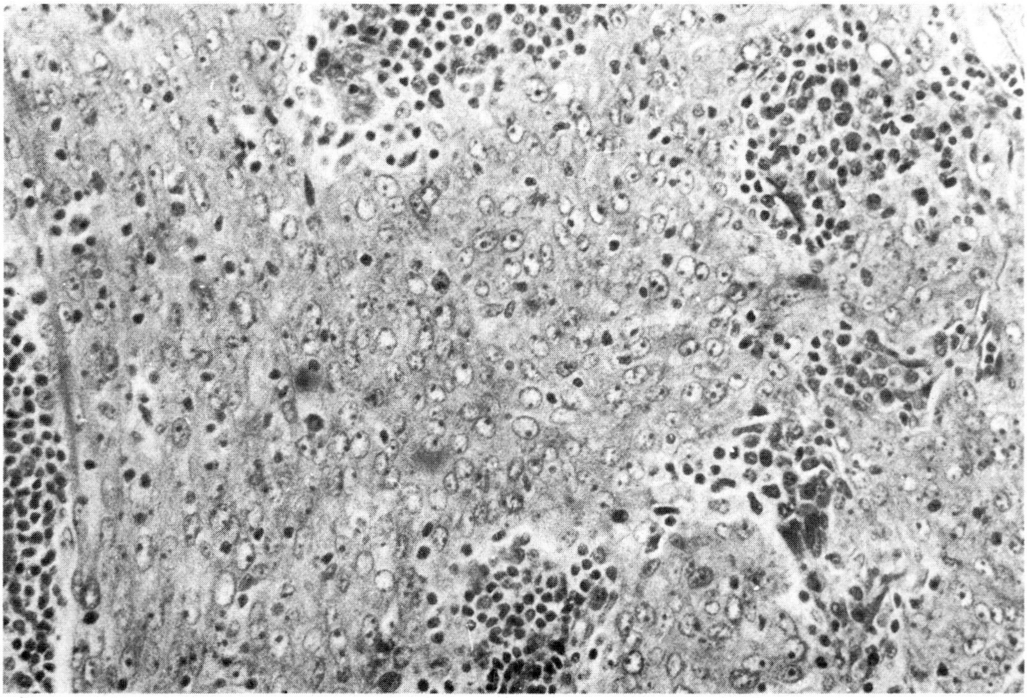

FIG. 9. 'NASOPHARYNGEAL' CARCINOMA

Cell borders are not definite, chromatin is scarce and the nuclei are clear and appear to be 'holed' x 225

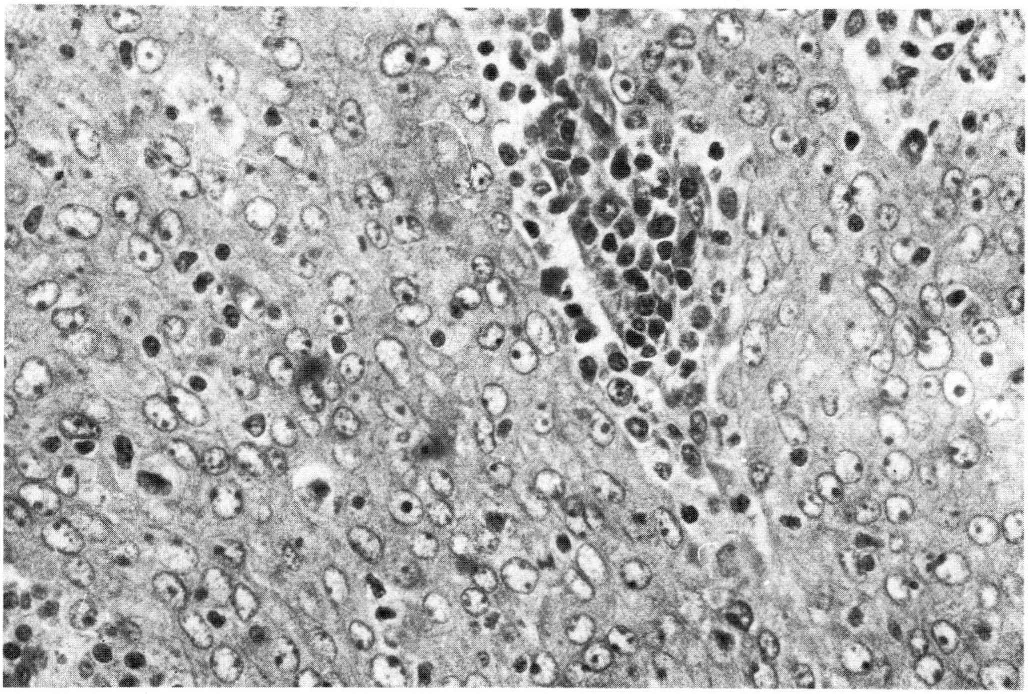

Table 1. Histological features of poorly-differentiated squamous-cell and 'nasopharyngeal' carcinomas

Histological feature	Poorly-differentiated squamous-cell	'Nasopharyngeal'
Basement-like membrane	+++	0
Syncytial pattern	0	+++
Stroma-tumour delineation	++	±
Keratinization	0	0
Staining of nuclei and cytoplasm	++	0
Cytoplasmic limits	++	0
'Holed' nuclei	±	+++

Children showed a predominance of this type of tumour, with 39 cases among the patients (51.3%), compared with only 45 cases among 370 adults (12.1%).

(4) *Anaplastic carcinoma.* These tumours retain only a vague epithelial structure; they can, however, be confused with sarcomas.

We found no cases of this histological type among children, and there were only 15 cases (4%) among the adults.

Table 2 shows the percentage distribution of these four histological types of NPC among the adult and young patients studied. It can be seen that the most frequent type for both age groups was poorly-differentiated squamous-cell carcinoma, comprising 71% of all the NPCs in our population. It occurred most frequently in adults (76%). 'Nasopharyngeal' carcinoma was the most common type found among children and was relatively rare among adults. Both well-differentiated squamous-cell and anaplastic carcinomas were seen only in adults.

Table 2. Percentage distribution of the four histological types of nasopharyngeal carcinoma among 370 adults and 76 children

	Well-differentiated squamous-cell %	Poorly-differentiated squamous-cell %	'Nasopharyngeal' %	Anaplastic %
Adults	7.8	76	12	4
Children	0	48	51	0

Table 3 shows the percentage distribution of histological types of NPC in children by T and N classifications. It can be seen that 'nasopharyngeal' tumours in this group are characteristically small and show lymphatic involvement. In comparison, poorly-differentiated squamous-cell carcinomas are generally larger but are less aggressive in terms of lymphatic spread. Comparable findings are seen in adults with regard to tumour size but not with regard to lymphatic involvement (Table 4).

Results of treatment in children after two years (Table 5) indicate that poorly-differentiated squamous-cell carcinomas do not respond as well to treatment as, and thus have a worse prognosis than, 'nasopharyngeal' tumours. These results include only those from the first two years, since in the following three years the number of patients was too small to draw any significant conclusions. The same prognostic indication could be seen among adults (Table 6), in whom survival was longest for those with 'nasopharyngeal' tumours. Again,

Table 3. Percentage distribution of histological types of nasopharyngeal carcinoma in children, by T and N classifications

	'Nasopharyngeal'	Poorly-differentiated squamous-cell
N0, N1, N2	16	27.5
N3	84	73
T2	19.5	16
T3	28	16
T4	52.5	68

Table 4. Percentage distribution of histological types of nasopharyngeal carcinoma in adults, by T and N classification

	'Nasopharyngeal'	Poorly-differentiated squamous-cell
N1, N2, N3	25	27
N3	75	73
T2	40.5	31
T3	16	22.5
T4	43.5	68

the results were questionable for the third, fourth and fifth years, since the number of cases was so very small.

The difference in behaviour of these two histological types of NPC is again apparent from a study of the percentages of recurrence and metastasis. Among children (Table 5), there was a low incidence of recurrence of 'nasopharyngeal' tumours, but metastases seemed to occur during the first year. Poorly-differentiated squamous-cell carcinomas recurred more frequently but were slower to metastasize. Almost analogous patterns were observed in adults (Table 6): recurrence of 'nasopharyngeal' tumours was more frequent during the second year, whereas recurrence of poorly-differentiated squamous-cell carcinomas was the same in the first and second years; on the other hand, metastases occurred later in patients with poorly-differentiated carcinomas than in those with the 'nasopharyngeal' type. It would

Table 5. Evolution of nasopharyngeal carcinoma by histological type in children

Evolution	'Nasopharyngeal' %	Poorly-differentiated squamous-cell %
2-year survival rate (actuarial method)	53.5	34.5
recurrence 0-1 yr	11	15
1-2 yrs	7	15
metastasis 0-1 yr	37	19
1-2 yrs	0	38

Table 6. Evolution of nasopharyngeal carcinoma by histological type in adults

	'Nasopharyngeal'	Poorly-differentiated squamous-cell %	Well-differentiated squamous-cell %
2-year survival rate (actuarial method)	40	36	0
recurrence 0-1 yr	14	18	40
1-2 yrs	25	18	100
metastasis 0-1 yr	17	18.5	13.5
1-2 yrs	18.5	23.5	

appear, therefore, that 'nasopharyngeal' tumours have a greater tendency to metastasize, and poorly-differentiated carcinomas are more likely to recur. In patients with well-differentiated squamous-cell carcinomas, recurrence is even more frequent, often leading to a destruction of the base of the skull, thus aggravating the course of the disease; however, this type of tumour rarely metastasizes. It would seem, then, that the more highly differentiated a tumour (in terms of epidermoid features), the worse the prognosis.

DISCUSSION

The validity of the histological classification outlined above seems to be supported by epidemiological, anatomical/clinical and treatment results.

Children never have well-differentiated squamous-cell carcinomas but often have the 'nasopharyngeal' type (Cammoun et al., 1974) and, less frequently, poorly-differentiated tumours. All reports on NPC in children and young people describe undifferentiated types of tumours, which often enter the category of lymphoepitheliomas (Brugère et al., 1975; De Stefani et al., 1973; McConnell, 1958; Picks et al., 1974; Schmauz & Templeton, 1972; Straka & Bluestone, 1972).

In adults, 'nasopharyngeal' tumours were rarest, and poorly- and well-differentiated squamous-cell carcinomas occurred in more than 84% of cases; 4% were anaplastic.

Patients with 'nasopharyngeal' carcinomas have small tumours, early lymphatic spread and a good prognosis. These findings are in agreement with those of de Stephani et al. (1973) with regard to lymphoepitheliomas. Poorly-differentiated squamous-cell carcinomas are macroscopically larger, less prone to lymphatic spread, have a tendency to recur after treatment and have a less favourable prognosis. Well-differentiated squamous-cell carcinomas have a very bad prognosis; this fact has been observed by other workers (Brugère et al., 1975; Hara, 1971).

We have noted that the more highly differentiated the carcinoma, the worse its prognosis; and Brugère et al. (1975) have confirmed this observation in a study in which the majority of patients were of North African origin. He pointed out that the undifferentiated forms have a better prognosis in spite of a higher incidence of metastasis. Hara (1971) has also noted the more favourable prognosis of undifferentiated carcinomas.

In a recent, unpublished study carried out in collaboration with Dr G.B. de-Thé, Epstein-Barr virus early antigen antibody titres were seen to vary with histological type of tumour (Table 7). Thus, the well-differentiated type was associated with a low antibody titre; on the other hand, adults with poorly-differentiated carcinomas had high antibody titres (there were no cases in children). The 'nasopharyngeal' type of carcinoma was associated with a high antibody titre in adults but with a very low one in children. This discrepancy could be explained by a varying role of the Epstein-Barr virus in different age groups.

In another study (Desgranges et al., 1977), the IgA immunoglobulin fraction specific to Epstein-Barr viral capsid antigen was more often found to be absent from the serum and saliva of children than of adults. A preliminary, immunological/histological study[1] has shown a relationship between histological type and the presence of IgA in the saliva:

[1] Unpublished data

thus, 'nasopharyngeal' carcinoma is more often associated with saliva negative for IgA.

Table 7. Geometric mean titres (GMT) of Epstein-Barr virus early antigen in nasopharyngeal carcinoma patients under and over the age of 20 yrs, by histological type

Group of patients	No. of patients	GMT	Confidence intervals[a]	Standard error
10-19 yrs 'Nasopharyngeal' carcinoma	18	68.6	29.5 159.3	0.61
20 yrs + 'Nasopharyngeal' carcinoma	24	201.6	108.2 375.7	0.45
Well-differentiated squamous-cell carcinoma	9	74.1	24.2 226.7	0.81
Poorly-differentiated squamous-cell carcinoma	109	243.4	183.6 322.8	0.20

[a] + 2 SE
- 2 SE

In conclusion, the classification proposed here is validated by its correlation with clinical, epidemiological, prognostic, virological and, perhaps, immunological findings. It is clear, on the basis of these results, that a classification based upon two histological types alone (i.e., well-differentiated squamous-cell carcinoma and undifferentiated squamous-cell carcinoma) should be rejected. The latter type includes, in our opinion, at least two morphological entities.

SUMMARY

Between April and December 1974, 485 cases of NPC were seen at the Salah Azaïz Institute in Tunis. A histological study was carried out according to a classification that comprises four types of tumour: well-differentiated squamous-cell carcinoma, poorly-differentiated squamous-cell carcinoma, 'nasopharyngeal' type carcinoma and an anaplastic type. Some correlation between these histological types and clinical, epidemiological, virological and prognostic features was found.

REFERENCES

Brugère, J., Eschwege, F., Schwaab, G., Micheau, C. & Cachin, Y. (1975) Les carcinomes du nasopharynx (cavum): aspects cliniques et évolutifs. *Bull. Cancer*, *62*, 319-330

Cammoun, M., Hoerner, G.V. & Mourali, N. (1974) Tumors of the nasopharynx in Tunisia, an anatomic and clinical study based on 143 cases. *Cancer*, *33*, 184-192

Desgranges, C., de-Thé, G., Ho, J.H.C. & Ellouz, R. (1977) Neutralizing EBV-specific IgA in throat washings of nasopharyngeal carcinoma (NPC) patients. *Int. J. Cancer*, *19*, 627-633

De Stefani, E., Suzman, P. & Oreggia, F. (1973) Carcinome du cavum: revision anatomo-clinique de 47 cas: problème du lymphoepithelioma. *Rev. Laryngol.*, *94*, 11-12

Hara, H.J. (1971) Malignant tumor of the nasopharynx. *Clin. Med.*, *78*, 30-35

McConnell, E.M. (1958) Nasopharyngeal carcinoma in children and young adults. *Brit. J. Cancer*, *12*, 195-201

Perez, C.A., Ackerman, L.V., Mill, W.B., Ogura, J.H. & Powers, W.E. (1969) Cancer of the nasopharynx: factors influencing prognosis. *Cancer*, *24*, 1-17

Picks, T., Maurer, H.M. & MacWilliam, N.D. (1974) Lymphoepithelioma in childhood. *J. Pediat.*, *84*, 96-100

Regaud, C. (1921) Discussion dans Reverchon, L. & Coutard, H. Lymphoepithelioma de l'hypopharynx traité par la roentgentherapie. *Bull. Soc. franç. Otorhinolaryngol.*, *34*, 209

Schmauz, R. & Templeton, A.C. (1972) Nasopharyngeal carcinoma in Uganda. *Cancer*, *29*, 610-621

Schmincke, A. (1921) Uber lymphoepitheliale Geschwülste. *Beitr. path. Anat.*, *68*, 161-170

Straka, J.A. & Bluestone, C.D. (1972) Nasopharyngeal malignancies in children. *Laryngoscope*, *82*, 807-816

UICC (1974) *TNM Classification of Malignant Tumours*, Geneva

HISTOPATHOLOGICAL TYPES OF NASOPHARYNGEAL CARCINOMA IN A LOW-RISK AREA: JAPAN

H. SUGANO & G. SAKAMOTO

Department of Pathology,
Cancer Institute,
1-37 Kami-Ikebukuro,
Toshima-ku,
Tokyo 170, Japan

S. SAWAKI

Department of Otolaryngology,
Yokohama City University Hospital,
3-46 Urafune-cho,
Minami-ku,
Yokohama 232, Japan

T. HIRAYAMA

Division of Epidemiology,
National Cancer Center Research Institute,
5-1 Tsukiji, Chuo-ku
Tokyo 104, Japan

INTRODUCTION

Nasopharyngeal carcinoma (NPC) is rare in Japan, but morbidity and mortality rates for this tumour have been increasing gradually (Hatori, 1966; Sawaki et al., 1976; Sugano et al., 1971). About 160 new NPC patients visit the major outpatient clinics annually. The morbidity rate for NPC in the peak age group, 60-70 years, was 0.794 per 100,000 population in males and 0.451 in females in 1970; the mortality rate was 0.517 per 100,000 population in males and 0.264 in females in 1965-69, while in 1970-74 it was 0.797 in males and 0.327 in females.

The male:female sex ratio is almost 2.0. The histopathology of NPC in Japan has been discussed by Ootsuka (1964), Miyagi (1967), Sugano et al. (1971) and Sawaki et al. (1975).

In this paper, the histopathological types of NPC in Japan are described and discussed. The study on which it is based is an analysis of biopsy material from 816 cases of Japanese NPC, divided into the following two groups:

Group 1: 85 NPC patients seen at the Cancer Institute during the 30 years between 1947 and 1976 and selected from 121 patients with nasopharyngeal tumours among 2 413 cases of malignant tumours of the upper respiratory tract. This group includes NPC patients in 'group 1' reported by Sugano et al. (1971).

Group 2: 731 NPC patients selected from 925 with nasopharyngeal tumours referred from outpatient clinics of otorhinolaryngological departments of all medical schools and major hospitals throughout Japan in the five years from 1969 to 1972. This group includes cases in 'group 3' reported by Sugano et al. (1971) and 84 patients in whom titres of antibody to anti-Epstein-Barr viral capsid antigen (VCA) were reported by Sawaki et al. (1975, 1976).

For comparison with the Japanese NPC biopsies, 201 were selected from 208 Taiwanese NPC biopsies. The cases from which they were taken were included in a series reported by Lynn et al. (1973). All of the cases were histopathologically confirmed and reviewed by two of the authors (H.S. and G.S.)

HISTOLOGICAL CLASSIFICATION OF NPC

According to the classification adopted by the Department of Pathology, Cancer Institute, NPCs are either well-differentiated or poorly-differentiated squamous-cell carcinomas. The former may be either keratinized or nonkeratinized squamous-cell carcinomas. The latter are either spindle-polygonal-cell carcinomas, transitional-cell carcinomas or lymphoepitheliomas.

Spindle-polygonal-cell carcinomas are those with spindle-and/or polygonal-shaped cells which are nonkeratinized and are similar in morphology to *in situ* or early squamous-cell carcinomas of the uterine cervix originating from the endocervix.

Transitional-cell carcinomas and lymphoepitheliomas have long been recognized as carcinomas peculiar to the nasopharynx (Chen et al., 1971; Schmincke, 1921; Shanmugaratnam & Muir, 1967; Yeh, 1962). Transitional-cell carcinomas are characterized by large vesicular nuclei with prominent nucleoli. Tumour cells are closely arranged and form bulky clumps. Lymphoepitheliomas are characterized by polygonal-shaped or reticular tumour cells with an abundant admixture of lymphocytes.

Keratin fibres, seen in the cytoplasm by electron microscopy, are useful as differential markers of squamous-cell carcinomas. They are observed more or less frequently in spindle-polygonal-cell carcinomas. The cytoplasm of transitional-cell carcinomas and lymphoepitheliomas shows no keratin fibres, although desmosomes are clearly demonstrable between adjacent cell membranes; however, a careful examination reveals tiny keratin fibres in some cells (Chen et al., 1971; Lin et al., 1969). This suggests that these two carcinomas are of a squamous nature, and from these morphological findings one may consider transitional-cell carcinomas and lymphoepitheliomas to be undifferentiated or anaplastic carcinomas of a squamous-cell series. If this is the case, spindle-polygonal-cell carcinoma can remain in the category of poorly-differentiated carcinomas.

One could classify NPCs into three categories: well-differentiated, poorly-differentiated and undifferentiated carcinomas. However, a considerable number of cases have a mixed histology; furthermore, repeated biopsies in the same patient often reveal different morphological patterns, varying from lymphoepithelioma or transitional-cell carcinoma to spindle-polygonal-cell carcinoma. It is reasonable, therefore, to consider that transitional-cell carcinomas and lymphoepitheliomas are also varieties of poorly-differentiated carcinoma and simply to use the term 'anaplastic carcinoma', instead of 'poorly-differentiated carcinoma'.

NPC IN RELATION TO OTHER MALIGNANT TUMOURS OF THE UPPER RESPIRATORY TRACT

In order to situate NPCs among other malignant tumours of the upper respiratory tract, 2 413 cases, from which those in Group 1 were taken, were analysed. As shown in Table 1, 2 139 were shown to be squamous-cell carcinomas, and 225 were malignant lymphomas. Other types of

Table 1. Histological types of malignant tumours of the upper respiratory tract in 2 413 patients seen at the Cancer Institute, Tokyo, 1947-1976

Histology	No. of tumours							
	Nasal cavity	Naso-pharynx	Oro-pharynx	Palatine tonsil	Hypo-pharynx	Larynx	Maxilla	Total
Squamous-cell carcinoma	62	85	8	85	196	1 203	500	2 139
Other carcinoma	7	2	2	0	0	1	15	27
Lymphoma	13	33	3	162	4	1	9	225
Other sarcoma	7	1	0	1	1	1	11	22
Total	89	121	13	248	201	1 206	535	2 413

carcinomas and sarcomas were few. An examination of the frequency of tumours in various organs showed that those of the nasopharynx accounted for 5%. Tumours of the oropharynx were very rare; however, carcinomas of the larynx and maxilla were highly frequent.

Almost all of the malignant tumours of the hypopharynx, larynx and maxilla were of squamous origin. The most frequent malignant tumour of the tonsil was lymphoma, and a relatively high occurrence of lymphomas was also observed in the nasopharynx. If the squamous-cell carcinomas occurring in each organ are divided into the subgroups described above (Table 2), it is clear that poorly-differentiated carcinomas occur most frequently (88%) among NPCs. Furthermore, among poorly-differentiated NPCs, transitional-cell carcinomas and lymphoepitheliomas are prevalent; in other organs, well-differentiated carcinomas predominate, and, when poorly-differentiated ones occur, most are spindle-polygonal-cell carcinomas.

Table 2. Histological types of squamous-cell carcinoma of the upper respiratory tract in 2 139 patients seen at the Cancer Institute, Tokyo, 1947-1976

Carcinoma	No. of tumours							
	Nasal cavity	Naso-pharynx	Oro-pharynx	Palatine tonsil	Hypo-pharynx	Larynx	Maxilla	Total
Well-differentiated								
keratinized	21	4	4	32	104	251	203	619
nonkeratinized	7	6	0	17	41	286	135	492
Poorly-differentiated								
spindle-polygonal-cell	30	48	3	31	50	666	152	980
transitional-cell	4	20	1	4	1	0	10	40
lymphoepithelioma	0	7	0	1	0	0	0	8
Total	62	85	8	85	196	1 203	500	2 139
	% of total							
Well-differentiated	45	12	50	58	74	45	68	52
Poorly-differentiated	55	88	50	42	26	55	32	48

CHARACTERISTICS OF NPC IN A LARGER SERIES

A detailed histological analysis of NPC was carried out in the larger series comprising Group 2. Of 925 histologically proven nasopharyngeal tumours, a vast majority (79.0%) were NPC (squamous-cell carcinomas) and malignant lymphomas (15.5%) (Table 3). Subclassification of the squamous-cell carcinomas (Table 4) shows that 13.3% were well-differentiated and 86.7% poorly-differentiated tumours. Of the

Table 3. Histological types of malignant tumours of the nasopharynx in 925 cases from throughout Japan, 1969-1972

Histology	No. of cases	% of total	% of subgroup
Carcinoma	758	81.9	
squamous cell	731		79.0
other	27		2.9
Sarcoma	167	18.1	
lymphoma	143		15.5
other	24		2.6

latter, almost half were spindle-polygonal-cell carcinomas; transitional-cell carcinomas and lymphoepitheliomas accounted for 40.9% of the NPC.

Table 4. Histological types of squamous-cell carcinoma of the nasopharynx in 731 patients from throughout Japan, 1969-1973

Carcinoma	No. of cases	% of total	% of poorly-differentiated
Well-differentiated	96	13.3	
Poorly-differentiated	635	86.7	
spindle-polygonal-cell	335		45.5
transitional-cell	195		26.6
lymphoepithelioma	105		14.3

A study of the age distribution of 758 of these NPC patients indicated that the peak age in both sexes was between 60-70 years. A ridit analysis (Fig. 1) showed that the ridit mean value decreases in older groups, especially in that of persons more than 60 years old. This value deviated significantly from the total mean at the 95% confidence limit.

Examination of the percentage distribution of histological types of tumours for different age groups (Fig. 2) shows that spindle-polygonal-cell carcinoma is the major NPC in all age groups. The frequency of transitional-cell carcinoma and lymphoepithelioma tends slightly to decrease in higher age groups, and that of well-differentiated carcinoma increases slightly. Thus, poorly-differentiated carcinomas, especially transitional-cell carcinomas and lymphoepitheliomas, were much more frequent in the younger age groups.

FIG. 1. AGE DISTRIBUTION OF NASOPHARYNGEAL CARCINOMA PATIENTS

Ridit analysis of age distribution of 758 nasopharyngeal carcinoma patients from throughout Japan, 1969-1973

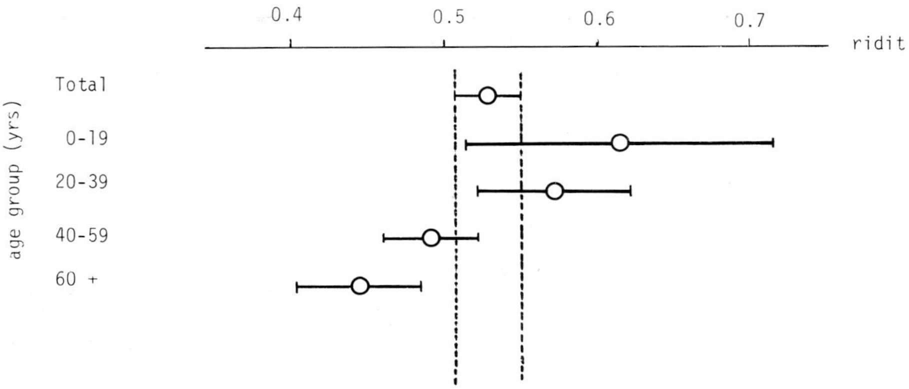

FIG. 2. HISTOLOGICAL TYPES OF NASOPHARYNGEAL CARCINOMA

Percentage distribution of histological types of nasopharyngeal carcinoma in those of 758 patients from throughout Japan, 1969-1973

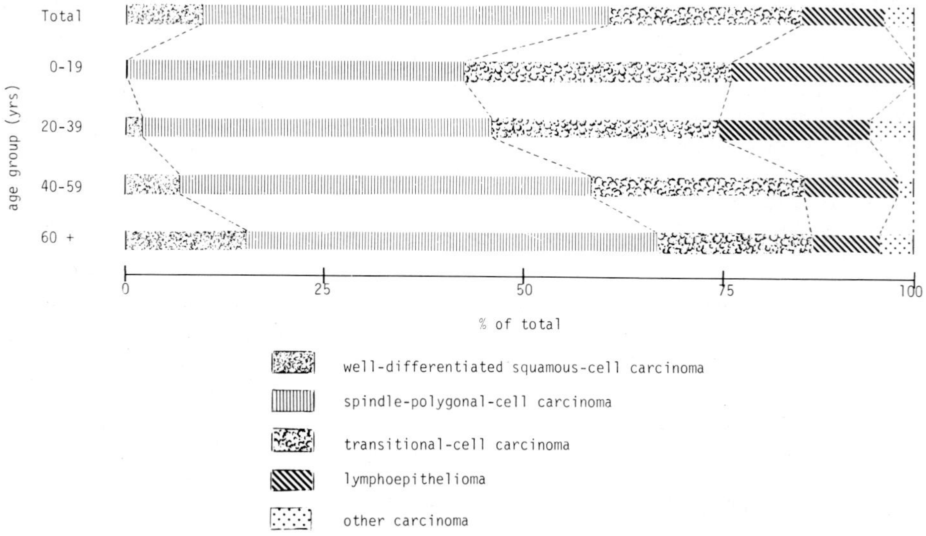

The sex ratio was almost the same for each subgroup of NPC, i.e., twice as high in males; the frequency of lymphoepithelioma tended to be even higher in males.

COMPARISON OF HISTOLOGICAL TYPES OF NPC IN A LOW-RISK AND A HIGH-RISK AREA

As described above, the majority of NPCs in Japan, a low-risk area, are poorly-differentiated carcinomas. There have been excellent reports concerning the histopathology of NPC in a high-risk area, Taiwan (Chen et al., 1971; Yeh, 1962), where a vast majority were also poorly-differentiated. We considered it important to determine whether the histology of NPCs in a low-risk area differs from that in a high-risk area and therefore carried out a comparative study of the histopathology of NPC in Taiwanese and Japanese patients.

The results obtained from biopsies of 208 Taiwanese cases of NPC in the Department of Pathology, Taiwan University between 1971 and 1973 were compared with those for the Japanese NPC described above as Group 2. As shown in Table 5, poorly-differentiated carcinomas predominated, and well-differentiated carcinomas were few in both groups, especially in Taiwanese; the incidence of the former was 95.6% in Taiwanese and 68.6% in Japanese. Analysis of the percentage distribution of subgroups within poorly-differentiated carcinoma shows that spindle-polygonal-cell carcinoma accounted for 52.8% in Japanese and for 23.1% in Taiwanese patients, whereas transitional-cell carcinomas and lymphoepitheliomas were more frequent (76.9%) in Taiwanese than in Japanese (47.2%). Of other malignancies, lymphoma was much more frequent in Japanese patients.

Table 5. Histological types of malignant tumours of the nasopharynx in 925 cases from a low-risk area, Japan, and in 208 cases from a high-risk area, Taiwan

	Japanese			Taiwanese		
	No. of cases	% of total	% of poorly-differentiated	No. of cases	% of total	% of poorly-differentiated
Squamous-cell carcinoma						
well-differentiated	96	10.4		6	2.9	
poorly-differentiated	635	68.6		199	95.6	
spindle-polygonal-cell	335	36.2	52.8	46	22.1	23.1
transitional-cell	195	21.1	30.7	110	52.8	55.3
lymphoepithelioma	105	11.3	16.5	43	20.7	21.6
Other carcinoma	27	2.9		2	1.0	
Lymphoma	143	15.5		1	0.5	
Sarcoma	24	2.6		0	0.0	

These figures clearly indicate that among NPCs in a high-risk area there is an extremely high frequency of poorly-differentiated carcinoma, especially of transitional-cell carcinoma and lymphoepithelioma, and a very low frequency of well-differentiated carcinoma. There is thus a considerable difference in the histology of NPC in a low-risk area from that in a high-risk area. In the high-risk area, almost all malignant tumours of the nasopharynx were NPC and poorly-differentiated, with a predominance of particular histological types.

HISTOLOGICAL TYPES OF NPC AND ANTI-VCA ANTIBODY TITRES

A close relationship between NPC and Epstein-Barr virus (EBV) has been reported by many scientists (de-Thé et al., 1969; Henle et al., 1970; Ito et al., 1969; Sugano, 1975; Sugano et al., 1970; zur Hausen et al., 1970). In an attempt to clarify the relationship of histological subgrouping to anti-VCA antibody titres, these were measured in 84 Japanese NPC patients, using Kawamura's modification of Henle's fluorescence antibody test (Sawaki et al., 1975). Geometric means of anti-VCA antibody titres in patients with various types of NPC and their ridit analysis are shown in Table 6 and Fig. 3, respectively. It can be seen that the mean titre was very high in patients with lymphoepitheliomas; in addition, 80% of these patients showed positive reactions, while positive rates for other types ranged from 33% (well-differentiated carcinoma) to 47% (spindle-polygonal-cell carcinoma and transitional-cell carcinoma). It is uncertain why both antibody titre and positive rate were so high in the lymphoepithelioma group. These results are interesting enough to anticipate that EBV genomes latent in cancer cells are different in different subgroups of NPC and may vary with the grade of differentiation of NPC. However, a ridit analysis did not show these data to be statistically significant.

Table 6. Anti-Epstein-Barr viral capsid antigen (VCA) antibody levels in 84 Japanese patients with nasopharyngeal tumours, by tumour type[a]

	Tumour type					
	Well-differentiated carcinoma	Spindle-polygonal-cell carcinoma	Transitional-cell carcinoma	Lympho-epithelioma	Other carcinoma	Lymphoma
Geometric mean titre	81	314	304	760	22	110
Positivity[b] (%)	33.3	47.4	47.4	80	0	40

[a] From Sawaki et al. (1975)
[b] ≥ 1:640 was considered to be positive.

In order to confirm these preliminary results, the relationship between histological subgrouping and anti-VCA antibody titres was examined in a still larger series of 205 Taiwanese NPC cases whose anti-VCA antibody titres had previously been examined by Lynn et al. (1973). These cases were classified by the same histological criteria.

FIG. 3. ANTI-EPSTEIN-BARR VIRAL CAPSID ANTIGEN TITRES IN JAPANESE NASOPHARYNGEAL CARCINOMA PATIENTS

Ridit analysis of anti-Epstein-Barr viral capsid antigen titres in 84 Japanese nasopharyngeal carcinoma patients, by histological type of tumour

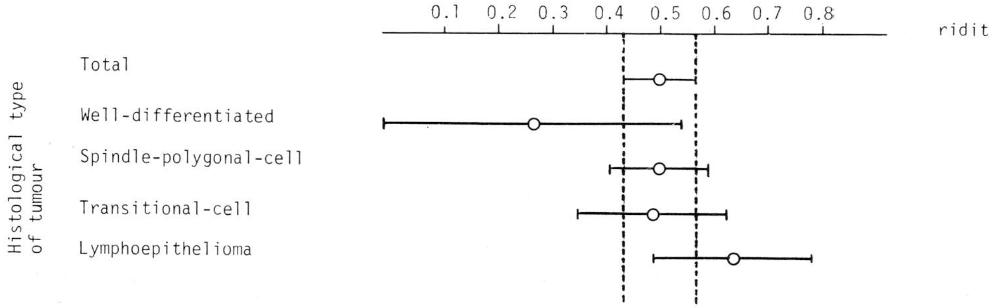

As shown in Table 7, the results did not support our findings obtained in Japanese NPC patients: geometric means of anti-VCA antibody titres and and positivity rates were almost the same in all subgroups of poorly-differentiated carcinoma. The mean titre in patients with well-differentiated carcinoma was low; however, the number of cases in this group was small, and these figures were not statistically significant.

Table 7. Anti-Epstein-Barr viral capsid antigen (VCA) antibody levels in 205 Taiwanese patients with nasopharyngeal carcinoma, by tumour type[a]

	Tumour type			
	Well differentiated carcinoma	Spindle-polygonal-cell carcinoma	Transitional cell carcinoma	Lympho-epithelioma
No. of cases	6	46	110	43
Geometric mean titre	156	320	350	259
Positivity[b] (%)	33.3	45.7	54.7	44.2

[a] Selected from cases reported by Lynn et al. (1973)

[b] ⩾ 1:640 was considered to be positive.

As reported by Lin et al. (1969), Chen et al. (1971) and Sugano (1975), electron microscope studies show that nuclear bodies, inclusion bodies in both the nuclei and the cytoplasm and tubular structures in the endoplasmic reticulum often occur in cells from lymphoepitheliomas, and these findings suggest that certain ultrastructural changes are induced by viral infection. It is possible to conclude from our study that anti-VCA antibody titres are different in patients with different histological types of NPC, i.e., low in those with well-differentiated carcinomas and high in those with lymphoepitheliomas. Further studies to pursue this possibility will be useful in understanding the nature of NPC.

SUMMARY

NPC in Japan was studied histopathologically by examining 816 NPCs from among 3 338 biopsies from patients with tumours of the nasopharynx and other parts of the upper respiratory system. In addition, a comparative study on NPC among Taiwanese and an immunoserological study were carried out.

When comparing histological types of malignant tumours of the upper respiratory tract, poorly-differentiated squamous-cell carcinoma predominated only in those of the nasopharynx. Malignant nasopharyngeal tumours in Japanese patients were characterized by two histological features: predominance of squamous-cell carcinoma, especially of the poorly-differentiated type, and a relatively high frequency of malignant lymphoma.

An analysis of 731 cases of NPC showed that a vast majority (86.7%) were poorly-differentiated and a minority (13.3%) well-differentiated squamous-cell carcinomas. The former included 45.8% spindle-polygonal-cell carcinomas, 26.6% transitional-cell carcinomas and 14.3% lymphoepitheliomas. Although the transitional-cell carcinomas and lymphoepitheliomas showed a peculiar morphology, it was confirmed that they are of a squamous nature.

A comparative study of the histology of NPCs in a high-risk area, Taiwan, and in a low-risk area, Japan, revealed considerable differences between the two groups. Well-differentiated carcinomas were infrequent in both groups but were more frequent in Japanese than in Taiwanese, while the frequency of poorly-differentiated carcinomas, especially transitional-cell carcinomas and lymphoepitheliomas, was much higher among Taiwanese.

A seroepidemiological study on the relation of anti-VCA antibody titres to histological type of tumour in 84 Japanese NPC patients revealed that the rate of positivity and the geometric mean of the titres were considerably higher in patients with lymphoepitheliomas. Although corresponding results have not yet been obtained in the 205 Taiwanese cases, a seropathological study along this line would appear to be important, since the results obtained in Japanese NPC cases may suggest that EBV genomes in NPC cells vary with the grade of differentiation of NPC.

ACKNOWLEDGEMENTS

The authors are deeply indebted to Professor S. Yeh, Professor W.S.J. Lin and Associate Professor S.W. How, Department of Pathology, and to Professor S.M. Tu and Dr T.C. Lynn, Department of Otorhinolaryngology, Taiwan University Hospital, for their cooperation, valuable discussion and generous permission to examine biopsy materials and to use serological data from Taiwanese cases; to Professor A. Kawamura and Dr K. Hamajima, Department of Immunology, Institute of Medical Science, The University of Tokyo, for their generous permission to use serological data from Japanese and Taiwanese cases; and to Dr A. Sakamoto, Department of Pathology, for his help in preparing the data on Group 1. These investigations were supported in part by grants from the Ministry of Education, Science and Culture and from the Ministry of Health and Welfare, the Government of Japan.

REFERENCES

Chen, H.-C., Yeh, S., Tu, S.-M., Hsu, M.-M., Lynn, T.-C. & Sugano, H. (1971) *Anaplastic carcinoma of the nasopharynx*. In: Nakahara, W., Nishioka, K., Hirayama, T. & Ito, Y., eds, *Recent Advances in Human Tumor Virology and Immunology*, Tokyo, University of Tokyo Press, pp. 237-267

de-Thé, G., Ambrosioni, J.C., Ho, H.-C. & Kwan, H.-C. (1969) Lymphoblastoid transformation and presence of herpes-type viral particles in a Chinese nasopharyngeal tumor cultured *in vitro*. *Nature (Lond.)*, *221*, 770-771

Hatori, H. (1966) [Statistics of malignant tumors of the epipharynx], *Jibi-Rinsho*, *59*, 581-584 (in Japanese)

Henle, W., Henle, G., Burtin, P., Cachin, Y., Clifford, P., de Schryver, A., de-Thé, G., Diehl, V., Ho, H.C. & Klein, G. (1970) Antibodies to Epstein-Barr virus in nasopharyngeal carcinoma, other head and neck neoplasms, and control groups. *J. nat. Cancer Inst.*, *44*, 225-231

Ito, Y., Takahashi, T., Kawamura, A., Jr & Tu, S.M. (1969) High anti-EB virus titer in sera of patients with nasopharyngeal carcinoma: a small-scale seroepidemiological study. *Gann*, *60*, 335-340

Lin, H.-S., Lin, C.-S., Yeh, S. & Tu, S.-M. (1969) Fine structure of nasopharyngeal carcinoma with special reference to the anaplastic type. *Cancer*, *23*, 390-405

Lynn, T.-C., Tu, S.-M., Hirayama, T. & Kawamura, A. (1973) Nasopharyngeal carcinoma and Epstein-Barr virus. *Jap. J. exp. Med.*, *43*, 121-133, 135-144

Miyagi, T. (1967) *Carcinoma of the nasopharynx and related organs in Japan based on mortality, morbidity and autopsy studies.* In: Muir, C.S. & Shanmugaratnam, K., eds, *Cancer of the Nasopharynx (UICC Monograph Series No. 1)*, Copenhagen, Munksgaard, pp. 29-32

Ootsuka, H. (1964) [On the so-called lymphoepithelioma of the nasopharynx]. *Saishin-Igaku*, *19*, 1708-1709 (in Japanese)

Sawaki, S., Sugano, H., Hirayama, T., Kawamura, A., Jr & Tachibana, T. (1975) Histopathological and immunological studies of nasopharyngeal carcinoma. *Chin. J. Microbiol.*, *8*, 73-81

Sawaki, S., Hirayama, T. & Sugano, H. (1976) Studies on nasopharyngeal carcinoma in Japan. *Gann Monogr.*, *18*, pp. 63-74

Schmincke, A. (1921) Über Lymphoepitheliale Geschwülste. *Beitr. Path. Anat.*, *68*, 161-170

Shanmugaratnam, K. & Muir, C.S. (1967) *Nasopharyngeal carcinoma: origin and structure.* In: Muir, C.S. & Shanmugaratnam, K., eds, *Cancer of the Nasopharynx (UICC Monograph Series No. 1)*, Copenhagen, Munksgaard, pp. 153-162

Sugano, H. (1975) *Potential viral etiology of human tumors.* In: Grundmamm, E., ed., *Handbuch der allgemeinen Pathologie* VI/6 *Tumors II, Viral and Chemical Carcinogenesis*, Berlin-Heidelberg-New York, Springer-Verlag, pp. 243-328

Sugano, H., Takada, M., Chen, H.-C. & Tu, S.-M. (1970) Presence of herpes-type virus in the culture cell line from a nasopharyngeal carcinoma in Taiwan. *Proc. Japan. Acad.*, *46*, 453-457

Sugano, H., Sawaki, S., Sakamoto, G. & Hirayama, T. (1971) *Carcinoma of the nasopharynx in Japan.* In: Nakahara, W., Nishioka, K., Hirayama, T. & Ito, Y., eds, *Recent Advances in Human Tumor Virology and Immunology*, Tokyo, University of Tokyo Press, pp. 229-235

Yeh, S. (1962) A histological classification of carcinoma of the nasopharynx with a critical review as to the existence of lympho-epitheliomas. *Cancer*, *15*, 895-920

zur Hausen, H., Schulte-Holthausen, H., Klein, G., Henle, W., Clifford, P. & Santesson, L. (1970) DNA in biopsies of Burkitt tumors and anaplastic carcinoma of the nasopharynx. *Nature (Lond.)*, *228*, 1056-1058

THE HISTOPATHOLOGICAL SPECTRUM OF NASOPHARYNGEAL CARCINOMA

L.H. WEILAND

Department of Surgical Pathology,
Mayo Clinic and Mayo Medical School,
Rochester, Minn., USA

The term nasopharyngeal carcinoma (NPC) includes a variety of malignant tumours. All are rare in the US (Cutler & Young, 1975). Adenocarcinomas are usually of a type which indicates an origin in the minor salivary glands of the area; they are not difficult to diagnose and will receive no further discussion. Of greater interest are those that arise from the epithelial cells lining the nasopharynx. This tissue varies from pseudostratified columnar epithelium to stratified squamous epithelium and has a unique relationship with the underlying lymphoid tissue. This intimate association of epithelium and lymphoid tissue is observed frequently, but the implications of the relationship evade complete understanding. It is common to see a blending of lymphoid elements and epithelium, which obscures the apparent basement membrane supporting the epithelial layer.

Most histopathological studies of NPC are based on biopsies of a primary tumour and may be accompanied by excisional biopsies of cervical lymph nodes containing metastatic tumour deposits. Data is therefore derived from multiple small biopsies that are subject to mechanical trauma and numerous other artefacts; it is inherently undesirable to judge the morphology of a tumour from small biopsy specimens, especially when it is known that the tumour may lack homogeneity. Custom and restrictions in post-mortem examinations usually preclude removal and examination of the nasopharynx. These problems make an accurate, consistent and meaningful classification difficult to establish. Therefore, results of studies relating to the percentages of different histopathological types are unreliable, and statistical studies on the prognosis of different varieties of NPC are likewise of questionable validity.

Because of its rarity, most pathologists in the US do not have the opportunity to become familiar with the micromorphological varieties of NPC. At the Mayo Clinic, a large referral institution, however, an average of 15 cases are seen each year for diagnosis and treatment. This rate has remained relatively constant for the past thirty years.

The desirability of establishing a simplified classification for NPC which is accurate and which minimizes inter- and intrapathologist variability is obvious. There is little doubt that the NPCs with which this paper is concerned originate in the epithelium of the nasopharynx (Gazzolo et al., 1972). Ultrastructural studies (Svoboda et al., 1967) on even the very poorly differentiated tumours have shown characteristic features of squamous cells, i.e., keratin production and desmosomes; tumours that have keratin production observable by light microscopy are thought to originate from the epithelial surface.

Since NPCs are squamous carcinomas and since some produce keratin that is easily recognized by light microscopy, the single most useful and consistently reproducible observation is whether the tumour is keratinizing or nonkeratinizing. This distinction can usually be made even with small biopsy specimens. Prognosis for NPC is dependent on the radiosensitivity of the tumour and is inversely related to the ability of the cells to produce keratin (Perez et al., 1969; Scanlon et al., 1967). Thus, separation of these two basic types of tumour has clinical usefulness.

KERATINIZING SQUAMOUS-CELL CARCINOMA

This type of NPC accounts for approximately 25% of squamous carcinomas. Although there may be a full spectrum of differentiation, the great majority are well differentiated and have abundant keratin production (Fig. 1). Both intracellular keratin and extracellular 'pearls' are commonly seen, and intracellular bridges are readily found.

FIG. 1. KERATINIZING SQUAMOUS CARCINOMA

The tumour has surface involvement and abundant keratin. H & E x100

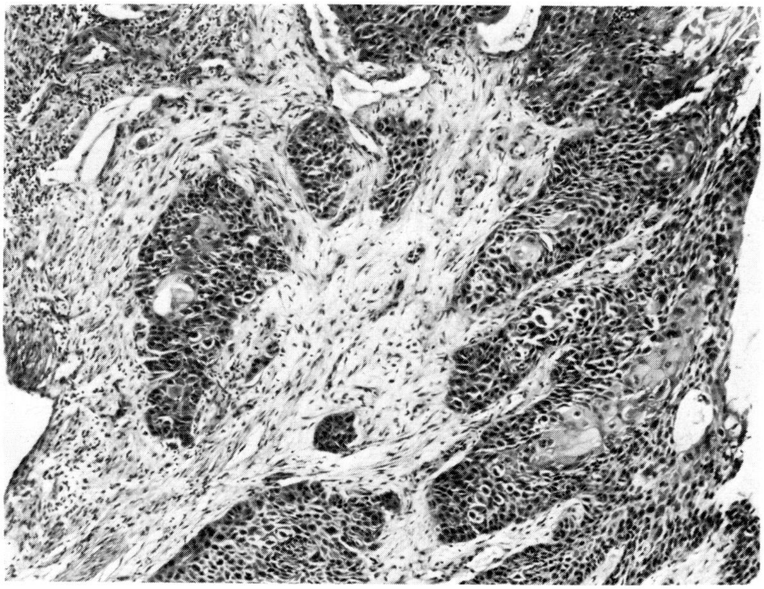

This tumour always occurs on the surface of the nasopharyngeal epithelium from which it originates. An apparent *in situ* component is frequently observed (Fig. 2). Non-neoplastic epithelium adjacent to the tumour is almost invariably stratified squamous in structure. The tissue reaction to infiltration of this tumour is predictably one of desmoplasia (Fig. 3) and may be marked. The inflammatory reaction which

FIG. 2. KERATINIZING SQUAMOUS CARCINOMA

An apparent *in situ* component is frequently present. H & E x160

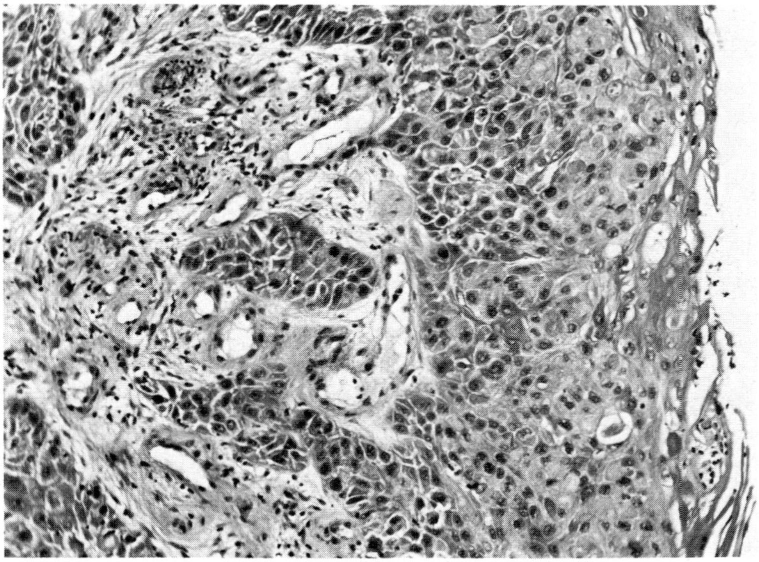

FIG. 3. KERATINIZING SQUAMOUS CARCINOMA

The response to invasion is marked desmoplasia. H & E x160

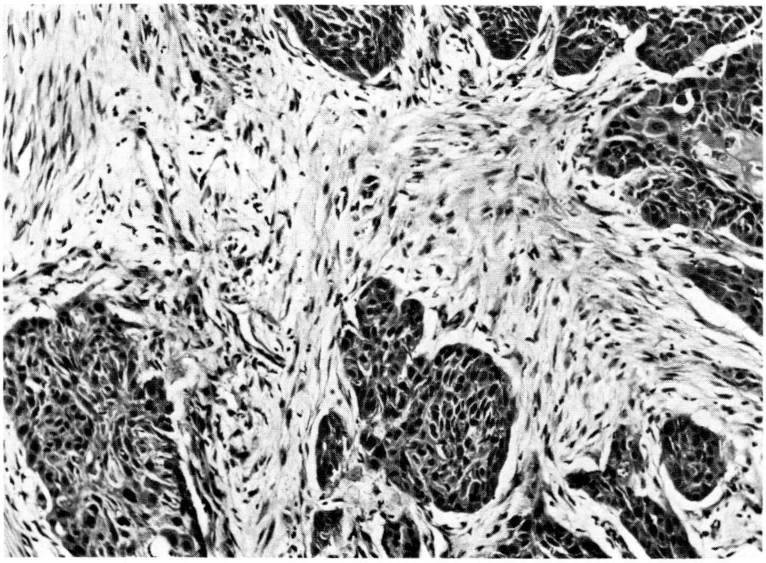

accompanies this fibroblastic activity is moderate and consists of polymorphonuclear leucocytes, lymphocytes and occasional plasma cells. Keratinizing squamous carcinomas have less tendency to pleomorphism than do the nonkeratinizing variety; the same keratin production and reactive desmoplasia of the primary tumour are found even in lymph node deposits.

In all probability, the keratinizing NPC is not unique to the nasopharynx. Microscopically, its features are similar or identical to those of tumours of the tongue, oral epithelium, oropharynx, larynx and other parts of the upper aerodigestive tract. If the nasopharynx were accessible to the surgeon's scalpel, this tumour would undoubtedly be infinitely more curable.

NONKERATINIZING SQUAMOUS CARCINOMA

Although this tumour also originates in the surface nasopharyngeal epithelium, it lacks the keratin production, the large cells and the growth pattern of the keratinizing type. Many variants of this tumour can be recognized microscopically (Yeh, 1962): these include lymphoepithelioma, transitional-cell carcinoma, clear-cell carcinoma, spindle-cell carcinoma and anaplastic carcinoma. Their different microscopic patterns have led previous investigators to consider some of these to be distinct tumour entities. Such considerations have created confusion in the medical literature and have resulted in the statement by Scanlon et al. (1967) that "there is probably no other single regional group of malignant lesions of the respiratory system with less agreement in the world literature with regard to the correct and proper classification". The demonstration (Svoboda et al., 1962) that even the undifferentiated tumours have ultrastructural characteristics of squamous tumours has done much to reduce the confusion. Proof that the cells are epithelial makes acceptable the concept that these different microscopic patterns are variants of nonkeratinizing squamous carcinomas, even though there is a natural reluctance to use the term 'squamous' when light microscopy fails to demonstrate the necessary features.

Of additional major importance in accepting this concept is an appreciation that the variants frequently coexist in the same tumour. Thus, if multiple areas of such a tumour are examined, some sections may have the appearance of lymphoepithelioma and others the appearance of anaplastic carcinoma. Yeh (1962) has considered such tumours to be combined-cell type.

Even though keratinizing and nonkeratinizing tumours arise from the same epithelium, the nonkeratinizing ones are less frequently observed microscopically to originate in the nasopharyngeal epithelium (Fig. 4), whereas surface epithelial involvement is readily found in keratinizing tumours (Fig. 2). This feature led Ewing (1929) to believe that the origin of nonkeratinizing tumours was the lymphoid reticulum. Multiple tissue sections, however, usually reveal that the tumour communicates

FIG. 4. NONKERATINIZING SQUAMOUS CARCINOMA

Involvement of the surface epithelium is seen less frequently than in keratinizing tumours. The overlying epithelium is typically pseudo-stratified columnar. H & E x250

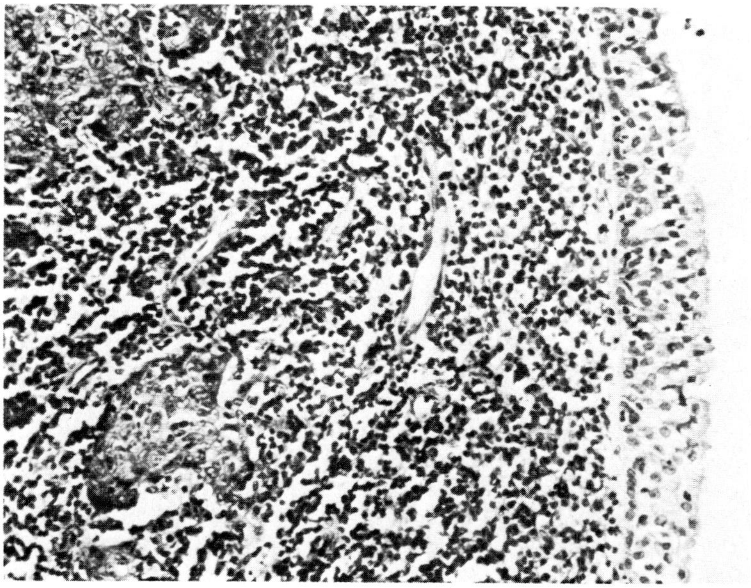

with the overlying epithelium. The non-neoplastic epithelium adjacent to and overlying the tumours is more frequently of a pseudostratified columnar than a stratified squamous type (Fig. 4). Likewise, it is unusual, and again in contrast with the keratinizing type, to find an apparent *in situ* component in nonkeratinizing tumours; when it is seen, proof that it represents true *in situ* carcinoma and not epithelial replacement from an underlying tumour is difficult to establish.

As stated previously, keratinizing tumours are similar in their microscopic features to other tumours in the upper aerodigestive tract and are probably not unique to the nasopharynx. The same cannot be said of the nonkeratinizing tumours of the nasopharynx, which are probably restricted to the nasopharynx and to the tissues of Waldeyer's ring, in which the epithelium has a unique and often intimate relationship with the lymphoid tissue that resides beneath it. This applies particularly to nasopharyngeal tumours that have an abundant lymphoid stroma. Virological studies should eventually clarify these differences with certainty. The other tissue in which such a relationship normally exists is the thymus gland: tumours of the thymus gland may have microscopic features strikingly similar to those of nonkeratinizing squamous carcinomas of the nasopharynx. Other tumours that arise in nonlymphoid tissue and that may have a similar blending of neoplasm and lymphoid stroma are medullary carcinomas of the breast and seminomas.

While the tissue reaction to infiltrating keratinizing tumours is always desmoplasia, reactions to nonkeratinizing tumours are variable: there might be a fibroblastic response, but this is not the most common; the usual reaction is one of mixed desmoplasia and inflammatory-cell reaction. The participating inflammatory cells consist of lymphocytes, plasma cells, histiocytes and polymorphonuclear leucocytes; these latter cells are frequently seen when necrosis is present. Those tumours that elicit no tissue reaction to invasion have a microscopic pattern of lymphoepithelioma. It is not unusual to find desmoplasia in only one portion of the tumour and not in adjacent areas; or, the primary tumour might elicit no tissue reaction, while a metastatic tumour in the cervical lymph nodes has marked desmoplasia. Caution is necessary in interpreting such findings in tissues that have been irradiated: in essence, they are invalid, since radiation-induced fibrosis might be identical microscopically to that which is tumour-elicited. The reason why some malignant tumours elicit striking fibroblastic tissue responses and, just as importantly, why others show a total absence of such responses requires elucidation. Permeation of lymphatic vessels by NPC must occur frequently, since in approximately 50% of patients metastatic tumour is present in cervical lymph nodes at the time of diagnosis (Cammoun et al., 1974); however, such invasion is seldom seen in biopsy specimens (Fig. 5).

FIG. 5. KERATINIZING SQUAMOUS CARCINOMA

Tumour growth within vascular channels is seen only rarely. H & E x250

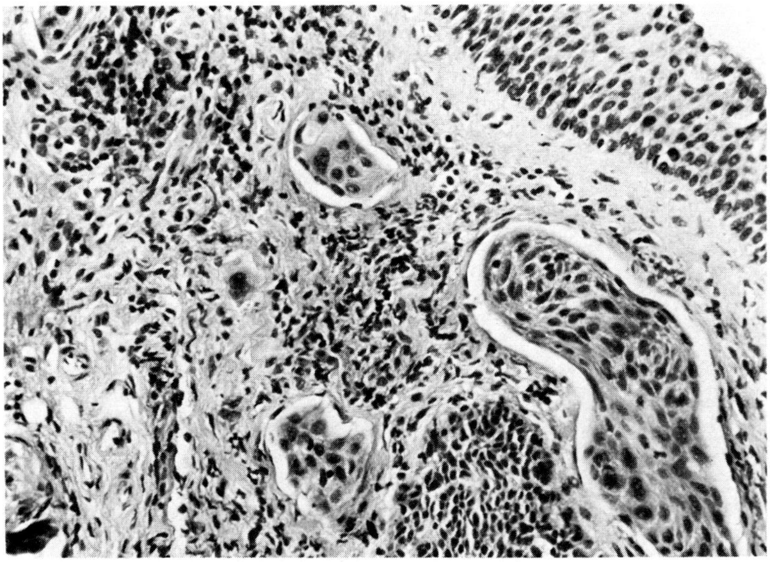

Lymphoepithelioma variant

An intriguing variant of nonkeratinizing squamous carcinoma, lymphoepithelioma, has unusual gross and microscopic features that occasionally cause it to be mistaken for malignant lymphoma. Both the gross and microscopic features can be attributed to the failure of this variant to elicit tissue desmoplasia (Fig. 6). Microscopically, the cells have little to suggest their epithelial and squamous origin, especially when the portion of the tumour under examination is growing in fine strands and single cells in the lymphoid stroma. The cells frequently lack the cytoplasmic outline that is usually associated with epithelial cells. Other cytological characteristics include a prominent nucleolus and pale vesicular nuclei; this latter feature may be accentuated artefactually by improper tissue processing.

FIG. 6. NONKERATINIZING SQUAMOUS CARCINOMA

A total absence of desmoplastic tissue reaction defines the lymphoepithelioma variant. H & E x250

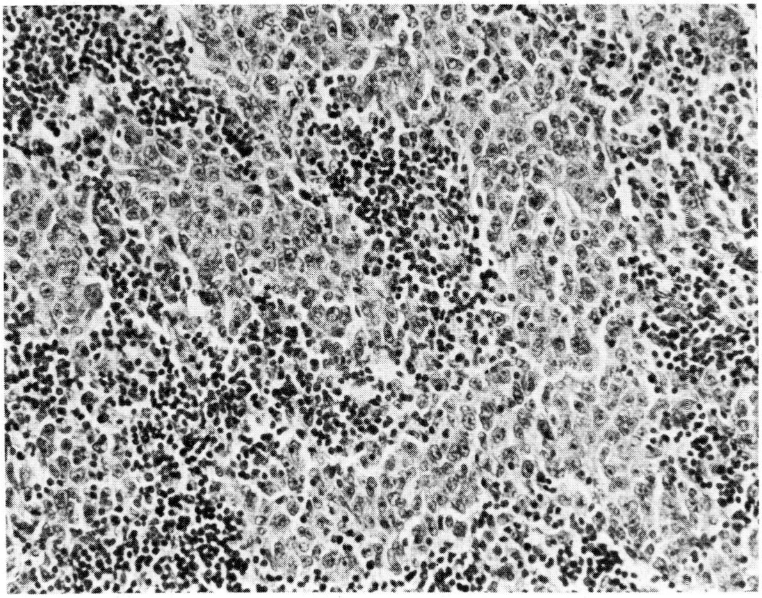

Transitional-cell carcinoma variant

The description of this variant derives from its resemblance to tumours originating in the epithelium of the urinary tract. It is rarely mistaken for anything other than an epithelial tumour since its growth tends to develop a frond-like pattern (Fig. 7). The tissue reaction to its invasion is usually desmoplastic but not of the marked degree seen in keratinizing squamous carcinomas.

FIG. 7. NONKERATINIZING SQUAMOUS CARCINOMA

Tumour growth featuring frond-like structures with fibrovascular stalks sets apart the transitional-cell carcinoma variants. They resemble epithelial tumours of the urinary bladder. H & E x250

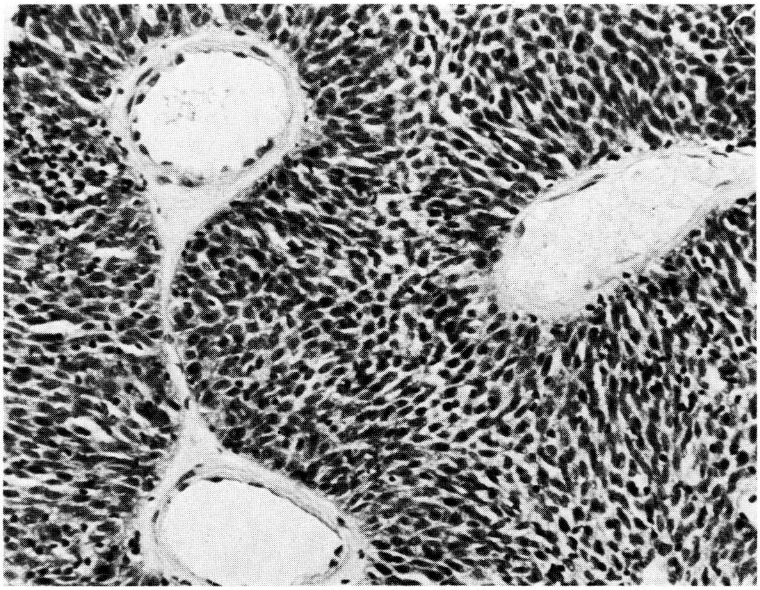

Spindle-cell carcinoma variant

When the cells of nonkeratinizing tumours have spindling morphology, they can be mistaken for sarcomas. Almost without exception, such spindling is a focal phenomenon within the tumour, other areas showing the usual polyhedral cell shape. Spindling is also a common artefact in biopsies that are obtained by removing tissue with small forceps.

Undifferentiated carcinoma variant

Nonkeratinizing squamous carcinomas whose growth pattern appears microscopically as sheets of undifferentiated cells without lymphoid stroma have often received the designation 'undifferentiated carcinoma'. Individually, the cells are similar or identical to those of the lymphoepithelioma variant. Although cell stratification may be observed, other evidence of their squamous nature is lacking.

SUMMARY

Nonglandular carcinomas of the nasopharynx originate in the epithelium of that anatomical region. Although numerous morphological patterns exist at the level observable by light microscopy, ultrastructurally, all have features of squamous-cell carcinoma. The most useful and consistent classification on the basis of light microscopy is that which separates keratinizing squamous carcinomas from nonkeratinizing carcinomas. Approximately 25% of tumours have abundant and easily recognized keratin. The nonkeratinizing types are more confusing, since many variants exist, both from tumour to tumour and, frequently, within the same tumour. Variable tissue reactions to infiltrating tumours, ranging from marked desmoplasia to complete absence of reaction, add to the confusion. The descriptive names applied to the variants of nonkeratinizing squamous carcinomas are well engraved in medical communications, and there is little chance that they will be abandoned.

REFERENCES

Cammoun, M., Hoerner, G.V. & Mourali, N. (1974) Tumors of the nasopharynx in Tunisia: an anatomic and clinical study based on 143 cases. *Cancer, 33*, 184-192

Cutler, S.J. & Young, J.L., Jr, eds (1975) Third National Cancer Survey: Incidence Data. *Nat. Cancer Inst. Monogr., 41*

Ewing, J. (1929) Lymphoepithelioma. *Amer. J. Pathol., 5*, 99-107

Gazzolo, L., de-Thé, G., Vuillaume, M. & Ho, H.C. (1972) Nasopharyngeal carcinoma. II. Ultrastructure of normal mucosa, tumor biopsies and subsequent epithelial growth *in vitro*. *J. nat. Cancer Inst., 48*, 73-86

Perez, C.A., Ackerman, L.V., Mill, W.B., Ogara, J.H. & Powers, W.E. (1969) Cancer of the nasopharynx: factors influencing prognosis. *Cancer, 24*, 1-17

Scanlon, P.W., Rhodes, R.E., Jr, Woolner, L.B., Devine, K.D. & McBean, J.B. (1967) Cancer of the nasopharynx: 142 patients treated in the 11 year period 1950-1960. *Amer. J. Roentgenol., 99*, 313-325

Svoboda, D.J., Kirchner, F.R. & Shanmugaratnam, K. (1967) *The fine structure of nasopharyngeal carcinomas*. In: Muir, C.S. & Shanmugaratnam, K., eds, *Cancer of the Nasopharynx (UICC Monograph Series No. 1)*, Copenhagen, Munksgaard, pp. 163-171

Yeh, S. (1962) A histological classification of carcinomas of the nasopharynx with a critical review as to the existence of lympho-epitheliomas. *Cancer*, *15*, 895-920

DIAGNOSIS AND DIFFERENTIAL DIAGNOSIS OF LYMPHOEPITHELIAL CARCINOMA IN LYMPH NODES: HISTOLOGICAL, CYTOLOGICAL AND ELECTRON-MICROSCOPIC FINDINGS

K. LENNERT & E. KAISERLING

Department of General Pathology and Pathologic Anatomy,
University of Kiel,
D 2300 Kiel 1, Federal Republic of Germany

T. MAZZANTI

Istituto di Anatomia et Istologia Patologica,
Ospedale Civile 'Umberto I',
60100 Ancona, Italy

For many years, we have diagnosed a particular type of carcinoma in cervical lymph nodes that allowed us to predict the presence of a primary tumour in the nasopharynx or tonsils. We call this lymph-node tumour a lymphoepithelial carcinoma or Schmincke's tumour. We present here some of the findings we have made in a series of such tumours collected at the Lymph Node Registry in Kiel between 1964 and 1976.

MATERIALS AND METHODS

The Lymph Node Registry series comprised 159 cases. A few other cases observed before 1964 or since 1976 were also considered, but only in certain respects.

As far as possible, we investigated all cases not only with haematoxylin-eosin staining but also with Giemsa and silver staining and with the periodic acid-Schiff (PAS) reaction. Imprints were available in five cases, and these were examined with Pappenheim staining and with PAS, nonspecific alpha-naphthyl acetate esterase and acid phosphatase. Reactions with other enzymes (alkaline phosphatase, naphthol-AS-D-chloroacetate esterase, peroxidase) are not discussed in detail here, because the tumour cells gave completely negative responses. In four cases, it was possible to do electron-microscopic studies.

RESULTS

A definite diagnosis of lymphoepithelial carcinoma was made in 120 cases; the other 39 diagnoses were only 'probable'. In most of the cases in which clinical information or additional biopsies were available, however, a primary tumour was found in the nasopharynx or, less often, in the tonsils. The ratio of nasopharyngeal to tonsillar tumours was about 1: 5 (on the basis of the 42 cases that had been diagnosed at that time). In no case was a primary tumour found outside the nasopharynx.

Zur Hausen[1] demonstrated the presence of Epstein-Barr virus in two of our cases by means of the hybridization technique. We thus felt it permissible to assume that the lymphoepithelial carcinoma observed by us is the same as the tumour under consideration at this conference. We would like to stress, however, that the following data are based mainly on a subtle morphological analysis of a tumour with a very characteristic appearance. Moreover, even though clinical information was incomplete, we were still able to recognize a characteristic clinical behaviour of this tumour.

Age and sex

The age distribution and sex ratio of our patients are shown in Figure 1. The age curve for all patients reveals a predominance of the disease in patients between 40 and 70 years of age, with a flat peak in the sixth decade. When the sexes are considered separately, however, only the curve for females shows a similar peak, whereas the curve for males reveals that men from 30 to 70 years of age are affected with almost equal frequency. As a result, the median age of female patients is somewhat higher (40 years) than that of males (36 years). The median age of all patients is 37.5 years, whereas the mean is 45.7 years. The ratio of male:female patients was 2.2:1.

Histology

Firstly, we would like to stress that the tumour is much easier to diagnose in Giemsa-stained sections than it is with haematoxylin-eosin staining. At first glance, there are strands and masses of medium-sized to large cells that appear to be cohesive and that have quite abundant, deep grey-blue cytoplasm. These grey-blue tumour cells can easily be distinguished from the blue lymphocytes and especially from the dark-blue plasma cells found between the tumour masses.

---

[1] Unpublished data

FIG. 1. AGE DISTRIBUTION AND SEX RATIO OF LYMPHOEPITHELIAL CARCINOMA PATIENTS

Age distribution and sex ratio of 155 patients with lymph-node metastases of lymphoepithelial carcinoma

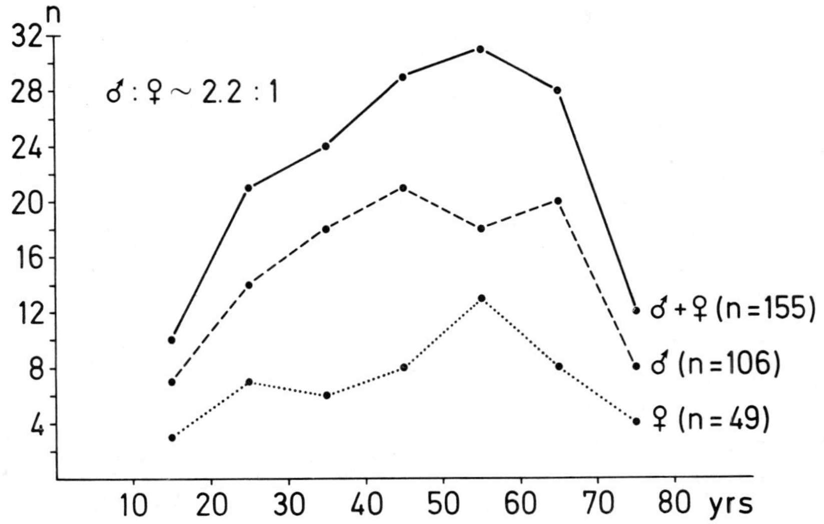

The nuclei of the tumour cells are also characteristic. Especially in the large-cell variant, they have very prominent basophilic nucleoli that often appear to be solitary, but are sometimes multiple (Fig. 2). The nucleoli are located centrally in the very clear nuclei. Sometimes the nuclear chromatin is hardly visible, as in Hodgkin and Sternberg-Reed cells; otherwise, it is very fine and irregularly distributed.

Among the tumour cells there are generally some, and occasionally many, lymphocytes. The means of distinguishing between a Schmincke-type and a Régaud-type of tumour by the number of lymphocytes was not substantiated by our observations and seems to be an artificial division.

Tumour-cell complexes are occasionally seen in the sinuses. They are surrounded by a variable number of reticulin and collagenous fibres, which often contain a large amount of hyalin material. The collagenous fibres are synthesized by fibroblasts (see section on ultrastructure), which sometimes form large strands and areas of connective tissue that may be somewhat similar to those seen in Hodgkin's disease.

FIG. 2. LYMPHOEPITHELIAL CARCINOMA WITH GIEMSA STAINING

a: At upper left, a tumour-cell complex (Ca); note the vesicular nuclei and the large nucleoli. On the right, an epithelioid-cell granuloma (Ep). x 350

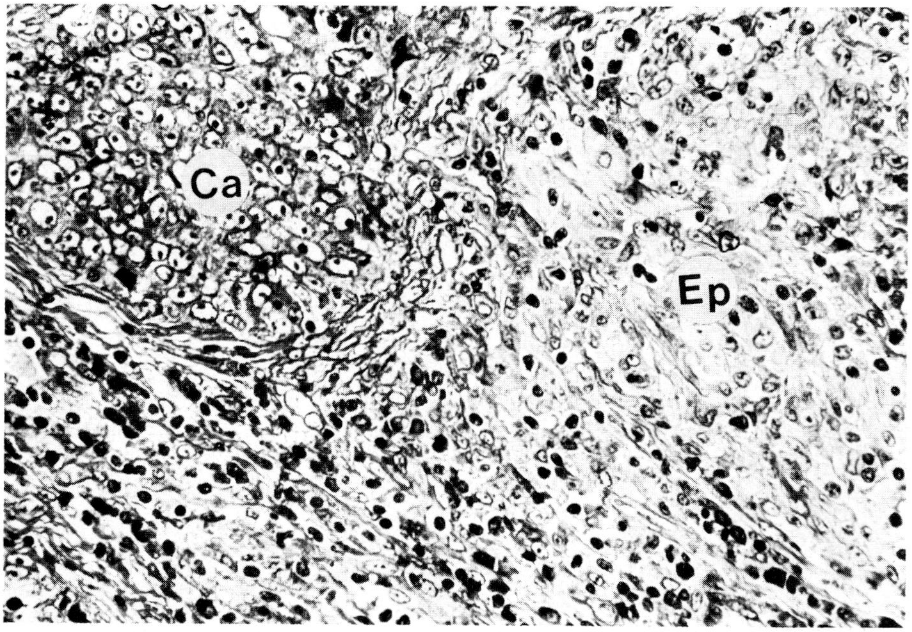

b: At the top, a tumour-cell mass. At the borders of the surrounding lymphatic tissue there are numerous mast cells (Mc), some histiocytes and plasma cells and many lymphocytes. x 560

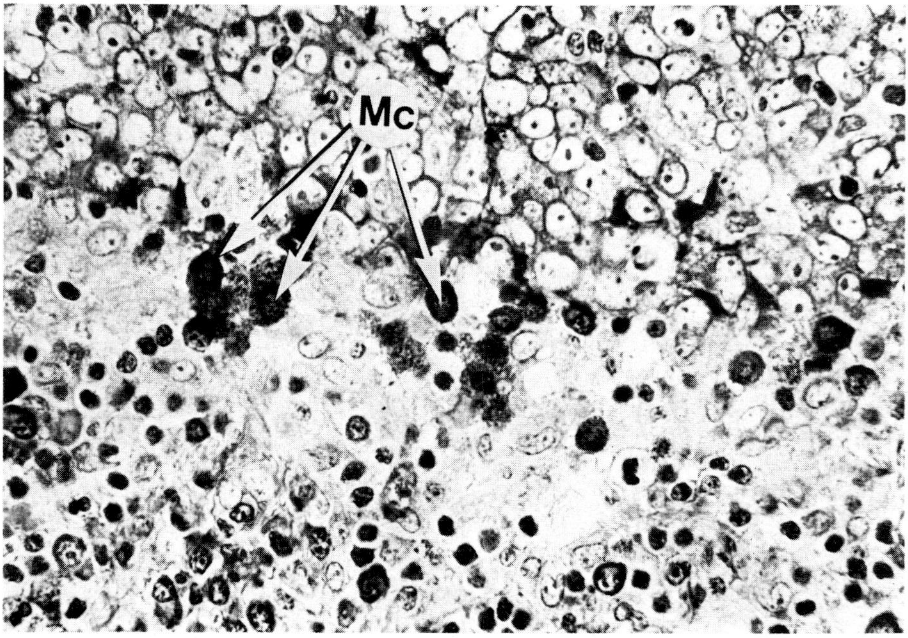

The areas between the tumour strands and masses contain lymphocytes and, often, numerous typical plasma cells and eosinophils. Plasmablasts are very rare; neutrophils are found in moderate numbers and are best seen with the chloroacetate esterase and PAS reactions. In 16% of our cases there was a marked increase in the number of mast cells (Fig. 2b), which were often small and immature. Only some mast cells were seen in 63% of the tumours, and hardly any were found in 21%.

Tuberculoid features, namely, epithelioid-cell granulomas (Figs 2a and 3), were seen in 17.8% of the lymph-node metastases, combined with caseation necrosis in 8.5% (Fig. 4; Rennke & Lennert, 1973). The granulomatous epithelioid-cell reaction was sometimes clearly related to the presence of tumour cells: we found sheets of epithelioid cells around tumour-cell complexes. The epithelioid-cell reaction appeared to progress until there were only a few isolated groups of tumour cells in the epithelioid-cell granuloma. Finally, only epithelioid cells were seen.

We made similar observations with regard to caseation necrosis. There were often 'ghosts', namely, amorphous, dark masses or pyknotic tumour cells left over from the tumour. These necrotic, casein-like tumour masses were surrounded by epithelioid cells. As in tuberculosis, the epithelioid cells were interspersed with increased numbers of fibres containing some hyalin material.

Tubercle bacilli were not found in any of the cases; we therefore interpreted the tuberculoid lesions to be analogues of the sarcoid-like lesions seen in other tumours. In contrast to the sarcoid-like lesions, however, the tuberculoid lesions were sometimes combined with caseation necrosis. To our knowledge, this combination has not been described in any other malignant tumour.

In one case, acute coagulation necrosis was found instead of caseation necrosis. It was identical with the hyperergic necrosis that sometimes occurs in hyperimmune reactions of lymph nodes, such as hydantoin lymphadenopathy. Dilated vessels were seen in the necrotic areas, and an enormous number of eosinophils were found in the surrounding lymphatic tissue.

Differential diagnosis

Lymphoepithelial carcinoma must be distinguished in particular from the following lymph-node lesions:

(1) Metastases from other carcinomas, particularly those of undifferentiated squamous-cell carcinoma

(2) Immunoblastic sarcoma

(3) Hodgkin's disease

(4) Tuberculosis and other tuberculoid lymph-node lesions (e.g., lues III)

FIG. 3. EPITHELIOID-CELL GRANULOMAS

Epithelioid-cell granulomas with remnants of tumour-cell complexes (X)

a: Giemsa, x 175

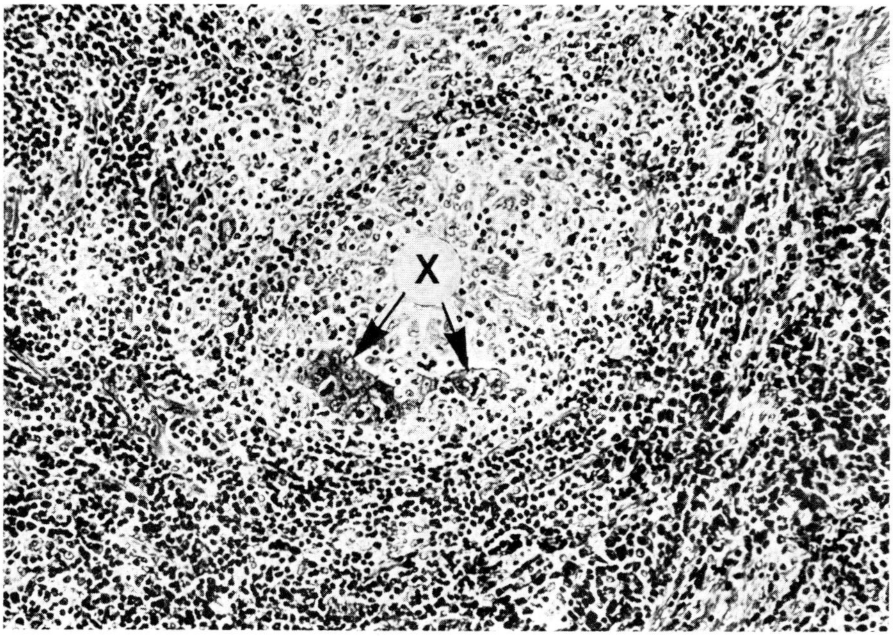

b: PAS, x 350

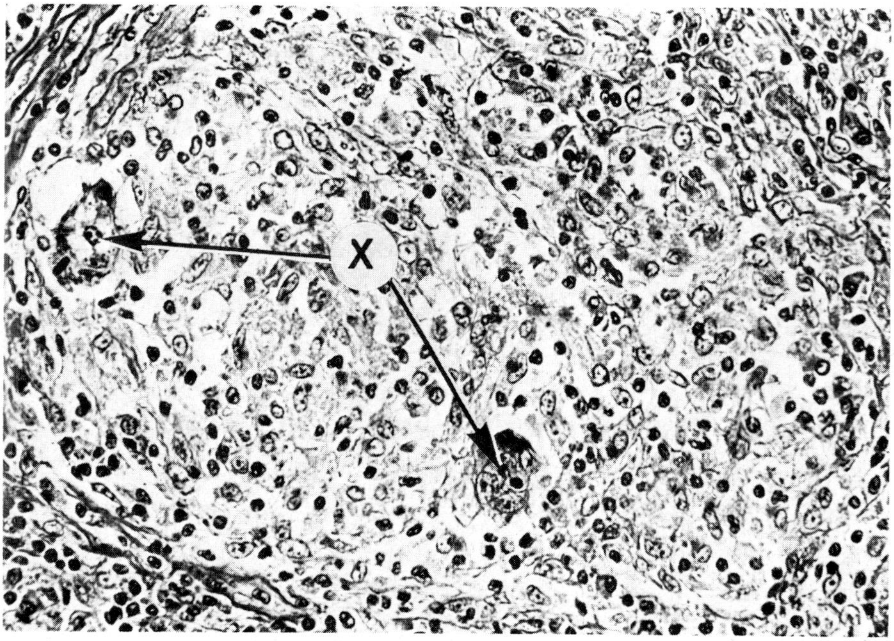

FIG. 4. CASEATION NECROSIS IN LYMPHOEPITHELIAL CARCINOMA

a: Note the epithelioid-cell granulation tissue surrounding the caseation necrosis. H & E, x 56

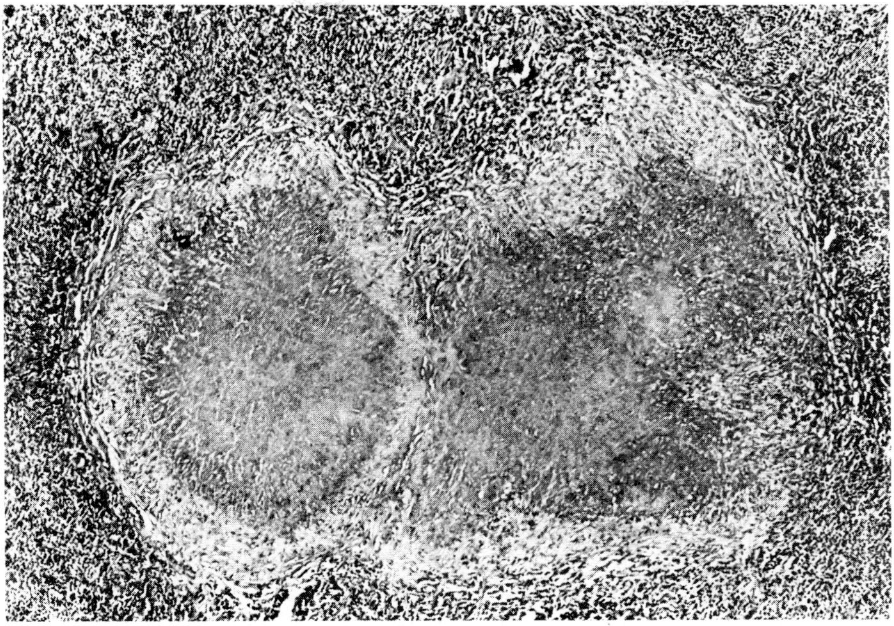

b: Note the remnants of large, dark tumour cells with silver staining (X). The necrotic area is surrounded by epithelioid-cell granulomas. Gomori, x 135

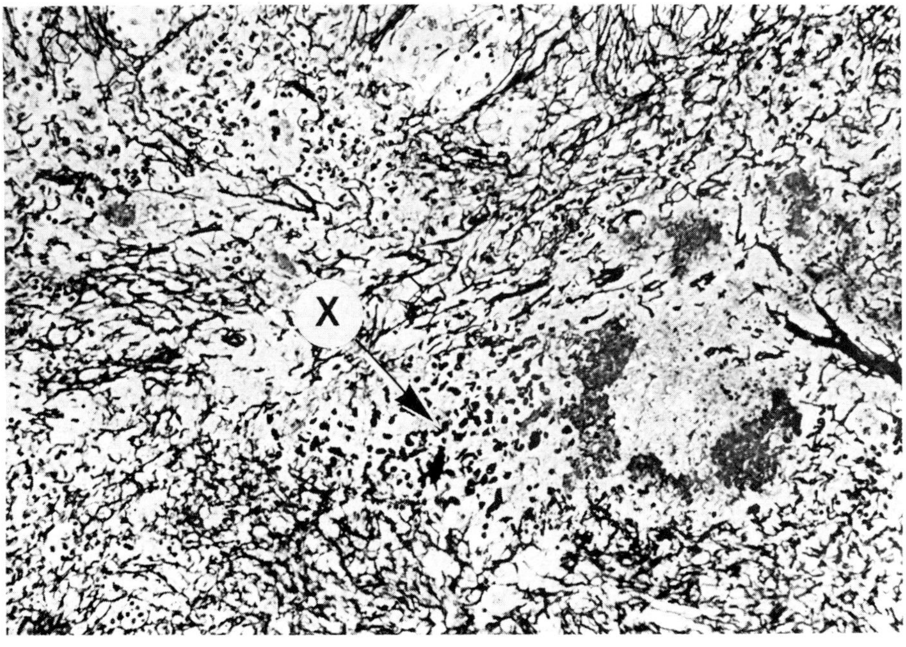

(1) In contrast to lymphoepithelial carcinoma, undifferentiated squamous-cell carcinoma only rarely shows a large increase in the number of plasma cells (Fig. 5) and never shows pronounced eosinophilia (Fig. 6). Nine percent of our squamous-cell carcinomas contained some epithelioid cells and Langhans' giant cells; in most instances, however, these cells were found in small clusters, or singly, and only rarely as granulomas. Caseation necrosis was never seen (Tables 1 and 2).

FIG. 5. PLASMA CELLS IN LYMPH-NODE METASTASES

Incidence of plasma cells in lymph-node metastases of lymphoepithelial carcinoma ('NPC') and of squamous-cell carcinoma (SCC). - Absence of plasma cells; +, ++, +++ plasma cells present in increasing numbers

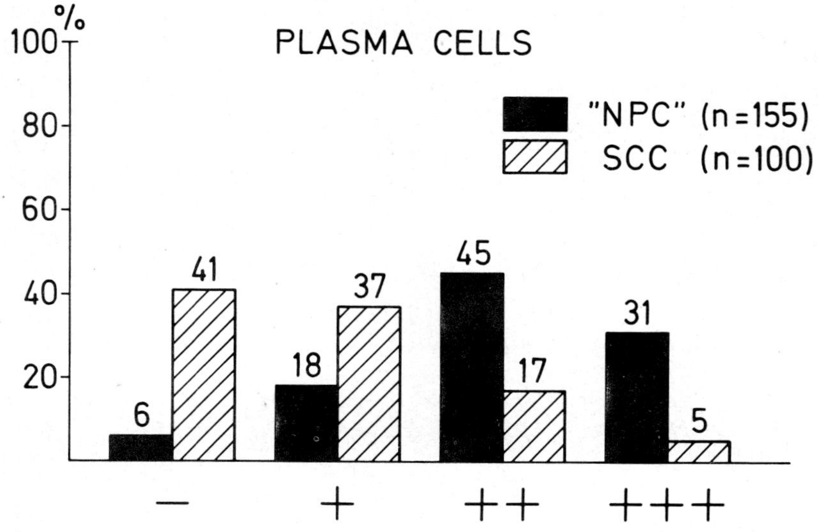

The PAS reaction is sometimes positive in squamous-cell carcinoma and nearly always negative in lymphoepithelial carcinoma.

(2) We began our immunoglobulin analyses of malignant lymphomas because we had sometimes been unable to distinguish lymphoepithelial carcinoma from the large-celled, basophilic lymphomas that we now identify as immunoblastic lymphomas (Lennert, 1973; Lukes & Collins, 1974; Stein et al., 1974). Immunoblastic lymphoma consists of large cells that are more basophilic, have a somewhat smaller rim of cytoplasm and are not as cohesive as the cells of lymphoepithelial carcinoma. Immunoblastic lymphoma also reveals a sarcomatous fibre pattern, and there is no proliferation with the appearance of lymphangiosis blastomatosa in the sinuses.

FIG. 6. EOSINOPHILS IN LYMPH-NODE METASTASES

Incidence of eosinophils in lymph-node metastases of lymphoepithelial carcinoma ('NPC') and of squamous-cell carcinoma (SCC). - Absence of eosinophils; +, ++, +++ eosinophils present in increasing numbers

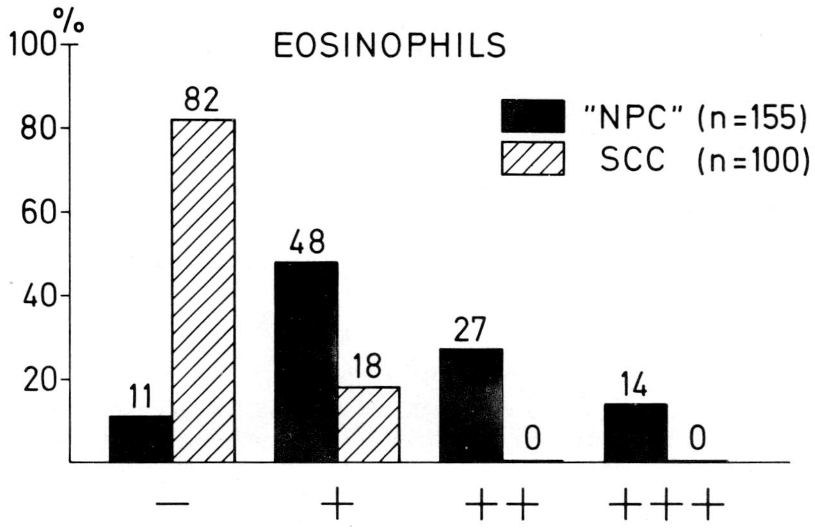

Table 1. Epithelioid cells and caseation necrosis in lymph-node metastases of lymphoepithelial carcinoma and squamous-cell carcinoma

	Lymphoepithelial carcinoma (n=155) %	Squamous-cell carcinoma (n=100) %
Epithelioid cells	17.8	9
Caseation necrosis	8.5	-

In contrast, lymphoepithelial carcinoma is, at least in its later stages, composed of compact sheets of tumour cells, and there are usually numerous plasma cells in the stroma. Fibrosis is conspicuous. Typical Marschalkó plasma cells are not found in immunoblastic lymphoma, and a small number of eosinophils are seen in only a few cases. Immunoblastic lymphoma occasionally shows epithelioid-cell clusters, or even granulomas, but it never reveals caseation necrosis.

Table 2. Caseous-tuberculoid reactions in 40 lymph nodes, with or without metastasis, from 11 patients with lymphoepithelial carcinoma (1966-1976)

	No. of lymph nodes	
Lymph nodes with carcinoma metastasis	28	
with epithelioid cells and caseation		13
with epithelioid cells, without caseation		9
no epithelioid cells		6
Lymph nodes without carcinoma metastasis	12	
with epithelioid cells and caseation		0
with epithelioid cells, without caseation		3
no epithelioid cells		9

(3) When there is marked fibrosis and eosinophilia, lymphoepithelial carcinoma is often misdiagnosed as Hodgkin's disease. The pathologist is misled chiefly by the occurrence of a few or solitary, huge, very clear nuclei and of giant nucleoli that appear to be 'vacuolated', as in Hodgkin cells (Fig. 7). The tumour cells may be interspersed with so many 'inflammatory cells' that the tumour complexes can hardly be distinguished and are therefore often misinterpreted as Hodgkin's sarcoma cells.

The misdiagnosis of Hodgkin's disease can be prevented by using appropriate histological techniques. We prefer a high-quality Giemsa stain, with which the sheets of grey-blue carcinoma cells are obvious at first glance.

(4) In one of our cases, caseous tuberculosis was diagnosed in a cervical lymph node four years before a second node was removed. Both lymph nodes showed numerous epithelioid-cell granulomas and large areas of caseation necrosis. Careful examination, however, especially of Giemsa-stained sections, revealed several small areas containing carcinoma cells. A blind biopsy from the nasopharynx then disclosed the primary tumour.

Cytology and cytochemistry

Rilke et al. (1975) have shown that cytological investigation of nasopharyngeal carcinomas provides at least the same, if not better, diagnostic results than biopsies. Biopsy specimens are often small and may be damaged by the surgical procedure; the cells, therefore, often show artificial changes. In smears or imprints, on the other hand, the cells are well preserved. Lymphoepithelial carcinoma, in particular, is relatively well characterized by its cytological features.

FIG. 7. LYMPHOEPITHELIAL CARCINOMA WITH AN APPEARANCE SIMILAR TO THAT SEEN IN HODGKIN'S DISEASE

Note the large, Hodgkin cell-like tumour cells with large, vacuolated nucleoli and numerous eosinophils and lymphocytes (section kindly provided by Prof. Dr S. Blümcke). H & E, x 560

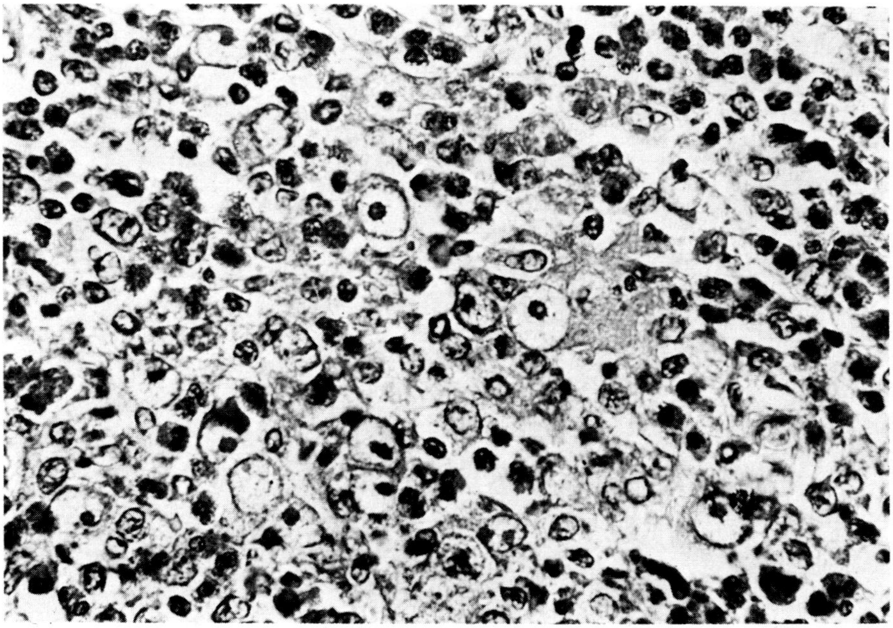

The tumour cells are large; some are huge (Fig. 8a). It is very often impossible to identify their cytoplasm; when it is visible, it is grey-blue to moderately basophilic. The cells are often poorly outlined, and some of the nuclei are therefore found in an amorphous, grey-blue mass. Small vacuoles are sometimes seen in the cytoplasm.

The nuclei are oval and have very prominent, blue nucleoli that are sharply delineated by chromatin, which is fine and distinctly 'reticular'. The nucleoli may be solitary, huge and round, or multiple, medium-sized and irregular in shape.

The tumour cells are sometimes arranged in strands and clusters and are then often difficult to recognize. Among them there are always many 'inflammatory cells', i.e., lymphocytes, plasma cells, eosinophils, neutrophils and mast cells. In addition, many histiocytes of all sizes and of variable phagocytic activity are always found. These cells are easy to identify with the acid phosphatase and nonspecific esterase reactions (Lennert, 1961).

FIG. 8. LYMPHOEPITHELIAL CARCINOMA IN IMPRINTS

a: Pappenheim staining. Note the large basophilic nucleoli and the (grey) poorly demarcated cytoplasm. x 875

b: Acid phosphatase reaction. Note the strong focal positivity in nearly all tumour cells. x 560

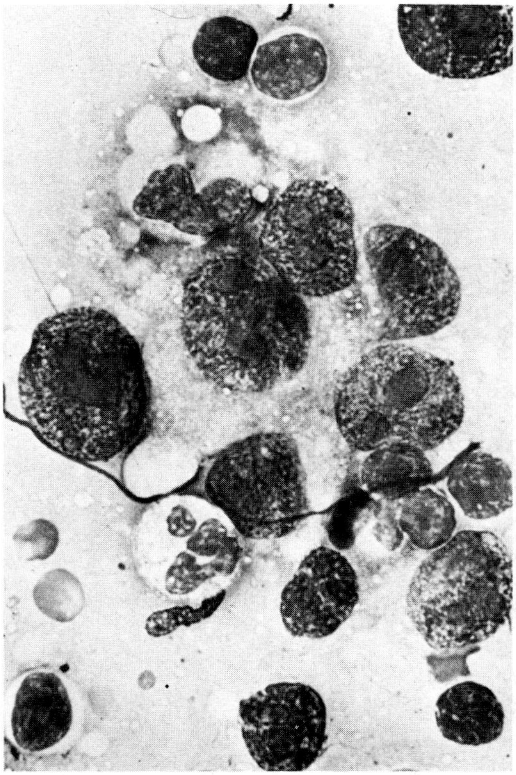

a

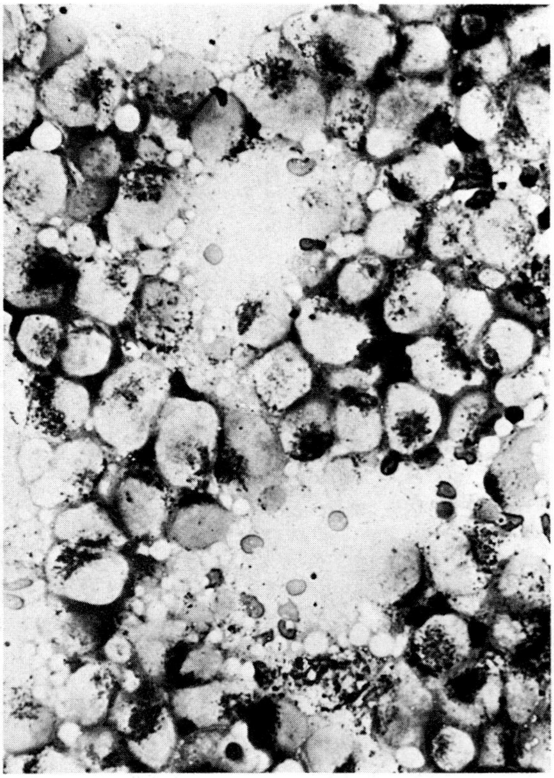

b

The tumour cells were either completely negative for all of the cytochemical reactions we applied (3/5) or showed predominantly focal, positive acid phosphatase and nonspecific esterase reactions (2/5; Fig. 8b). The enzyme activity was evident as small or large granules, often accumulated on one side of the nucleus (Golgi body with lysosomes?). The PAS reaction was negative in all but one of the cases we investigated.

Ultrastructure

It is not possible to present here all of the electron-microscopic findings, and we describe only the data that contribute to the interpretation of the light-microscopic findings, to differential diagnoses and to a basic understanding of lymphoepithelial carcinoma.

The tumour cells contain monoribosomes and moderate numbers of polyribosomes, corresponding to the grey-blue cytoplasm seen in Giemsa-stained sections and in imprints. The Golgi body may be large and surrounded by lysosome-like granules; this finding is probably equivalent to the positive acid phosphatase and nonspecific esterase reactions. The enzyme-negative cells are probably the tumour cells that show a paucity of organelles on electron microscopy. Glycogen deposits are found occasionally, as predicted by PAS staining.

Tumour cells from all cases studied by electron microscopy contained keratin fibrils and were connected by a few closely packed desmosomes. Furthermore, hook-shaped cytoplasmic processes of the tumour cells were frequently interdigitated. These features coincide with the interpretation of the cells as squamous cells, but the tumour cells were not connected by the intercellular bridges usually seen in typical squamous-cell carcinoma (Mori & Lennert, 1969).

In lymphoepithelial carcinoma, lymphocytes are always found among the tumour cells, whereas this is usually not the case in typical squamous-cell carcinoma. The lymphocytes have irregularly shaped, sometimes cleaved, nuclei, and they often contain lysosomes. They never transform into large blast cells. The 'polymorphonuclear' lymphocytes that contain lysosomes are also seen in large numbers, together with numerous plasma cells, in the surrounding tissue. We assume that at least most of these lymphocytes are the T lymphocytes demonstrated by Jondal & Klein (1975) to be the main lymphocytic components of lymphoepithelial carcinoma.

Some fibroblasts with a large amount of rough endoplasmic reticulum are found around the carcinoma-cell complexes. These cells produce large numbers of collagenous fibres, and conspicuous bundles of collagenous fibres ultimately surround the carcinoma cells. This is not found in typical squamous-cell carcinoma.

SUMMARY AND CONCLUSIONS

(1) Lymphoepithelial carcinoma, which occurs in the nasopharynx and palatine tonsils, is a special variant of squamous-cell carcinoma with a non-neoplastic lymphocytic component.

(2) The morphology of lymphoepithelial carcinoma is very characteristic, if not specific. Therefore, whenever lymphoepithelial carcinoma is diagnosed in a cervical lymph node, the clinician must try to find the primary tumour in the nasopharynx or tonsils, by blind biopsy if necessary.

(3) The 'inflammatory' component of lymphoepithelial carcinoma is often very conspicuous. Tuberculoid lesions, with or without caseation necrosis, and marked eosinophilia and plasmacytosis are highly characteristic and help to confirm the diagnosis.

(4) The 'inflammatory' component, including the lymphocytes among and around the tumour cells, is not fully understood; but, it would appear that T lymphocytes are responsible for all, or most, of the cellular reactions against the tumour.

REFERENCES

Jondal, M. & Klein, G. (1975) Classification of lymphocytes in nasopharyngeal carcinoma (NPC) biopsies. *Biomedicine, 23*, 163-165

Lennert, K. (1961) *Lymphknoten. Diagnostik in Schnitt und Ausstrich.* In: Lubarsch, O., Henke, F., Rössle, R. & Uehlinger, E., eds, *Handbuch der speziellen pathologischen Anatomie und Histologie I/3 A*, Bandteil A, *Cytologie und Lymphadenitis*, Berlin-Göttingen-Heidelberg, Springer

Lennert, K. (1973) *Pathologisch-histologische Klassifizierung der malignen Lymphome.* In: Stacher, A., ed., *Leukämien und maligne Lymphome*, München-Berlin-Wien, Urban & Schwarzenberg, pp. 181-194

Lukes, R.J. & Collins, R.D. (1974) A functional approach to the classification of malignant lymphoma. *Recent Res. Cancer Res., 46*, 18-30

Mori, Y. & Lennert, K. (1969) *Electron Microscopic Atlas of Lymph Node Cytology and Pathology*, Berlin-Heidelberg-New York, Springer

Rennke, H. & Lennert, K. (1973) Käsig-tuberkuloide Reaktion bei Lymphknotenmetastasen lymphoepithelialer Carcinome (Schmincke-Tumoren). *Virchows Arch. A. 358*, 241-247

Rilke, F., Pilotti, S., Clemente, C. & Molinari, R. (1975) Le diagnostic cytologique et les corrélations cyto-histologiques des tumeurs épithéliales malignes du rhinopharynx. *Bull. Cancer, 62*, 287-294

Stein, H., Kaiserling, E. & Lennert, K. (1974) Evidence for B-cell origin of reticulum cell sarcoma. *Virchows Arch. A, 364*, 51-67

A HISTOPATHOLOGICAL STUDY OF LYMPHOID TISSUE REACTION TO METASTATIC NASOPHARYNGEAL CARCINOMA IN NUDE MICE

H.-C. CHEN, A. KAWAMURA, Jr, M. MURATA, K. HAMAJIMA & M. OSONO

Department of Immunology

K. SUZUKI & K. SUDO

Laboratory of Experimental Animals,
Institute of Medical Science,
University of Tokyo,
Shirokanedai, Minato-ku,
Tokyo 108, Japan

INTRODUCTION

The growth of human malignant tumours in nude mice is usually characterized by local growth at the site of transplantation, with preservation of the original architecture but with no stromal mononuclear cell infiltration or distant metastasis (Kuga et al., 1975; Povlson & Rygaar, 1971). However, as we have pointed out previously (Kawamura et al., 1976), when a nasopharyngeal carcinoma (NPC) is transplanted into nude mice by inoculation with cultured NPC cells, the histological picture of the transplanted tumour may be different from that of the original one.

Still more surprising is the occurrence of metastases into the regional nodes during serial passages of the transplanted NPC; the response of the lymphoid tissue to the metastatic tumour is also a highly unusual one. The present study was undertaken to obtain information relevant to the effects of the interaction of reticulo-endothelial cells and tumour cells on the outcome of lymphatic metastasis.

MATERIALS AND METHODS

Animals

Eight-week old BALB/c (nu/nu) nude mice of both sexes, bred and maintained under specific pathogen-free conditions at the Laboratory of Experimental Animals, Institute of Medical Science, University of Tokyo, were used. Five mice were used as controls.

Transplanted materials

Seven cultured cell lines derived from human NPC were used for heterotransplantation.

Inoculation

Each 0.1 ml of cultured cell suspension was adjusted to 1-2 x 10^7 cells in 1 ml of culture medium and injected subcutaneously into the back and nuchal region of one mouse. When the transplanted tumours had grown to about 10-15 mm in diameter, they were removed aseptically for serial passage at intervals of 28-30 days.

Light microscope studies

After the animals had been sacrificed, all of the visceral organs, including brain and tumours, were fixed in formalin. Paraffin sections were stained with haematoxylin-eosin. Periodic acid-Schiff, Masson's trichrome and Foot's stains were also used.

RESULTS

The number of primary takes of the cultured NPC cell lines was 2/7 (28.5%). NPC-204, grown in nude mice, had been successively transplanted for 33 passages up to the time of reporting; serial passages of NPC-501 were interrupted at the 14th generation because of extensive necrosis of tumour tissue. Lymphatic metastases occurred during the periods between the 11th and 14th generations and the 24th and 30th generations with NPC-204 and between the 9th and 14th generations with NPC-501. Only the regional nodes were involved. Stromal mononuclear-cell infiltration was seen during the periods of metastasis.

Lymph nodes

The T-cell areas were replaced with relatively well-developed reticulum cells and were well differentiated from the B-cell areas by the presence of aggregates of lymphocytes. During the first several passages (pre-metastatic phase), the response to the serially transplanted tumours was the appearance of large numbers of wandering macrophages floating in the dilated sinuses of the medulla (Fig. 1).

FIG. 1. A LYMPH NODE IN THE PRE-METASTATIC PHASE

Wandering macrophages are abundant in the medullary sinuses. T-cell areas are well differentiated from B-cell areas by aggregates of lymphocytes. x 200

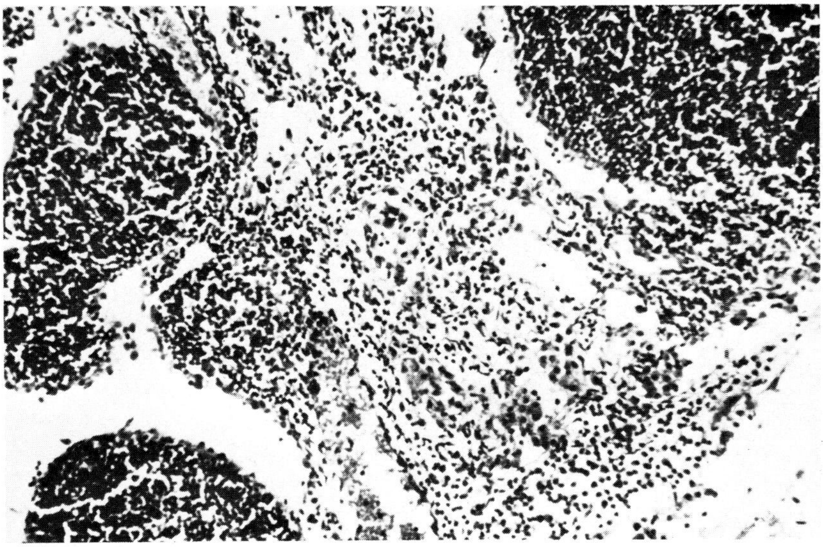

Subsequently, with the gradual disappearance of the wandering macrophages from the sinuses, T-cell areas became crowded with Thy 1-2 and surface immunoglobulin (S-Ig)-negative lymphocytes (null cells?), whereas there was almost no formation of secondary lymph follicles (Fig. 2). At this point, discrete tumour cells could be seen to be migrating *via* the lymphatic canaliculi deep into the subcortical areas, after free passage through the subcapsular sinuses. Nevertheless, metastases were formed from clumps of tumour cells rather than from individual, embolic tumour cells. There were three ways in which tumour-cell clumps lodged and spread further until the node was completely taken over (metastatic phase).

(1) The tumour-cell clumps were first confined to the subcapsular cortical sinuses and thereafter spread deeply into the medulla, as is usually seen in human cancers (Fig. 3). Unexpectedly, the metastatic NPC did not always behave in this way in the nude mice.

(2) Metastases arose more frequently from tumour-cell clumps lodged in the subcortical areas (Fig. 4), rather than from those in the subcapsular areas. The process of spread was signified by

FIG. 2. A LYMPH NODE IN THE EARLY STAGE OF METASTASIS, SHOWING DIFFUSE HYPERPLASIA OF LYMPHOCYTES WITH LOSS OF DEMARCATION BETWEEN T-CELL AND B-CELL AREAS. x 100

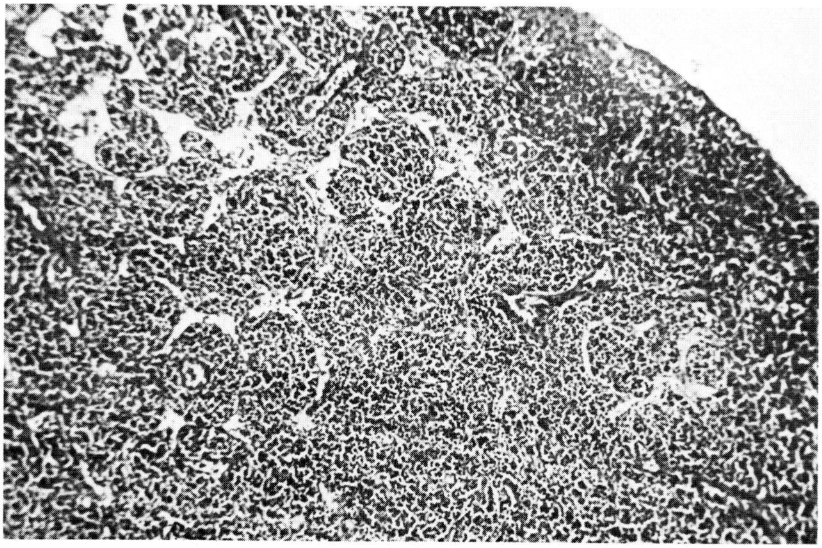

FIG. 3. TUMOUR CELLS IN A LYMPH NODE SPREADING FROM THE SUBCAPSULAR SINUSES DOWNWARDS TOWARDS THE MEDULLA

A few ill-defined aggregates of lymphocytes are scattered in the right third of the figure. x 100

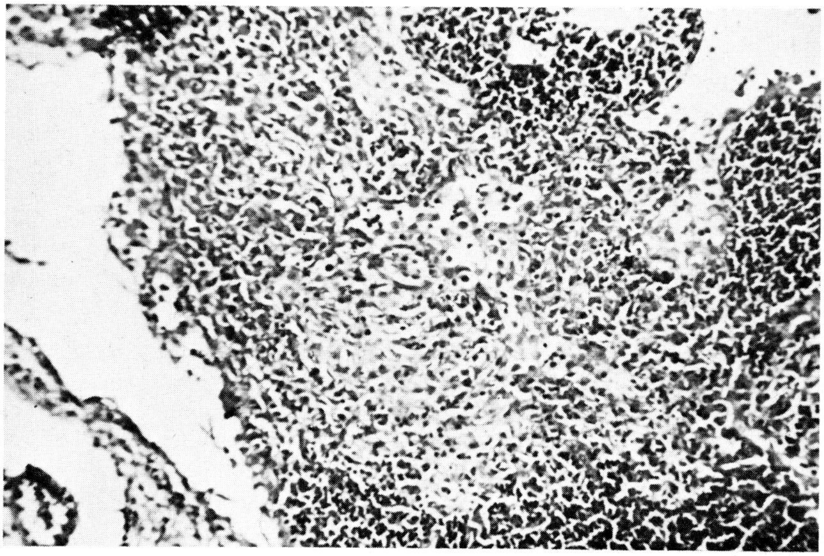

expansive proliferation of the clumped tumour cells upwards into the cortex and downwards toward the medulla (Fig. 5).

FIG. 4. A CLUMP OF TUMOUR CELLS IN THE SUBCORTICAL AREA OF A LYMPH NODE SURROUNDED BY LYMPHOCYTES AND DEBRIS. x 200

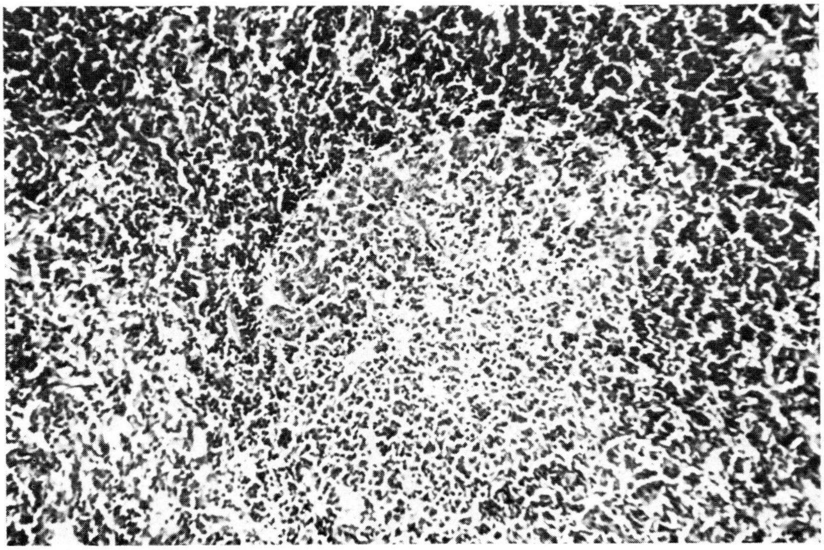

FIG. 5. A MASS OF TUMOUR CELLS IN A REGIONAL LYMPH NODE SPREADING UPWARDS AND DOWNWARDS FROM THE SUBCORTICAL AREA. x 100

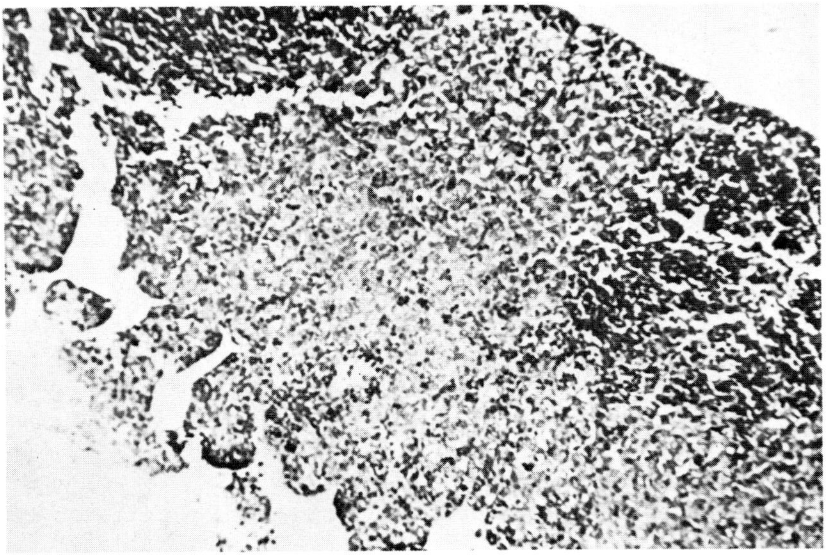

(3) The embolic tumour cells did not always give rise to metastases in regional lymph nodes. Aggregates of cellular and nuclear debris might have represented dissolution of tumour cells; these limited foci were often crowded with lymphocytes and, later on, with epithelioid cells and monocytes. Granulomas can form an effective temporary barrier and in this way change the mode of metastasis, which is governed largely by the flow of lymph. Thus, there was little direct spread from regional nodes into neighboring nodes in which granuloma formation was not uncommon. The occasional involvement of nodes scattered with granulomas was due to retrograde metastasis *via* a reverse pathway from the hilus into the medulla (Figs 6 & 7).

FIG. 6. A LARGE GRANULOMA FORMED IN A LYMPH NODE ADJOINING A REGIONAL NODE. x 200

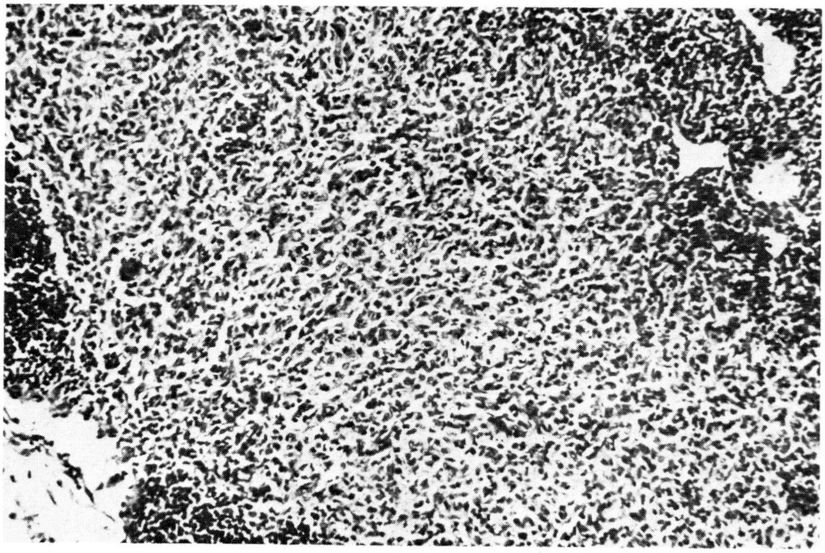

By the end of the metastatic phase, granulomas gradually became reduced in their size and eventually disappeared. During the post-metastatic phase, a large number of wandering macrophages appeared in the sinuses, as in the pre-metastatic phase. The T-cell areas were diffusely infiltrated with plasma cells, some of which apparently contained Russell-fuchsin bodies in their cytoplasm (Fig. 8).

Spleen

In nude mice deficient in T cells, the sheaths around the central and trabecular arteries and the trabecular vein were replaced by

FIG. 7. TWO GRANULOMAS FORMED IN THE SUBCORTICAL AREA OF A LYMPH NODE, WITH RETROGRADE METASTASIS FROM THE HILUS. x 100

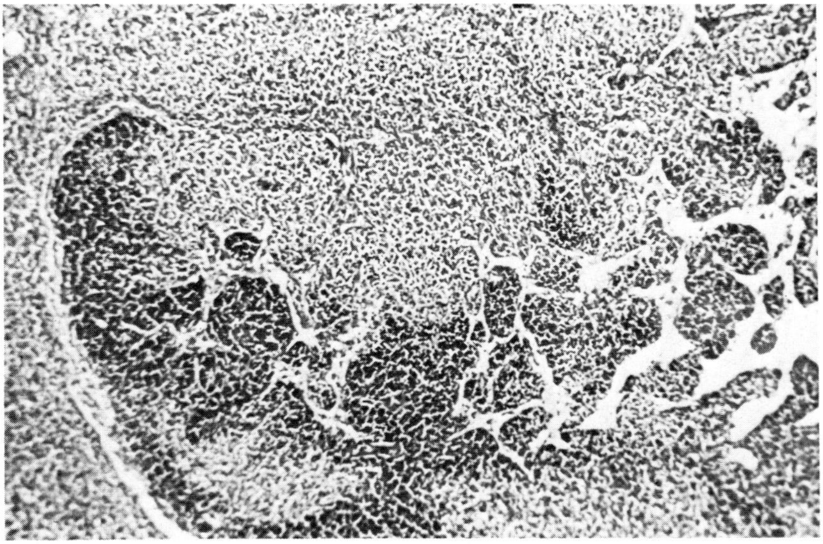

FIG. 8. A REGIONAL LYMPH NODE IN THE POST-METASTATIC PHASE

Wandering macrophages are floating in the medullary sinuses. x 400.

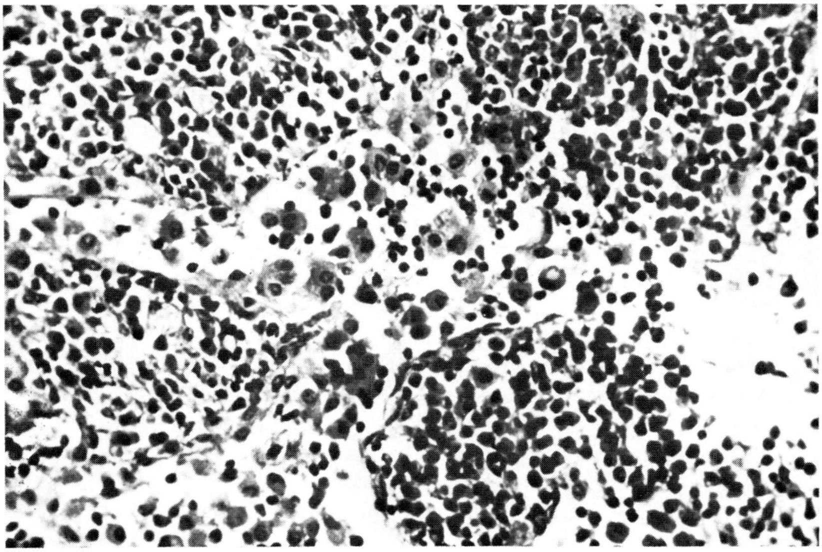

strands of reticulum cells intermingled with monocytic or histiocytic splenic cells (Fig. 9). Functionally, the spleens of such mice affected haematopoiesis in the bone marrow, allowing a few large, multinucleated megakaryocytes to escape into the sinuses of the red pulp of the spleen.

FIG. 9. SPLEEN OF A CONTROL NUDE MOUSE

T-cell area around the central artery is replaced by reticulum cells intermingled with monocytes. x 200

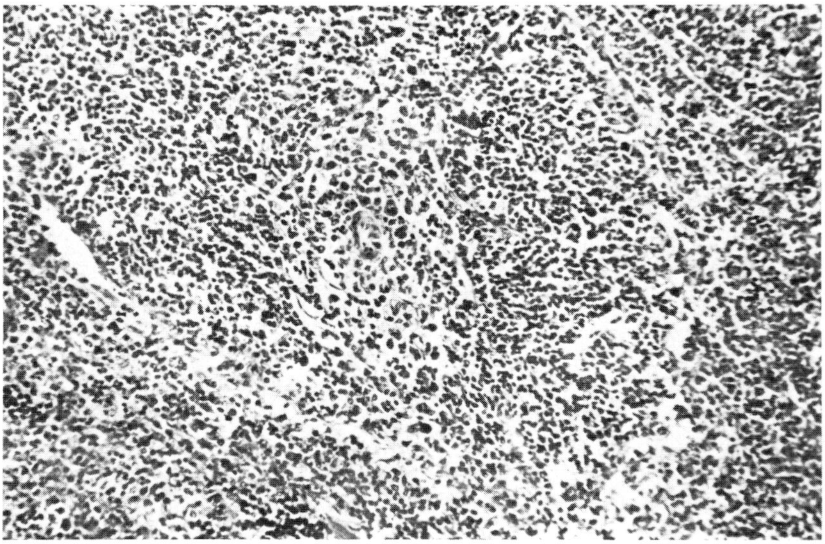

Like the lymph nodes, the spleen had a remarkable capacity of reacting to the transplanted tumours, and diffuse hyperplasia of lymphocytes occurred throughout the red and white pulps during the pre-metastatic phase (Fig. 10). Enlargement of the spleen was a common occurrence during the metastatic phase. The most important change was a proliferation of the reticulin in the splenic cords, which gradually replaced the normal, net-like framework. Eventually, the splenic cords collapsed (Fig. 11), and fibrotic, hyalinized septa embedded with sclerotic venules were formed in all directions (Fig. 12). The Malpighian bodies became atrophic and often fused together in a nodule surrounded by well-formed septa (Fig. 13). Simultaneously, the megakaryocytes underwent pyknosis and cytolysis, and giant, histiocytic cells appeared in the vicinity of tubercle-like granulomas of unknown origin (Figs 14 & 15). With time, the sclerotic changes in the spleen gradually disappeared, and groups of plasmacytoid cells and monocytes resembling splenic cells appeared, especially in the T-cell areas (Fig. 16).

FIG. 10. SPLEEN IN PRE-METASTATIC PHASE

Diffuse hyperplasia of lymphocytes results in loss of demarcation between the red and white pulps. x 100

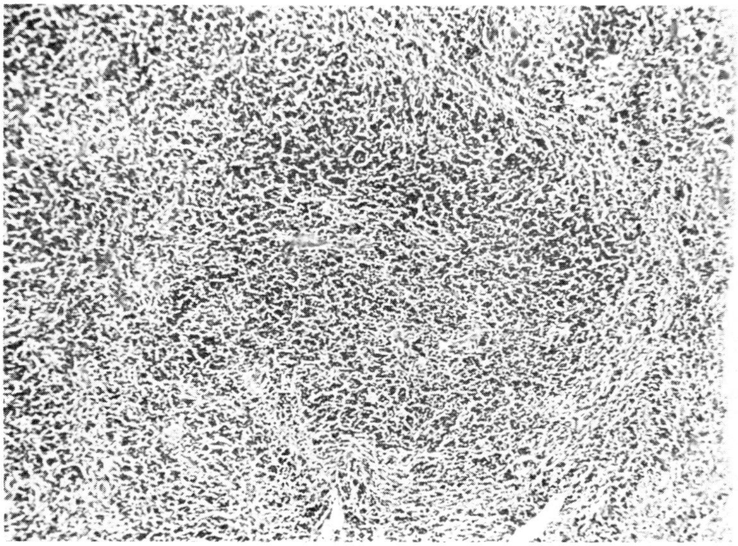

FIG. 11. COLLAPSED SPLENIC CORDS AROUND A MALPIGHIAN BODY

Many megakaryocytes are scattered throughout the red pulp. x 200.

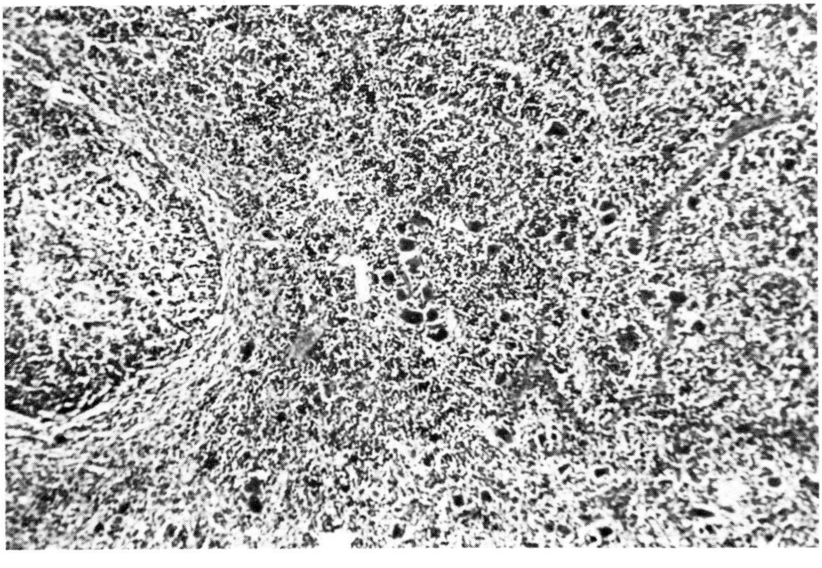

FIG. 12. COLLAPSED SPLENIC CORDS FUSED AND HYALINIZED, WITH FORMATION OF SEPTA IN THE RED PULP.

Thick-walled venules are embedded in the septa. x 200.

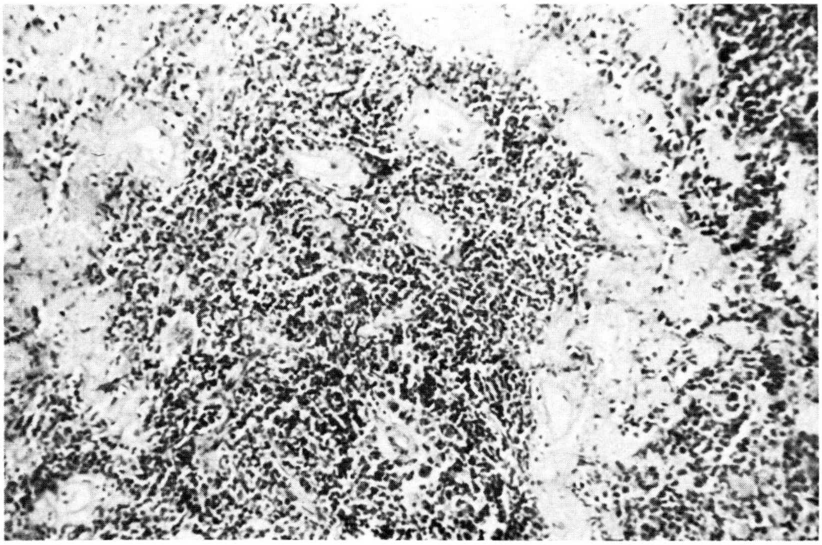

FIG. 13. APPROACH OF ATROPHIED MALPIGHIAN BODIES RESULTING FROM SCLEROTIC CHANGES WITH FORMATION OF SEPTA. x 200.

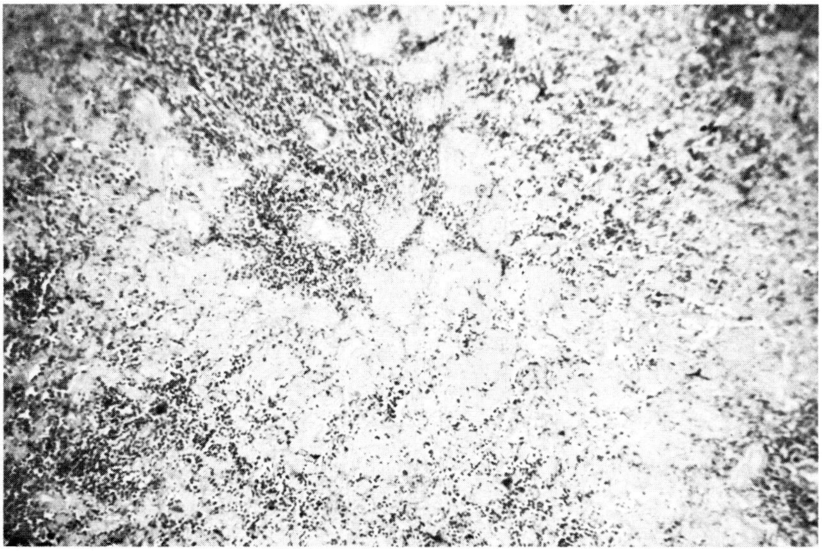

FIG. 14. AN ILL-DEFINED GRANULOMA IN THE EXTENSIVELY ALTERED RED PULP OF THE SPLEEN x 100

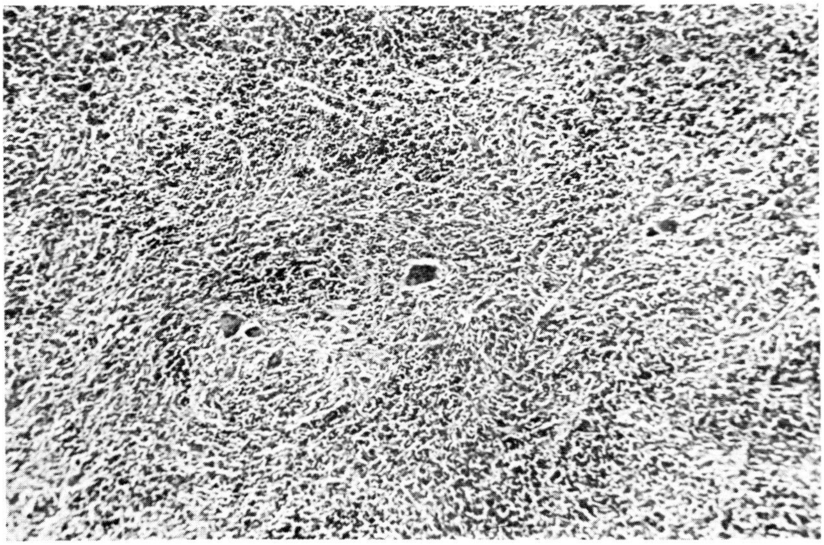

FIG. 15. MAGNIFICATION OF GRANULOMA SHOWN IN FIGURE 14, WITH MEGAKARYOCYTES IN VARYING DEGREES OF DEGENERATION. x 200.

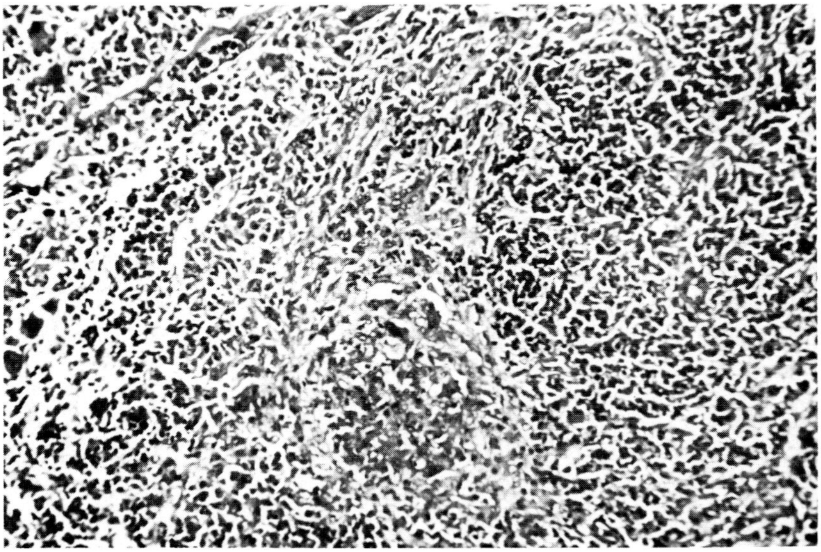

FIG. 16. SPLEEN IN POST-METASTATIC PHASE

Proliferation of monocytes and plasmacytoid cells in the white pulp. x 400.

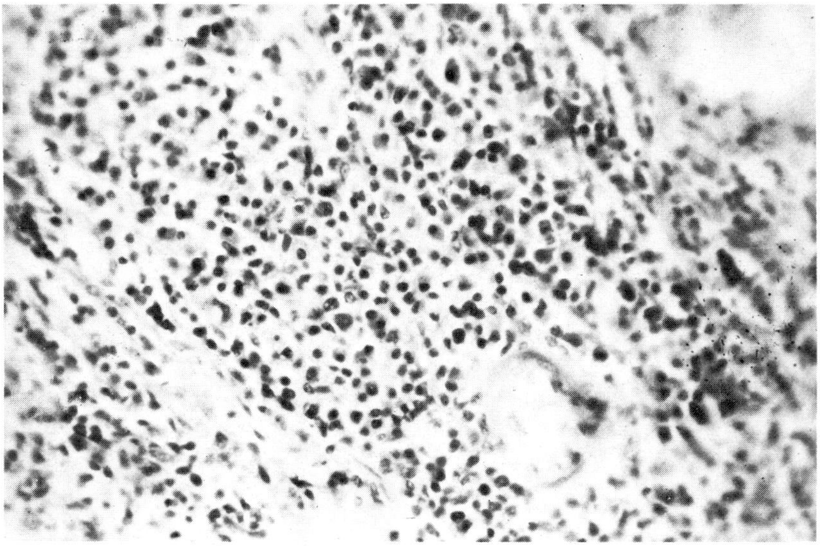

These marked changes occurred in the spleen despite the absence of tumour cells, in sharp contrast to events in the regional nodes, and should be regarded as a defense reaction of the reticuloendothelial system.

Bone marrow

Although the bones are partly destroyed by direct invasion of transplanted tumour cells, metastases did not occur in bone marrow. The bone marrow itself probably served as a supply centre, regulating the rate at which lymphocytes and monocytes were released into the spleen and the lymph nodes. Firstly, the number of lymphoid cells gradually decreased, accompanied by enhanced granulopoiesis (Fig. 17). At the peak of the metastatic phase, granulopoietic foci underwent necrobiosis, and megakaryocytes were degenerated to varying degrees (Fig. 18). During the post-metastatic phase, monocytic cells and, probably, stem cells dominated the picture.

FIG. 17. BONE MARROW IN PRE-METASTATIC PHASE

Granulopoiesis is marked; megakaryocytes appear to be normal. x 200.

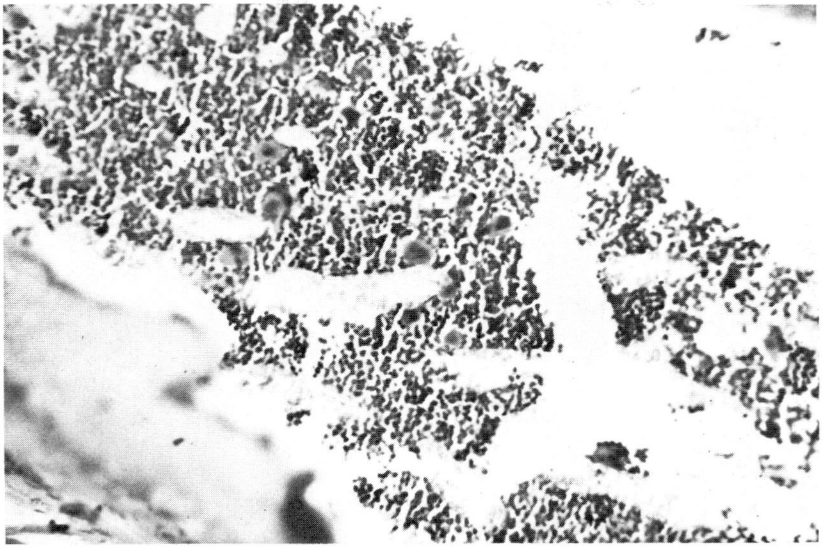

FIG. 18. BONE MARROW IN METASTATIC PHASE

Granulocytes are undergoing focal necrobiosis; megakaryocytes are degenerated. x 100.

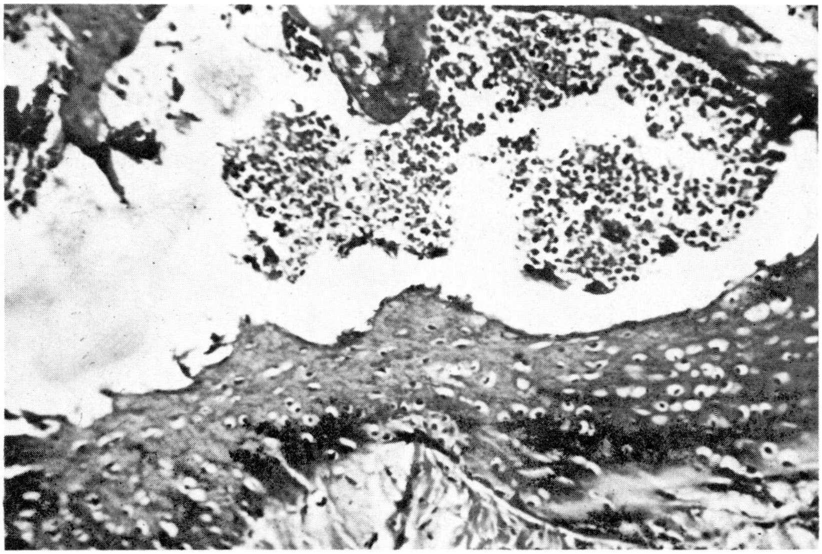

DISCUSSION

One of the major functions of the lymphoreticular system is regulation of the rate of growth of transplanted tumours (Prehn & Lappé, 1971). Nude mice may be congenitally athymic and deficient in the T cells that are essential to the rejection of allografts and tumours (Zembala et al., 1973); however, the deficiency of T cells in the homozygous nude mice used in this study does not necessarily mean a complete absence of their function. A few Thy 1-2 antigen-positive T cells occur, comprising from 3-8% of the total lymphocyte population, and we have found enormous numbers of S-Ig-positive cells congregated in the B-cell areas of the spleen and lymph nodes. A parallel to this situation, which corresponds to immunological tolerance (Klein & Klein, 1966), is that in which transplanted human NPCs attain the ability to grow locally after transfer, for several successive generations, without metastasis, under the surveillance of macrophages instead of T cells. Serial passages of tumours in nude mice enhance the migration of macrophages into the lymph nodes, in contrast to the spleen, where a gradual decrease in the number of splenic cells (Pearsall & Weiser, 1970) and a proliferation of lymphocytes is seen. Indeed, metastases never occur when the T-cell areas of the regional lymph nodes are occupied by well-developed reticulum cells and when large numbers of wandering macrophages are on guard in the sinuses of the lymph nodes. This is probably the reason for the low incidence of metastasis observed in general in nude mice (Klein et al., 1974).

Like human NPCs, which have a strong tendency to metastasize into the lymph nodes of the neck (Tu, 1971), their laboratory counterparts metastasize to the regional lymph nodes after serial passages in nude mice. Hyperplasia of the lymphocytes in the regional nodes does not occur until a number of viable tumour cells have migrated into the lymphatic canaliculi; eventually the whole node is completely replaced by proliferative lymphocytes (antigen-activated?), thus simultaneously inhibiting the entry of wandering macrophages (migration inhibition factor?) (Evans & Alexander, 1971). With this progressive decrease in the numbers of wandering macrophages, stromal mononuclear cell infiltration into the transplanted tumours becomes prominent, and, finally, the regional nodes are invaded by the metastatic NPC.

Metastasis is a complicated biological phenomenon which is influenced by a multitude of events. It has been suggested by Makidono et al. (1976) that two factors are necessary in the relationship between host and tumour for the development of metastasis. The first is loss of or decrease in tumour-specific antigens in the cell populations in the metastatic foci; however, this does not always occur. The second is an imbalance of immune responses to the tumour, resulting in deficient protection against its growth. According to the observation of Fidler (1974), the incidence of experimental metastasis can be enhanced or decreased by *in vitro* incubation of the tumour cells with various concentrations of normal nonspecifically sensitized, specifically sensitized and/or immunized syngeneic lymphocytes. Other experimental evidence strongly supports the thesis that 'immunosuppression' by thymectomy and irradiation facilitates metastasis (Gershon et al., 1968; Treves et al., 1974). In view of our observation that loss of lymphocytes from the bone marrow and spleen causes diffuse sclerotic changes in the spleen, the concept of 'immunosuppression' seems to be the most acceptable.

It is obvious that the rapid and abundant proliferation of lymphocytes that occurs in regional lymph nodes invaded by embolic cancer cells must be an immune response to the metastatic NPC cells. Two populations of lymphocytes were seen: S-Ig-positive B cells and large numbers of both Thy 1-2- and S-Ig-negative cells (null cells?). Most of the latter were transferred from the spleen and bone marrow, although their appearance was different from that of the original cells.

Clumps of tumour cells are first confined to the subcortical areas of the lymph node and then grow and spread into the entire node. This means of spreading is different from that of human metastases, and it is our opinion that this occurs as a result of the defective surveillance system, as reflected by the decrease in numbers of wandering macrophages.

Why do tumour-cell clumps survive to produce metastases with general involvement of regional lymph nodes? If this situation is comparable to a low dosage of immune spleen cells, the depressed immune reaction actually assists the growth of nascent metastatic NPC cells (Prehn, 1972). Furthermore, it has been shown that serum factors can block cell-mediated cytotoxity *in vitro* (Basham & Currie, 1974; Chieco-Bianchi et al., 1974; Steele et al., 1975). It is also possible, however, that suppressor T cells, probably few in number in nude mice, may play some role in stimulating tumour growth (Kirkwood & Gershon, 1974; Okubo et al., 1974). Whatever the mechanism, it is interesting that lymphocytes, mostly transferred from spleen and bone marrow, must first come into contact with emigrating tumour cells and can then stimulate tumour growth in regional lymph nodes.

The embolic tumour cells may be destroyed by a non-phagocytic mechanism, presumably through cell-contact interaction (Granger & Weiser, 1964; Tsoi & Weiser, 1968). Certainly, there is evidence that tumour cells as well as lymphoid cells may be destroyed, since occasionally clumps of nuclear debris containing a few viable tumour cells can be found. There is further evidence to suggest that T cells mediate antibody-independent cytotoxicity (Britton et al., 1973; Dennert & Lennox, 1973; Zighelboim et al., 1974), but their effect appears to be small. It has recently been suggested that null cells are responsible for antibody-dependent cytotoxicity (Greenberg et al., 1973). There is increasing evidence that macrophages, in conjunction with either non-immune or immunized lymphocytes, are the key effector cells in the inhibition of tumour-cell growth, acting by a non-phagocytic mechanism which requires cell contact (Evans & Alexander, 1972; Piessens et al., 1975; Shin et al., 1972; Temple et al., 1973; Zarling & Tevethia, 1973; Zembala et al., 1973). It has been pointed out (Scornik & Cosenza, 1974) that adherent as well as non-adherent spleen cells, mostly macrophage-like, are usually more effective in inducing cytotoxity than either the original, unseparated spleen-cell population or the peritoneal macrophages. In addition, they point out that spleen cells from nude mice are as effective as normal spleen cells in inducing antibody-dependent cytotoxity. Thus, it is plausible to assume that in nude mice macrophages, especially those derived from the spleen, serve not only in a surveillance system for controlling the spread of transplanted tumours but also to kill the tumour cells.

In regional lymph nodes, widespread hyperplasia of lymphocytes occurs upon the arrival of migrating tumour cells during the early phase of metastasis, since large numbers of lymphocytes are required completely to destroy the tumour-cell clumps (Pearsall & Weiser, 1968). At this point, some of the lymphocytes aggregated around the tumour cells may be killed, and some may survive, probably having acquired antibodies. The sensitized lymphocytes might then inhibit migration of macrophages and, instead, aggregate them, especially in sites rich in antigen (Lolekha et al., 1970; Pels & Otter, 1974), due to the interaction of the antigen with antibody adhering to the surface of the macrophages. This would account for the formation of granulomas in the lymph nodes and spleen, although the spleen is always free from metastatic tumour cells. The granulomas serve as a barrier or defense line and are often seen scattered throughout the subcortical areas of lymph nodes or in the red pulp of the spleen, despite the absence of inflammatory agents. They serve as a powerful barrier against invasion by tumour cells from the cortical sinuses but are useless against retrograde metastasis from the hilus of the lymph node.

The sensitized lymphocytes can potentially cause blastogenesis of non-sensitized lymphocytes, as manifested by a proliferation of plasma-cytoid cells in the T-cell areas during the post-metastatic phase, although there is no evidence of an increase in immunoglobulins in the serum. These may be variants of lymphoblasts, or they may belong to the histiocyte-macrophage family of cells (Binet & Mathé, 1962). It is nevertheless certain that metastasis from transplanted NPCs cannot occur in nude mice when the functioning of macrophages has been well preserved.

SUMMARY

In attempts to heterotransplant human NPCs into nude mice, using seven cultured cell lines, we have succeeded in growing a carcinoma simplex, composed of Epstein-Barr virus-determined nuclear antigen-positive and Epstein-Barr virus genome-positive cancer cells, at the injected site with two of the cell lines. These originated from a spindle-cell carcinoma (Chinese NPC-204) and from a combined-cell carcinoma (Chinese NPC-501), respectively. During the first few passages, wandering macrophages were prevalent and increased in number in response to the presence of the tumours. In conjunction with a gradual decrease in the number of wandering macrophages in the medullary sinuses, diffuse hyperplasia of lymphocytes occurred in regional lymph nodes. As a result of the release of lymphocytes and macrophages into the peripheral lymph nodes, the spleen underwent extensive change, as manifested by the collapse of the splenic cords and the formation of septa studded with granulomas. Under these conditions of immunosuppression, lymphatic metastases were observed during the periods between the 11th and 14th generations and the 24th and 30th generations with NPC-204 and between the 9th and 14th generations with NPC-501.

The neighbouring lymph nodes, like the spleen, were often studded with epithelioid-cell granulomas, formed by the aggregation of macrophages around nuclear debris in the subcortical areas. We assume that the clumps of debris are the remnants of metastatic cancer cells which were probably killed by macrophages or by sensitized lymphocytes. If the lymph nodes contain a barrier of granulomas, they are not invaded by tumour cells from the cortical sinuses, except in the rare case of retrograde metastasis from the hilus. It would appear that macrophages can replace T lymphocytes, which are found in very small numbers in the nude mice used in this study, in killing tumour cells and, furthermore, in protecting the lymph nodes from the spread of metastases. Metastasis cannot occur in these nude mice when their lymphoreticular system, especially that of the spleen, is working in a stable balance.

ACKNOWLEDGEMENT

This study was supported in part by Grant-in-Aids for Scientific Research from the Ministry of Education, Science and Culture, and the Ministry of Public Health and Welfare, Japan.

REFERENCES

Basham, C. & Currie, G.A. (1974) Development of specific cell-dependent antibody during growth of syngeneic rat sarcoma. *Brit. J. Cancer, 29*, 189-198

Binet, J.L. & Mathé, G. (1962) Optical and electron microscope studies of the immunologically competent cells during the reaction of graft against the host. *Ann. N. Y. Acad. Sci., 99*, 426-431

Britton, S., Perlmann, H. & Perlmann, P. (1973) Thymus-dependent and thymus-independent effector functions of mouse lymphoid cells. Comparison of cytotoxity and primary antibody formation *in vitro*. *Cell. Immunol., 8*, 420-434

Chieco-Bianchi, L., Sends, F., Aoki, T. & Barrera, O.L. (1974) Immunologic tolerance to antigens associated with murine leukemia viruses: T-cell unresponsiveness? *J. nat. Cancer Inst., 52*, 1345-1350

Dennert, G. & Lennox, E.S. (1973) Phagocytic cells as effectors in a cell-mediated immunity system. *J. Immunol., 111*, 1844-1854

Evans, R. & Alexander, P. (1971) Rendering macrophages specifically cytotoxic by a factor released from immune lymphoid cells. *Transplantation, 12*, 227-229

Evans, R. & Alexander, P. (1972) Mechanism of immunologically specific killing of tumor cells by macrophages. *Nature (Lond.), 236*, 168-170

Fidler, I.J. (1974) Immune stimulation inhibition of experimental metastasis. *Cancer Res., 34*, 491-498

Gershon, R.K., Carter, R.L. & Kondo, K. (1968) Immunologic defenses against metastasis: impairment by excision of an allotransplanted lymphoma. *Science, 159*, 646-647

Granger, G.A. & Weiser, R.S. (1964) Homograft target cells: specific destruction *in vitro* by contact interaction with immune macrophages. *Science, 145*, 1427-1429

Greenberg, A.H., Hudson, L., Shen, L. & Roitt, I.M. (1973) Antibody-dependent cell-mediated cytotoxicity due to a 'null' lymphoid cell. *Nature (New Biol.), 242*, 111-113

Kawamura, A., Jr, Chen, H.-C., Murata, M., Hamajima, K., Suzuki, K., Sudo, K., Takada, M., Saito, Y. & Sawaki, S. (1976) Hetero-transplantation of cultured cells and biopsies derived from naso-pharyngeal carcinoma into thymus-less (nude) mice. I. Growth and antigenic properties of heteroplanted tumors and their histo-pathological findings. *Japan. J. exp. Med., 46*, 351-362

Kirkwood, J.M. & Gershon, R.H. (1974) A role for suppressor T cells in immunological enhancement of tumor growth. *Progr. exp. Tumor Res. (Basel)*, *19*, 157-164

Klein, E. & Klein, G. (1966) Immunological tolerance of neonatally infected mice to the Moloney leukemia virus. *Nature (Lond.)*, *209*, 163-165

Klein, G., Giovanella, B.C., Lindahl, T., Fialkow, P.J., Singh, S. & Stehlin, J.S. (1974) Direct evidence for the presence of Epstein-Barr virus DNA and nuclear antigen in malignant epithelial cells from patients with poorly differentiated carcinoma of the nasopharynx. *Proc. nat. Acad. Sci. (Wash.)*, *71*, 4737-4741

Kuga, N., Yoshida, K., Seido, T., Oboshi, S., Koide, T., Shimosato, Y. & Nomura, T. (1975) Heterotransplantation of cultured human cancer cells and human cancer tissue into nude mice. *Gann*, *66*, 547-560

Lolekha, S., Dray, S. & Gotoff, S.P. (1970) Macrophage aggregation *in vitro:* a correlate of delayed hypersensitivity. *J. Immunol.*, *104*, 296-304

Makidono, R., Nomoto, K. & Takeya, K. (1976) Enhanced development of metastatic foci in thymectomized, irradiated, and bone marrow-reconstituted mice. *Gann*, *67*, 645-649

Okubo, S., Oettgen, H.F., Caiazza, S.S. & Ovary, Z. (1974) Enhancement of tumor growth by graft-*versus*-host-reaction. *Proc. nat. Acad. Sci. (Wash.)*, *71*, 4264-4266

Pearsall, N.N. & Weiser, R.S. (1968) The macrophages in allograft immunity. II. Passive transfer with immune macrophages. *J. Reticuloendoth. Sci.*, *5*, 121-133

Pearsall, N.N. & Weiser, R.S. (1970) *Macrophage*, Philadelphia, Lea & Febiger, p. 11

Pels, E. & Otter, W.D. (1974) The role of cytophilic factor from challenged immune peritoneal lymphocytes in specific macrophage cytotoxity. *Cancer Res.*, *34*, 3089-3094

Piessens, W.F., Churchill, W.H., Jr & David, J.R. (1975) Macrophages activated *in vitro* with lymphocyte mediators kill neoplastic but not normal cells. *J. Immunol.*, *114*, 293-299

Povlsen, C.O. & Rygaard, J. (1971) Heterotransplantation of human adenocarcinomas of the colon and rectum to the mouse mutant nude. A study of nine consecutive transplantations. *Acta path. microbiol. scand.*, *79A*, 159-169

Prehn, R.T. (1972) The immune reaction as a stimulator of tumor growth. *Science*, *176*, 170-171

Prehn, R.T. & Lappé, M.A. (1971) An immunostimulation therapy of tumor development. *Transplant. Rev.* *7*, 26-54

Scornik, J.C. & Cosenza, H. (1974) Antibody-dependent cell-mediated cytotoxity. III. Two functionally different effector cells. *J. Immunol.*, *113*, 1527-1532

Shin, H.S., Kaliss, N., Borenstein, D. & Gately, M.K. (1972) Antibody-mediated suppression of grafted lymphoma cells. II. Participation of macrophages. *J. exp. Med.*, *136*, 375-380

Steele, G., Jr, Sjögren, H.O., Rosengren, J.E., Lindström, C., Larsson, A. & Leandoer, L. (1975) Sequential studies of serum blocking activity in rats bearing chemically induced primary bowel tumors. *J. nat. Cancer Inst.*, *54*, 959-967

Temple, A., Loewi, G., Davies, P. & Howard, A. (1973) Cytotoxity of immune guinea-pig cells. II. The mechanism of macrophage cytotoxity. *Immunology*, *24*, 655-669

Treves, A.J., Carnaud, C., Trainin, N., Feldman, M. & Cohen, I.R. (1974) Enhancing T lymphocytes from tumor-bearing mice suppress host resistance to a syngeneic tumor. *Europ. J. Immunol.*, *4*, 722-727

Tsoi, M.-S. & Weiser, R.S. (1968) Mechanisms of immunity to sarcoma I allografts in C57BL/Ks mouse. I. Passive transfer studies with immune peritoneal macrophages in X-irradiated hosts. *J. nat. Cancer Inst.*, *40*, 25-36

Tu, S.-M. (1971) *Recent advances in human tumor virology and immunology*. In: Nakahara, W., Nishioka, K., Hirayama, T. & Ito, Y. eds, *Clinical Characteristics of Nasopharyngeal Carcinoma in Taiwan*, Tokyo, University of Tokyo Press, pp. 221-228

Zarling, J.M. & Tevethia, S.S. (1973) Transplantation immunity to simian virus 40-transformed cells in tumor-bearing mice. II. Evidence for macrophage participation at the effector level of tumor cell rejection. *J. nat. Cancer Inst.*, *50*, 149-157

Zembala, M., Ptak, W. & Hanczakowska, M. (1973) The role of macrophages in the cytotoxic killing of tumor cells *in vitro*. I. Primary immunization of lymphocytes *in vitro* for target cell killing and the mechanism of lymphocyte-macrophage cooperation. *Immunology*, *25*, 631-644

Zighelboim, J., Bonavida, B. & Fahey, J.L. (1974) Heterogenous populations of cytotoxic cells in the peritoneal cavity of BALB/c mice immunized with allogenic EL 4 leukemia cells. *Cell. Immunol.*, *12*, 280-289

ANIMAL MODELS FOR NASOPHARYNGEAL CARCINOMA

D.V. ABLASHI & J.M. EASTON

Viral Oncology Program,
National Cancer Institute,
Bethesda, Md., USA

R. GLASER

Department of Microbiology and
Specialized Cancer Research Center,
Milton S. Hershey Medical Center,
Hershey, Penn., USA

INTRODUCTION

The study of nasopharyngeal carcinoma (NPC) is receiving attention because of the complex interaction of genetic, viral and other environmental factors which may be involved in the etiology of this disease (Ablashi et al., 1976a). In this paper, we review animal models for NPC; the first models to be discussed are naturally occurring tumours of the mouth, pharynx and nose in domestic animals, with particular reference to dogs (Brodey, 1961; Cohen et al., 1964; Dorn & Priester, 1976; Madewell et al., 1976). The second model is an experimental system in which somatic-cell hybrids containing the Epstein-Barr virus (EBV) genome were studied in athymic nude mice (Ablashi et al., 1976b; Glaser, 1975; Glaser et al., 1977).

SPONTANEOUS MALIGNANCIES OF MOUTH, PHARYNX, NOSE & PARANASAL SINUSES IN DOMESTIC ANIMALS

Dorn & Priester (1976) studied 469 oropharyngeal malignancies diagnosed in dogs, cats, horses and cattle; 84% were in dogs. Madewell et al. (1976) studied 300 cases of primary neoplasms of the nose and paranasal sinuses; significant numbers were observed in dogs, horses and cats. Table 1 gives the estimated crude incidence rates for these neoplasms: dogs had the highest rates for both sites, followed by cats and horses. Of interest are the data of Cohen et al. (1964), who reported a prevalence rate of 34 per 10,000 for canine oral and pharyngeal cancer; this rate is much higher than that described by Dorn & Priester (1976). Table 2 shows the relative frequency of neoplasms in domestic animals by histological type. Squamous-cell carcinomas occurred most frequently at both sites in cats and horses;

Table 1. Estimated crude rates for neoplasms per 100,000 patient years by species for oropharyngeal and nasal-paranasal sinus sites[a]

Species	Site: Mouth and pharynx	Nose and paranasal sinuses
Canine	130	81
Feline	45	39
Equine	28	26
Bovine	3	2

[a] From Madewell et al. (1976) and Dorn & Priester (1976)

in dogs, squamous-cell carcinomas ranked second in incidence for the mouth and pharynx and third in incidence for the nose and paranasal sinuses. The number of squamous-cell carcinomas in dogs is still quite significant, however, and supports the use of this animal as a model for human NPC.

Table 3 gives a further breakdown of canine squamous-cell carcinomas by site. Of particular importance is the number of carcinomas of the tonsil. Cohen et al. (1964) found that the oral and pharyngeal neoplasm most frequently observed in dogs (site and type) was tonsillar carcinoma, and an unusual predominance of males was found to have this neoplasm. The tonsil resembles the human nasopharynx in that lymphoid tissue is covered by a layer of epithelium; in addition, lymphoepitheliomas have been found to occur in the human tonsil as well as in the human nasopharynx (Ash et al., 1964). Thus, tonsillar carcinoma in dogs will prove to be an interesting natural model for human NPC.

Table 4 shows the estimated relative risk values by age for intranasal neoplasms in domestic animals. Oropharyngeal relative risk values were similar. In general, the relative risk values tended to increase with age: in dogs, the highest relative risk occurred in the 10-14 year age group. Cohen et al. (1964), however, found that the average age for all canine oropharyngeal cancer cases was 9.8 years;

Table 2. Relative frequency of neoplasms in domestic animals by histological type[a]

Species	Mouth and pharynx	Number	Nose and paranasal sinuses	Number
Canine	1. Melanoma	147	1. Adenocarcinoma	56
	2. SQUAMOUS-CELL CARCINOMA	115	2. Carcinoma (NOS)[b]	40
	3. Fibrosarcoma	85	3. SQUAMOUS-CELL CARCINOMA	29
			4. Chondrosarcoma	23
(Total)[c]		(469)		(245)
Feline	1. SQUAMOUS-CELL CARCINOMA	32	1. SQUAMOUS-CELL CARCINOMA	15
	2. Fibrosarcoma	11	2. Adenocarcinoma	9
	3. Odontogenic cancer	2	3. Carcinoma (NOS)	2
(Total)		(50)		(35)
Equine	1. SQUAMOUS-CELL CARCINOMA	14	1. SQUAMOUS-CELL CARCINOMA	6
	2. Melanoma	5	2. Fibroma	4
	3. Odontogenic cancer	5	3. Carcinoma (NOS)	3
(Total)		(29)		(22)
Bovine	1. Odontogenic cancer	2	1. Fibrosarcoma	1
(Total)		(2)		(1)

[a] From Madewell et al. (1976) and Dorn & Priester (1976)

[b] Not otherwise specified

[c] Totals include all histological types, including those not listed

Table 3. Numbers of canine squamous-cell carcinomas of the mouth, pharynx, nose and paranasal sinuses by site[a]

Site	Number
Mouth and pharynx	(115)
Gingivae-alveolae	34
Tonsil	28
Mouth, general	24
Lip	7
Palate	3
Other	19
Nose and paranasal sinuses	(29)
Nose	18
Paranasal sinuses	11

[a] From Madewell et al. (1976) and Dorn & Priester (1976)

Table 4. Estimated relative risk by age, intranasal neoplasms[a]

Age (yrs)	Species: Canine	Feline	Equine
0 - 3	0.1	0.1	0.2
4 - 6	1.0	1.0	1.0
7 - 9	2.5	2.5	1.5
10 -14	5.0	15.0	0.8
> 15	2.0	14.0	8.0

[a] From Madewell et al. (1976) and Dorn & Priester (1976)

they reported that this may have been because their cases originated in an industrialized metropolitan area. Exposure to environmental carcinogens, particularly air pollutants, could have a significant bearing on the relatively high occurrence of tonsillar carcinoma found by these authors. It is possible that carcinogens that gain access to the tonsillar crypts are not removed by the cleansing action of saliva (Brodey, 1961).

Table 5 gives the estimated relative risks of oropharyngeal and intranasal neoplasms in different breeds of dogs; these varied both with breed and site. Although clinical reports have suggested that

Table 5. Estimated relative risks of oropharyngeal and intranasal neoplasms in selected breeds of dogs[a]

Breed	Site: Mouth and pharynx	Nose
All breeds combined	1.0	1.0
Keeshond	ND	7.2[b]
German short-haired pointer	2.8[b]	1.5
Cocker spaniel	1.8[b]	0.6
Collie	1.4	2.1[b]
Mixed breed	0.8	1.2
Beagle	0.5[b]	1.2
Miniature/toy poodle	ND	0.4[b]
Dachshund	0.3[b]	0.6

[a] From Madewell et al. (1976) and Dorn & Priester (1976)

[b] Values differ significantly from R = 1 ($P<0.05$)

ND = not determined

intranasal neoplasms are more frequent in dogs with long noses, the data reviewed here do not support this theory. The variation in incidence of these cancers in different breeds of dog is similar to the variation in incidence of NPC in different human populations (Ho, 1972). These data could thus provide interesting information about the role of genetics in the variation in incidence of NPC.

We are not aware that virological investigations have been carried out on the tumours described above. Since EBV is considered to be an important etiological factor in NPC and in Burkitt's lymphoma, and since transforming virus has been isolated from throat washings of patients with these tumours, it is important that such virological studies be undertaken. Particular emphasis should be placed on tonsillar carcinomas and on squamous-cell carcinomas.

INDUCTION OF TUMOURS IN ATHYMIC NUDE MICE WITH LYMPHOID AND EPITHELIAL CELLS CONTAINING THE EBV GENOME

We will now describe the use of a laboratory model for NPC, i.e., tumours induced in nude mice by human epithelial somatic-cell hybrids containing the EBV genome (Ablashi et al., 1976b; Glaser, 1975; Glaser et al., 1977). EBV is known to be associated naturally with lymphoblastoid cell lines and not with those that have a non-lymphoblastoid morphology. However, it has been possible to prepare non-lymphoblastoid somatic-cell hybrids which contain the EBV genome; one of the parental lines of these hybrids is lymphoblastoid and contains EBV. The parental lymphoblastoid line described in these experiments is HR-1; hybridization with the D98 line (a HeLa variant) resulted in the formation of the epithelial D98/HR-1 line, which contains the EBV genome. We attempted to induce tumours in nude mice because these animals are almost completely deficient in immunological responses mediated by T-lymphocytes. Nude mice can accept heterotransplants of many human tumours, and this phenomenon has been exploited in a number of studies of human cancer (Giovanella et al., 1974; Klein et al., 1974).

Table 6 shows tumour induction with D98, HR-1 and D98/HR-1 cells (original inoculum), tumour cells and cell lines derived from tumours. The D98/HR-1 cells had the highest percentage of tumour 'takes', and they induced tumours more rapidly than did the HR-1 parental cells. Tumours induced by the D98 parental cell line were smaller than those induced by cells of the other two lines. These results indicate that tumours induced by the D98/HR-1 cells were more aggressive than those induced by the two parental cell lines. The greater aggressiveness of the hybrid epithelial cells may be related to their association with EBV.

Tumours induced by cell lines were histologically identical, regardless of whether they were induced by cells from the lines themselves, from tumours induced by these cells, or from cell lines

Table 6. Induction of tumours in nude mice with D98/HR-1 and D98 cells[a]

Inoculum	Percentage of takes			Time of appearance of first tumour (days)			Average size of tumour at necropsy[b] (cm^3)			Tumour type
	A	B	C	A	B	C	A	B	C	
D98/HR-1 cells	80	80	90	14	11	26	3.1	3.5	3.2	Undifferentiated carcinoma
HR-1 cells	30	50	55	36	23	35	4.5	4.9	4.5	Poorly differentiated lymphoma
D98 cells	50	80	ND	22	15	ND	0.8	1.1	ND	Carcinoma

[a] From Ablashi et al. (1976b)

[b] Animals were sacrificed 70 days after inoculation.

A = cell lines B = cells from tumours C = cell lines derived from tumours

ND = not determined

derived from tumours. Tumours induced by HR-1 cells were poorly differentiated lymphomas; those induced by D98 cells were carcinomas, and those induced by the D98/HR-1 hybrid cells were undifferentiated carcinomas (Glaser et al., 1977). Histological examination of the undifferentiated carcinomas showed that broad masses of tumour cells formed densely-packed aggregates containing a large number of mitoses. Cells varied in size, shape and staining characteristics (Glaser et al., 1977). Such tumours, induced in nude mice by HR-1 and D98/HR-1 cells, could serve as EBV-carrying models for Burkitt's lymphoma and anaplastic NPC in humans.

Table 7 shows that the vast majority of HR-1 cells contained EBV nuclear antigen (EBNA). The sharp reduction of the number of EBV genome equivalents in the HR-1 tumours suggests that virus production was 'turned off'. Almost all of the cells from the line derived from the HR-1 tumour contained EBNA, but the number of cells containing viral capsid antigen (VCA) or early antigen (EA) had declined in comparison with that in the original inoculum. This is reflected in the number of EBV genome equivalents in such cells. No mouse chromosomes were found in this line; the modal number of chromosomes was 47.

Table 8 shows that the vast majority of D98/HR-1 cells contained EBNA but that VCA and EA were not detectable; VCA and EA could, however, be induced by iododeoxyuridine (IUdR). In D98/HR-1 cells, the EBV genomes are latent and are associated stably with the host cells. Approximately 80% of the cells in imprint preparations from tumours induced by D98/HR-1 cells also contained EBNA. However, the number of EBV genome equivalents in tumour cells was sharply reduced. An early *in vitro* passage of a cell line derived from a tumour showed some recovery of viral genomes, and full recovery occurred with a later passage. Preliminary data also suggest that the chromosomes in these cells were all human and were comparable with the original D98/HR-1

Table 7. Genetic characteristics of HR-1 cells and tumours[a]

	Antigens			Hybridization data EBV genomes/cell[b]		Modal number of chromosomes
	EBNA	VCA	EA	cRNA	DNA-DNA reassociation	
HR-1 cells	90%	10-15%	ND	600	ND	47
Tumours, or imprints from tumours, induced by HR-1 cells	80%	ND	ND	19	20	
Cell line (early and later passage) derived from HR-1 tumour	90%	2%	0.5-1.0%	170	ND	47

[a] From Ablashi et al. (1976b)

[b] For controls, Simpson cells (EBV genome-negative) were used: 217 counts/50 μg DNA were subtracted from all values.

EBNA = Epstein-Barr virus nuclear antigen

VCA = Epstein-Barr virus capsid antigen

EA = Epstein-Barr virus early antigen

cRNA = complementary RNA

ND = not determined

Table 8. Characteristics of D98/HR-1 cells and tumours[a]

	Antigens			Hybridization data EBV genomes/cell[b]		Modal number of chromosomes
	EBNA	VCA	EA	cRNA	DNA-DNA reassociation	
D98/HR-1 cells	90%	None	None	44	ND	84-90
D98/HR-1 cells (IUdR treatment followed by normal incubation)	90%	8-10%	10-30%	ND	ND	
Tumour, or imprints from tumours, induced by D98/HR-1 cells	80%	None	None	2-3	4.5	
Cell culture (early passage) derived from tumour induced by D98/HR-1 cells	90%	None	None	5-6	8.2	
Cell culture (later passage) derived from tumour induced by D98/HR-1 cells	90%	None	None	43	ND	80-91
Cell culture derived from tumour induced by D98/HR-1 cells (IuDR treatment followed by normal incubation)	90%	8-10%	10-30%	ND	ND	

[a] From Ablashi et al. (1976b)

[b] For controls, Simpson cells (EBV genome-negative) were used: 217 counts/50 μg DNA were subtracted from all values.

EBNA = Epstein-Barr virus nuclear antigen

EA = Epstein-Barr virus early antigen

VCA = Epstein-Barr virus capsid antigen

IUdR = iododeoxyuridine

cRNA = complementary RNA

ND = not determined

cells. No evidence has been found that C-type particles are present in the D98/HR-1 cells.

Passage in nude mice may therefore influence the number of EBV genomes in both the productive and the nonproductive states; thus, the passage of HR-1 and D98/HR-1 cells in nude mice might serve as models for the study of EBV genome regulation in Burkitt's lymphoma and NPC (Ablashi et al., 1976b; Glaser et al., 1977). This is important because there are at present no established epithelial cell lines that have been derived from NPC (Trumper et al., 1976).

TUMOURS IN NUDE MICE AS MODELS FOR THERAPY

Recent studies by Woodruff & Warner (1977) suggest use of the nude mouse tumour model for therapy. These investigators successfully treated two murine lymphomas in nude mice by local injections of *Corynebacterium parvum*. The lymphoid and epithelial tumours described here carry the EBV genome and can consistently and rapidly be induced in nude mice; thus, they could serve as inexpensive and useful models for the evaluation of antiviral and antitumour drugs (O'Connor, 1976).

CONCLUSIONS

It is hoped that the naturally-occurring and experimental animal models for NPC described here will be of use to scientists. These models may be useful, independently or collectively (Woodruff & Warner, 1977), for study of the respective roles of genetics, viruses and other environmental factors in the etiology of NPC and may also be useful for immuno- and/or chemotherapy.

SUMMARY

Animal models for nasopharyngeal carcinoma have been reviewed. One group of models occurs naturally, and the other is the result of laboratory experimentation. Naturally occurring tumours of the mouth, pharynx and nose in domestic animals, particularly dogs, are of great interest. The numbers of squamous-cell carcinomas found in these regions in dogs are significant; the most frequently observed canine oral and pharyngeal neoplasm may be carcinoma of the tonsil. The tonsil resembles the human nasopharynx in that both have lymphoid tissue covered with epithelium; thus, tonsillar carcinoma in dogs may provide an interesting natural model for human NPC. The relative risks of oropharyngeal and intranasal neoplasms vary with breed of dog and this variation resembles that in the incidence of NPC in different human populations. It is of particular importance that virological studies be carried out on these tumours.

The laboratory model for NPC involves induction of tumours in nude mice with D98/HR-1, an epithelial somatic-cell hybrid containing the EBV genome. Parental HR-1 cells used in the same way could serve as a model for Burkitt's lymphoma. Passage of these cells in nude mice apparently influences the EBV genome content of the induced tumours. In addition to their use in studies of EBV genome regulation in NPC and Burkitt's lymphoma, tumours induced by these cell lines could be used in the evaluation of antineoplastic and antiviral sub stances of possible benefit in the treatment of NPC or Burkitt's lymphoma.

ACKNOWLEDGEMENTS

We thank Dr M. Nonoyama for the nucleic acid hybridization assays and Dr W. Priester of the National Cancer Institute, USA, for his suggestions and for providing some of the data on spontaneous tumours of the mouth, pharynx, nose and paranasal sinuses in domestic animals. Part of the investigations on nude mouse tumours was supported by contract number N01-CP5 3516 and grant number CA 15038-02 from the National Cancer Institute, USA (R. Glaser). R. Glaser is also the recipient of a Leukemia Society of America, Inc. Scholar Award. We also thank Dr J.B. Moloney of the National Cancer Institute, USA, and Dr G.B. de-Thé of the International Agency for Research on Cancer, Lyon, France, for motivating us to review and discuss animal models for nasopharyngeal carcinoma for this symposium.

REFERENCES

Ablashi, D.V., Easton, J.M. & Guégan, J.H. (1976a) Herpesviruses and cancer in man and subhuman primates. *Biomedicine, 24*, 286-305

Ablashi, D.V., Glaser, R., Easton, J.M., Nonoyama, M. & Armstrong, G.R. (1976b) Athymic nude mice: induction of tumors containing Epstein-Barr virus using Burkitt's-related cell lines. *Proc. Int. Soc. exp. Hemat., 4*, 163

Ash, J.E., Beck, M.R. & Wilkes, J.D. (1964) Tumors of the upper respiratory tract and ear. Armed Forces Inst. of Pathology (Washington, DC), pp. 56-57

Brodey, R.S. (1961) *A clinico-pathological study of 200 cases of oral and pharyngeal cancer in the dog.* In: *The Newer Knowledge About Dogs*, New York, NY, Gaines Dog Research Center, pp. 5-11

Cohen, D., Brodey, R.S. & Chen, S.M. (1964) Epidemiologic aspects of oral and pharyngeal neoplasms of the dog. *Amer. J. vet. Res.*, *25*, 1776-1779

Dorn, C.R. & Priester, W.A. (1976) Epidemiologic analysis of oral and pharyngeal cancer in dogs, cats, horses and cattle. *J. Amer. vet. Med. Assoc.*, *169*, 1202-1206

Giovanella, B.C., Stehlin, J.S. & Williams, L.J., Jr (1974) Heterotransplantation of human malignant tumors in 'nude' thymusless mice. II. Malignant tumors induced by injection of cell cultures derived from human solid tumors. *J. nat. Cancer Inst.*, *52*, 921-930

Glaser, R. (1975) *Expression and regulation of the Epstein-Barr virus early antigen components in Burkitt-epithelial hybrid cells.* In: *Proceedings of the International Workshop on EBV Production, Concentration and Purification.* Lyon, International Agency for Research on Cancer, *Internal Report No. 75003*, pp. 225-235

Glaser, R., Ablashi, D.V., Nonoyama, M., Henle, W. & Easton, J.M. (1977) Enhanced oncogenic behavior of human and mouse cells following cellular hybridization with Burkitt tumor cells. *Proc. nat. Acad. Sci. (Wash.)* (in press)

Ho, J.H.C. (1972) Nasopharyngeal carcinoma (NPC). *Advanc. Cancer Res.*, *15*, 57-85

Klein, G., Giovanella, B.C., Lindahl, T., Fialkow, P.J., Singh, S. & Stehlin, J.S. (1974) Direct evidence for the presence of Epstein-Barr virus DNA and nuclear antigen in malignant epithelial cells from patients with poorly differentiated carcinoma of the nasopharynx. *Proc. nat. Acad. Sci. (Wash.)*, *71*, 4737-4741

Madewell, B.R., Priester, W.A., Gillette, E.L. & Snyder, S.P. (1976) Neoplasms of the nasal passages and paranasal sinus in domestic animals as reported by 13 veterinary colleges. *Amer. J. vet. Res.*, *37*, 851-856

O'Connor, T.E. (1976) Approaches to antiviral chemotherapy: a status report. *Advanc. Pathobiol.*, *5*, 151-158

Trumper, P.A., Epstein, M.A. & Giovanella, B.C. (1976) Activation *in vitro* by BUdR of a productive EB virus infection in the epithelial cells of nasopharyngeal carcinoma. *Int. J. Cancer*, *17*, 578-587

Woodruff, M.F.A. & Warner, M.L. (1977) Effect of *Corynebacterium parvum* on tumor growth in normal and athymic (nude) mice. *J. nat. Cancer Inst.*, *58*, 111-116

DISCUSSION SUMMARY

M. CAMMOUN

Institut Salah Azaiz,
Tunis, Tunisia

It was pointed out that the number of cases of nasopharyngeal carcinoma in children was too small for any conclusion to be drawn with regard to predominant histological type.

The suggestion that nasopharyngeal carcinomas could be classified as either well-differentiated, non-keratinizing squamous-cell or poorly-differentiated non-keratinizing squamous-cell types was criticized on the basis that lymphoepitheliomas and certain undifferentiated carcinomas were also found in the nasopharynx. The Pathologist Group (Head and Neck) of the European Organization for Research and Treatment of Cancer had designated such tumours 'undifferentiated carcinomas of the nasopharyngeal type'. They recommended that nasopharyngeal carcinomas be classified as 'undifferentiated carcinoma of the nasopharyngeal type' or 'squamous-cell carcinoma (well-, mildly- or poorly-differentiated)'.

The need was stressed for a histological classification on which all apthologists present could agree, so that correlations could be made between histological types and virological, immunological and treatment results.

CLINICAL ASPECTS OF NASOPHARYNGEAL CARCINOMA

STAGE CLASSIFICATION OF NASOPHARYNGEAL CARCINOMA: A REVIEW

J.H.C. HO

Medical and Health Department
Institute of Radiology and Oncology,
Queen Elizabeth Hospital,
Kowloon, Hong Kong

INTRODUCTION

The extent of a cancer in a patient is best described by the extent of its primary tumour, the extent of involvement of the regional lymph nodes and the clinically demonstrated presence or absence of metastases. Although the spread of cancer is a continuous process, there is a practical need to classify cancer cases into groups according to certain stages, for the following purposes:

1. To guide treatment planning
2. To give some indication of prognosis
3. To help in the evaluation and comparison of treatment results, especially those from different centres
4. To facilitate cancer research

In order to achieve the latter two goals, general agreement on the stage classification to be adopted is essential. At present, a number of stage classifications of nasopharyngeal carcinomas (NPC) are used, but none has yet received general acceptance.

STAGE CLASSIFICATIONS

Geist & Portman (1952) were the first to produce a stage classification of NPC, as follows:

I. Tumor limited to nasopharynx;
no palpable nodes and no neurological signs

II. Palpable cervical nodes;
no other evidence of metastases or extension and no neurological signs

III. Local invasion of orbit, sinuses or base of skull; neurological signs; general carcinomatosis

The attraction of this system lies in its simplicity. It is easy to remember and is consequently more likely to find acceptance in centres where the tumour is encountered only occasionally. It is unsatisfactory in that stages II and III both cover too wide a range of involvement to serve any useful purpose.

In 1962, the International Union Against Cancer (UICC) recommended a TNM (Tumor Node Metastases) stage classification of malignant tumours, which was revised in a second edition published in 1974 (UICC, 1974):

Anatomical regions of the nasopharynx:

Postero-superior wall - Extends from the level of the junction of the hard and soft palates to the base of the skull

Lateral wall - Including the fossa of Rosenmüller

Inferior wall - Consists of the superior surface of the soft palate

Note: The margin of the choanal orifices, including the posterior margin of the nasal septum, is included in the nasal fossae.

T - Primary tumour

T1S Pre-invasive carcinoma (carcinoma *in situ*)

T0 No evidence of primary tumour

T1 Tumour limited to one region

T2 Tumour extending into two regions

T3 Tumour extending beyond nasopharynx without bone involvement

T4 Tumour extending beyond nasopharynx with bone involvement

N - Regional lymph nodes

NO No palpable nodes

N1 Movable homolateral nodes

N2 Movable contralateral or bilateral nodes

N3 Fixed nodes

M - Distant metastases

MO No evidence of distant metastases

M Distant metastases present.

In this classification, the apparent extent of the disease is stated, but no attempt is made to classify the extent into stages. The main criticism of this scheme is, however, in its classification of the extent of the primary tumour and of regional lymph node involvement. It is not always possible to ascertain the limits of the primary tumour within the nasopharynx, since, even for the expert, examination of this area is sometimes notoriously difficult. Furthermore, a carcinoma may occur submucosally in the nasopharynx and thus not be visible; the diagnosis in such cases is established by biopsy, which, however, does not indicate the extent of the tumour. Also, in the UICC classification, the fossa of Rosenmüller, a frequent site of origin of the primary tumour, is included as part of the lateral wall, when in fact it is formed partly by the lateral wall and partly by the posterior wall. Primary tumours often originate in the posterior wall of the fossa, which is actually an extension of the posterior wall of the nasopharynx. In practice, therefore, the suggested classification of the primary tumour into T1 and T2 may be neither possible nor accurate, and, from the point of view of treatment planning and prognostication, it has little significance.

The difference between T3 and T4 in this classification is the presence or absence of bone involvement, the detection of which depends on the thoroughness of the radiographical investigation. The common practice of taking only the submentovertical (axial) and lateral projections of the skull is not sufficient for this purpose; even with the most thorough investigation, a certain amount of bony involvement, which nearly always accompanies the involvement of certain cranial nerves *via* the natural foramina at the base of skull, may be overlooked. T4 should, therefore, include involvement of cranial nerves; since this implies evidence of intracranial entry, such a classification would indicate an even graver prognosis than mere bone involvement.

With regard to regional lymph node involvement, the UICC classification was designed primarily as a guide for surgical treatment by block dissection. It is not suitable as a guide for radiation therapy, which is now the main treatment used for cervical nodal metastases in NPC.

In the second edition of the UICC TNM classification (UICC, 1974), the following statement was made with regard to cervical lymph nodes:

> "It is recognised that the level of involvement of cervical lymph nodes has a bearing on both treatment and prognosis. Although it is not possible at present to incorporate these levels in the N classification, it is recommended that they should always be recorded. Four levels are defined:
>
> Level 1. Lymph nodes palpable in the submandibular and/or submental regions.
>
> Level 2. Lymph nodes palpable distal to level 1. and confined to the region above the skin crease at or just below the level of the thyroid notch.
>
> Level 3. Lymph nodes palpable distal to level 2. and confined to the anterior cervical triangle including those deep to the sternomastoid muscle.
>
> Level 4. Lymph nodes palpable distal to level 3. and confined to the posterior cervical triangle below the skin crease at or just below the thyroid notch."

The American Joint Committee for Cancer Staging and End Results Reporting (1976) recommended the following staging for nasopharyngeal cancers:

Primary tumor

T1S Carcinoma *in situ*

T1 Tumor confined to one site of nasopharynx (posterior) superior wall or lateral wall) or no tumor visible (positive biopsy only)

T2 Tumor involving two sites of the nasopharynx

T3 Extension of tumor into nasal cavity or oropharynx

T4 Tumor invasion of skull and/or cranial nerve involvement

Cervical nodes (midline nodes considered to be homolateral)

NO No clinically positive node

N1 Single clinically positive homolateral node less than 3 cm in diameter

N2 Single clinically positive homolateral node 3 cm to 6 cm in diameter or multiple clinically positive homolateral nodes, none over 6 cm in diameter

N3 Massive homolateral node(s), bilateral nodes or contralateral node(s)

Stage grouping

Stage I	T1, N0, M0
II	T2, N0, M0
III	T3, N0, M0
	T1 or T2 or T3, N1, M0
IV	T4, N0, M0
	Any T, N2, M0
	Any T, any N, M1

It is felt that stages I and II could well be combined, for reasons stated earlier, and that stage IV covers too wide a range of involvement to be of value for guiding treatment or prognosis. Certainly, patients with T4, N2 or even N3 involvement without metastases (M0) should not be included in the same category as those with M1, who are usually dead within three years of diagnosis. In our experience, at least a quarter of patients with T4, N0-1 tumours could be expected to be alive five years after radiation therapy; this also applies to patients with N2 or with N3 bilateral or contralateral but not massive nodal involvement.

Since the nasopharynx is a midline organ with bilateral lymphatic drainage, and since nodal fixation does not preclude radiation therapy as it does block dissection, the cervical nodes should be treated bilaterally and according to the level of involvement; it is this that determines prognosis, regardless of the mobility of the nodes or of the side(s) involved. That this is the case is shown in Tables 1-3.

Table 1. Patients with nasopharyngeal carcinoma with mobile nodes: 5-year absolute survival rates by laterality (1965-1967)

Stage[a]	Initial no. of cases		No. of cases alive at 5 years (%)		
	Unilateral	Bilateral	Unilateral	Bilateral	Probability & significance
II (T1 or T2, N1)	62	16	40 (64.5)	7 (43.8)	0.14 (NS)
III (T1 or T2, N2)	31	33	11 (35.5)	12 (36.4)	0.94 (NS)
IV (T1 or T2, N3)	8	19	1 (12.5)	5 (26.3)	0.43 (NS)
Total	101	68	52 (51.5)	24 (35.3)	0.04 (S)

[a] Ho, 1970

NS - not significant; S - significant

Table 2. Patients with nasopharyngeal carcinoma with unilateral nodes: 5-year absolute survival rates by nodal mobility (1965-1967)

Stage[a]	Initial no. of cases		No. of cases alive at 5 years (%)		
	Mobile	Fixed	Mobile	Fixed	Probability & significance
II (T1 or T2, N1)	62	20	40 (64.5)	8 (40.0)	0.055 (NS)
III (T1 or T2, N2)	31	63	11 (35.5)	19 (30.2)	0.60 (NS)
IV (T1 or T2, N3)	8	46	1 (12.5)	5 (10.9)	0.89 (NS)
Total	101	129	52 (51.5)	32 (24.8)	0.00003 (S)

[a] Ho, 1970

NS - not significant; S - significant

Table 3. Five-year absolute survival and relapse-free rates of nasopharyngeal carcinoma patients with cervical nodal involvement by level regardless of mobility or laterality of involvement (1965-1968)

Stage[a]	Initial no. of cases	No. of cases alive at 5 yrs (%)	Probability & significance(s)	No. relapse-free	Probability & significance(s)
II (T1 or T2, N1)	102	55 (53.9)		49 (48.0%)	
			N1/N2 P = 0.0001 S		N1/N2 P = 0.0004 S
III (T1 or T2, N2)	183	56 (30.6)		50 (27.3%)	
			N2/N3 P = 0.0003 S		N2/N3 P = 0.000004 S
IV (T1 or T2, N3)	161	23 (14.3)		13 (8.1%)	

[a] Ho, 1970

The stage classification used in these tables is the revised classification of Ho (1970), which evolved as a result of successive analyses of results of treatment since 1965. This classification is as follows:

T - *Primary tumour*

T1 Tumour confined to the nasopharynx (space behind the choanal orifices and nasal septum and above the posterior margin of the soft palate in the resting position)

T2 Tumour extended to the nasal fossa, oropharynx or adjacent muscles or nerves below the base of the skull

T3 Tumour extending beyond T2 limits and subclassified as follows:

T3a Bone involvement below the base of the skull (including floor of sphenoid sinus)

T3b Involvement of base of skull

T3c Involvement of cranial nerve(s)

T3d Involvement of orbit, laryngopharynx (hypopharynx) or infratemporal fossa

N - *Regional lymph nodes* (Figs 1 & 2)

N0 No palpable nodes (excluding nodes thought to be benign)

N1 Node(s) wholly in upper cervical level, bounded below by the neck crease extending laterally and backwards from or just below the thyroid notch (laryngeal eminence)

N2 Palpable node(s) between the crease and the supraclavicular fossa, the upper limit being a line joining the upper margin of the sternal end of the clavicle and the apex of an angle formed by the lateral surface of the neck and the superior margin of the trapezius

N3 Palpable node(s) in the supraclavicular fossa and/or skin involvement in the form of carcinoma *en cuirasse* or satellite nodules above the clavicles

In addition, the apparent extent of the disease as a whole was classified into stages as a guide to prognosis and treatment:

I. Tumour confined to the nasopharynx (T1, N0, M0)

II. Tumour extending to nasal fossa, oropharynx or adjacent muscles or nerves below the base of the skull (T2) and/or N1 involvement

FIG. 1. PATIENT WITH NASOPHARYNGEAL CARCINOMA:
FRONT VIEW OF NECK SHOWING REGIONAL LYMPH NODE LEVELS

Thyroid notch and skin crease between N1 and N2 levels is indicated by the arrow. This patient has N2 involvement on the right side, since the nodal swelling extends below the crease.

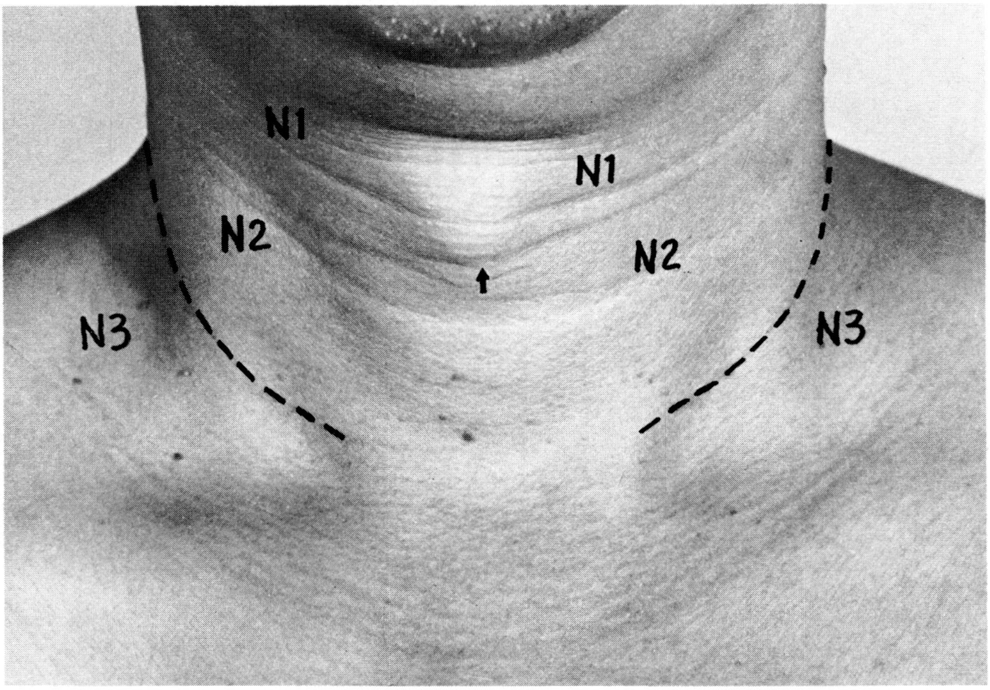

III. Tumour extending beyond T2 limits or with bone involvement (T3) and/or N2 involvement

IV. N3 involvement, irrespective of the stage of the primary tumour

V. Haematogenous metastasis and/or involvement of the skin or lymph node(s) below the clavicles (M1)

The size of an involved node has an important bearing on prognosis: a large metastatic node may metastasize directly *via* the blood stream. That the level of involvement is also important has already been shown in Tables 1-3. By the time both sides are involved, there are frequently palpable nodes at a lower level (this applies also to fixed

FIG. 2. PATIENT WITH NASOPHARYNGEAL CARCINOMA:
SIDE VIEW OF NECK SHOWING REGIONAL LYMPH NODE LEVELS

Note nodal swelling extending below skin crease.

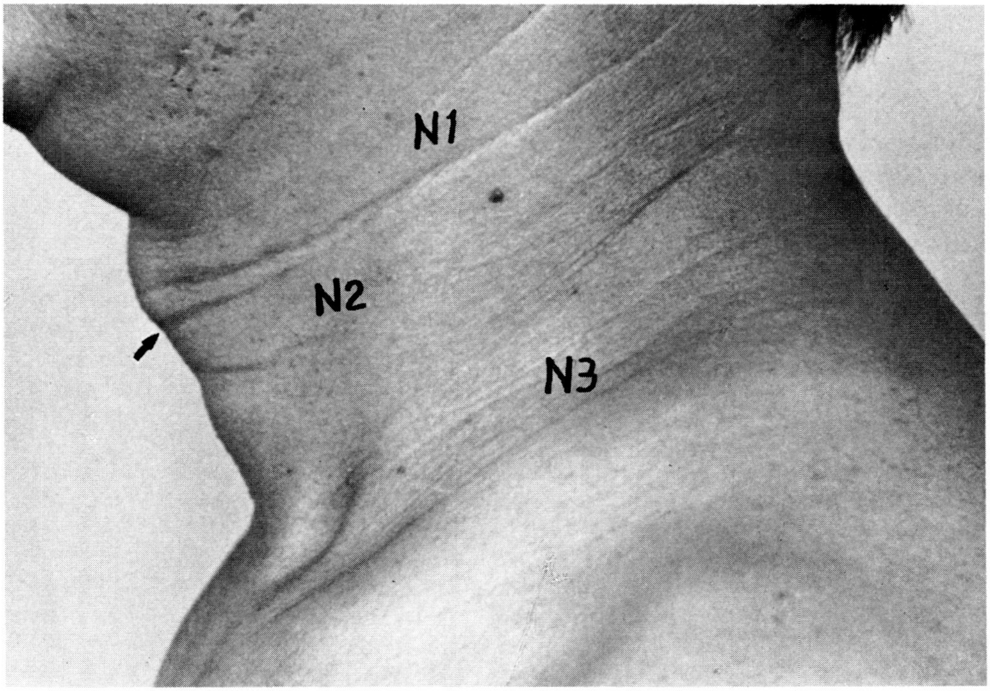

nodes). This may partly explain why patients with bilateral nodal involvement have a significantly poorer prognosis than those with unilateral involvement (Table 1) and those with fixed nodes a poorer prognosis than those with mobile ones (Table 2). Ho's N classification takes size into account by requiring palpation and observation as to whether any of the nodes have enlarged so as to encroach upon a lower level. A decision can more easily be made on this basis than on whether a node is 3 cm or less in diameter, for instance. Occasionally the skin crease between levels 1 and 2 may be indistinct; however, this is usually seen on one side only, and hence little difficulty is encountered in tracing it.

TREATMENT RESULTS IN RELATION TO STAGE CLASSIFICATION

Scanlon et al. (1967) reported on 141 patients with NPC, of which 119 had keratinizing squamous or undifferentiated carcinomas, who were treated during the 11-year period 1950-1960 at the Mayo Clinic and

Foundation. They had been classified by stage of disease according to the TNM system formulated by the American Joint Committee for Cancer Staging and End Results Reporting in May, 1965. The authors found the classification to be inadequate and expressed the opinion that T2 (tumour confined to the nasopharynx) and T3 (tumour extended outside the nasopharynx) without nodal involvement should not be included in the same stage (II) since T3 carries a definitely poorer prognosis. Furthermore, they felt that the N classification should not be based primarily on the presence or absence of palpable lymph nodes and their degree of fixation, which was sometimes particularly difficult to ascertain, without concern for the number involved and the extent of involvement.

Chen & Fletcher (1971) reported the following stage classification, in use at the M.D. Anderson Hospital, Houston, Texas:

Primary tumour

T1 Primary tumour invisible but biopsy-positive, or tumour less than 1 cm in greatest diameter

T2 Tumour more than 1 cm in diameter but confined to the nasopharynx

T3 Tumour extending beyond nasopharynx, but no evidence of invasion of base of skull or cranial nerves

T4 Tumour, regardless of size, involving base of skull and/or cranial nerves

Cervical lymph nodes

N0 No palpable lymph node

N1 Single lymph node < 3 cm

N2A Single lymph node > 3 cm

N2B Multiple nodes confined to one side, movable

N3A Fixed unilateral node(s)

N3B Bilateral nodes

Stage grouping

Stage I. T1, N0

II. T2, T3 or T4, N0

III. N1, N2A or N2B, irrespective of T

IV. N3A or N3B, irrespective of T.

They reported better absolute (or crude) five-year survival rates for patients with stage III than for those with stage II: 37.5% for 16 stage II patients and 44.9% for 49 stage III patients; 76 stage IV patients (squamous-cell carcinomas and lymphoepitheliomas combined) had a five-year survival rate of 27.6%. There was also poor correlation between the various stages of N involvement and survival, possibly because levels of involvement were disregarded. Patients with T4 tumours had a poor survival rate, similar to ours, but they were grouped within stage II as long as there was no nodal involvement.

In China, where NPC is prevalent, the classification of clinical stages of the disease used is that in the TNM system adopted at the Second Chinese National Conference on Cancer held in Shanghai in 1965. It is as follows:

Primary tumour

T0 No visible primary tumour in the nasopharynx

T1 Primary tumour involving one wall of the nasopharynx

T2 Primary tumour involving two or more walls of the nasopharynx

T3 Primary tumour extending beyond the nasopharynx, involving one of the following groups of structures: (1) the contiguous soft tissues or the neighboring sinuses or cavities, (2) the bone of the base of the skull, or (3) cranial nerves I, II, III, IV, V_1 and/or VI

T4 As T3, but involving two or more groups of structures

Regional lymph nodes

N0 No palpable lymph nodes in the neck

N1 Freely movable lymph nodes in the upper cervical region on one or both sides, diameter under 3 cm

N2 Entirely or partially fixed lymph nodes in the cervical region on one or both sides, diameter under 8 cm

N3 Cervical lymph node enlargement, together with involvement of cranial nerve IX, X, XI or XII and a sympathetic ganglion

N4 Cervical lymph node enlargement, over 8 cm in diameter, or with involvement of the supraclavicular fossa

Distant metastases

M0 Absence of distant metastasis

M1 Presence of distant metastasis

Stage grouping

I. T1, NO, MO

II. TO-1, N1, MO; T2, NO-1, MO

III. TO-3, N2, MO; T3, NO-2, MO

IV. TO-4, N4, MO; T4, NO-4, MO; TO-4, NO-4, M1

On the basis of this stage classification, the Chung San Medical College Tumor Hospital Department of Radiology (1974), in Canton, reported absolute (or crude) survival rates of 61.3% for 31 stage I patients, 55.0% for 269 with stage II, 45.8% for 330 with stage III and 23.6% for 72 with stage IV; disease-free rates of 45.2% were reported for those with stage I, 42.6% for stage II, 35.8% for stage III and 19.4% for stage IV.

The main criticism of this classification is that M1 should not be included in stage IV since it carries a hopeless prognosis, whereas patients with some of the T and N combinations in stage IV may be curable.

Figure 3 shows ten-year cumulative actuarial survival and relapse-free curves for 467 patients treated, some by orthovoltage and some by megavoltage radiation therapy, in Hong Kong in 1965 by stage of tumour, according to the classification of Ho (1970); Figure 4 shows five-year cumulative actuarial survival and relapse-free curves for 616 patients with stages I to III of the disease treated only by megavoltage radiation therapy during 1969-1971.

FIG. 3. PERCENTAGES OF 467 PATIENTS WITH NASOPHARYNGEAL CARCINOMA TREATED AT QUEEN ELIZABETH AND QUEEN MARY HOSPITALS, HONG KONG IN 1965, SURVIVING AND RELAPSE-FREE THROUGHOUT, BY STAGE OF DISEASE

(HO, 1970)

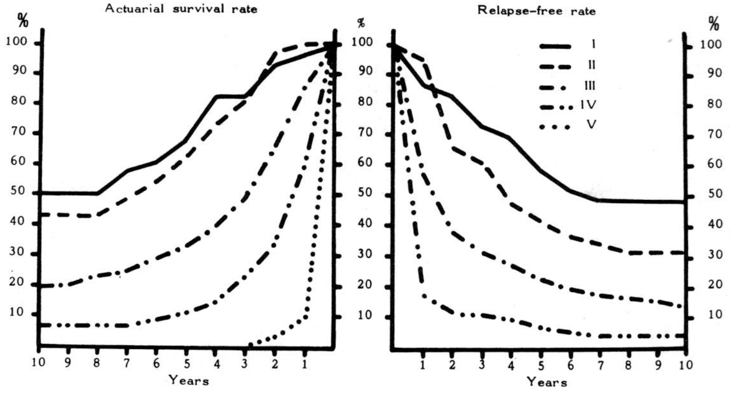

FIG. 4. RESULTS OF TREATMENT OF STAGES I, II AND III NASOPHARYNGEAL CARCINOMA PATIENTS WITH 4.5 MeV X-RAYS IN HONG KONG, 1969-1971: PERCENTAGES SURVIVING AND RELAPSE-FREE, BY STAGE OF DISEASE (HO, 1970)

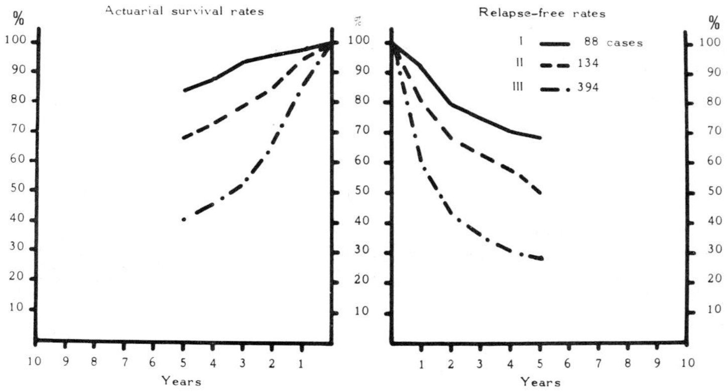

Table 4 shows the 5-year actuarial survival and relapse-free rates for patients treated in 1965 and in 1969-1971. There was good correlation between stage and prognosis in both series, although the modality and method of treatment were not identical in the two groups.

Table 4. Five-year actuarial survival rates and relapse-free rates[a] by stage of disease[b]

Stage \ Year	Actuarial survival rate - %		Relapse-free rate (%)	
	1965	1969-1971	1965	1969-1971
I	67.9	83.9	17/29 (58.6)	60/88 (68.2)
II	62.2	67.9	16/38 (42.1)	67/134 (50.0)
III	32.9	48.3	55/242 (22.7)	114/394 (28.9)
IV	11.0		9/128 (7.0)	

[a] Relapse-free after the first and only course of radiation therapy

[b] Ho, 1970

The same stage classification was used by Henle et al. (1970, 1973) and by de-Thé et al. (1975) in their studies of the spectra and titres of antibodies to Epstein-Barr virus-related antigens in NPC; they found that the geometric mean titres increased stepwise with the stage of disease, which may be taken to reflect tumour burden.

SUMMARY

Various stage classifications of NPC have been described and discussed. Treatment results have been reported for the various stages for only four of these classifications; the correlation between stage and treatment results was best in the classification of the author.

ACKNOWLEDGEMENTS

The author is grateful to Miss May Fong for collecting data, to Mr C.M. Lam for statistical calculations, to Mrs P. Liu for typing the manuscript, to Mr R. Abesser for drawing the figures and to Mr K.W. Leung for photographic assistance.

REFERENCES

The American Joint Committee for Cancer Staging and End Results Reporting (1976) *Staging of cancer at head and neck sites.* In: Task Force on Head and Neck Sites, eds, *Preliminary Handbook on Classification and Staging*, pp. 61-72

Chen, K.Y. & Fletcher, G.H. (1971) Malignant tumors of the nasopharynx. *Radiology*, *99*, 165-171

Chung San Medical College Tumor Hospital Department of Radiology (1974) [Radiotherapy of nasopharynx cancer] *Chin. med. J.*, *11*, 687-692 [in Chinese] de-Thé, G., Ho, J.H.C., Ablashi, D.V., Day, N.E., Macario, A.J.L., Martin-Berthelon, M.C., Pearson, G. & Sohier, R. (1975) Nasopharyngeal carcinoma. IX. Antibodies to EBNA and correlation with response to other EBV antigens in Chinese patients. *Int. J. Cancer*, *16*, 713-721

Geist, R.M., Jr & Portman, U.V. (1952) Primary malignant tumors of nasopharynx. *Amer. J. Roentgenol.*, *68*, 262-271

Henle, W., Henle, G., Ho, H.C., Burtin, P., Cachin, Y., Clifford, P., de Schryver, A., de-Thé, G., Diehl, V. & Klein, G. (1970) Antibodies to Epstein-Barr virus in nasopharyngeal carcinoma, other head and neck neoplasms and control groups. *J. nat. Cancer Inst.*, *44*, 225-231

Henle, W., Ho, J.H.C. & Kwan, H.C. (1973) Antibodies to Epstein-Barr virus related antigens in nasopharyngeal carcinoma: comparison of active cases and long term survivors. *J. nat. Cancer Inst.*, *51*, 361-369

Ho, J.H.C. (1970) *The natural history and treatment of nasopharyngeal carcinoma.* In: Lee-Clark, R., Cumley, R.W., McCay, J.E. & Copeland, M., eds, *Proceedings of the X International Cancer Congress*, Vol. 4, Chicago, Yearbook Medical Publishers, pp. 1-14

Scanlon, P.W., Rhodes, R.E., Jr, Woolner, L.B., Devine, K.D. & McBean, J.B. (1967) Cancer of the nasopahrynx: 142 patients treated in the 11-year period 1950-1960. *Amer. J. Roentgenol.*, *99*, 313-325

UICC (1974) TNM Classification of Malignant Tumours, 2nd ed., Geneva

NASOPHARYNGEAL CARCINOMA IN CHILDREN AND ADOLESCENTS IN TUNISIA: CLINICAL ASPECTS AND THE PARANEOPLASTIC SYNDROME

R. ELLOUZ, M. CAMMOUN, R. BEN ATTIA & J. BAHI

Department of Head and Neck Surgery,
Salah Azaïz Institute,
Tunis, Tunisia

INTRODUCTION

It is well recognized that nasopharyngeal carcinoma (NPC) occurs relatively frequently in Tunisia (Ellouz et al., 1975; Zaouche, 1970), and this is confirmed by recent studies at our Institute. The Salah Azaïz Institute, which is the National Cancer Institute of Tunis, opened in 1969. It is the only centre that specializes in cancer treatment in this small country in the extreme northern part of Africa that has a population of about 5 million people.

This paper describes in particular the incidence of NPC among youths in their second decade of life, i.e., between 10 and 19 years of age. The clinical symptomatology described in our earlier publications (Cammoun et al., 1973; Ellouz et al., 1975) is briefly reiterated; however, emphasis is laid on the epidemiological, clinical/anatomical and evolutionary characteristics of this cancer that are particular to young people.

MATERIALS AND METHODS

Of a total of 485 cases of NPC observed at the Salah Azaïz Institute between March 1969 and December 1974 (less than six years), 82 (17%) were in children and adolescents of less than 19 years of age. All of the patients were Tunisians, of the Moslem religion; all underwent clinical, radiological and histological examinations.

Curative treatment was carried out for 58 of the 82 young patients; 11 received palliative treatment; nine with advanced stages of the disease were not treated; and four were lost to follow-up before any treatment.

Treatment consisted of external radiotherapy by telecobalt to the rhinopharynx and cervical lymph nodes. The tumour and involved nodes received 7,500 rads, with 5,500 rads directed to apparently healthy cervical nodes. A few cases underwent conventional radiotherapy at 200 kV with additional telecobalt. One patient received chemotherapy for local recurrence, and another underwent cervical lymphadenectomy after radiotherapy.

RESULTS

Age and sex distribution

In our series, the youngest patient was 10 years old and the oldest 19; the age-sex distribution curve (Fig. 1) shows a peak incidence of NPC in males at 15 years. The disease occurred more often in males, the sex ratio being 3.5:1 (58 males, 24 females).

FIG. 1. AGE AND SEX DISTRIBUTION

Age and sex distribution of 82 Tunisian children with nasopharyngeal carcinoma

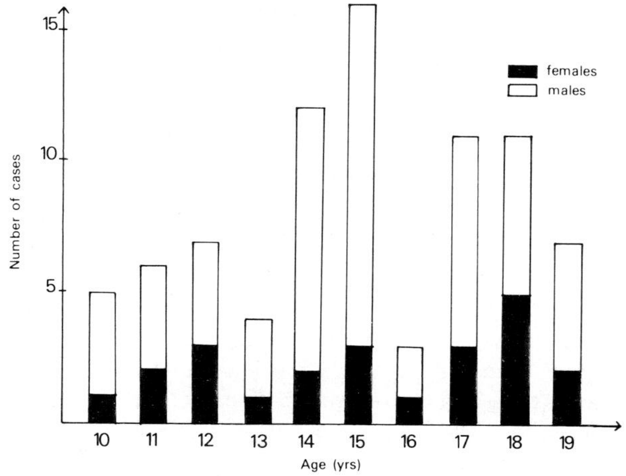

Geographical distribution

A study of the geographical incidence of NPC in Tunisia revealed no significant differences (Fig. 2). It was noticed, however, that a fairly large number of children with NPC came from north-eastern Tunisia (28.5% of all NPC cases), while the incidence in each of the other regions was only about 17%.

FIG. 2. GEOGRAPHICAL DISTRIBUTION

Geographical distribution of nasopharyngeal carcinoma in children and adults in Tunisia; % - no. of cases in children/total no. of NPC cases in each region

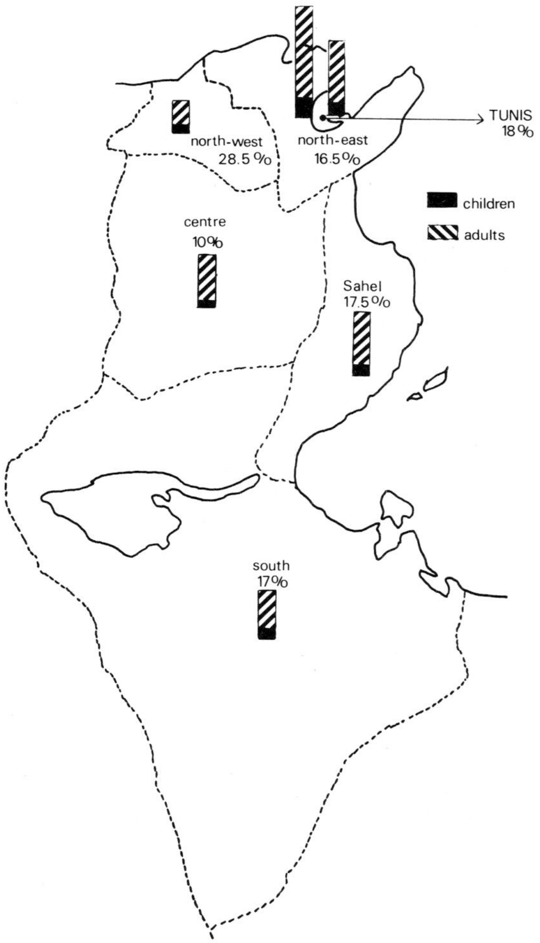

Clinical observations

The interval between the first symptom and the date of the first consultation is much more difficult to determine in children than in adults, but the average delay was estimated to be five months. The first sign is usually enlarged lymph nodes (in 83% of cases), either as an isolated adenopathy or associated with other signs (Table 1).

Table 1. First symptom of nasopharyngeal carcinoma seen in 82 Tunisian children

Symptom	No. of patients (%)	
Lymph-node enlargement	27 (33)	(83)
Lymph-node enlargement + other signs	41	
Other	14	

It is often difficult to specify the primary tumour site in children, because the nasopharynx is not easy to see. In some cases, we could only take a blind biopsy after bidigital evaluation of the tumour's topography. The distribution of tumour sites in our series is shown in Table 2.

Table 2. Distribution of primary tumour site in 82 Tunisian children

Primary tumour site	No. of patients
Lateral wall	16
Anterior wall	1
Roof	6
Entire nasopharyngeal region	40
Posterior wall	1
Unknown	18

The extent of the tumour (Table 3) was evaluated by both clinical and routine X-ray examinations. Neurological signs, seen in 22 cases (27%), were due essentially to involvement of the V and VI cranial nerves. Trismus was seen in 34 cases (41.5%); and 40 patients presented with bone involvement (49%). 81 patients revealed cervical adenopathy at the first examination, which was most often high

Table 3. Local and regional extension of nasopharyngeal tumours in 82 Tunisian children

Extension of tumour	No. of patients	(%)
Neurological signs	22	(27)
Trismus	34	(41)
Bone involvement	40	(49)
Lymph node involvement		
unilateral	34	
bilateral	41	

and bilateral; five had supraclavicular lymph-node involvement.

Classification of the tumours according to the TNM system (UICC, 1974) showed (Table 4) that none were T1 and only one was N0. On the other hand, there were large numbers of T4 (47 cases) and N3 (63 cases) tumours. Distant metastases appeared to be particularly common in children: three cases were observed at first examination before any treatment.

Table 4. Distribution of nasopharyngeal tumours in 82 Tunisian children by TN classification (UICC, 1972)

	No. of patients						
	T0	T1	T2	T3	T4	TX	Total
N0					1		1
N1				1	7		8
N2			3	1	4		8
N3			11	14	35	3	63
NX			1			1	2
Total			15	16	47	4	82

The histopathological classification adopted by our group is described elsewhere[1]. The distribution of our cases according to this system was as follows: well-differentiated squamous-cell carcinoma: non-existent in children; poorly-differentiated squamous-cell carcinoma: 37 cases (45%); and 'nasopharyngeal' carcinoma: 39 cases (47.5%).

[1] See p. 13

Six of the cases in our series could not be classified.

Rates of survival

The five-year survival rate, calculated according to the actuarial method, was 32.5% in our series of children, while that in adults was only 20%; the two-year survival rates were 37% and 24%, respectively. The essential factors that influence prognosis are histological type of tumour, local extent of the tumour and the degree of lymphatic involvement. Two-year survival rates in children and adults in our series in relation to these parameters are shown in Table 5.

Table 5. Two-year survival rates of Tunisian children and adults with nasopharyngeal carcinoma by tumour characteristic

Tumour characteristic	% of patients surviving at 2 yrs	
	Children	Adults
Histological type		
'Nasopharyngeal'	53.0	32.5
Poorly-differentiated	34.0	24.5
Tumour spread[a]		
T2	54.0	25.5
T3	51.0	29.0
T4	25.0	18.0
Lymph-node involvement[a]		
N1	37.5	36.0
N2	35.5	18.0
N3	35.5	18.0

[a] UICC, 1974

A calculation of two-year survival rates in relation to histological type of tumour showed these to be 53% for children with 'nasopharyngeal' tumours and 34% for those with poorly-differentiated squamous-cell carcinomas. In adults, the respective rates were 32.5% and 24.5%. It can, therefore, be concluded that prognosis is better for 'nasopharyngeal' carcinoma and for young patients.

Children with lesions limited to the soft tissue of the nasopharynx (T2) had a two-year survival rate of 54%, while only 25% survived at this time when the tumour extended to the base of the skull or was accompanied by neurological signs (T4). These survival rates were markedly lower in adults: 25.5% for those with T2 tumours, and 18% for those with T4. Extensive tumour lesions, therefore, appear to indicate a bad prognosis.

With regard to degree of lymphatic involvement, survival at two years was 37.5% for children with N1 tumours and 35.5% for those with N2 and N3 tumours; relatively fewer N1 tumours were found, however, than N2 and N3. Although lymph-node involvement does not appear to play an important role in survival in young patients, in adults it appears to influence prognosis, since survival was very poor for those with N2 and N3 tumours.

Disease evolution: recurrence, metastasis and the paraneoplastic syndrome

Failure to cure is due to local recurrences and to metastases. Compared to adults, younger patients surviving at two years more frequently had distant metastases (37% *vs*. 20.5%) than local recurrences (18.5 *vs*. 24%), perhaps due to the large number of 'nasopharyngeal' tumours seen in children. The relationship of recurrence and metastases to extent of tumour and to degree of lymph-node involvement is shown in Table 6.

Table 6. Relationship of rates of recurrence and metastasis of nasopharyngeal carcinomas in Tunisian children and adults to extent of primary tumour and degree of lymph-node involvement

Tumour	% of children with		% of adults with	
characteristic[a]	Recurrence	Metastasis	Recurrence	Metastasis
T1	-	-	42	10
T2	15	30	24.5	26
T3	7.5	45	25	27.5
T4	39	36	37	14.5
N0	-	-	35	6
N1	37.5	25	39	0
N2	14	28	25	25
N3	24	42	26	27

[a] UICC, 1974

The rate of recurrence does not appear to be related to the extent of the primary tumour, except in patients with T4 tumours (15% in T2 and 39% in T4); however, the incidence of metastasis was found to correspond closely to the degree of lymph-node involvement (25% in N1 and 42% in N3).

Metastases occurred with equal frequency (37%) in children with the 'nasopharyngeal' type of tumour as in those with poorly-differentiated squamous-cell carcinomas; however, the latent periods differed for the two histological types, with all the metastases of the 'nasopharyngeal' tumours appearing during the first year of follow-up (Table 7).

Table 7. Sites of metastases of nasopharyngeal carcinomas in Tunisian children during 2 yrs of follow-up, by histological type

Year of follow-up	Metastases from 'Nasopharyngeal' tumours	Poorly-differentiated tumours
1st	5 bone 1 lung 1 lung + bone 1 lung + liver 1 lung + liver + bone 1 bone + liver	4 bone 1 lung
2nd	none	2 lung 2 bone 1 lung + bone

Metastatic sites, in descending order of frequency, were bone, lung and liver; patients often had multiple metastases.

Of great interest to us is the paraneoplastic syndrome, which occurs in children and only exceptionally in adults. We found 12 cases among our series of 82 children (14.5%); in a series of 403 adult NPC cases, two occurred, both in young patients (21 and 30 years old). This syndrome, which involves hypertrophic pulmonary osteoarthropathy, periostitis, clubbing and gynecomastia, was frequently seen in association with pulmonary or mediastinal metastases (Table 8). This finding is in agreement with that of Arce et al. (1973) who reported a paraneoplastic syndrome in a 17-year old NPC patient with pulmonary metastasis. Endocrine studies in four patients revealed generalized lowering of pituitary function. After autopsy, one patient was found to have metastases in the lung, liver and para-aortic lymph node.

DISCUSSION

Epidemiology

A search of the literature showed only a few reports of NPC in children and adolescents. Our series of 82 cases of NPC in patients up to 19 years of age over a six-year period is probably the most important; these represented 17% of our total series of NPC cases.

Table 8. Characteristics of 12 young, Tunisian nasopharyngeal carcinoma patients with paraneoplastic syndrome

Age (yrs)	Sex	Tumour histology[a]	Stage[b]	Delay (mths)	Other metastasis
19	M	NP	T2 N3	24	lung + bone
15	M	NP	T3 N3	17	lung
17	M	NP	T4 N3	7	liver
15	M	NP	TX NX	unknown	lung
12	F	NP	T4 N3	before treatment	lung + bone
14	F	PD	T4 N3	5	lung + bone
15	M	PD	T4 N3	14	lung
18	M	PD	T4 N3	20	lung
18	F	PD	T4 N1	24	lung + bone
10	M	PD	T3 N3	24	0
19	F	PD	T2 N3	15	lung
13	M	PD	T2 N3	unknown	lung

[a] NP- 'nasopharyngeal' tumour; PD - poorly-differentaited squamous-cell carcinoma

[b] UICC, 1974

At the present time, it would be difficult to establish the general incidence of NPC in Tunisia. Nevertheless, we know that the incidence rate (adjusted to the age structure of the world population per 100,000 inhabitants and by year) of all NPC is about 4 (Muir, 1971). We also know that in Tunisia NPC is the most frequent cancer of the upper respiratory tract (485 cases out of 1370, or 35%).

In collaboration with the National Children's Institute, we carried out a survey between 1969-1974 of malignant tumours in children and adolescents up to 20 years of age. Of a total of 582 malignant tumours, 84 (14%) were diagnosed as NPC by the pathology department of our institute (Cammoun et al., 1976). NPC is thus the most frequent cancer found in Tunisian patients under 20 years of age; and, apart from xeroderma pigmentosum, which is a particular problem, it represents almost the totality of malignant epithelial tumours of the head and neck region in Tunisian children.

Few such cases have been reported in the literature. A series of 27 cases of squamous-cell carcinoma of the head and neck region were observed over a period of 15 years by Schwaab et al. (1975) at the Head and Neck and Pediatric Departments of the Gustave Roussy Institute; 20 of these were NPC. One-third of the patients were of North African origin (Algerian, Moroccan, Tunisian).

The high frequency of NPC in children is shown not only by the crude age distribution curve of our series (Fig. 3) but also by the curve obtained by plotting specific rate by age (Fig. 4). The double peaks seen in these two figures have also been noted in high-risk areas.

FIG. 3. AGE DISTRIBUTION

Age distribution of 485 Tunisian patients with nasopharyngeal carcinoma

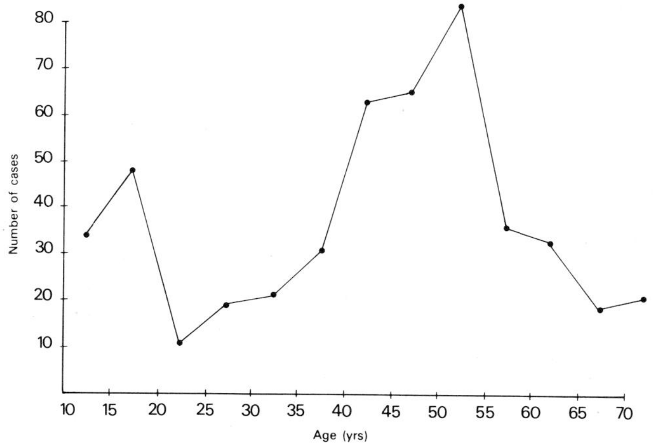

Only a few cases have been reported from south-east Asia: 13 out of 1000 cases in Formosa (Yeh, 1962), 8 out of 974 in Singapore (Muir, 1967) and 2 out of 211 in Hong Kong (Choa & Genge, 1974). Schmauz & Templeton (1972) estimated the frequency in these high-risk areas to be 2%.

Some workers have also noted a relatively high frequency of this cancer among children in countries at low risk (Europe and the USA). Already in 1929, Ewing (cited by McConnell, 1958) pointed out that NPC occurred frequently in patients 10-20 years of age. The series of

FIG. 4. AGE-SPECIFIC INCIDENCE RATE OF NASOPHARYNGEAL CARCINOMA

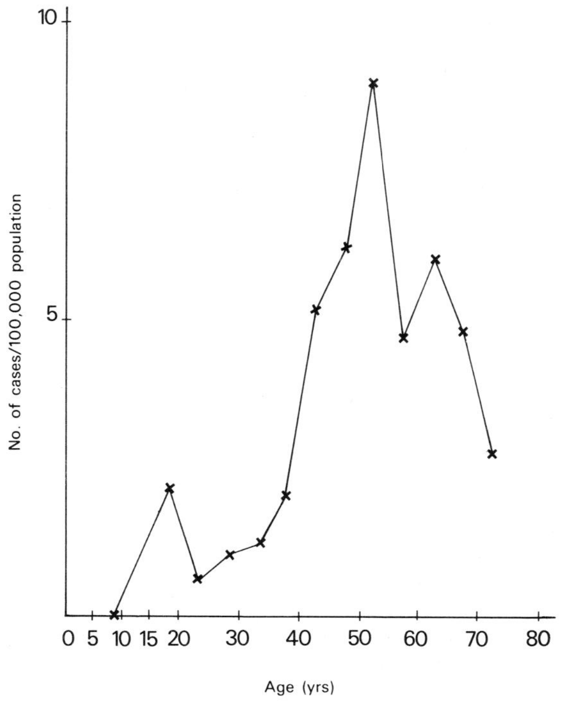

Martin & Blady (1940) seemed to confirm this impression, since 9% of their cases were in children. McConnell (1958) reported seven cases in young English patients, four of whom were less than 15 years old. More recently, Nishiyama et al. (1967) reported two further cases, and Stier et al. (1973), one other. Creely et al. (1973) reaffirmed that NPC occurs relatively frequently in patients between 10 and 20 years of age (with bimodal age distribution). The literature review carried out by Straka & Bluestone (1972) of nasopharyngeal malignancies in children covered 166 cases, including 6 of their own; however, histological information was very poor, and the exact number of NPC is not known.

Relatively high incidences of NPC have been reported in Uganda (Schmauz & Templeton, 1972); Kenya (Clifford, 1970), Nigeria (Martinson, 1968) and the Sudan (El Hassan et al., 1968), which, like Tunisia, are intermediate risk areas.

The percentage frequencies of NPC in areas of high, low and intermediate risk are shown in Table 9, from which it would appear that non-Mongoloid children are more often affected than are Chinese children.

Table 9. Percentage frequencies of nasopharyngeal carcinoma in children in areas of different degrees of risk

Area	Risk	% frequency
Southern China	High	2
Europe USA	Low	2-9
Tunisia Uganda	Intermediate	17
Kenya Nigeria The Sudan		10-20

Treatment results

Younger patients respond better to therapy than adults. This has also been pointed out by Brugère et al. (1975) at the Gustave Roussy Institute. It may be explained by the fact that the young patient who does not develop early metastasis is less subject to tumour recurrence than are adults.

Prognosis

Factors that influence prognosis include the following:

(1) Extent of tumour spread determines the frequency of recurrence; the more extensive the tumour, the greater the chances of recurrence.

(2) Degree of lymph-node involvement determines the frequency of metastasis.

(3) Different histological types have different prognoses. The 'nasopharyngeal' type, which is most prevalent in children, is more radiosensitive than are the other types. Well-differentiated squamous-cell carcinoma, non-existent in children, has a very poor prognosis, recurs frequently and rarely metastasizes.

Etiology and pathogenesis

Several comments are relevant to these topics.

North Africans and Southern Chinese have little in common in terms of race and environment. African and Caucasian children appear to be much more at risk than Chinese children. The race factor, therefore, far from becoming a common denominator, serves only further to divide these two populations.

The occurrence of NPC at the age of puberty (the average age of our patients was 15 years) suggests an endocrine factor.

NPC is an epithelial malignancy that occurs in young people, in whom epithelial cancers are rare. Its occurrence may be due to a genetic predisposition of the nasopharyngeal mucosa, which is sensitized by an unknown exogenous factor (like ultra-violet rays in xeroderma pigmentosum) that intervenes early in life. If this is so, the factor intervenes much later in Southern Chinese than in Africans or Europeans. According to a study in progress by de-Thé[1], the IgA immunoglobulin factor specific to Epstein-Barr viral capsid antigen is more often absent from the serum and saliva of children than those from adults. However, complete results are needed before final conclusions can be drawn.

We do not believe that environmental factors (food, smoking, incense, etc.) satisfactorily explain the relatively high frequency of NPC in Tunisia.

Conclusion

The high incidence of NPC in children, its characteristic histological type, its frequent metastases (in conjunction with the paraneoplastic syndrome), its relatively favourable prognosis and several preliminary immunological and serological observations lead us to believe that NPC in children may be a different disease from that in adults and that they comprise two different etiological and pathogenetic entities.

SUMMARY

Of 485 cases of NPC collected from the files of our institute between March 1969 and December 1974, 82 (17%) were in children and adolescents (0-19 years old). This relatively high frequency of NPC in young people was not suggested by reports from high-incidence areas (Southern China, for example) but appears to be a characteristic feature of areas of intermediate incidence (Uganda, Kenya, Sudan, Tunisia). NPC is the tumour that occurs most frequently in young people between 1 and 20 years old in Tunisia, showing a peak in those 16 years of age. The male:female sex ratio was 3:1.

Advanced stages of the disease occured frequently; no clinical anomalies were noted in this age group. The 'nasopharyngeal' type of

[1] Unpublished data

carcinoma was the histological form seen most frequently; poorly-differentiated squamous-cell carcinomas were not uncommon; and well-differentiated squamous-cell carcinomas were not seen in this series.

The five-year survival rate was 32.5% for children and only 20% for adults. This can perhaps be explained by the fact that the 'nasopharyngeal' type of tumour has a better prognosis than other histological types, and, compared to adults, younger patients more frequently have distant metastases (37%) than local recurrences (18.5%).

A paraneoplastic syndrome, consisting of hypertrophic pulmonary osteoarthropathy with occasional generalized lowering of pituitary function, was seen in 12 of the patients. This syndrome has been described only in children, and no cases were found in our series of adult NPC patients.

Epidemiological, clinical and histological aspects suggest that NPC in young people is different from that found in adults.

REFERENCES

Arce, B., Stejfa, M., Mansouri, M., Hamidou, B. & Rocek, V. (1973) Ostéo artropatia hypertrofiante pneumica como complication de un carcinoma de nasopharyngé con metastasis pulmonar. *Rev. Cuba. Med.*, *12*, 73-80

Brugère, J., Eschwege, F., Schwaab, G., Micheau, C. & Cachin, Y. (1975) Les carcinomes du nasopharynx (cavum): aspects cliniques et évolutifs. *Bull. Cancer*, *62*, 319-330

Cammoun, M., Ellouz, R. & Ben Attia, R. (1973) Les carcinomes nasopharyngés chez l'enfant et l'adolescent: étude anatomo-clinique de 43 observations. *Cah. O.R.L.*, *8*, 617-628

Cammoun, M., Houissa, T., Ellouz, R., Ben Jilani, S., Ben Attia, R., Tabbane, F. & Ben Alaya, M. (1976) Le cancer de l'enfant en Tunisie: fréquence relative des différents types histologiques; à propos de 582 observations. *Tunis. med.*, *5*, 765-771

Choa, G. (1974) Nasopharyngeal carcinoma. *J. Laryngol.*, *88*, 145-158

Clifford, P. (1970) A review on the epidemiology of nasopharyngeal carcinoma. *Int. J. Cancer*, *5*, 287-309

Creely, J.J., Jr, Lyons, G.D., Jr & Trail, M.L. (1973) Cancer of the nasopharynx: a review of 114 cases. *Sth. med. J. (Bgham, Ala)*, *66*, 405-409

El Hassan, A.M., Milosov, B., Daoud, E.A. & Kashaw, A. (1968) *Malignant diseases of the upper respiratory tract in the Sudan.* In: Clifford, P., Linsell, C.A. & Tinns, G.L., eds, *Cancer in Africa*, New York, International Publications Service, pp. 307-314

Ellouz, R., Cammoun, M., Zaouche, A. & Ben Attia, R. (1975) Les cancers du rhinopharynx en Tunisie: aspects épidémiologiques et anatomocliniques. *Bull. Cancer, 62*, 295-306

Martin, H.E. & Blady, J.V. (1940) Cancer of the nasopharynx. *Arch. Otolaryngol., 32*, 692-727

Martinson, F.D. (1968) Cancer of the nasopharynx in Nigeria. *J. Laryng., 12*, 1119-1128

McConnell, E.M. (1958) Nasopharyngeal carcinoma in children and young adults. *Brit. J. Cancer, 12*, 195-201

Muir, C.S. (1967) A historical vignette. In: Muir, C.S. & Shanmugaratnam, K., eds, *Cancer of the Nasopharynx (UICC Monograph Series No. 1)*, Copenhagen, Munksgaard, pp. 13-17

Muir, C.S. (1971) Nasopharyngeal carcinoma in non-Chinese populations, with special reference to South-East Asia and Africa. *Int. J. Cancer, 8*, 351-363

Nishiyama, R.H., Batsakis, J.G. & Weaver, D.K. (1967) Nasopharyngeal carcinomas in children. *Arch. Surg. (Chicago), 94*, 214-217

Schmauz, R. & Templeton, A.C. (1972) Nasopharyngeal carcinoma in Uganda. *Cancer, 29*, 610-621

Schwaab, G., Carlier, J.C., Brugère, J. & Schweisguth, O. (1975) Les épithéliomas épidermoïdes de la région cervico-faciale chez l'enfant: à propos de 27 cas. *Cah. O.R.L., 10*, 519-523

Stier, J., Huh, C.H. & Lapidot, A. (1973) Squamous carcinoma of nasopharynx in a child. *Bull. N.Y. Acad. Med., 49*, 610-612

Straka, J.A. & Bluestone, C.D. (1972) Nasopharyngeal malignancies in children. *Laryngoscope, 82*, 807-816

Yeh, S. (1962) A histological classification of carcinoma of the nasopharynx with a critical review as to the existence of lymphoepitheliomas. *Cancer, 15*, 895-920

UICC (1974) *TNM Classification of Malignant Tumours*, Geneva

Zaouche, A. (1970) Les tumeurs malignes de la sphère otorhinolaryngologie en Tunisie (Thesis, Faculté de Médecine, Paris, France)

CLINICAL ASPECTS AND NATURAL HISTORY OF NASOPHARYNGEAL CARCINOMA IN WESTERN EUROPE

Y. CACHIN, G. SCHWAAB, H. SANCHO-GARNIER & P. MARANDAS

Institut Gustave Roussy,
Villejuif, France

The clinical aspects of nasopharyngeal carcinomas, their mode of invasion and their natural history have been the subject of few systematic studies in Western Europe, due to the relative infrequency of these tumours in this area of the world (1.3 per 100,000 in France). The results of three studies, two retrospective and one prospective, are analysed below.

The retrospective studies come from two large European cancer centres, the Institut Gustave Roussy (IGR, Villejuif, France; 1959-1976, 326 cases) and the Istituto Nazionale dei Tumori (INT, Milan, Italy; 1958-1972, 118 cases). The prospective study, performed with statistical controls in 1974-1975 at the instigation of the Institut Gustave Roussy, includes data on 188 patients in 19 different medical centers (16 in France, 1 in Italy, 1 in Greece and 1 in Tunisia). Data from Western Europe only comprise that for 143 patients from the 17 centres in France and Italy. An epidemiological study of this group of patients has been presented elsewhere[1]. The present, clinical study considers only information about these 143 patients.

The results presented do not take into account the geographic origin of the patients involved. However, although this is an analysis of nasopharyngeal carcinomas in Western Europe, certain demographic phenomena make it less restrictive:

(1) Certain of the centres have ties with other countries; for example, IGR has ties with North Africa and the Caribbean.

(2) The INT (Milan) accepts many patients from southern Italy.

(3) Important population migrations have affected the groups referred to these centres; for example, 1 million Algerians,

---

[1] See p. 241

Moroccans and Tunisians currently work in France; and 1.5 million Frenchmen were repatriated from North Africa when three countries in that region became independent; some of these were of Jewish and others of European stock.

(4) Of the patients at IGR, only 36% of those with nasopharyngeal carcinomas (120/326) were born in France, i.e., in Western Europe.

CLINICAL DATA

Presenting symptoms

Patients with nasopharyngeal carcinomas seek medical attention for an isolated symptom, a complex of symptoms or cervical adenopathy. In 26% of the cases in the IGR study and in 31% of those in the prospective study, the presenting symptom was an isolated one; it was either rhinological (nasal obstruction or epistaxis) or otological (deafness, tinnitus or earache). Less frequently, the complaint was neurological (migraine or other headache); and, on occasion, ocular symptoms or a trismus presented (Table 1).

Table 1. Presenting symptoms of patients with nasopharyngeal carcinomas

	% of patients	
	IGR study	prospective study
Single symptom	26	31
Multiple symptoms	36	31
Cervical lymph nodes only	29	38
Not specified	9	-

Multiple symptoms were present in 36% of the cases in the IGR study and in 31% of those in the prospective study. There appears to be a correlation between the presence of multiple complaints and the occurrence of palpable nodes: adenopathy was found in 30% of patients with multiple symptoms (IGR) but in only 6% of those with an isolated presenting symptom.

Cervical adenopathy in the absence of other symptoms constituted the initial symptom in 29% of patients in the IGR group and in 38% of those in the prospective study group (44/115). In 2/3 of these cases the nasopharyngeal tumour was evident at the time of the initial evaluation; in the remaining 1/3 the primary tumour was found only months or years later.

In some of the cases in both studies, no presenting complaint was identified. The delay between the onset of symptoms and the time the patient first sought medical advice was noted for 112 cases in the prospective study group (Fig. 1). On average, the patient delay amounted to 10 months, but 50% of cases were first seen after less than five months. One patient waited six years before seeking medical evaluation.

FIG. 1. DELAY BETWEEN ONSET OF SYMPTOMS AND INITIAL MEDICAL EVALUATION (PATIENT DELAY), 112 CASES

• 92 patients not treated previously
x 20 patients treated previously

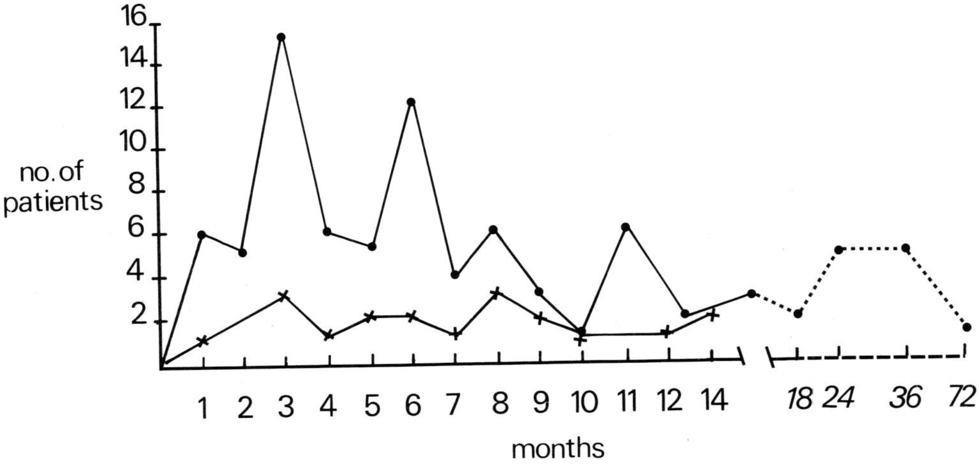

Initial extent of tumour by TNM classification

When the patients already treated at the time of referral were excluded from the IGR group (88 patients, or 27%), the distribution of tumour extent by TNM classification was tabulated for the remaining 238 (Table 2). Of this group, 46% had tumours limited to the soft tissues of the nasopharynx (T1 & T2), 16% had extension to the oro-pharynx or to the nasal fossae (T3), and 38% had osteolytic lesions in the basilar region of the skull, with or without neurological deficits (T4). The INT group showed different percentages (T1 & T2 = 60%, T3 = 14% and T4 = 18%), but this study was confined to 102 cases of highly undifferentiated carcinoma (Table 3).

Table 2. Distribution of tumour extent by TNM classification of carcinomas of the nasopharynx seen at the Institut Gustave Roussy between 1959-76, 238 cases

Initial extent of tumour[b]	% of patients with nodal involvement at first examination[a]					
	N0	N1	N2	N3	Total	%
TX		1	1		2	
T1	1	3	0	8	12	5
T2	16	16	12	54	98	41
T3	12	7	4	16	39	16
T4	31	6	9	41	87	38
Total	60	33	26	119	238	
%	25	14	11	50		

[a] N0 - no palpable nodes
N1 - movable homolateral nodes
N2 - movable contralateral or bilateral nodes
N3 - fixed nodes

[b] TX - impossible to assess
T1 - limited to one region
T2 - extending into two regions
T3 - extending beyond nasopharynx, without bone involvement
T4 - extending beyond nasopharynx, with bone involvement

Certain additional information about the mode of tumour extension was obtained from the cases in the prospective study:

(1) Only a single region of the nasopharynx was involved in 21% of cases. This consisted of the lateral wall in 6 cases, the posterior wall in 14 and the superior wall in 4.

Table 3. Distribution of tumour extent by TNM classification of poorly differentiated carcinomas of the nasopharynx seen at the Istituto Nazionale dei Tumori between 1958-72, 102 cases

	No. of cases
T0	6
T1	26
T2	34
T3	14
T4	18
TX	4
Total	102

T0 - no evidence of primary tumour
T1 - limited to one region
T2 - extending into two regions
T3 - extending beyond nasopharynx, without bone involvement
T4 - extending beyond nasopharynx, with bone involvement

(2) Several regions of the nasopharynx were involved simultaneously, without extension beyond the nasopharynx, in 28% of cases.

(3) Neurological signs, indicating invasion of the basilar region of the skull, were present in 26 cases (22%) (Table 4). In more than half of these (15/26) only a single nerve was involved; however, two nerves were involved in five patients, and three or more in six patients. The nerve most frequently involved was the abducens, the 6th cranial nerve (18 cases).

Table 4. Cranial nerve involvement in 26 cases from a prospective study of carcinomas of the nasopharynx

Cranial nerve	No. of cases		
	Single nerve	Multiple nerves	Total
III	1	5	6
IV		4	4
V	1	6	7
VI	10	8	18
VII	2	2	4
IX		3	3
X	1	3	4

Degree of nodal involvement at the time of initial evaluation (Table 5)

In the IGR study, 25% of patients had no palpable nodes when first examined (N0). This figure rose to 35% for patients with T4 lesions; another 25% had movable nodes (N1 & N2), and 50% had fixed nodes (N3). The latter were usually located high in the neck, in the upper spinal accessory area or behind the angle of the mandible.

Table 5. Cervical nodal involvement at the time of initial evaluation of carcinomas of the nasopharynx

	Total no. of patients	% of patients with nodal involvement at first examination[a]		
		N0	N1 & N2	N3
IGR retrospective study	236	25	25	50
Cooperative prospective study	92	26	23	51

[a] N0 - no palpable nodes
N1 - movable homolateral nodes
N2 - movable contralateral or bilateral nodes
N3 - fixed nodes

The degree of nodal involvement noted in the INT study cannot be compared with that in the IGR results, since the classification system used was quite different. The unusual finding of 20% of supraclavicular adenopathies in this group of patients should, however, be noted.

The prospective study confirmed the findings of the IGR retrospective study: N0 in 26%, N1 & N2 in 23% and N3 in 51%.

Existence of metastases at the time of initial evaluation

In the IGR study, metastases were found in 14 patients at the time of initial evaluation (8 to bone, 3 to lungs and 3 elsewhere), to make a total of 6%. Only two patients in the prospective study (2%) were found to have metastases.

Serological data at the time of initial evaluation (IGR 1976)

A comparison was made between the titres of antibodies to antigens of the Epstein-Barr virus in patients with nasopharyngeal carcinomas and those in patients with other head and neck carcinomas. The study group was composed of 50 patients, 31 with highly undifferentiated carcinomas of the nasopharyngeal type and 19 with well-differentiated squamous-cell carcinomas. The control group was composed of 49 patients with non-nasopharyngeal carcinomas of the upper respiratory and digestive tracts.

A significant difference was found between the antibody titres to Epstein-Barr virus in patients with nasopharyngeal carcinomas and those with carcinomas elsewhere in the upper respiratory and digestive tracts. This difference was particularly great for early antigen and viral capsid antigen.

We have a project currently underway to compare antibody levels in patients with highly undifferentiated carcinomas of the nasopharyngeal type with those in patients with well-differentiated carcinomas, by examination of serological with clinical and histopathological data.

TREATMENT

Treatment protocols

The treatment protocol at the IGR has varied over the years. From 1959-1969, treatment for T1 & T2 tumours was a bimodal radiotherapy consisting of 4500 rads telecobalt and 4000 rads contact curietherapy with Ir 192 wires. Patients with N0 were treated with 4500 rads telecobalt to the cervical nodal regions; those with palpable nodes had complementary neck dissection. Treatment for T3 & T4 tumours was telecobalt alone (7000 to 7500 rads), with eventual complementary neck dissection. Since 1970 all patients at the IGR have been treated solely with external radiotherapy (7000 to 7500 rads) by means of telecobalt; electrons are used in the posterior cervical region to reduce cord doses.

At the INT, treatment has always consisted of telecobalt alone (6000 to 7000 rads), but only recently have the treatment fields included the entire neck. Both institutes have kept the dose delivered to the lower cervical region in the range of 5000-5500 rads for patients with N0.

Immediate results of treatment

The immediate results of treatment are not specified in the INT study. At the IGR, of 238 cases not previously treated, 179 were treated with curative intent, 36 were treated for palliation only, and 18 were given no treatment. In five cases, the treatment given was not specified. Ninety percent of the 179 patients treated with curative intent showed complete regression of the primary tumour (Table 6). Of 96 patients with palpable adenopathies who received the complete dose of radiotherapy, 78% showed complete regression of these nodes, and 22% had persistent adenopathy.

With the treatment protocol used at the IGR between 1959-1969, 36 of 38 T1 & T2 patients with palpable nodes, or 95%, who received

Table 6. Immediate results of treatment of 179 nasopharyngeal carcinomas at the Institut Gustave Roussy with curative intent

	No. of patients	% of patients receiving	
		Co^{60}, 7500 rads	Co^{60}, 4500 rads
Nasopharyngeal tumour disappeared	179	90	
Adenopathy disappeared	96	78	
	38		95

4500 rads telecobalt to the cervical region had complete regression of their cervical adenopathy. Thirty of these patients then underwent unilateral or bilateral neck dissection (for a total of 43 operative specimens); histological persistence of the tumour was noted, despite the clinical regression, in 16 cases (37%), and tumour remnants were noted in 8 cases (19%). Absence of tumour involvement was confirmed in the remaining 19 cases (44%) (Table 7). Carcinomas of the nasopharynx are, therefore, relatively radiosensitive, even to a moderate dose of 4500 rads; this does not, however, imply a parallel radiocurability, since persistent disease was documented histologically in 56% of these patients, even though clinically apparent disease was present in only 5%.

Table 7. Immediate results of treatment of 30 nasopharyngeal carcinomas at the Institut Gustave Roussy by Co^{60} 4500 rads + radical neck dissection

		% of cases
Adenopathy disappeared		95
Histologically		
Microscopic invasion persisted	37	56
Tumour remnants (keratin pearls)	19	
No histological invasion	44	

Survival

For the groups of patients followed for sufficiently long periods, the survival after treatment was as follows (Table 8): at the IGR the three-year survival rate was 40% (69/173), and the five-year survival rate was 30% (39/132). When one considers only the determinant

Table 8. Long-term results for patients with nasopharyngeal carcinoma

		% of patients surviving	
		3 years	5 years
Institut Gustave Roussy,	All cases	40	30
all histological types	Determinant group (complete treatment)	49	37
Istituto Nazionale dei Tumori highly undifferentiated carcinomas only		51	43

group, those patients treated with curative intent, the three-year survival increases to 49% (68/139) and the five-year survival to 37% (38/102). A similar level of survival was noted for those patients who had received prior treatment elsewhere.

At the INT, results of treatment of 102 cases of highly undifferentiated carcinomas were a three-year survival rate of 51% and a five-year survival of 43%. It must be stressed that this series contained no patients with well-differentiated carcinomas, whose prognosis is worse.

An improvement in the long-term results for both groups has been noted since the radiation fields have been extended to include the entire neck as well as the nasopharynx. Neither study allows any comment on the role of systematic chemotherapy.

Outcome of treated patients

The two most important causes of treatment failure are local recurrence (or continued local development of the primary disease) and distant metastases. It is important to note that all of the figures presented below are drawn from clinical examinations alone, the number of autopsies being too small to provide useful information.

1. *Local recurrences*. At the IGR, local tumour invasion was clinically documented in 71 of 122 patients who died (58%), either as an isolated finding (23%) or associated with nodal recurrence or distant metastases or both (Table 9). At the INT, local recurrence or continued evolution was documented in 26% of cases. In true recurrences, the average time for reappearance of the tumour was 11 months.

2. *Nodal recurrences (cervical) (Table 9)*. Among the 122 patients in the IGR series who died, 43 had nodal recurrences (35%). Almost all had a local recurrence as well, and in only three cases was the nodal recurrence an isolated finding. The proportion of patients with nodal recurrences in the INT study was similar (31%).

Table 9. Clinical manifestations established in 122 deceased patients with nasopharyngeal carcinoma at the Institut Gustave Roussy[a]

Clinical manifestation	No. of patients	% of total
Nasopharyngeal involvement	71	58
only	28	23
+ lymph-node involvement	23	
+ lymph-node involvement + metastasis	16	
+ metastasis	4	
Lymph-node involvement	43	35
only	3	
+ nasopharyngeal involvement	23	
+ nasopharyngeal involvement + metastasis	16	
+ metastasis	1	
Metastasis	46	37
only	25	20
+ nasopharyngeal involvement	4	
+ nasopharyngeal involvement + lymph-node involvement	16	
+ lymph-node involvement	1	
Intercurrent disease	2	
Haemorrhage	2	
Not specified	18	

[a] Since patients often showed more than one clinical manifestation, they may be included more than once in this table.

3. *Distant metastases.* Forty-six of the 122 patients in the IGR series who died had distant metastases (37%). In 19 of these, there was an associated local or nodal recurrence, but in 25 cases the metastasis was the sole pathological finding (20%) (Table 9). Distant metastases were demonstrated at some time during the course of their disease in 29% (30/103) of the patients in the INT series.

The most frequent sites of involvement by distant metastases were the bony skeleton, the lungs and pleura and the extracervical nodes (Table 10). However, the relative frequency of involvement varied from centre to centre: the figures presented here are drawn from 65 patients

Table 10. Sites of distant metastases in patients with nasopharyngeal carcinoma

Centre	% of patients with metastases in			
	Bone	Lung	Lymph nodes (extracervical)	Other organs (liver, brain, etc.)
IGR	44	37	26	14
INT	36	15	35	14

in the IGR series and 30 patients in the INT series who, at some time in the course of their disease, developed distant metastases.

Bony metastases represented 44% of the total in the IGR series and 36% of those in the INT series. Sixty different metastatic sites were found in the 29 IGR patients with bony lesions: vertebral lesions accounted for 32, pelvic lesions for 10 and rib lesions for 7.

Pleuro-pulmonary metastases were more frequent in the IGR series than in the INT series (37% *versus* 15%). Extracervical nodal metastases, divided evenly among the axillary, mediastinal and sub-diaphragmatic regions, represented 26% of the metastases in the IGR series and 35% of those in the INT series. Metastases to other areas (liver, brain, subcutaneous tissues) were rarer.

Several further observations were made concerning the metastatic spread of nasopharyngeal carcinomas:

(a) The length of time from initial treatment to the appearance of metastases was from 0 to 30 months, with an average of 10 months (figures from the INT study).

(b) In a group of 30 patients in the IGR study, lymphangiography was performed routinely as part of the initial evaluation. In only one of these patients were pathologic abdomino-pelvic nodes identified (in a patient who already had demonstrable bony and pulmonary metastases). In two other cases the lymphangiograms were considered to be suspicious.

(c) Of a group of 16 patients at the IGR with highly undifferentiated carcinomas of the nasopharyngeal type, four had bone-marrow invasion, as demonstrated by biopsy and a positive bone scan. In two (T4 N2*b* and T3 N3), metastases were present; in the two others (T2 N1*b* and T2 N2*b*), there were no metastases at the time of initial evaluation, but these appeared after the end of treatment (Table 11).

(d) Of a group of 18 patients at the IGR with highly undifferentiated carcinomas of the nasopharyngeal type, seven had positive bone scans (total body scan with technetium pyrophosphate), either before treatment (three cases) or during treatment (four cases). Bone pain was present in six of these patients, and positive marrow biopsies were obtained in four of the six patients (Table 12).

Table 11. Positive bone-marrow biopsies among 16 patients with highly undifferentiated carcinomas of the nasopharyngeal type

TNM classification[a]	Bone-marrow biopsy	Bone scan	Functional signs
T4 N2*b* M1	+	+	+
T3 N3 M1	+	+	+
T2 N1*b* M0	+	+	+
T2 N2*b* M0	+	+	+

[a] T2 - tumour extending into two regions
T3 - tumour extending beyond nasopharynx, without bone involvement
T4 - tumour extending beyond nasopharynx, with bone involvement

N1*b* - movable homolateral nodes considered to contain growth
N2*b* - movable contralateral or bilateral nodes considered to contain growth

M0 - no evidence of distant metastases
M1 - distant metastases present

(e) The percentage of patients with distant metastases in the IGR group was much higher among patients with highly undifferentiated carcinomas than among those with well-differentiated carcinomas (31% *versus* 15%).

(f) If autopsies had been performed systematically on all deceased patients in these series, the number of distant metastases would probably have been much higher.

4. *Multiple cancers*. Second primary tumours are rarely seen in association with nasopharyngeal carcinomas: only eight cases were identified among the IGR series of 326 patients (1%). Furthermore, only three of these second primary tumours were located in the upper respiratory or digestive tracts. In contrast, 7% of other tumours of the upper respiratory and digestive tracts are associated with second cancers in the same region.

Table 12. Positive bone scans among 18 patients with highly undifferentiated carcinomas of the nasopharyngeal type

TNM classification[a]	Bone-marrow biopsy	Bone scan	Functional signs
T4 N2*b* M1	+	+	+
T4 N2*b* M1		+	+
T3 N3 M1	+	+	+
T4 N2*b* M0	-	+	0
T4 N3 M0	-	+	+
T2 N2*b* M0	+	+	+
T2 N1*b* M0	+	+	+

[a] T2 - tumour extending into two regions
T3 - tumour extending beyond nasopharynx, without bone involvement
T4 - tumour extending beyond nasopharynx, with bone involvement

N1*b* - movable homolateral nodes considered to contain growth
N2*b* - movable contralateral or bilateral nodes considered to contain growth
N3 - fixed nodes

M0 - no evidence of distant metastases
M1 - distant metastases present

PROGNOSTIC FACTORS

Prognostic factors in nasopharyngeal carcinoma are indicated by examination of the two retrospective studies (Table 13). Age and sex play no role in prognosis, but the degree of nodal involvement probably does. The IGR study shows that the three-year survival was 59% for patients with nodes graded N0, 44% for those with N1 & N2 and 35% for those with N3.

Degree of tumour extent and histological type constitute more definite prognostic indicators. The three-year survival (IGR) was 53% for patients with T1 & T2 tumours, 35% for those with T3 tumours and 25% for those with T4 tumours. Five-year survival is better for patients with undifferentiated carcinomas than for those with well-differentiated ones (39% *versus* 23% at the IGR, 43% *versus* 13% at the INT). If one studies the cause of death of these patients, one finds

Table 13. Prognostic factors in patients with nasopharyngeal carcinomas at the Institut Gustave Roussy (IGR) and the Istituto Nazionale dei Tumori (INT)

		% of patients surviving	
		IGR	INT
Lymph node involvement (3-year survival)[a]	N0	59	
	N1 & N2	44	
	N3	38	
Extent of naso-pharyngeal tumour (3-year survival)[b]	T1 & T2	53	
	T3	35	
	T4	25	
Histological type (5-year survival)	undifferentiated carcinoma or lymphoepithelioma	39	43
	well-differentiated carcinoma	23	13

N0 - no palpable nodes
N1 - movable homolateral nodes
N2 - movable contralateral or bilateral nodes
N3 - fixed nodes

T1 - tumour limited to one region
T2 - tumour extending into two regions
T3 - tumour extending beyond nasopharynx, without bone involvement
T4 - tumour extending beyond nasopharynx, with bone involvement

that those with well-differentiated tumours more frequently die of local and nodal extension than do those with undifferentiated carcinomas. Even though distant metastases are less frequent in patients with well-differentiated carcinomas (15% *versus* 31%), their prognosis is worse, probably because of the lower radiosensitivity and lower radiocurability of these tumours.

COMMENTS

Cancers of the nasopharynx are considered to be part of the group of cancers of the upper respiratory and digestive tract that are, in general, a relatively uniform group of tumours, derived from structures with common anatomical and physiological features and linked by etiological factors which act as local irritants, such as tobacco and alcohol.

Within this group, the nasopharyngeal carcinomas must be viewed as a special entity, as must, in certain ways, tumours of the paranasal sinuses. Tobacco and alcohol appear to play no role in their etiology. An important percentage are characterized histologically as highly undifferentiated carcinomas of the nasopharyngeal type, a classification which is practically specific to this region.

A possible explanation for the origin of this unique tumour is that carcinomas of this region develop in contact with the lymphoid tissue of the pharyngeal tonsil. However, this histological form is almost never seen at the level of the palatine tonsils, although the same mingling of epithelial and lymphoid elements is also present in this area. The natural history of these carcinomas, especially of the undifferentiated ones, is characterized by a tendency to frequent metastases to regional nodes and to distant sites (in particular, to extracervical nodes, to bones and to the lungs) and by a high degree of radiosensitivity, not always paralleled by radiocurability.

In conclusion, it can be stated, especially with regard to the highly undifferentiated nasopharyngeal carcinomas, that:

(1) The natural history of nasopharyngeal carcinomas is similar on the one side to that of the squamous-cell carcinomas and on the other to that of the lymphomas.

(2) It can be assumed that the characteristics that separate these tumours from other cancers of the upper respiratory and digestive tracts are related in some way to the different etiologies.

ANALYTICAL ASPECTS OF SYMPTOMS OF NASOPHARYNGEAL MALIGNANCIES

S. SAWAKI

Department of Otolaryngology,
Yokohama City University,
Yokohama 232, Japan

H. SUGANO

Department of Pathology,
Cancer Institute Tokyo,
Tokyo 170, Japan

T. HIRAYAMA

Division of Epidemiology,
National Cancer Research Institute,
Tokyo 104, Japan

INTRODUCTION

The nasopharynx is a site that cannot be inspected easily and is known as a clinical blind spot. When a tumour develops in this area, the subjective signs are poor and do not become evident until the tumour has developed considerably. So-called early diagnosis is thus very difficult. In some cases, a neck swelling is the first indication that persuades a patient to consult a surgeon; needless to say, this sign is an advanced symptom of the disease. Cranial nerve symptoms indicate that the tumour has invaded the base of the skull; such cases are sometimes wrongly diagnosed as systemic nervous disease, especially in Japan, where the incidence of this cancer is very low.

Obtaining a definite diagnosis depends firstly on the patient's complaints. These can be divided into aural, nasal, pharyngeal, ophthalmic, neurological and cervical lymph node symptoms. In this paper we report a statistical analysis of the frequencies of these symptoms in Japanese patients.

MATERIALS AND METHODS

Data from 766 cases of nasopharyngeal malignancies observed throughout Japan between 1968 and 1973 were analysed. Histological slides from these cases were examined by a single pathologist and classified according to a uniform standard (Table 1).

Table 1. Histological classification of 766 cases of nasopharyngeal malignancies

Histological type	No. of cases		
Carcinoma			641
squamous-cell carcinoma		618	
well-differentiated	46		
undifferentiated	310		
transitional-cell	197		
lymphoepithelioma	65		
adenocarcinoma		23	
Malignant lymphoma			125
malignant lymphoma		62	
reticulum-cell sarcoma		63	

The clinical records were analysed with regard to symptoms, which were divided into initial ones and those observed during the clinical course of the disease, and statistical analyses were made accordingly. The frequencies of symptoms, such as cervical lymph-node metastasis, were related to histological type of malignancy.

RESULTS

In general, the frequencies of the complaints at the patient's first visit were significantly different for each histological type of tumour; this was not true of aural and cervical symptoms (Fig. 1). Patients with lymphomas most commonly had nasal and pharyngeal complaints, due to the way in which massive development of this tumour takes place. It was assumed that ophthalmic and neurological symptoms are more prevalent in patients with carcinomas because of the infiltrating invasion seen with this type of tumour.

FIG. 1. COMPARATIVE FREQUENCIES OF SYMPTOMS

Frequencies of various symptoms in patients with nasopharyngeal carcinoma (CA) or lymphoma (LY)

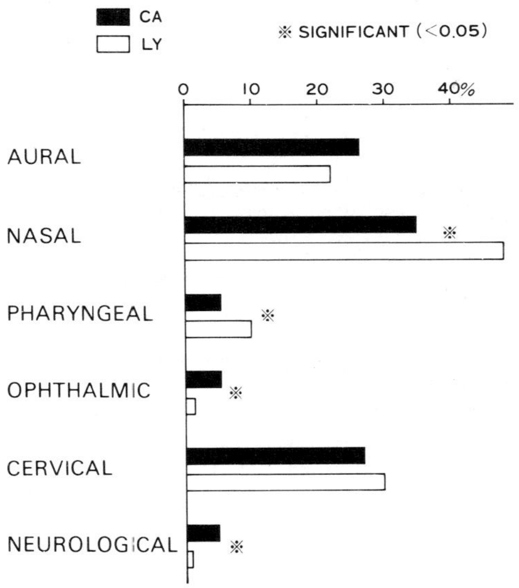

Aural symptoms

The vast majority of aural symptoms were unilateral hearing impairment and a 'full' sensation in the ear. Some patients suffered from tinnitus and otalgia caused by obstruction of the Eustachian tube orifice of the nasopharynx by the tumour.

The frequencies of these complaints as initial symptoms were about 10%, and the frequency of each symptom increased throughout the clinical course of the disease. However, no significant difference was observed between the two kinds of malignancies with regard to this sign (Fig. 2).

The covariance of aural symptoms and tumour location, whether lateral, posterior, superior or inferior, was examined by ridit analysis. The frequency of aural symptoms was low in patients with carcinomas in a superior location, but no difference was observed among patients with the four different locations of lymphomas (Fig. 3).

FIG. 2. FREQUENCIES OF AURAL SYMPTOMS

Frequencies of aural symptoms, as initial complaints and as observed during the clinical course of the disease, in patients with nasopharyngeal carcinoma (CA) or lymphoma (LY)

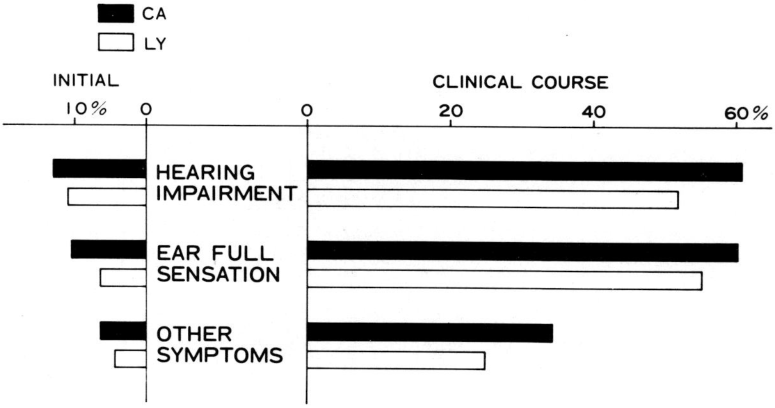

FIG. 3. RIDIT ANALYSIS OF COVARIANCE OF AURAL SYMPTOMS

Ridit analysis of covariance of aural symptoms with tumour location in patients with nasopharyngeal carcinoma (CA) or lymphoma (LY)

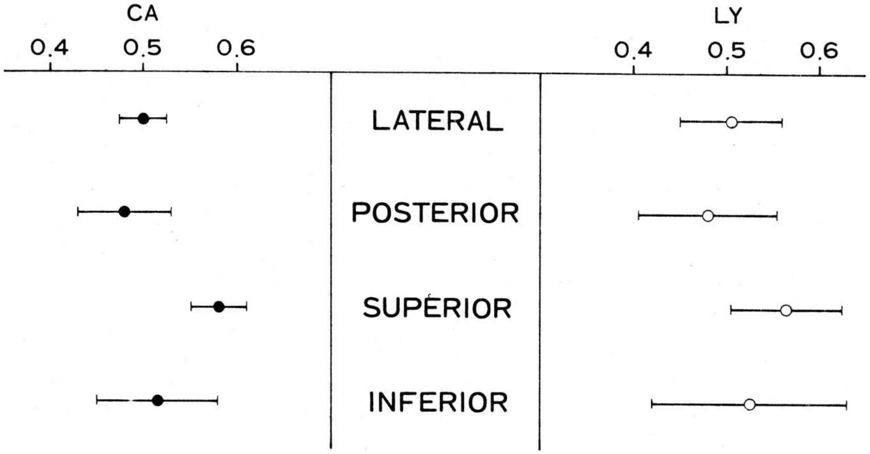

Nasal symptoms

Nasal obstruction occurs at a relatively early stage of lymphoma. In patients with carcinomas, nasal bleeding occurs, due to the fact that these tumours readily result in surface erosion. The difference in the frequencies of these two symptoms disappears during later stages of the disease (Fig. 4).

FIG. 4. FREQUENCIES OF NASAL SYMPTOMS

Frequencies of nasal symptoms, as initial complaints and as observed during the clinical course of the disease, in patients with nasopharyngeal carcinoma (CA) or lymphoma (LY)

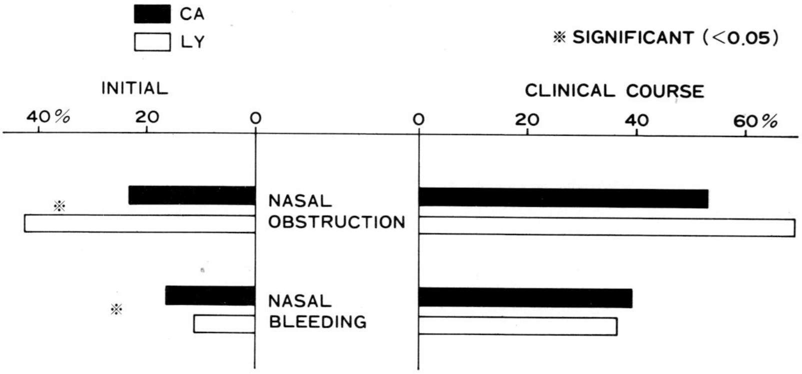

Nasal obstruction was observed more frequently in tumours of either histological type that were located posteriorly than in those located inferiorly (Fig. 5); no difference in the frequency of nasal bleeding was observed among patients with the four different locations of both malignancies.

Pharyngeal symptoms

Complaints related to the pharynx are a sensation of the presence of a foreign body and a mild sore throat. These signs are slightly more prevalent in patients with lymphoma, probably because of the massive growth of lymphomas as compared with carcinomas.

Ophthalmic symptoms

A major ophthalmic symptom was dysfunction of eye movements. Patients also complained of double vision, which is due to abductor paralysis resulting from cranial nerve involvement (Fig. 6). Both complaints occurred more frequently in patients with carcinoma (Fig. 7).

FIG. 5. RIDIT ANALYSIS OF COVARIANCE OF NASAL SYMPTOMS

Ridit analysis of covariance of nasal symptoms with tumour location in patients with nasopharyngeal carcinoma (CA) or lymphoma (LY)

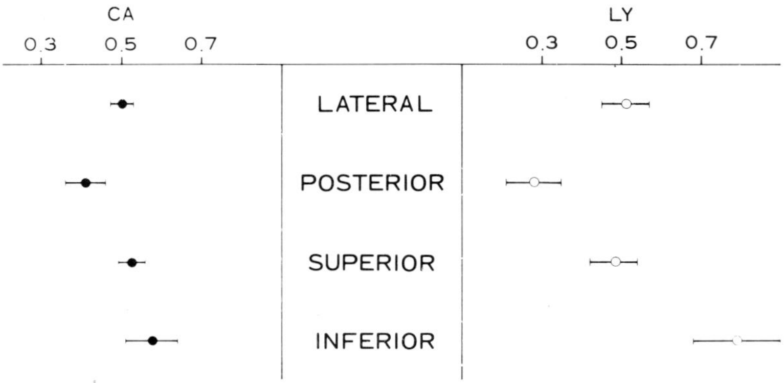

FIG. 6. LEFT ABDUCTOR PARALYSIS IN A NASOPHARYNGEAL CARCINOMA PATIENT

Left abductor paralysis in a 34-year old female with a nasopharyngeal carcinoma

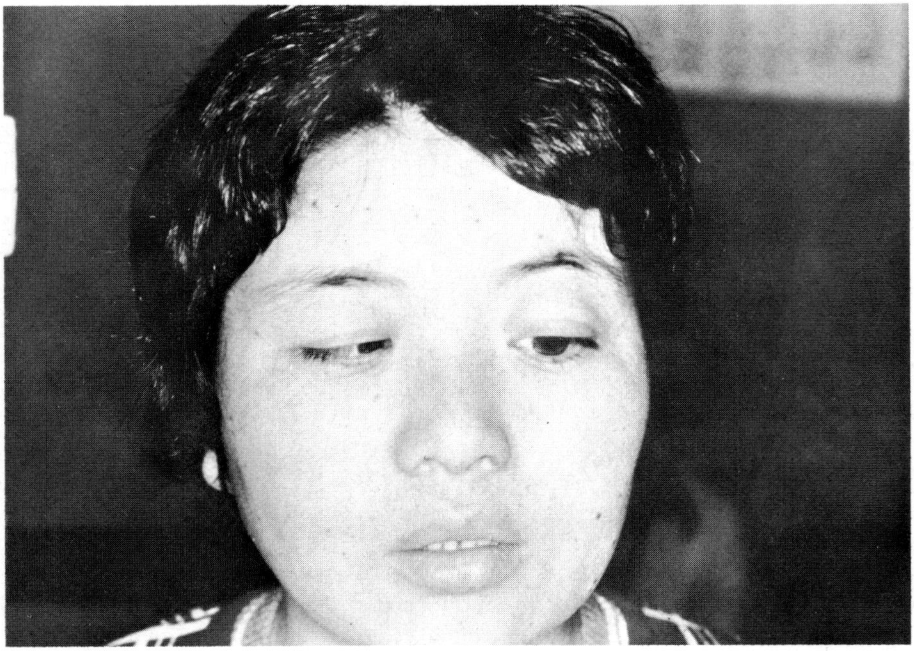

FIG. 7. FREQUENCIES OF OPHTHALMIC SYMPTOMS

Frequencies of ophthalmic symptoms in patients with nasopharyngeal carcinoma (CA) or lymphoma (LY)

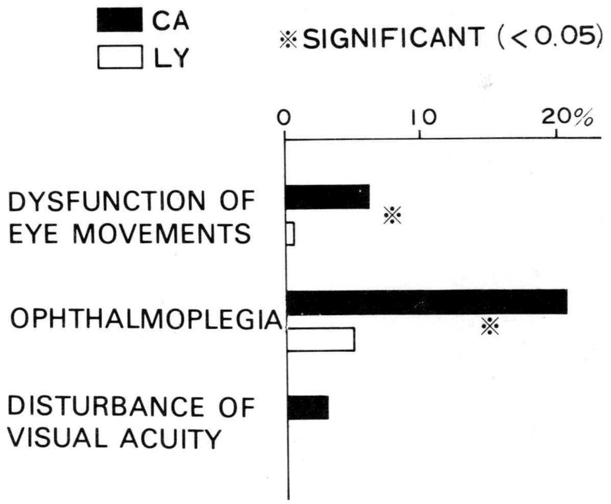

A small number of patients complained of disturbances of visual acuity; X-ray examination showed bony destruction of the optic canal (Fig. 8).

Cranial nerve symptoms

Cranial nerve symptoms cannot serve as an indication for early diagnosis; unfortunately, however, they are the only initial symptoms in some cases. The sixth nerve is the most often affected, and the fifth next most frequently (Fig. 9). When the third to sixth nerves are involved, the symptom is known as the petrosphenoidal syndrome; when the ninth to the twelfth nerves are involved, the condition is known as the retroparotidian or foramen jugular syndrome. Ridit analysis of the covariance between tumour location and cranial nerve involvement (Fig. 10) showed no intimate relation with either of the two major syndromes, indicating that the mid- or posterior portion of the skull base may be affected whatever the location of the primary tumour.

A significant difference in the frequency of cranial nerve involvement was observed between patients with carcinoma and those with lymphoma but not among those with different histological

FIG. 8. BONY DESTRUCTION OF LEFT OPTIC CANAL

Bony destruction of the left optic canal in a 34-year old female with a nasopharyngeal carcinoma complaining of distrubance of visual acuity

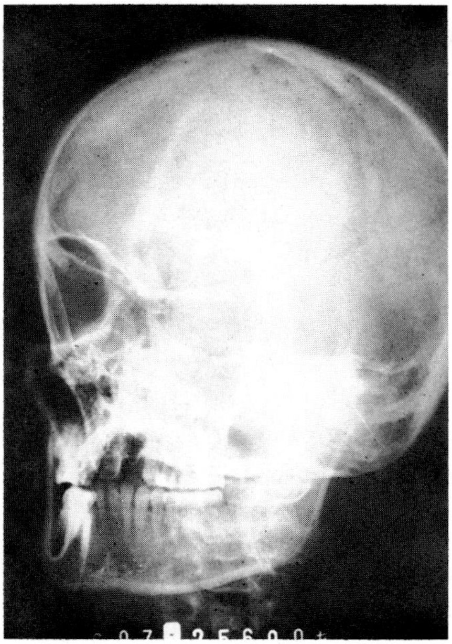

FIG. 9. CRANIAL NERVE INVOLVEMENT

Cranial nerve involvement in 771 cases of nasopharyngeal carcinoma

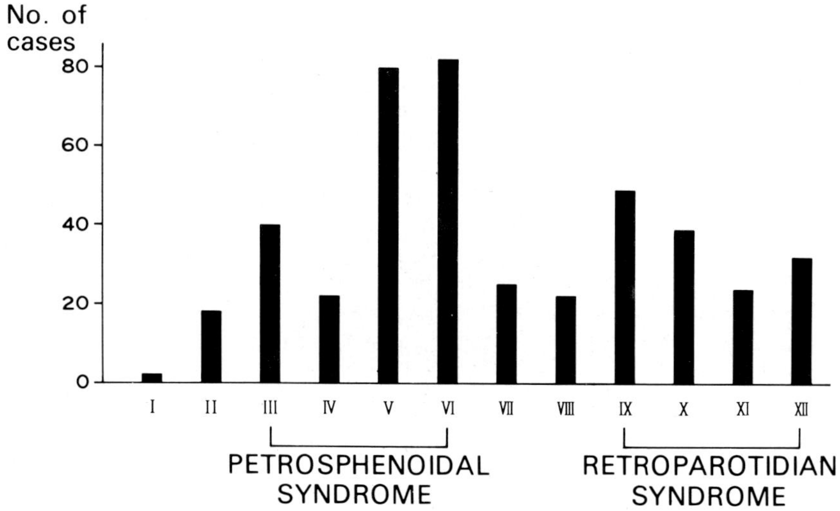

FIG. 10. RIDIT ANALYSIS OF COVARIANCE OF THE MAJOR CRANIAL NERVE SYNDROMES

Ridit analysis of covariance of the two major cranial nerve syndromes with tumour location in patients with nasopharyngeal malignancies

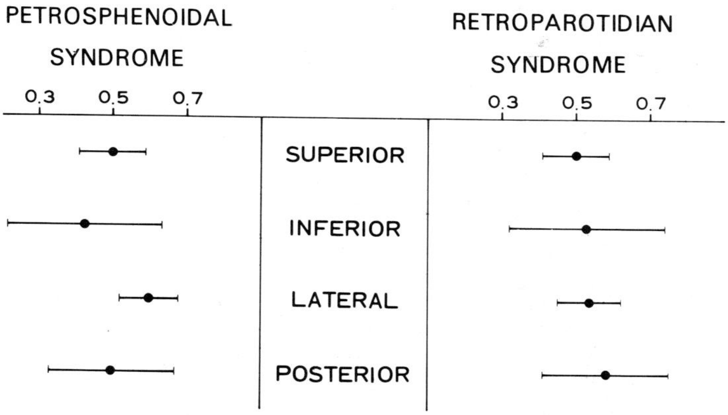

subclassifications of carcinoma nor among those with different degrees of differentiation of squamous-cell carcinoma (Fig. 11).

FIG. 11. FREQUENCIES OF CRANIAL NERVE INVOLVEMENT

Frequencies of cranial nerve involvement in patients with different histological types of nasopharyngeal malignancy

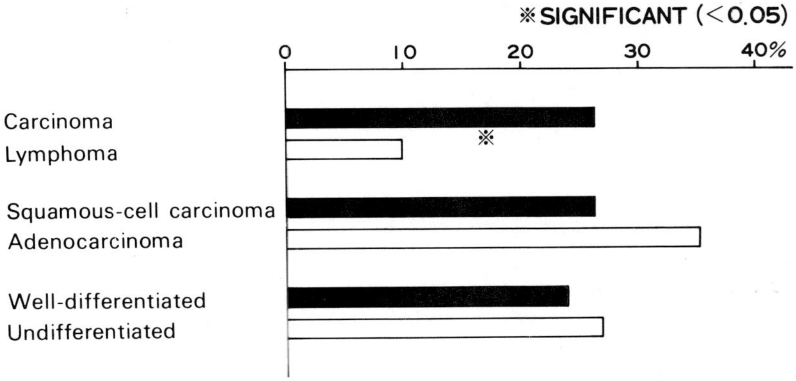

The cranial nerves are involved as a result of destruction of the base of the skull by the tumour such as can be observed from a computerized tomograph (Fig. 12).

FIG. 12. COMPUTERIZED TOMOGRAPH OF THE BASE OF THE SKULL

Computerized tomograph of the base of the skull of a 20-year old male with a nasopharyngeal carcinoma, showing destruction of the right spenoidal bone

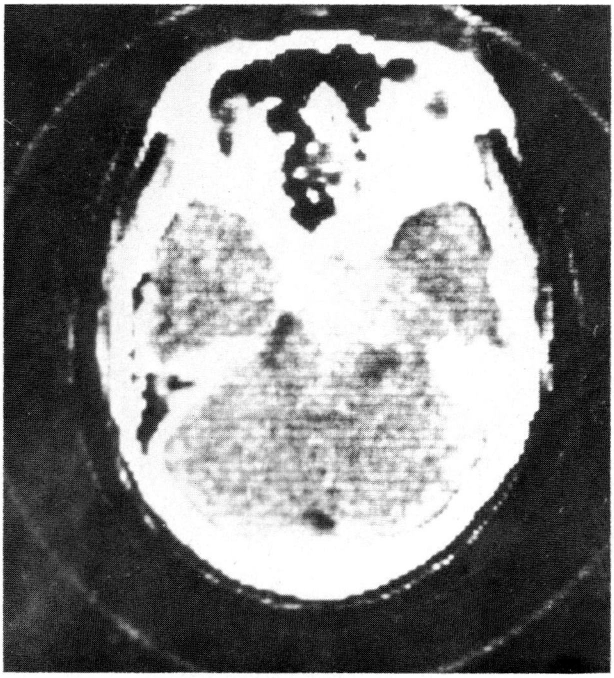

Headache was a complaint of 8% of patients with carcinoma and 3% of those with lymphoma; this difference was significant. In patients with carcinoma, the frequency of this symptom increased to 40%, while in those with lymphoma it increased to 30% during clinical progress of the disease. Its cause is mainly intracranial involvement of the trigeminal nerve and it thus constitutes one of the cranial nerve symptoms. In a few cases it may be caused by an increase in intracranial pressure as a result of tumour invasion.

Cervical lymph node symptoms

Lymph-node metastasis is obviously not an early symptom of these malignancies. However, in many cases a neck swelling is the first sign observed and is a fairly frequent symptom. Such patients often consult general surgeons, and the swelling may be incised unless a careful inspection is made to identify the site of the primary tumour.

Lymph-node metastases were palpable in 20% of carcinoma and 30% of lymphoma patients at their first visit. About half of them were palpable in both sides of the neck. The frequency of this symptom increased to 67% in patients with either type of tumour during clinical progress of the disease (Fig. 13).

FIG. 13. FREQUENCIES OF LYMPH-NODE METASTASIS

Frequencies of lymph-node metastasis in patients with nasopharyngeal carcinoma (CA) or lymphoma (LY), as an initial symptom and as observed during the clinical course of the disease

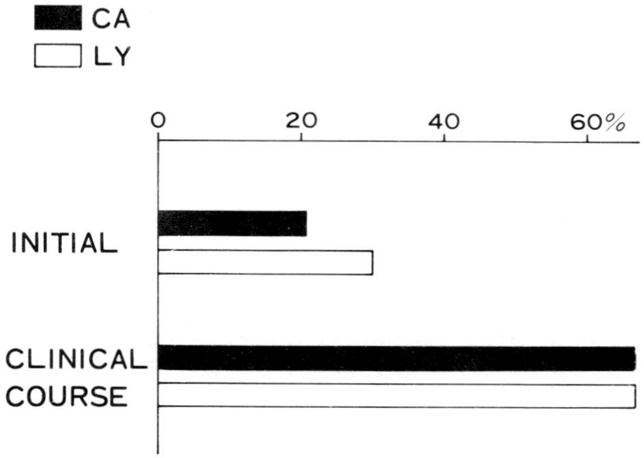

Low frequencies of lymph-node metastases were observed in the initial stages in patients with well-differentiated squamous-cell carcinoma or adenocarcinoma. In later stages, those with well-differentiated carcinoma showed an increased frequency of this symptom, and, of patients with different histological types of nasopharyngeal malignancy, only those with adenocarcinoma showed a low frequency, significantly different from that in other patients (Fig. 14).

DISCUSSION

Diagnosis of cancer in a particular organ is dependent on the complaints reported by the patient. In the case of nasopharyngeal malignancies, direct symptoms are rare and only those in adjoining

FIG. 14. RIDIT ANALYSIS OF COVARIANCE OF LYMPH-NODE METASTASIS

Ridit analysis of covariance of lymph-node metastasis, as an initial symptom and as observed during the clinical course of the disease, with histological type of tumour in patients with nasopharyngeal malignancies

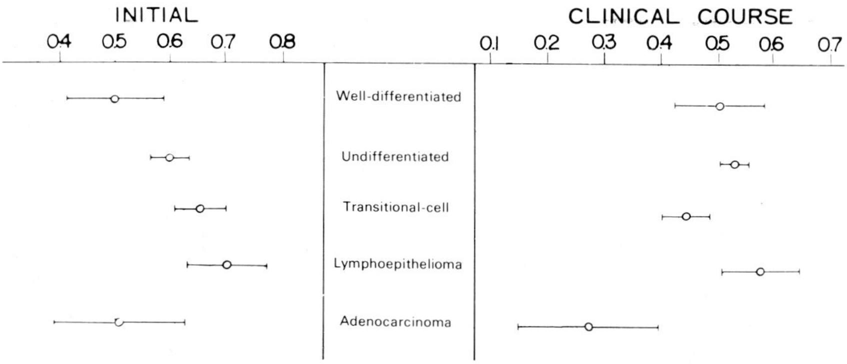

organs, such as the ear, nose or eye, are observed; however, even otolaryngologists often overlook the presence of such tumours. It is thus important that these symptoms be analysed carefully.

The frequencies of the various symptoms are reported differently by different workers (Table 2). Cervical lymph-node symptoms would appear to be the most prevalent, however, it is difficult to make direct comparisons of these frequencies since the cases reported were in different clinical stages of the disease.

Textbooks of otolaryngology emphasize aural symptoms as initial signs of nasopharyngeal malignancies, although they do not occur very frequently. On the other hand, care must be taken in diagnosing the illness of a patient with unilateral aural symptoms, such as tinnitus, a 'full' sensation in the ear or hearing impairment as conductive deafness, since these may be the initial signs of a nasopharyngeal tumour.

Nasal obstruction is rather more prevalent in patients with early stages of lymphoma, and nasal bleeding is more frequently observed in those with carcinoma. This difference is due to the ways in which these two kinds of tumours develop and also accounts for the different frequencies of aural symptoms in patients with these two tumour types. On the whole, carcinoma patients initially have both aural and nasal symptoms, as a result of the infiltrative development of this tumour,

Table 2. Frequencies of various symptoms of nasopharyngeal malignancies as reported by different workers

Reference	No. of cases	Frequency of symptom (%)			
		Aural	Nasal	Cervical lymph node	Neurol-ogical
Moloney, 1957	87	31	44	69	33
Scanlon, 1958	88	35	28	47	
Bloom, 1961	57	40	44	28	45
Wang et al., 1962	115	27	22	38	13
Godfredsen, 1965	673	50	55	75	
Hara, 1969	72	30	28	40	
Perez et al., 1969	79	19	21	32	15

while lymphoma patients have increased frequencies of both signs as the tumour mass grows with time.

Pharyngeal symptoms are slight and occur only rarely as signs of nasopharyngeal malignancies; they cannot, therefore, serve as indications for early diagnosis in many cases. The nasopharynx must thus be considered a special area, even though it is a part of the pharynx.

Many nasopharyngeal tumour patients first consult an ophthalmologist to complain of double vision caused by abductor nerve paralysis. Needless to say, this is not an early symptom but indicated that the tumour has already invaded the intracranial cavity. However, such nerve paralysis can be cured by radiation therapy if the tumour has not spread widely. The attention of ophthalmologists must be called to this sign so that they can be alerted to the possibility of a tumour.

Cranial nerve symptoms are also not early signs of these malignancies, although many patients notice them as the initial symptom. The frequencies with which the different nerves are involved differ: the abductor nerve is most often affected, and the trigeminal and glossopharyngeal nerves next. This tendency has been well documented (Table 3).

Combined involvement of several cranial nerves is not infrequent. Many of these syndromes, such as those of Vernet, Jackson, Avellius, Schmidt, etc., are distinguished according to which combination of nerves is affected by the tumour; however, the major division into petrosphenoidal and retroparotidian syndromes proposed by Ackerman & del Regato (1970) is more convenient. The affected area can easily be estimated by examination of the involved nerves.

Table 3. Frequencies of involvement of different cranial nerves in nasopharyngeal malignancies, as reported by various workers[a]

Reference	No. of cases/ Total	Cranial nerve I	II	III	IV	V	VI	VII	VIII	IX	X	XI	XII	S
		No. of cases												
Mekie et al. (1954)	54/120	3	11	16	8	16	31	12	5	10	7	6	19	-
Scanlon et al. (1958)	37/88	-	1	5	4	10	29	6	0	10	8	3	9	-
Lederman (1961)	58/218	1	9	20	17	35	31	7	2	13	20	17	13	-
Bloom (1963)	26/57	2	4	11	6	19	14	7	6	14	5	4	8	8
Clifford & Beecher (1964)	31/85	-	8	10	9	13	17	8	7	8	6	7	13	
Total	206/568	6	33	62	44	93	122	40	20	55	46	37	62	8
Tu (1965)	373/915		38	80	91	190	227	39	8	109	89	60	167	30
Tu (1970)	192/820	1	10	32	28	145	129	14	1	45	52	20	67	8

[a] From Tu, 1971

Neck swellings are another diagnostic indication; however, most patients with swellings of the cervical lymph node consult general surgeons, who frequently make an incision for a biopsy. It should be noted that a careless incision of such a metastasis may cause spread of tumour cells to another site in the body, thus making prognosis poor. Martin (1944) warned that 20% of unknown neck masses originate from the nasopharynx.

Usually, lymph-node swelling occurs on the same side as that on which the primary tumour is located. However, many patients have bilateral swellings, and, in some cases, the lymph nodes are palpable on just the opposite side of the neck. Lymph-node swelling is generally observed in the upper half of the neck, such as in the inframandibular region; in a few cases it spreads into the lower half, such as the supraclavicular region. Prognosis in the latter case is poor.

A prominent characteristic of nasopharyngeal carcinoma is that the metastases invade distant organs, and especially the bones. However, this appears in a later stage of the disease and has no relevance for diagnosis.

One of the pitfalls in diagnosis of these malignancies is the age factor: many physicians believe that cancer is a disease of adults, whereas many young people suffer from nasopharyngeal cancer. Nasopharyngeal carcinoma differs even from other head and neck tumours, such as laryngeal and maxillary cancers, in its age distribution, and physicians should be cautious in analysing the symptoms of such cases, especially in younger persons.

If a nasopharyngeal tumour is suspected, an inspection is usually made by posterior rhinoscopy. However, this technique is not always easy and in some cases is hindered by the gagging reflex or by an elongated uvula. For detailed observation, the nasopharyngo-fiberscope is recommended. If the patient is cooperative, smaller tumours can easily be detected with this instrument, since the tube is flexible and the illumination is very bright.

For a definitive diagnosis, a biopsy is indispensable. This procedure is not always simple: a specimen may be taken from elsewhere besides the tumour, indicating a false-negative result; on the other hand, the specimen may not be quantitatively sufficient for histological diagnosis, and a repeat biopsy becomes necessary.

Hopp (1958) recommended cytological diagnosis from a smear taken from the nasopharyngeal wall; and in some cases, a needle biopsy of a cervical lymph node is performed. However, these procedures cannot always assure a definite diagnosis of a nasopharyngeal malignancy. The well-known increase in anti-Epstein-Barr viral capsid antigen-antibody titres in most patients with nasopharyngeal carcinoma equally cannot be taken as a measure of diagnosis.

SUMMARY

The various symptoms of 766 patients with nasopharyngeal malignancies (641 carcinomas and 125 malignant lymphomas, confirmed histologically) were analysed statistically from the viewpoint of early diagnosis. These can be divided into aural, nasal, pharyngeal, ophthalmic, cervical lymph node and cranial nerve symptoms. The frequencies of these symptoms were compared in patients with tumours of different histopathological classifications: the nasopharyngeal malignancies were divided into carcinoma and malignant lymphoma, and the carcinomas were subclassified according to their degree of differentiation.

On the whole, lymphoma patients more often had nasal and pharyngeal symptoms, and carcinoma patients ophthalmic and cranial nerve symptoms. It is considered that this difference is due to the different ways in which the two kinds of tumour develop.

The frequencies of the symptoms naturally increased with the clinical course of the disease; the frequencies of the symptom both as an initial sign and as observed during the clinical course of the disease were examined.

Nasopharyngeal malignancies are not indicated by localized symptoms but become evident when adjoining organs, such as the ear or nose, give some sign of abnormality. In not a few cases, a neck swelling is the initial sign; and in some patients, cranial nerve involvement is the first symptom.

Since a patient may not understand the significance of his symptom and may consult a general surgeon, physician, ophthalmologist and/or paediatrician, these specialists should be alerted to the recognition of this disease.

ACKNOWLEDGEMENTS

The authors are deeply indebted to many doctors throughout Japan who made available the clinical records and histological slides of their cases of nasopharyngeal malignancies. These investigations were carried out in part with the support of grants from the Ministry of Health and Welfare, the Government of Japan.

REFERENCES

Ackerman, L.V. & del Regato, J.A. (1970) *Cancer-Diagnosis, Treatment and Prognosis*, 4th ed., St. Louis, Mo., Mosby, pp. 254-276

Bloom, S.M. (1961) Cancer of the nasopharynx; with special reference to the significance of the histopathology. *Laryngoscope, 71*, 1207-1260

Bloom, S.M. (1963) Management of malignant neoplasms of the nasopharynx. *Eye Ear Nose Throat Monthly, 42*, 37-39

Clifford, P., & Beecher, J.L. (1964) Nasopharyngeal cancer in Kenya: clinical and environmental aspects. *Brit. J. Cancer, 18*, 25-43

Godfredsen, E. (1965) Diagnostic and prognostic roles of ophthalmoneurologic signs and symptoms in malignant nasopharyngeal tumors. *Amer. J. Ophthal., 59*, 1063-1069

Hara, H.J. (1969) Cancer of the nasopharynx. Review of the literature. Report of 72 cases. *Laryngoscope, 79*, 1315-1329

Hopp, E.S. (1958) Cytologic diagnosis and prognosis in carcinoma of the mouth, pharynx and nasopharynx. *Laryngoscope, 68*, 1281

Lederman, M. (1961) *Cancer of the Nasopharynx: Its Natural History and Treatment.* Springfield, Ill., Charles C. Thomas Co.

Martin, H. (1944) Cervical lymph node metastasis as the first symptom of cancer. *Surg. Gyn. Obst.*, *78*, 133

Mekie, D.E.C. & Lawley, M. (1954) Nasopharyngeal carcinoma: clinical analysis of 120 cases. *Arch. Surg.*, *69*, 841-848

Moloney, T. (1957) Malignant tumors of the nasopharynx. *Laryngoscope*, *67*, 1297

Perez, C.A., Ackerman, L.V., Mill, W.B., Ogura, J.H. & Powers, W.E. (1969) Cancer of the nasopharynx: factors influencing prognosis. *Cancer*, *24*, 1-17

Scanlon, P.W. et al. (1958) Malignant lesions of nasopharynx. *Ann. Otol.*, *67*, 1005-1021

Tu, S.M. (1965) *Nasopharyngeal carcinoma in Taiwan.* In: Eighth International Congress Series, *113*, 184-185

Tu, S.M. (1971) *Clinical characteristics of nasopharyngeal carcinoma in Taiwan.* In: Nakahara, W., Nishioka, K., Hirayama, T. & Ito, Y., eds, *Recent Advances in Human Tumor Virology and Immunology*, Tokyo, University of Tokyo Press, pp. 221-228

Wang, C.C., Little, J.B. & Schulz, M.D. (1962) Cancer of the nasopharynx. Its clinical and radiotherapeutic considerations. *Cancer*, *15*, 921-926

EPIDEMIOLOGY OF NASOPHARYNGEAL CARCINOMA

DESCRIPTIVE AND ANALYTICAL EPIDEMIOLOGY OF NASOPHARYNGEAL CANCER

T. HIRAYAMA

Epidemiology Division,
National Cancer Center Research Institute,
Tsukiji-5, Chuo-ku,
Tokyo, Japan

DESCRIPTIVE EPIDEMIOLOGY

The most recent edition of *Cancer Incidence in Five Continents* (Waterhouse et al., 1976) confirms the fact that nasopharyngeal cancer (NPC) is rare in most countries in the world, with an age-adjusted incidence rate of less than 1 per 100,000. Patterns of its occurrence are outlined in Table 1.

Table 1. Patterns of occurrence of nasopharyngeal cancer

Item	Observation	Key references
Time trend	Stable in most areas Downward trend in US Chinese, especially in 3rd generation	Fraumeni & Mason, 1974; Buell, 1974
Intercountry variation	Marked variation, reflecting ethnic susceptibility	Waterhouse et al., 1976
Migration	High risk in migrants from southern China (highest in Cantonese, followed by Teochew and Hokkien)	Ho, 1972; Shanmugaratnam, 1973; Shanmugaratnam & Tye, 1970
Clustering within countries	Marked intracountry variation, by district (China, Japan), by ethnic group (Hawaii, California), by place of birth (Israel)	Waterhouse et al., 1976; Sawaki et al., 1976; Hirayama[a]
Urban:rural ratio	Males: 2.17; females: 1.66	Hoover et al., 1975
Socio-economic status (high:low ratio)	Males: 1.10; females: 1.28; 2-fold risk in low income Chinese	Hoover et al., 1975; Buell, 1965
Marital status	Higher risk in unmarried persons	Lin et al., 1973a

[a] This paper

Time trend

The time trend of the NPC incidence rate is stable in most areas. However, the mortality rate from NPC is rapidly on the increase in certain countries such as Japan, probably because of better descriptions in death certificates, since there was no increase in the morbidity rate during the same period.

Sex

In most countries, the incidence is twice as high in males as in females. The uniformity of the sex ratio is one of the important characteristics of NPC epidemiology.

Race

There have been numerous reports concerning the different risks and patterns of NPC in different ethnic groups (Andrews & Michaels, 1968; Belamaric, 1969; Booth et al., 1968; Brown et al., 1976; Chadli et al., 1976; Dharmalingam & Wong, 1973; Ellouz et al., 1975; Har-Kedar et al., 1974; Huong et al., 1969; Khor et al., 1975; Lanasa & Putney, 1974; Mallen & Shandro, 1974; Marsden, 1964; Martinson, 1968; McCallum, 1974; Miyaji, 1967; Muir, 1962, 1971, 1972, 1975; Muir & Oakley, 1967; Muir & Shanmugaratnam, 1967; Muir et al., 1968; Naumov, 1973; Pantangco et al., 1970; Papavasiliou, 1974; Quisenberry & Reimann-Jasinski, 1967; Schaefer et al., 1975; Schmauz & Templeton, 1972; Snow, 1975; Strelka & Barta, 1974; Tran et al., 1963).

Age-standardized incidence rates for NPC in males and females from 81 registries throughout the world are shown in Figure 1, and Table 2 shows age-adjusted incidence rates for NPC in Chinese living in selected geographical regions. It is apparent that significant difference exist among Chinese according to their origin. Chinese of southern origin have a uniquely high risk, the incidence rates per 100,000 being 10-20 in males and 5-10 in females; the inhabitants of Kwangtung show the highest frequency (Ho, 1976).

In the Singapore Chinese population over a five-year period (1968-1972), age-standardized incidence rates were 18.4 per 100,000 person years for males and 7.0 for females. The rates for the specific Chinese communities were 14.1 and 4.7 for Hokkien, 18.3 and 6.2 for Teochew, 29.1 and 11.0 for Cantonese, 14.2 and 3.3 for Hainanese, 12.6 and 4.8 for Hakka, 10.6 and 8.6 for Foochow, 6.2 and 10.3 for Shanghainese and 8.1 and 0.0 for Henghua. It is evident that although all of the specific Chinese communities in Singapore have high risks for NPC, only the Cantonese group have risks significantly higher than those of the rest of the Chinese population. NPC incidence rates for the other major racial groups in Singapore were 4.7 and 0.6 for Malays and 0.9 and 0.0 for Indians (Shanmugaratnam et al.[1]).

[1] See p. 191

FIG. 1. AGE-STANDARDIZED INCIDENCE RATES FOR NASOPHARYNGEAL CANCER (standardized to the world population) from 81 registries throughout the world (Waterhouse et al., 1976)

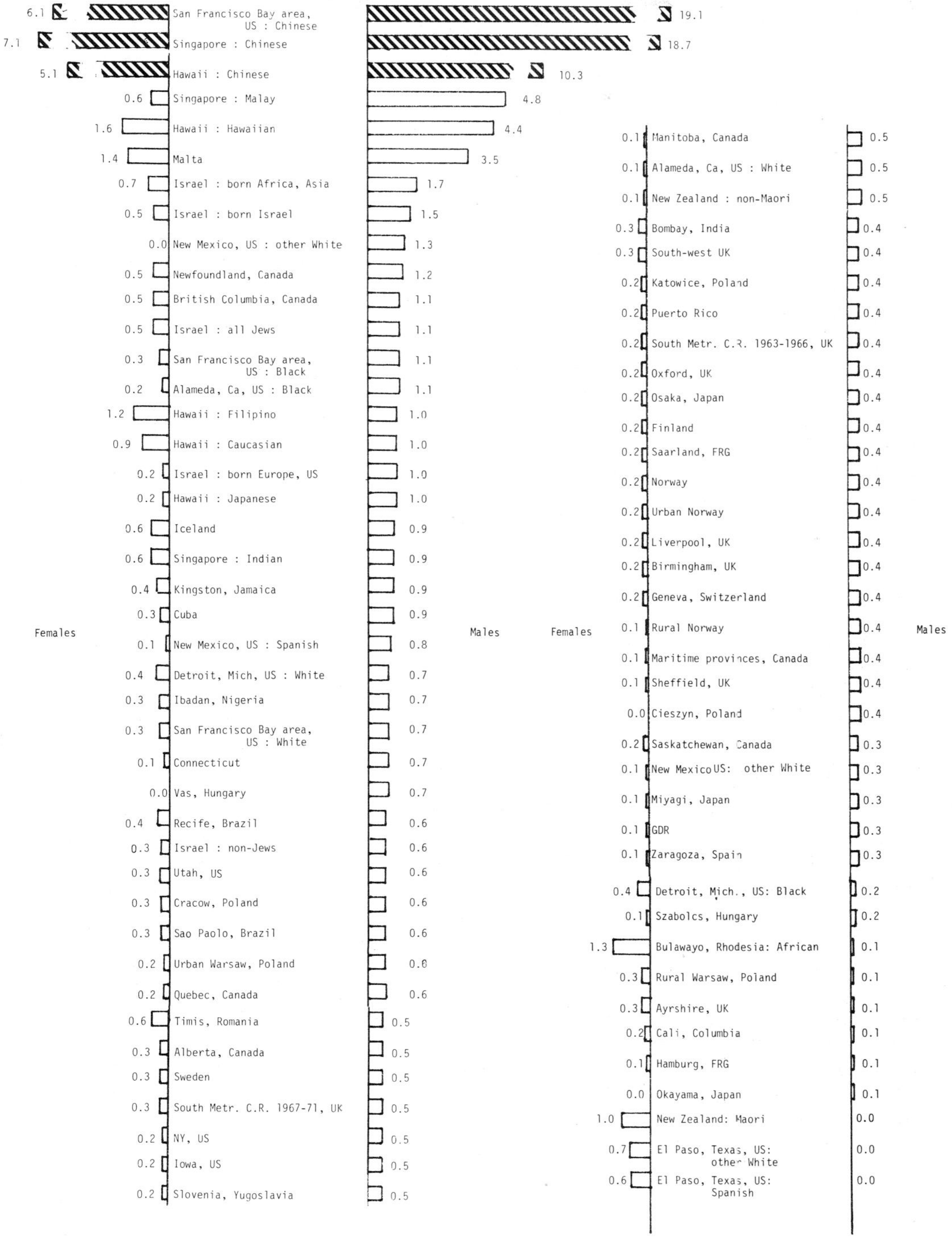

Table 2. Age-adjusted incidence rates per 100,000 per annum for nasopharyngeal cancer in selected Chinese populations

Geographical region	Males	Females	
Hong Kong	24.3	10.2	Ho, 1972
Singapore	18.7	7.1	Waterhouse et al., 1976
Cantonese	29.4	10.3	Shanmugaratnam, 1973
Teochew	17.4	5.9	"
Hokkien	13.7	4.0	"
Taiwan			
Mainlanders	11.4	11.7	Lin et al., 1973a
Taiwanese	5.9	2.8	"
Japan	6.8	3.0	Sawaki & Hirayama, 1977
Hawaii	10.3	5.1	Waterhouse et al., 1976
California	19.1	6.4	"
Eskimos	9.6	3.8	Lanier et al., 1976
Hawaiians	4.4	1.6	Waterhouse et al., 1976

In the State of Selangor, Malaysia, age-adjusted incidence rates among Chinese males and females were 17.3 and 7.3 per 100,000; among Malay males and females, the rates were 2.5 and 0.3, and that among Indian males, 1.1. Estimated incidence rates are highest among the Cantonese, lowest among the Hokkien/Teochew and intermediate in the Khek population (Armstrong et al., 1974).

It is interesting to note the unusually high incidence in Eskimos and Hawaiians. An intermediate risk is observed among non-Chinese in Vietnam, the Philippines, Indonesia, Singapore and Thailand. A higher risk has also been recorded among Tunisians and in Africans.

Effect of part-Chinese ancestry: Ho (1971) reported that, in Hong Kong, 'Macaonese' (descendants of Portuguese settlers in Macao who intermarried with Chinese from Kwangtung) had a much higher frequency of NPC than the rest of the non-Chinese population; Garnjana-Goochorn & Chantarakul (1967) reported that, in Thailand, Thais of part-Chinese ancestry have a relative frequency of NPC that is intermediate between those of Thais and Chinese. The greater the admixture of southern Chinese blood in a given ethnic group, the more likely it is that the NPC incidence rate in that group will be raised.

Trend in NPC incidence rate in Chinese migrants: The risk for first generation migrant southern Chinese does not appear to be altered by geographical factors (Anon., 1974); this applies to migrants to south-east Asia, California (Buell, 1973) and Australia (Booth et al., 1968). However, a decline in mortality from NPC has been reported in Chinese Americans of both sexes over the period 1950-1969 (Fraumeni & Mason, 1974); and it has been observed that second and third generation American-born Chinese have a lower risk than first generation Orient-born Chinese (Buell, 1973, 1974).

Shanmugaratnam & Tye (1970), however, failed to detect any difference in risk between Singapore-born and China-born Chinese. The discrepancy is very likely due to the fact that Chinese born in south-east Asia tend to lead a way of life (food habits, etc.) that more closely resembles that of China-born Chinese than do American-born Chinese.

Age

The incidence in both sexes begins to rise after the age of 20-24 and reaches a plateau at between 45 and 54 years of age. When the logarithm of the mortality is plotted against the logarithm of the age, the power of the age that provides the best fit to a straight line is approximately 2-4: US white (males, 3.94; females, 2.92) US Black (males, 2.13; females, 2.50) and Chinese (males, 4.61; females, 2.38), in age groups 20-59 over 1950-1969 (Fig. 2).

FIG. 2. MORTALITY RATE BY AGE GROUP AND AGE-SPECIFIC MORTALITY RATES FOR NASOPHARYNGEAL CANCER - 1950-1969

Calculated on the basis of Mason et al. (1976) and 'Vital Statistics, 1950-1969, Japan'

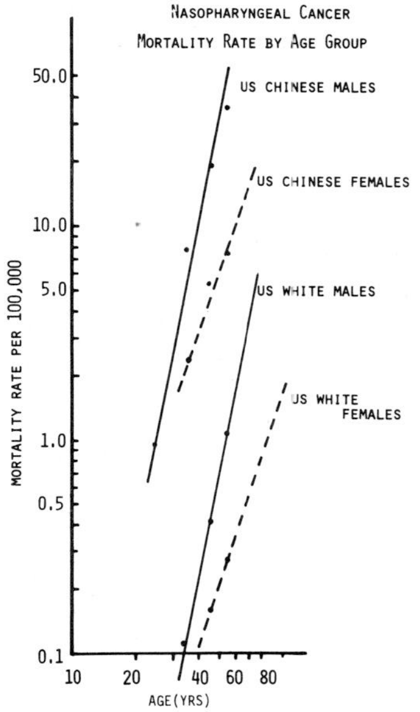

AGE-SPECIFIC MORTALITY RATES FOR NASOPHARYNGEAL CANCER
1950-1969

	AGE GROUP (YRS)	US WHITE	BLACK	CHINESE	JAPANESE
Males	0-	0.02	0.00	0.00	0.01
	10-	0.03	0.05	0.25	0.10
	20-	0.05	0.20	0.95	0.13
	30-	0.11	0.55	7.80	0.24
	40-	0.41	1.05	19.85	0.65
	50-	1.07	-1.05	35.65	1.02
	60-	1.60	1.10	23.80	1.22
	70-	1.49	-0.77	15.33	0.80
Females	0-	0.01	0.00	0.00	0.03
	10-	0.02	0.05	0.00	0.04
	20-	0.03	0.05	0.00	0.08
	30-	0.05	0.05	2.35	0.12
	40-	0.16	0.20	5.25	0.25
	50-	0.27	0.30	7.55	0.53
	60-	0.34	0.35	10.35	0.57
	70-	0.63	0.30	1.50	0.49

VALUE OF b IN $Y = aX^b$

	US WHITE	BLACK	CHINESE	JAPANESE
MALE	3.94	2.13	4.61	2.58
FEMALE	2.92	2.50	2.61	2.38

age 20-59

A similar trend occurs in the age-specific incidence rates in Singapore and in Japan (Fig. 3). The slope of the log-log linear curve was again steeper in males than in females. These figures are definitely lower than those for other cancers, suggesting that two hits are probably enough for NPC to occur, according to the multi-hit theory.

FIG. 3. NASOPHARYNGEAL CANCER INCIDENCE RATE BY AGE GROUP

Nasopharyngeal cancer incidence rate by age group and value of b in $Y = aX^b$ for Chinese in Singapore and Japanese in Japan

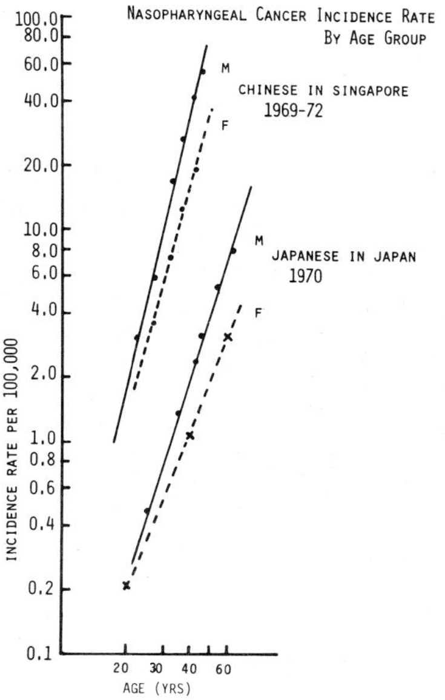

VALUE OF b IN $Y = aX^b$

	CHINESE IN SINGAPORE		JAPANESE IN JAPAN	
	1950-61	1969-72	1970	1975
M	2.79	3.80	3.01	2.79
F	2.54	3.59	2.48	2.02
AGE SPAN (YRS)	20 - 54		20 - 69	

NPC in childhood and adolescence: In Tunisia, out of 485 cases of NPC collected between March 1969 and December 1974, 82 (17%) were in children and adolescents (0-19 years old) (Ellouz et al[1]). This relatively high frequency of NPC in young persons seems to be a characteristic feature in areas of intermediate incidence (Uganda, Kenya, the Sudan, Tunisia). The age distribution showed a peak at 16 years of age. The additional peak in adolescence appears to be lacking in Chinese in USA (Fig. 4).

[1] See p. 115

FIG. 4. CUMULATIVE INCIDENCE RATE FOR NASOPHARYNGEAL CANCER IN CHINESE IN SINGAPORE AND IN USA (HAWAII, CALIFORNIA)

(from Doll et al., 1966, 1970; Waterhouse et al., 1976)

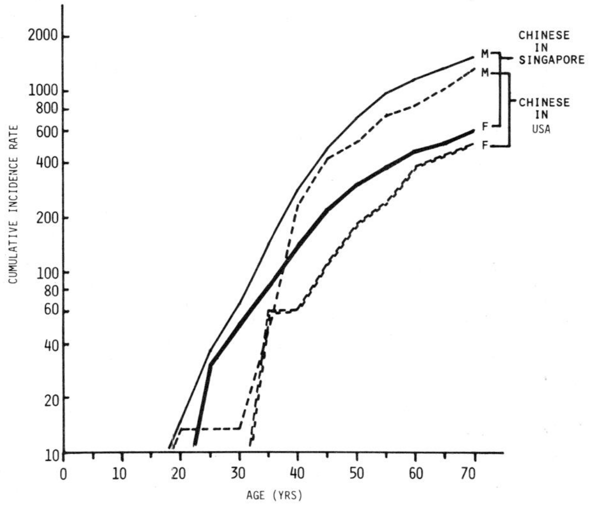

ANALYTICAL EPIDEMIOLOGY

Environmental factors

A number of environmental factors have been found to be related to NPC in case-control studies conducted in various areas. Environmental agents for which suspicion is supported by a certain amount of evidence are listed in Table 3.

In Taiwan, 442 patients with NPC were identified, and 343 of them were interviewed during an 18-month period. Similar interviews were conducted with 1017 persons without the disease who lived in the same neighborhoods as the patients and who served as controls. Smoking was significantly associated with NPC risk: calculation of relative risk indicated that persons who smoked more than 20 cigarettes a day had over twice the risk of those who had never smoked. Working under poorly ventilated conditions was also found to be associated with an NPC risk that was more than twice as great as in those without this experience. Certain nasal symptoms and the use of herbal drugs and nasal balms or oils were also associated with an elevated NPC risk.

Table 3. Environmental agents suspected of being related to nasopharyngeal cancer (NPC)

Agent		Observation	Key references
Virus		Elevated antibody titres to Epstein-Barr virus (EBV)-related antigens; EBV-DNA detected within NPC cells	Anderson et al.[a]; de Schryver et al., 1969, 1970, 1972; Desgranges et al., 1975; de-Thé, 1972a, b, 1975, 1976; de-Thé & Geser, 1974; de-Thé et al., 1969, 1970, 1975; Gunven et al., 1970; Henderson, 1974; Henderson et al., 1974; Henle et al., 1970; Hirayama et al., 1971; Ito et al., 1969; Kawamura, 1971; Kawamura et al., 1970, 1971; Klein et al., 1970; Lenoir & de-Thé[b]; Lin et al., 1971, 1973a, b; Lynn et al., 1973a, b; Nishioka et al., 1971; Old et al., 1966; zur Hausen, 1973; zur Hausen et al., 1970
Chemicals	Tobacco	2-3 fold risk in smokers	Balakrishnan et al., 1976; Lin et al., 1973a
	Drugs	2-3 fold risk in frequent users of herbal drugs and nasal balms	Lin, 1973a
	Diet	Nitrosamines from dry-salted fish High risk in areas of low animal protein intake, low fruit intake and high salted fish intake in Japan	Ho, 1972 Hirayama[c]
	Occupation	Exposure to fumes and smoke in whites	Henderson et al., 1976
	Air pollution	2-3 fold risk in poorly ventilated areas	Clifford, 1970, 1972; Lin, 1973b

[a] See p. 231
[b] See p. 377
[c] This paper

In Singapore, interviews were carried out with a total of 379 Singapore Chinese patients with NPC and with two groups of controls - 595 patients with diseases of the ear, nose and throat other than NPC and 1,044 patients with diseases other than cancer or otorhinolaryngical disease. NPC patients differed significantly from both groups of controls in that they had stronger associations with a personal history of nasal illnesses, a family history of nasal illnesses, use of Chinese medicines for the nose and throat and exposure to smoke from antimosquito coils (Shanmugaratnam et al.[1]).

In California, interviews with 156 patients and 267 controls revealed that an increased risk of NPC was significantly associated with a prior history of ear, nose or throat disease (relative risk = 1.8) or occupational exposure to fumes (relative risk = 2.0), smoke (relative risk = 3.0) or chemicals (relative risk = 2.4). Among Chinese, other Asians and Mexican-Americans, an increased risk was also associated with foreign birthplace (relative risk = 2.1), probably

[1] See p. 199

reflecting childhood exposure to carcinogens in inhaled smoke. In Chinese patients, the risk associated with foreign birthplace and occupational exposure increased among those with HLA-A2 and less than two antigens at the B locus, suggesting a genetic variation in susceptibility (Henderson et al., 1976).

In Hong Kong, a case-control study was undertaken with hospitalized Cantonese NPC patients (Geser et al.[1]). One age- and sex-matched control was selected for each NPC case from hospitalized patients with cancers other than NPC. A total of 150 NPC patients and 150 controls were interviewed. Factors that were found to be positively associated with NPC were as follows: belonging to the four lowest occupational classes; practising Buddhism or ancestor worship and having religious altars in the house; and having a history of previous illnesses of the ear or nose after the age of 15 years. Factors that were found to be negatively associated with NPC were the eating of bread and tinned food and the use of spices.

A study of weaning habits disclosed that salted fish was given to babies just after weaning more often in households with an NPC case than in control households. A multivariant analysis showed that a traditional lifestyle and the consumption of salted fish during weaning are independent risk factors for NPC.

Host factors

Epidemiological evidence with regard to host susceptibility is summarized in Table 4.

Table 4. Host susceptibility with regard to nasopharyngeal carcinoma (NPC)

Item	Observation	Key references
Sex	Risk 2-3 times higher in males	Waterhouse et al., 1976
Age	Log-log linear rise up to middle age, thereafter decline (prior adolescent exposure? Cessation of continued exposure? Susceptible to exhaust?) Additional peak in adolescents in some countries	Balakrishnan, 1975; Henderson, 1974; Ho, 1976
Race	Highest risk in Chinese of southern origin; intermediate risk among non-Chinese, especially of mixed blood, in Vietnam, Philippines, Indonesia, Singapore, Thailand. Risk also high in Tunisians, Eskimos, Hawaiians and Africans	Waterhouse et al., 1976; Muir, 1972; Zippin et al., 1962; Cammoun et al., 1971; Blot et al., 1975
Heredity	Familial aggregation in Uganda, China and Hong Kong and in persons with Burkitt's lymphoma and in those with A2-sin 2 haplotype (Chinese NPC)	Williams & de-Thé, 1974; Kerr et al., 1975; Liang, 1964; Ho, 1972; Joncas et al., 1975; Simons et al., 1976; Simons & Chan[a]
Predisposing morbid conditions	Prior ear, nose and throat disease Paranasal sinusitis Immunological disorders	Henderson et al., 1976; Lin et al., 1973b Yata & Tachibana, 1973

[a] See p. 271

[1] See p. 213

Family: A significantly higher frequency of NPC was observed in close blood relatives of patients with the disease than in those of patients suffering from other cancers. The report of a southern Chinese family with nine cases of NPC, affecting three successive generations (Ho, 1971, 1972) is of particular epidemiological interest.

HLA: Immunogenetic studies of NPC are of long-standing (Hawkins et al., 1974; Seow et al., 1964), and the HLA gene system has been thought to offer the best prospect for study. The hypothesis of a genetic predisposition to NPC has been supported by HLA studies in Chinese but not in other ethnic groups (Betuel et al., 1975). HLA-A2 at locus A and Singapore 2 at locus B have been shown to be associated with NPC in Singapore, Malaysian and Hong Kong Chinese, and there is evidence of a similar association in American Chinese patients (Simons et al., 1973, 1974a, b, 1976). According to Simons et al., the co-occurrence of A2-Singapore 2 is associated with increased susceptibility to NPC, but only in older patients (> 30 years). Furthermore, the A2-Singapore 2 phenotype is a marker of poor survival. By contrast, HLA-A2 in the absence of Singapore 2 is associated with longer survival (> 5 years). BW17 appear both to be a risk factor in newly diagnosed, young patients (< 30 years) and to be associated with poor survival. These points must be confirmed by carefully planned, future studies.

Specific agents

Nitrosamines: As described above, the consumption of salted fish during weaning is reported by Geser et al.[1] to be an independent risk factor for NPC in Hong Kong. They report that Cantonese salted marine fish, frequently not gutted, contains appreciable quantities of *N*-nitrosodimethylamine. Volatile *N*-nitrosodimethylamine has been detected in all samples of salted tested by Huang et al.[2], at levels ranging from 1-35 μg/kg, but no volatile nitrosamine was detected in any other salt-preserved food product.

A high intake of salted fish was revealed in a survey of 1,000 consecutive Chinese patients, 500 with NPC and 500 with other cancers at the Queen Elizabeth Hospital, Hong Kong (Ho, 1975). Only two patients in the latter group could recall not having eaten salted fish in any form: one was a vegetarian and the other a native of central China. One of Ho's two Caucasian patients with NPC also had a history of consumption of salted fish.

In Northern China, where NPC incidence is low, salted fish is seldom, if ever, consumed. Ho also reported that, until recently, 'boat' people in Hong Kong and Canton (a known high-risk group) would rather eat cheap salted fish than their fresh catch, which they could sell for a good price. Furthermore, their food often lacked sources

[1] See p. 223

[2] See p. 309

of vitamin C, such as fresh fruits and vegetables, because these could not be preserved for the long periods when they were at sea.

Huang et al.[1] have also reported that of 20 inbred WA albino rats fed with salted fish alternating with mouse chow, and 20 with mouse chow alone for a period of 1.5-2 years, 20-25% of the treated animals developed carcinomas in the nasal fossa, the posterior part of which may be considered to be the anatomical analogue of the human nasopharynx. None of the animals fed with mouse chow alone developed any tumour. This experiment is of interest and importance but naturally needs further confirmation.

Epstein-Barr virus: A consistently close serological association has been found between NPC and Epstein-Barr herpes virus (EBV). Patients in Africa, Hong Kong, Taiwan, Sweden, France, the US and other countries all show high serological reactivity to EBV-associated antigens.

During an 18-month retrospective study on NPC in Taiwan, sera collected from 321 NPC patients, age-and sex-matched with 817 neighborhood controls, 701 members of NPC families and 1081 members of neighborhood control families were titrated for antibodies to EBV capsid antigen (VCA). Antibody titres were found to be higher in NPC patients than in any of the three control groups, geometric means being 342, 72, 68 and 63, respectively. Similar results were obtained in a seroepidemiological study conducted in Japan (Sawaki et al., 1976).

Recently, it was reported by Klein and coworkers[2] that 60 of 61 biopsies from patients with confirmed undifferentiated NPC contained EBV genome equivalents. This finding is important, since it suggests a causal association between EBV and NPC.

NEED FOR STUDIES ON INTERACTION OF SELECTED RISK FACTORS

The seroepidemiological case-control studies in Taiwan reported here indicate that both different birthplace and abnormal response to EBV antigens significantly affect the risk for NPC. When these two factors are combined, the risk is altered even more (Fig. 5). The effect of other environmental chemicals, such as cigarette smoking, which were shown to be significant in this study, might explain selected known epidemiological phenomena such as sex difference in incidence (Fig. 6). The NPC risk was observed to be highest when these three factors, anti-EBV antibody titre, cigarette smoking and different birthplace, representing viral, chemical and genetic factors, respectively, were combined (Fig. 7).

[1] See p. 315

[2] See p. 347

FIG. 5. ESTIMATED AGE-ADJUSTED INCIDENCE RATE FOR NASOPHARYNGEAL CARCINOMA BY GROUP OF ORIGIN AND BY ANTI-VIRAL CAPSID ANTIGEN (VCA) TITRE IN MALES IN TAIWAN

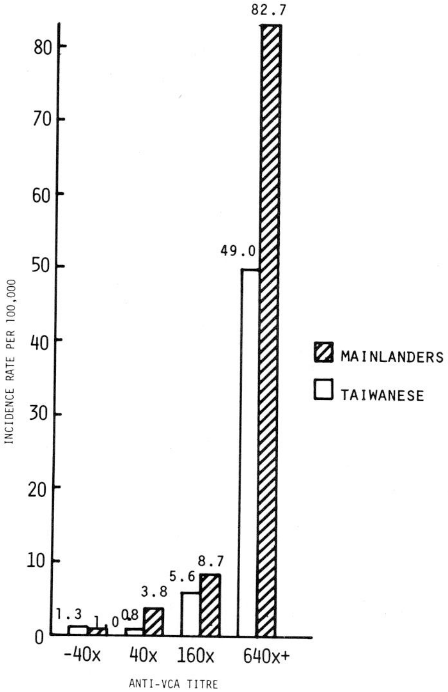

NEED FOR STUDIES ON THE EFFECT OF DIET AND NUTRITION

Recently, the etiological role of diet and nutrition has been studied intensively with regard to cancers at many sites, including breast, colon, pancreas, prostate, corpus uteri, kidney, blood, stomach, oesophagus, mouth and pharynx, cervix, etc., but apparently not yet for NPC.

A relatively high positive correlation (correlation coefficient r = 0.711) was observed between the ratio of salted fish intake (daily intake of salted fish:daily intake of raw fish) and the age-adjusted NPC incidence rate in nine districts in Japan (Table 5). A positive correlation (r= 0.579) was also observed with the proportion of Chinese in each district. On the other hand, negative correlations

FIG. 6. ESTIMATED AGE-ADJUSTED INCIDENCE RATE FOR NASOPHARYNGEAL CARCINOMA BY SEX, BY SMOKING HABITS AND BY ANTI-VIRAL CAPSID ANTIGEN (VCA) TITRE IN TAIWAN

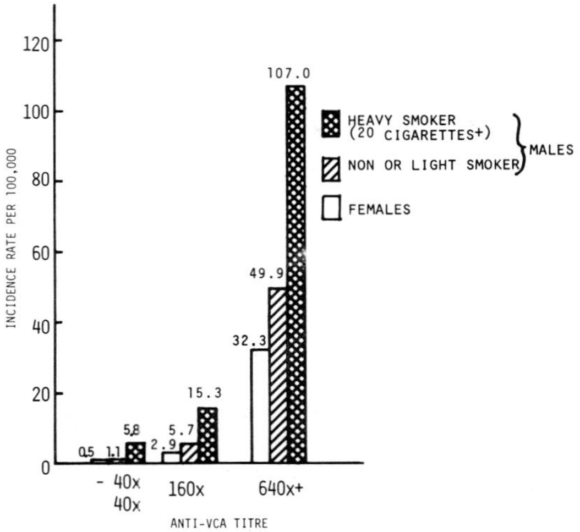

FIG. 7. ESTIMATED AGE-ADJUSTED INCIDENCE RATE FOR NASOPHARYNGEAL CARCINOMA BY SMOKING HABITS, GROUP OF ORIGIN AND ANTI-VIRAL CAPSID ANTIGEN (VCA) TITRE IN MALES IN TAIWAN

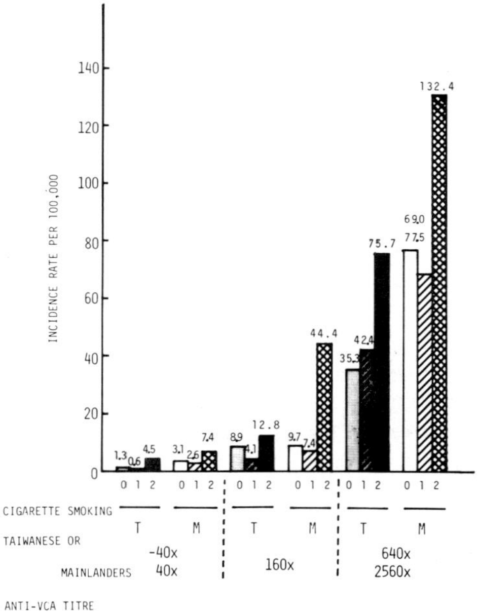

Table 5. Age-adjusted incidence rate per 100,000 for nasopharyngeal cancer (NPC) by district in Japan, 1968-1975

District	Adjusted incidence rate	Expected incidence rate[a]	Daily food intake		Ratio salted fish/ raw fish (1970)	Number of Chinese per 100.000 (1965)
			Animal protein (1970) (g)	Fruits 1970 (g)		
Hokkaido	0.072	0.069	39.9	97.4	0.24	10
Tohoku	0.102	0.128	33.5	65.6	0.30	9
Kanto	0.155	0.172	33.7	74.8	0.36	71
Hokuriku	0.173	0.151	29.1	62.0	0.29	6
Tokai	0.150	0.121	33.8	83.9	0.30	11
Kinki	0.178	0.168	36.9	93.2	0.39	95
Chugoku	0.087	0.090	34.8	92.6	0.16	12
Shikoku	0.106	0.121	32.3	83.5	0.27	6
Kyushu	0.117	0.121	32.9	65.6	0.18	25
Correlation coefficient with NPC incidence		0.881	-0.419	-0.303	0.711	0.579

[a] Multiple linear regression

were observed between the age-adjusted NPC incidence rate and the daily intake of fruit (r= 0.303) and between NPC and the daily intake of animal protein (r= 0.419). When the effects of these two nutritional factors were excluded, the partial correlation coefficients between the age-adjusted NPC incidence rate and ratio of salted fish intake was calculated to be 0.797. The partial correlation coefficient between the age-adjusted NPC incidence rate and the proportion of Chinese was 0.878. The multiple correlation coefficient between the age-adjusted NPC incidence rate and these four factors (ratio of salted fish intake, animal protein intake, fruit intake and proportion of Chinese) was 0.881.

In short, the NPC incidence rate appeared to be lower in districts in which intake of animal protein and/or consumption of fruit is high. The rate tended to be higher with an increase in the ratio of salted fish intake and/or with the proportion of Chinese in the district. The definitive reason for the uniquely high risk in southern Chinese should, however, be further investigated by taking into careful consideration the interactions of known host and environmental risk factors, as listed in tables 1, 3 and 4.

SUMMARY

Information concerning the descriptive and analytical epidemiology of NPC that has been reported mainly since the first international symposium on the subject in Singapore in 1964 are reviewed. NPC is rare in most countries in the world, with an age-adjusted incidence rate of less than 1 per 100,000, and the incidence rate is twice as high in males as in females. Chinese of southern origin have a uniquely high risk, the incidence rates per 100,000 being 10-20 in males and 5-10 in females. The greater the admixture of southern Chinese blood in a given ethnic group, the more likely it is that the NPC incidence rate in that group will be raised. The incidence in both sexes begins to rise after the ages of 20-24 and reaches a plateau at between 45 and 54. When the logarithm of mortality and morbidity is plotted against the logarithm of the age, the power of the age that provides the best fit to a straight line on a log-log graph is approximately two to four. These figures are lower than for other cancers.

Seroepidemiological case-control studies indicate that both different birthplace and abnormal response to EBV antigen significantly enhance the risk for NPC; when these two factors are combined, the relative risk appears to rise further. The effect of other environmental chemicals, such as from cigarette smoking, shown to be significant in several retrospective studies, could explain in part epidemiological phenomena such as sex difference in incidence.

The definitive reason for the uniquely high risk in southern Chinese should be further investigated by taking into account the interactions of host factors (birthplace, HLA, etc.) and environmental factors (EBV, chemical carcinogens including nitrosamines, excessive intake of salted fish, nutritional deficiencies, etc.).

REFERENCES

Andrews, P.A.J. & Michaels, L. (1968) Nasopharyngeal carcinoma in Canadian bush pilots. *Lancet, ii*, 85-87

Anon. (1974) Cancer in Chinese migrants. *Lancet, i*, 1027

Armstrong, R.W., Kutty, M.K. & Dharmalingam, S.K. (1974) Incidence of nasopharyngeal carcinoma in Malaysia, with special reference to the state of Selangor. *Brit. J. Cancer, 30*, 86-94

Balakrishnan, V. (1975) An additional younger-age peak for cancer of the nasopharynx. *Int. J. Cancer, 15*, 651-657

Balakrishnan, V., Gangadaran, P. & Nagaraj Rao, D. (1976) *Some epidemiological aspects of nasopharyngeal cancer.* In: Shanmugaratnam, K., Nambiar, R., Tan, K.K. & Chan, L.K.C., eds, *Liver Cancer: Cancer Problems in Asian Countries*, Singapore, Singapore Cancer Society, pp. 268-274

Belamaric, J. (1969) Malignant tumors in Chinese: a report based on biopsy and autopsy material from Chinese in Hong Kong. *Int. J. Cancer, 4*, 560-573

Betuel, H., Camoun, M., Colombani, J., Day, N.E., Ellouz, R. & de-Thé, G. (1975) The relationship between nasopharyngeal carcinoma and the HL-A system among Tunisians. *Int. J. Cancer, 16*, 249-254

Blot, W.J., Lanier, A., Fraumeni, J.F., Jr & Bender, T.R. (1975) Cancer mortality among Alaskan natives, 1960-69. *J. nat. Cancer Inst., 55*, 547-554

Booth, K., Cooke, R., Scott, G. & Atkinson, L. (1968) *Carcinoma of the nasopharynx and oesophagus in Australian New Guinea, 1958-1965.* In: Clifford, P., Linsell, C.A., Timms, G.L., eds, *Cancer in Africa*, Nairobi, East African Publishing House, pp. 319-322

Brown, T.M., Heath, C.W., Lang, R.M., Lee, S.K. & Whalley, B.W. (1976) Nasopharyngeal cancer in Bermuda. *Cancer, 37*, 1464-1468

Buell, P. (1965) Nasopharyngeal cancer in Chinese of California. *Brit. J. Cancer, 19*, 459-470

Buell, P. (1973) Race and place in the etiology of nasopharyngeal cancer: a study based on California death certificates. *Int. J. Cancer, 11*, 268-272

Buell, P. (1974) The effect of migration on the risk of nasopharyngeal cancer among Chinese. *Cancer Res., 34*, 1189-1191

Cammoun, M., Hoerner, G.V. & Mourali, N. (1974) Tumors of the nasopharynx in Tunisia: an anatomic and clinical study based on 143 cases. *Cancer, 33*, 184-192

Chadli, A., Hafsia, M. & Maamouri, M.T. (1976) Carcinoma of the cavum: statistical and pathological study over a period of 20 years. *Arch. Anat. Cytol. Pathol., 24*, 13-22

Clifford, P. (1970) A review on the epidemiology of nasopharyngeal carcinoma. *Int. J. Cancer, 5*, 287-309

Clifford, P. (1972) Carcinogens in the nose and throat: nasopharyngeal carcinoma in Kenya. *Proc. roy. Soc. Med., 65*, pp. 682-686

de Schryver, A., Friberg, S., Jr, Klein, G., Henle, W., Henle, G., de-Thé, G., Clifford, P. & Ho, H.C. (1969) Epstein-Barr virus-associated antibody patterns in carcinoma of the post-nasal space. *Clin. exp. Immunol., 5*, 443-459

de Schryver, A., Klein, G. & de-Thé, G. (1970) Surface antigens on lymphoblastoid cells derived from nasopharyngeal carcinoma. *Clin. exp. Immunol.*, *7*, 161-171

de Schryver, A., Klein, G., Henle, G., Henle, W., Cameron, H., Sanfesson, L. & Clifford, P. (1972) EB-virus associated serology in malignant disease, antibody levels to viral capsid antigens (VCA), membrane antigens (MA) and early antigens (EA) in patients with various neoplastic conditions. *Int. J. Cancer*, *9*, 353-364

Desgranges, C., Wolf, H., de-Thé, G., Shanmugaratnam, K., Cammoun, N., Ellouz, R., Klein, G., Lennert, K. & zur Hausen, H. (1975) Nasopharyngeal carcinoma. X. Presence of Epstein-Barr genomes in separated epithelial cells of tumors from Singapore, Tunisia and Kenya. *Int. J. Cancer*, *16*, 7-15

de-Thé, G. (1972a) The etiology of nasopharyngeal carcinoma. *Pathobiol. Annu.*, *2*, 235-254

de-Thé, G. (1972b) *Virology and immunology of nasopharyngeal carcinoma: present situation and outlook - a review.* In: Biggs, P.M., de-Thé, G. & Payne, L.N., eds, *Oncogenesis and Herpesviruses (IARC Scientific Publications No. 2)*, Lyon, pp. 275-284

de-Thé, G. (1975) Epidemiology in the study of the role of viruses in human cancers. *Bull. Cancer*, *62*, 151-160

de-Thé, G. (1976) Epstein-Barr virus behavior in different populations and implications. *Cancer Res.*, *36*, 692-695

de-Thé, G. & Geser, A. (1974) Nasopharyngeal carcinoma: recent studies and outlook for a viral etiology. *Cancer Res.*, *34*, 1196-1206

de-Thé, G., Ambrosioni, J.C., Ho, H.C. & Kwan, H.C. (1969) Lymphoblastoid transformation and presence of herpes-type viral particles in a Chinese nasopharyngeal tumour culture *in vitro*. *Nature (Lond.)*, *221*, 770-771

de-Thé, G., Ho, H.C., Kwan, H.C., Desgranges, C. & Favre, M.C. (1970) Nasopharyngeal carcinoma (NPC). I. Types of cultures derived from tumour biopsies and non-tumorous tissues of Chinese patients with special reference to lymphoblastoid transformation. *Int. J. Cancer*, *6*, 189-206

de-Thé, G., Day, N., Geser, A., Ho, J.H., Simons, M.J., Sohier, R., Tukei, P. & Vonka, V. (1975) Epidemiology of the Epstein-Barr virus infection and associated tumors in man. *Bibl. Haemat.*, pp. 216-220

Dharmalingam, S.K. & Wong, S.H. (1973) Nasopharynx cancer in West Malaysia: incidence, 1963-1965. *Australas. Radiol.*, *17*, 261-265

Doll, R., Payne, P. & Waterhouse, J., eds (1966) *Cancer Incidence in Five Continents, A Technical Report*, Berlin-Heidelberg, New York, Springer

Doll, R., Muir, C. & Waterhouse, J., eds (1970) *Cancer Incidence in Five Continents, Vol. II*, Berlin-Heidelberg-New York, Springer

Ellouz, R., Cammoun, M., Zaouche, A. & Ben Attia, R. (1975) Cancers of the rhinopharynx in Tunisia: epidemiological and anatomoclinical aspects. *Bull. Cancer, 62*, 295-306

Fraumeni, J.F., Jr & Mason, T.J. (1974) Cancer mortality among Chinese Americans, 1950-69. *J. nat. Cancer Inst., 52*, 659-665

Garnjana-Goochorn, S. & Chantarakul, N. (1967) *Nasopharyngeal cancer at Siriraj Hospital, Dhonburi, Thailand.* In: Muir, C.S. & Shanmugaratnam, K., eds, *Cancer of the Nasopharynx (UICC Monograph Series No. 1)*, Copenhagen, Munksgaard, pp. 33-37

Gunven, P., Klein, G., Henle, W. & Clifford, P. (1970) Epstein-Barr virus in Burkitt's lymphoma and nasopharyngeal carcinoma. *Nature (Lond.), 228*, 1053-1056

Har-Kedar, I., Chaitchik, S. & Hercberg, A. (1974) Nasopharyngeal carcinoma at the Tel-Hash-Qmer Hospital, Israel: a 20-year survey (1951-1970). *Clin. Radiol., 25*, 403-407

Hawkins, B.R., Simons, M.J., Goh, E.H. & Chia, K.B. (1974) Immuno-genetic aspects of nasopharyngeal carcinoma. II. Analysis of ABO, rhesus and Mnss red cell systems. *Int. J. Cancer, 13*, 116-121

Henderson, B.E. (1974) Nasopharyngeal carcinoma: present status of knowledge. *Cancer Res., 34*, 1187-1188

Henderson, B.E., Louie, E., Bogdanoff, E., Henle, W., Alena, B. & Henle, G. (1974) Antibodies to herpes group virus in patients with nasopharyngeal and other head and neck cancers. *Cancer Res., 34*, 1207-1210

Henderson, B.E., Louie, E., Soohoo Jing, J., Buell, P. & Gardner, M.B. (1976) Risk factors associated with nasopharyngeal carcinoma. *New Engl. J. Med., 295*, 1101-1106

Henle, W., Henle, G., Burtin, P., Cachin, Y., Clifford, P., de Schryver, A., de-Thé, G., Diehl, V., Ho, H.C. & Klein, G. (1970) Antibodies to Epstein-Barr virus in nasopharyngeal carcinoma, other head and neck neoplasms and control groups. *J. nat. Cancer Inst., 44*, 225-231

Hirayama, T., Nishioka, K., Kawamura, A. & Lin, T.M. (1971) *The natural history of HTV infection and its clinical, immuno-logical, and oncological manifestations.* In: Nakahara, W., Nishioka, K., Hirayama, T. & Ito, Y., eds, *Recent Advances in Human Tumor Virology and Immunology*, Tokyo, University of Tokyo Press, pp. 317-335

Ho, H.C. (1971) *Genetic and environmental factors in nasopharyngeal carcinoma.* In: Nakahara, W., Nishioka, K., Hirayama, T. & Ito, Y., eds, *Recent Advances in Human Tumor Virology and Immunology*, Tokyo, University of Tokyo Press, pp. 275-295

Ho, H.C. (1972) *Current knowledge of the epidemiology of nasopharyngeal carcinoma - a review.* In: Biggs, P.M., de-Thé, G. & Payne, L.N., eds, *Oncogenesis and Herpesviruses (IARC Scientific Publications No. 2)*, Lyon, pp. 357-366

Ho, H.C. (1975) Epidemiology of nasopharyngeal carcinoma. *J. roy. Coll. Surg. (Edinb.), 20*, (No 4), 223-235

Ho, H.C. (1976) *Epidemiology of nasopharyngeal carcinoma.* In: Hirayama, T., ed., *Cancer in Asia*, Baltimore, University Park Press, pp. 49-61

Hoover, R., Mason, T.J., Mckay, F.W. & Fraumeni, J.F., Jr (1975) *Geographic patterns of cancer mortality in the United States.* In: Fraumeni, J.F., ed., *Persons at High Risk of Cancer*, New York, Academic Press, pp. 343-360

Huong, B.Q., Buu-Hoi, N.P., Duong, P.N., Te, N.H. & Hoang, D.D. (1969) Nasopharyngeal cancers in Vietnam: epidemiology, clinical aspects, possible etiologic factors. *Ann. Otolaryngol. (Paris), 86*, 267-268

Ito, Y., Takahashi, T., Kawamura, A., Jr & Tu, S.M. (1969) High anti-EB viral titer in sera of patients with nasopharyngeal carcinoma: a small-scaled seroepidemiological study. *Gann, 60*, 335-340

Joncas, J.H., Rioux, E., Robitaille, R. & Wastiaux, J.P. (1975) Multiple cases of lymphoepithelioma and Burkitt's lymphoma in a Canadian family. *Bibl. Haemat.*, pp. 224-226

Kawamura, A., Jr (1971) *Present status of studies on nasopharyngeal carcinoma.* In: Nakahara, W., Nishioka, K., Hirayama, T. & Ito, Y., eds, *Recent Advances in Human Tumor Virology and Immunology*, Tokyo, University of Tokyo Press, pp. 209-215

Kawamura, A., Jr, Takada, M., Gotoh, A., Hamajima, K., Sanpe, T., Murata, M., Ito, Y., Takahashi, T., Yoshida, T.O., Hirayama, T., Tu, S.M., Liu, C.H., Yang, C.S. & Wang, C.H. (1970) Seroepidemiological studies on nasopharyngeal carcinoma by fluorescent antibody techniques with cultured Burkitt lymphoma cells. *Gann, 61*, 55-71

Kawamura, A., Hamajima, K., Murata, M., Goto, A., Takeda, M., Nishioka, K., Tachibana, T., Hirayama, T., Yoshida, T.O., Imai, K., Ito, Y., Yang, C.S., Chu, C.T., Wang, C.H., Ho, S.W., Tu, S.M., Liu, C.H. & Lin, T.M. (1971) Studies on nasopharyngeal carcinoma and Burkitt lymphoma by immunofluorescence. *Ann. N.Y. Acad. Sci., 177*, 250-267

Kerr, W.A., Allen, K.L., Haynes, D.R. & Sellars, S.L. (1975) Familial nasopharyngeal chordoma. *S. Afr. med. J., 49*, 1584

Khor, T.H., Tan, B.C., Chus, E.J. & Chia, K.B. (1975) Tumours of the nasopharynx, Singapore, 1969-1971: the presenting picture. *Singapore med. J., 16*, 236-243

Klein, G., Geering, G., Old, L., Henle, G., Henle, W. & Clifford, P. (1970) Comparison of the anti-EBV titer and the EBV associated membrane reactive and precipitating antibody levels in the sera of Burkitt lymphoma and nasopharyngeal carcinoma patients and controls. *Int. J. Cancer*, *5*, 185-194

Lanasa, J.J., Jr & Putney, F.J. (1974) Nasopharyngeal malignancy in childhood. *Sth. med. J. (Bgham, Ala.)*, *67*, 1363-1364

Lanier, A.P., Bender, T.R., Blot, W.J., Fraumeni, J.F., Jr & Hurlburt, W.B. (1976) Cancer incidence in Alaska natives. *Int. J. Cancer*, *18*, 409-412

Liang, P.C. (1964) Studies on nasopharyngeal carcinoma in the Chinese: statistical and laboratory investigations. *Chin. med. J.*, *83*, 373-390

Lin, T.M., Hsu, M.M., Chen, K.P., Chiang, T.C., Jung, P.F. & Hirayama, T. (1971) Morbidity and mortality of cancer of the nasopharynx in Taiwan. *Gann*, *10*, 137-144

Lin, T.M., Chen, K.P., Lin, C.C., Hsu, M.M., Tu, S.M., Chiang, T.C., Jung, P.F. & Hirayama, T. (1973a) Retrospective study on nasopharyngeal carcinoma. *J. nat. Cancer Inst.*, *51*, 1403-1408

Lin, T.M., Yang, C.S., Chiou, J.F., Tu, S.M., Lin, C.C., Liu, C.H., Chen, K.P., Ito, Y., Kawamura, A. & Hirayama, T. (1973b) Seroepidemiological studies on carcinoma of the nasopharynx. *Cancer Res.*, *33*, 2603-2608

Lynn, T.C., Tu, S.M., Hirayama, T. & Kawamura, A. (1973a) Nasopharyngeal carcinoma and Epstein-Barr virus. I. Factors related to the anti-VCA antibody. *Jap. J. exp. Med.*, *43*, 121-133

Lynn, T.C., Tu, S.M., Hirayama, T. & Kawamura, A. (1973b) Nasopharyngeal carcinoma and Epstein-Barr virus. II. Clinical course and the anti-VCA antibody. *Jap. J. exp. Med.*, *43*, 135-144

Mallen, R.W. & Shandro, W.G. (1974) Nasopharyngeal carcinoma in Eskimos. *Can. J. Otolaryngol.*, *3*, 175-179

Marsden, A.T.H. (1964) The pathology of carcinoma of the nasopharynx. *Med. Proc.*, *10*, 183-187

Martinson, F.D. (1968) Cancer of the nasopharynx in Nigeria. *J. Laryngol.*, *82*, 1119-1128

Mason, T.J., McKay, F.W., Hoover, R., Blot, W.J. & Fraumeni, J.F., Jr (1976) *Atlas of Cancer Mortality among US Non-Whites, 1950-1969*, DHEW Publication No (NIH)76-1201, US Department of Health, Education and Welfare - National Institutes of Health, Washington DC, US Government Printing Office

McCallum, D. (1974) Carcinoma of the nasopharynx: a review of 20 patients. *J. Laryngol. Otol.*, *88*, 843-849

Miyagi, T. (1967) *Cancer of the nasopharynx and related organs in Japan based on mortality, morbidity and autopsy studies.* In: Muir, C.S. & Shanmugaratnam, K., eds, *Cancer of the Nasopharynx (UICC Monograph Series No. 1)*, Copenhagen, Munksgaard, pp. 29-32

Muir, C.S. (1962) Cancer of the buccal cavity and nasopharynx in Singapore. *Brit. J. Cancer, 16*, 583-591

Muir, C.S. (1971) Nasopharyngeal carcinoma in non-Chinese populations with special reference to South-East Asia and Africa. *Int. J. Cancer, 8*, 351-363

Muir, C.S. (1972) *Nasopharyngeal carcinoma in non-Chinese populations.* In: Biggs, P.M., de-Thé, G. & Payne, L.N., eds, *Oncogenesis and Herpesvirus (IARC Scientific Publications No. 2)*, Lyon, pp. 367-371

Muir, C.S. (1975) Epidemiology of cancer of the cavum. *Bull. Cancer, 62*, 251-264

Muir, C.S. & Oakley, W.F. (1967) Nasopharyngeal cancer in Sarawak (Borneo). *J. Laryngol., 81*, 197-207

Muir, C.S. & Shanmugaratnam, K. (1967) *The incidence of nasopharyngeal carcinoma in Singapore.* In: Muir, C.S. & Shanmugaratnam, K., eds, *Cancer of the Nasopharynx (UICC Monograph Series No. 1)*, Copenhagen, Munksgaard, pp. 47-53

Muir, C.S. Evans, M.D.E. & Roche, P.J.L. (1968) Cancer in Sabah (Borneo): a preliminary survey. *Brit. J. Cancer, 22*, 637-645

Naumov, G.P. (1973) Malignant neoplasms of nasopharynx in Tunisia. *Vestn. Otorinolaringol., 35*, 84-87

Nishioka, K., Tachibana, Y., Hirayama, T., de-Thé, G., Klein, G., Takada, M. & Kawamura, A., Jr (1971) *Immunological studies on the cell membrane receptors of cultured cells derived from nasopharyngeal cancer, Burkitt's lymphoma and infections mononucleosis.* In: Nakahara, W., Nishioka, K., Hirayama, T. & Ito, Y., eds, *Recent Advances in Human Tumor Virology and Immunology*, Tokyo, University of Tokyo Press, pp. 401-420

Old, L.J., Boyse, E.A., Oettgen, H.F., de Harven, E., Geering, G., Williamson, B. & Clifford, P. (1966) Precipitating antibody in human serum to an antigen present in cultured Burkitt's lymphoma cells. *Proc. nat. Acad. Sci. (Wash.), 56*, 1699-1704

Pantangco, E.E., Basa, G.F. & Canlas, M. (1970) A survey of nasopharyngeal tumors among Filipinos: a report of 203 cases. *J. Philipp. med. Ass., 46*, 60-73

Papavasiliou, C.G. (1974) Cancer of the nasopharynx, incidence, clinical course and results of therapy: a report from Greece. *Clin. Radiol., 25*, 409-414

Quisenberry, W.B. & Reimann-Jasinski, D. (1967) *Ethnic differences in nasopharyngeal cancer in Hawaii.* In: Muir, C.S. & Shanmugaratnam, K., eds, *Cancer of the Nasopharynx (UICC Monograph Series No. 1)*, Copenhagen, Munksgaard, pp. 77-81

Sawaki, S., Hirayama, T. & Sugano, H. (1976) *Studies on nasopharyngeal carcinoma in Japan.* In: Hirayama, T., ed., *Cancer in Asia*, Baltimore, University Park Press, pp. 63-74

Schaefer, O., Hildes, J.A., Medd, L.M. & Cameron, D.G. (1975) The changing pattern of neoplastic disease in Canadian Eskimos. *Can. med. Ass. J.*, *112*, 1399-1409

Schmauz, R. & Templeton, A.C. (1972) Nasopharyngeal carcinoma in Uganda. *Cancer*, *29*, 610-621

Seow, L.J., Kwa, S.B. & Teoh, C.K. (1964) A preliminary survey of ABO blood group frequency in nasopharyngeal carcinoma in Chinese patients. *Singapore med. J.*, *5*, 93-95

Shanmugaratnam, K. (1973) Ethnic and dialect group variations in cancer incidence. *Singapore med. J.*, *14*, 69

Shanmugaratnam, K. & Tye, C.Y. (1970) A study of nasopharyngeal cancer among Singapore Chinese with special reference to migrant status and specific community (dialect group). *J. chron. Dis.*, *23*, 433-441

Simons, M.J., Kwa, S.B., Day, N.E., Wee, G.B., Hawkins, B.R., de-Thé, G.B. & Shanmugaratnam, K. (1973) *Immunogenetic studies of Southeast Asian ethnic groups with high and low-risk for nasopharyngeal carcinoma.* In: Nakahara, W., Hirayama, T., Nishioka, K. & Sugano, H., *Analytical and Experimental Epidemiology of Cancer*, Tokyo, University of Tokyo Press, pp. 171-193

Simons, M.J., Wee, G.B., Day, N.E., Morris, P.J., Shanmugaratnam, K. & de-Thé, G.B. (1974a) Immunogenetic aspects of nasopharyngeal carcinoma. I. Differences in HL-A antigen profiles between patients and control groups. *Int. J. Cancer*, *13*, 122-134

Simons, M.J., Day, N.E., Wee, G.B. Shanmugaratnam, K., Ho, H.C., Wong, S.H., Ti, T.K., Yong, N.K., Darmalingam, S. & de-Thé, G. (1974b) Nasopharyngeal carcinoma. V. Immunogenetic studies of Southeast Asian ethnic groups with high and low risk for the tumor. *Cancer Res.*, *34*, 1192-1195

Simons, M.J., Wee, G.B., Goh, E.H., Chan, S.H., Shanmugaratnam, K., Day, N.E. & de-Thé, G. (1976) Immunogenetic aspects of nasopharyngeal carcinoma. IV. Increased risk in Chinese of nasopharyngeal carcinoma associated with a Chinese-related HLA profile (A2, Singapore 2). *J. nat. Cancer Inst.*, *57*, 977-980

Snow, J.B., Jr (1975) Carcinoma of the nasopharynx in children. *Ann. Otol. Rhinol. Laryngol.*, *84*, 817-826

Strelka, J. & Barta, T. (1974) Geopathology of malignant nasopharyngeal neoplasms. *Cs. Otolaryngol.*, *23*, 165-169

Tran, H.T., Loi, L.V., Trin, F., Kim, F. & Nhon, L.S. (1963) Malignant tumors of the nasopharynx. *Vestn. Otorinolaringol., 25*, 41-44

Waterhouse, J., Muir, C., Correa, P. & Powell, J., eds (1976) *Cancer Incidence in Five Continents, Vol. III (IARC Scientific Publications No. 15)*, Lyon

Williams, E.H. & de-Thé, G. (1974) Familial aggregation in nasopharyngeal carcinoma. *Lancet, ii*, 295-296

Yata, J. & Tachibana, T. (1973) *The significance of lymphocytes in the etiology of Epstein-Barr-virus associated tumors: implications for serological epidemiology.* In: Nakahara, W., Hirayama, T., Nishioka, K. & Sugano, H., *Analytical and Experimental Epidemiology of Cancer*, Tokyo, University of Tokyo Press, pp. 161-169

Zippin, C., Tekawa, I.S., Bragg, K.U., Watson, D.A. & Linden, G. (1962) Studies on heredity and environment in cancer of the nasopharynx. *J. nat. Cancer Inst., 29*, 483-490

zur Hausen, H., Schulte-Holthausen, H., Klein, G., Henle, G., Clifford, P. & Santesson, L. (1970) EBV DNA in biopsies of Burkitt tumors and anaplastic carcinomas of the nasopharynx. *Nature (Lond.), 228*, 1056-1058

zur Hausen, H. (1973) *The significance of nucleic acid homology studies for etiology and epidemiology of human tumors.* In: Nakahara, W., Hirayama, T., Nishioka, K. & Sugano, H., *Analytical and Experimental Epidemiology of Cancer*, Tokyo, University of Tokyo Press, pp. 153-160

VARIATIONS IN NASOPHARYNGEAL CANCER INCIDENCE AMONG SPECIFIC CHINESE COMMUNITIES (DIALECT GROUPS) IN SINGAPORE

K. SHANMUGARATNAM

Department of Pathology,
University of Singapore,
Outram Road,
Singapore 3, Singapore

INTRODUCTION

The exceptionally high incidence of nasopharyngeal carcinoma (NPC) in China and among emigrant Chinese populations in many countries is well documented; the incidence levels are especially high in Chinese from the southern provinces of China (Ho, 1972; Shanmugaratnam, 1971). Reports from California have suggested that, although the incidence and mortality rates for NPC among US-born Chinese are significantly lower than among China-born Chinese, they are still considerably higher than among Caucasian populations in the US (Buell, 1965, 1974; Zippin et al., 1962). The essential racial differences in incidence are, however, to a large extent independent of geography. In Singapore, the age-standardized incidence levels are high among Chinese (18.7 per 100,000 per year for males and 7.1 for females), intermediate in Malays (4.8 and 0.6, respectively) and low in Indians (0.9 and 0.0, respectively) (Shanmugaratnam, 1976).

Significant differences in incidence of NPC have been reported among certain Chinese communities or dialect groups: reports from China have shown higher relative frequencies of the tumour among the Cantonese (Hu & Yang, 1959; Jung & Yu, 1963; Liang, 1964); the incidence rates are significantly higher among the Cantonese and Tanka (boat people) in Hong Kong (Ho, 1967, 1972) and among the Cantonese in Singapore (Shanmugaratnam, 1973). Previous reports of differences in cancer incidence among Chinese dialect groups in Singapore, based on a three-year period (1968-1970) of comprehensive cancer registration (Shanmugaratnam, 1973; Shanmugaratnam & Wee, 1973), were restricted to

Hokkiens, Teochews and Cantonese, who constitute the three major Chinese dialect groups in Singapore; the numbers of cases in the other dialect groups, namely, Hainanese, Hakka, Foochow, Shanghainese and Henghua, were too small for analysis. The relative incidence rates for NPC in Cantonese in comparison with the pooled Hokkien and Teochew groups were found to be 2.033 for males and 2.245 for females, both significant at $P \simeq 0.01$. It was the purpose of this study to extend this analysis over a five-year period of cancer registration (1968-1972) and to include two additional dialect groups, namely, the Hainanese and Hakka.

MATERIALS AND METHODS

The Singapore Cancer Registry

The island republic of Singapore, situated in the centre of the Malayan archipelago, comprises the main island of Singapore and several offshore islands and has a total area of 584 km^2. Singapore has a good standard of medical service, with centralized services for pathology, radiotherapy and death registration.

Comprehensive, population-based cancer registration covering the whole of the Republic of Singapore began on 1 January 1968. The Singapore Cancer Registry derives information on cancer cases from all sections of the medical profession, hospital records from all government hospitals, pathology reports of all biopsy and necropsy examinations and all death certificates issued in Singapore.

Population

A total of 2,074,507 persons (1,062,127 males and 1,012,380 females) were enumerated at the 1970 census of population, comprising 76% Chinese, 15% Malays, 7% Indians and 2% others. Only 33% of the population belonged to the age group of 30 years and over.

The Chinese in Singapore are mostly derived from the south-eastern Chinese provinces of Fukien and Kwangtung and comprise several specific communities or dialect groups. The dialect group status of a person was ascertained from the person concerned and checked by reference to his National Registration Identity Card, which is held by all persons aged 12 years and over. In both the national census and cancer registry files, the ethnic/dialect group of persons with mixed parentage is given as that of the father. The overwhelming majority of adult Chinese in Singapore (96% of 2,028 hospital patients aged 20 years and over interviewed between 1966 and 1968) are off-spring of within-dialect marriages (Shanmugaratnam, 1973).

The major dialect groups in Singapore according to the 1970 census are Hokkien, derived from Fukien province (42.2% of the Chinese population), Teochew, from the Teochew district of Kwangtung province (22.3%), Cantonese, from the other parts of Kwangtung (17.0%), Hainanese, from the island of Hainan off the southern Chinese coast

(7.3%), Hakka, who are of northern Chinese origin (although those in Singapore are derived mainly from prefectures lying north and south of the Kwangtung-Fukien boundary) (7.0%) and others (4.1%) (Arumainathan, 1973).

The majority of the Singapore Chinese population are Singapore-born. The proportion of immigrants is higher among those aged 30 years and over: in 1970, foreign-born immigrants comprised 23.4% of the total Chinese population, with 7.9% in the 0-29 year age group, 46.8% in the 30-59 year age group and 86.2% in the 60 year and over age group (Arumainathan, 1973).

A total of 729 new cases of NPC (517 males, 212 females) were diagnosed among the Singapore Chinese population during the five-year period between 1 January, 1968 and 31 December, 1972. The diagnosis was confirmed histologically for the majority (682 cases, 93.6%). Age-specific incidence rates for each of the dialect groups and for the Chinese population as a whole were calculated on the basis of the 1970 census of population. Incidence rates for NPC, age-standardized to the world population (UICC, 1970), were calculated for each ethnic and major Chinese dialect group in Singapore and compared with the rates for the total Chinese population.

RESULTS AND DISCUSSION

The results of the above analyses are shown in Table 1.

There have been several earlier studies in Singapore on dialect group differentials in the incidence of NPC. In the first study, Mekie & Lawley (1954) analysed 119 Chinese patients seen at the Singapore General Hospital between 1947 and 1953. These comprised 34 Cantonese (28.6%), 33 Hokkien (27.7%), 18 Hainanese (15.1%), 12 Hakka (Khek) (10.1%), 17 Teochew (14.3%) and 5 others (4.2%). The authors stated that the percentages of Hainanese and Hakka (Khek) patients in their series were significantly higher than those reported in the 1947 census of population (7.2% and 5.5%, respectively). Since the Hakka community is a relatively heterogeneous group and of northern Chinese origin, this finding has been used as an argument against the hypothesis of a genetic predisposition to the disease. We have been unable to confirm the statistical significance of these differences. In other studies, Hakka (Khek) patients were shown to be at relatively lower risk than the rest of the Chinese population. Mekie & Lawley (1954) also noted that the percentages of Hokkien and Teochew in their study were considerably lower than those in the general Chinese population. They made no observations regarding the Cantonese.

These authors made no separation of cases by sex in their analysis, and this would constitute a source of bias in view of significant differences in the sex ratios of the various dialect groups due to differences in migratory patterns. Throughout the 19th century,

Table 1. Incidence of nasopharyngeal cancer among ethnic groups and Chinese dialect groups in Singapore (1968-1972)

	Males			Females		
	No. of cases	Rate[a]	Ratio[b]	No. of cases	Rate[a]	Ratio[b]
Chinese dialect groups						
Hokkien	159	14.1	0.75	52	4.7	0.66
Teochew	112	18.3	0.98	42	6.2	0.87
Cantonese	146	29.1	1.56	82	11.0	1.55
Hainanese	38	14.2	0.76	8	3.3	0.46
Hakka (Khek)	24	12.6	0.67	10	4.8	0.68
Other dialects	19	12.2	0.65	6	6.0	0.85
Dialect unknown	19	-	-	12	-	-
Ethnic groups						
Chinese	517	18.7	1.00	212	7.1	1.00
Malays	23	4.8	0.26	3	0.6	0.08
Indians	4	0.9	0.05	0	0.0	0.00

[a] Incidence rate per 100,000 per year, age-standardized to world population (Doll et al., 1970)

[b] Ratio of incidence rate in each ethnic and Chinese dialect group to that in the total Chinese population

immigration to Singapore was principally of males in the working age groups. Following the depression during the early 1930s, strict controls were imposed on the immigration of Chinese men; however, since Chinese women were exempted from such controls, there was a net immigration of some 200,000 Chinese women, virtually all Cantonese, between 1934-38 into the combined territories of Malaya and Singapore (Ginsberg & Roberts, 1958). In subsequent censuses of population, the Cantonese were the only dialect group in which women outnumbered men. The emigration of Hainanese women, on the other hand, was particularly restricted, leading to a marked excess of males in this community. The sex ratios in the censuses held in 1947 and 1957 were 1.13 and 1.06, respectively, for Hokkien, 1.21 and 1.07 for Teochew, 0.82 and 0.81 for Cantonese, 1.80 and 1.29 for Hainanese and 1.30 and 1.15 for Hakka (Chua, 1964; del Tufo, 1949). The sex ratio differentials were more marked in the age groups in which most cases of NPC occurred; in the 1957 census the male:female ratios for persons aged 35 years and over were 1.05 for Hokkien, 1.07 for Teochew, 0.62 for Cantonese, 1.76 for Hainanese and 1.22 for Hakka (Chua, 1964). Furthermore, it is evident that the enumeration of the Hakka (Khek) population in the earlier censuses may have been inaccurate (del Tufo, 1949). In the analysis of Mekie & Lawley (1954), such inaccuracies and the differences between the sex ratio in their series of NPC patients (3:1) and those in the various dialect group populations may have spuriously inflated the risks among Hainanese and Hakkas and obscured a higher risk in Cantonese.

The next investigation was a hospital-based, case-control study in which Shanmugaratnam & Tye (1970) analysed dialect group differences in incidence of NPC separately for Singapore-born and for China-born Chinese. They reported (a) that Cantonese have a relatively higher risk (1.7 ×, $P < 0.01$) for NPC compared with all other groups, (b) that Hokkiens have a relatively lower risk (0.6 ×, $P < 0.01$), (c) that these patterns for Cantonese and Hokkiens persist among both immigrants and Singapore-born Chinese, (d) that a higher risk for Hainanese is observed only among those born in China and (e) that Hakkas may have a lower-than-average relative risk.

The present report, based on comprehensive cancer registration, shows that while all of the specific Chinese communities or dialect groups in Singapore have high risks for NPC, only the Cantonese have a risk significantly higher than that for the rest of the Chinese population. This finding is not due to differences in the use of hospital facilities by the various Chinese dialect groups in Singapore. Such a bias is, indeed, most unlikely, because the dialect group differences observed in the Cancer Registry have not occurred across the board but have varied in extent and type for different cancer sites; for example, the incidence levels of oesophageal and stomach cancers are significantly higher among the Hokkiens and Teochews than among the Cantonese (Shanmugaratnam, 1973). We are therefore confident that the dialect group differentials reported in this paper represent real differences in risk.

It is beyond the scope of this paper to examine in any detail the genetic and cultural differences that may be related to these cancer risk differentials. The hypothesis that the development of NPC is due to the action of some environmental carcinogen(s) in genetically susceptible persons has been strengthened by the demonstration of case-control differences in HLA antigen profiles. Simons et al. (1974, 1976) have shown that NPC patients have increased frequencies of HLA antigen A_2 in the first locus (relative risk, 2.24) and of unidentified antigens ('blank') in the second locus (relative risk, 2.60). They reported that the first locus HLA-A_2 and the second locus 'blank' appeared to act together (HLA-A_2 blank haplotype) in determining NPC risk in Cantonese patients, who are at highest risk, whereas they appeared to act independently in Hokkiens and Teochews, who are at a relatively lower risk. There is an indication, therefore, that differences in incidence of NPC in the dialect groups may be related to the strength of the associations between these HLA antigens.

The Chinese dialect groups in Singapore are not merely linguistic groups but are specific communities with cultural differences that may be related to their patterns of cancer incidence. Some of the traditional differences in occupation, economic status and areas of residence that were obvious some 30 years ago are much less evident today as a result of changes in life styles consequential to industrialization and massive relocations due to public housing programmes. However, there are still important differences, particularly in use of food items and their preparation, that may be relevant to patterns of cancer incidence.

SUMMARY

A total of 729 cases of NPC (93.6% confirmed histologically) were diagnosed among the Singapore Chinese population during a five-year period (1968-1972). Age-standardized incidence rates for the total Chinese population were 18.4 per 100,000 per year for males and 7.0 for females; the respective rates for the specific Chinese communities were 14.1 and 4.7 for Hokkien, 18.3 and 6.2 for Teochew, 29.1 and 11.0 for Cantonese, 14.2 and 3.3 for Hainanese, 12.6 and 4.8 for Hakka and 12.2 and 6.0 for the other dialect groups. It is evident that all of the Chinese communities in Singapore have high risks for NPC; only the Cantonese have risks significantly higher than that for the rest of the Chinese population. NPC incidence rates for males and females of the other major racial groups in Singapore were 4.7 and 0.6 for Malays and 0.9 and 0.0 for Indians, respectively.

ACKNOWLEDGEMENTS

Mrs W.K. Quah, Mrs C.L. Yap and Miss L.W. Quek provided secretarial assistance. This investigation was supported in part by IARC Collaborative Research Agreement RA/67/009.

REFERENCES

Arumainathan, P. (1973) *Report on the Census of Population 1970 Singapore*, Singapore, Government Printing Office

Buell, P. (1965) Nasopharynx cancer in Chinese of California. *Brit. J. Cancer, 19*, 459-470

Buell, P. (1974) The effect of migration on the risk of nasopharyngeal cancer among Chinese. *Cancer Res., 34*, 1189-1191

Chua, S.C. (1964) *State of Singapore. Report on the Census of Population, 1957*. Singapore, Government Printer

del Tufo, M.V. (1949) *Malaya, Comprising the Federation of Malaya and the Colony of Singapore. A Report on the 1947 Census of Population*, Kuala Lumpur, Government Printer

Doll, R., Muir, C.S. & Waterhouse, J., eds (1970) *Cancer Incidence in Five Continents*, Vol. II, Geneva, International Union Against Cancer

Ginsberg, N. & Roberts, C.F. (1958) *Malaya*, Seattle, University of Washington Press, p. 251

Ho, H.C. (1967) *Nasopharyngeal carcinoma in Hong Kong*. In: Muir, C.S. & Shanmugaratnam, K., eds, *Cancer of the Nasopharynx (UICC Monograph Series No. 1)*, Copenhagen, Munksgaard, pp. 58-63

Ho, J.H.C. (1972) Nasopharyngeal carcinoma (NPC). *Advanc. Cancer Res., 15*, 57-92

Hu, C.H. & Yang, C. (1959) A decade of progress in morphologic pathology. *Chin. med. J., 79*, 409-422

Jung, P.F. & Yu, C. (1963) Nasopharyngeal carcinoma in China. *Postgrad. med. J., 33*, 77-82

Liang, P.C. (1964) Studies on nasopharyngeal carcinoma in the Chinese: statistical and laboratory investigations. *Chin. med. J., 83*, 373-390

Mekie, D.E.C. & Lawley, M. (1954) Nasopharyngeal carcinoma: clinical analysis of 120 cases. *Arch. Surg., 69*, 841-848

Shanmugaratnam, K. (1971) Studies on the etiology of nasopharyngeal carcinoma. *Int. Rev. exp. Path., 10*, 361-413

Shanmugaratnam, K. (1973) Cancer in Singapore - ethnic and dialect group variations in cancer incidence. *Singapore med. J., 14*, 69-81

Shanmugaratnam, K. (1976) *Cancer incidence in Singapore 1968-1972*. In: Waterhouse, J., Muir, C., Correa, P. & Powell, J., eds, *Cancer Incidence in Five Continents*, Vol. 3 (*IARC Scientific Publications No. 15*), Lyon, pp. 280-291

Shanmugaratnam, K. & Tye, C.Y. (1970) A study of nasopharyngeal cancer among Singapore Chinese with special reference to migrant status and specific community. *J. chron. Dis., 23*, 433-441

Shanmugaratnam, K. & Wee, A. (1973) *'Dialect group' variations in cancer incidence among Chinese in Singapore*. In: Doll, R. & Vodopija, I., eds, *Host-Environmental Interactions in the Etiology of Cancer in Man* (*IARC Scientific Publications No. 7*), Lyon, pp. 67-82

Simons, M.J., Wee, G.B., Day, N.E., Morris, P.J., Shanmugaratnam, K. & de-Thé, G.B. (1974) Immunogenetic aspects of nasopharyngeal carcinoma. I. Differences in HL-A antigen profiles between patients and control groups. *Int. J. Cancer, 13*, 122-134

Simons, M.J., Wee, G.B., Goh, E.H., Chan, S.H., Shanmugaratnam, K., Day, N.E. & de-Thé, G. (1976) Immunogenetic aspects of nasopharyngeal carcinoma. IV. Increased risk in Chinese of nasopharyngeal carcinoma associated with a Chinese-related HLA profile (A_2, Singapore 2). *J. nat. Cancer Inst., 57*, 977-980

Zippin, C., Tekawa, I.S., Bragg, K.U., Watson, D.A. & Linden, G. (1962) Studies on heredity and environment in cancer of the nasopharynx. *J. nat. Cancer Inst., 29*, 483-490

ETIOLOGICAL FACTORS IN NASOPHARYNGEAL CARCINOMA: A HOSPITAL-BASED, RETROSPECTIVE, CASE-CONTROL, QUESTIONNAIRE STUDY

K. SHANMUGARATNAM

Department of Pathology,
University of Singapore
Outram Road,
Singapore 3, Singapore

C.Y. TYE

Department of Social Medicine and Public Health,
Institute of Health,
Outram Hill,
Singapore 3, Singapore

E.H. GOH & K.B. CHIA

Ear, Nose & Throat Department and
Department of Radiotherapy,
Singapore General Hospital,
Outram Road,
Singapore 3, Singapore

INTRODUCTION

Epidemiological evidence suggests that the development of nasopharyngeal carcinoma (NPC) is due in most cases to the action of environmental factors in genetically susceptible persons (Ho, 1972b; Shanmugaratnam, 1971). The existence of a genetic susceptibility, as indicated by the high risks for Chinese populations living in different countries (Ho, 1967, 1972a; Martin & Quan, 1951; Shanmugaratnam, 1967, 1971) and by reports of familial clustering (Ho, 1972a), has been further demonstrated by the observation of significant differences between the HLA antigen profiles of NPC patients and those of persons without this tumour (Simons et al., 1974, 1976). That environmental factors play a role is supported by reports of differences in incidence and mortality rates for the disease between US- and China-born Chinese (Buell, 1965, 1974; Zippin, 1962).

The hypothesis that infection by the Epstein-Barr virus (EBV) is an important factor in the etiology of NPC is based largely on the fact that patients with the disease have consistently shown substantially higher mean titres of antibodies against various EBV-related antigens (Henle et al., 1970; Klein et al., 1970) and on the demonstration of EBV genomes in the tumour cells (Wolf et al., 1973; zur Hausen et al., 1970).

The proposal that the consumption of salted fish may be etiologically related to NPC (Ho, 1972b) is supported by the demonstration of nitrosamines in this food item (Fong & Chan, 1973; Fong & Walsh, 1971). Hypotheses that the use of snuffs (Hou-Jensen, 1964) and the inhalation of smoke from burning incense (Sturton et al., 1966) and cooking fuels (Clifford & Beecher, 1964) may be etiologically involved have been supported by the demonstration of carcinogenic hydrocarbons in these materials (Cooper & Campbell, 1955; Schoental & Gibbard, 1967).

There have been few epidemiological studies to test these hypotheses. Three case-control, questionnaire studies have been reported to date, in Singapore (Shanmugaratnam & Higginson, 1967), in Taiwan (Lin et al., 1973) and in California (Henderson et al., 1976). The first study in Singapore, with 63 patients and with 63 controls matched crudely by race, sex and 20-year age groups, was essentially a pilot study designed to explore a wide variety of suspected factors. The present investigation was undertaken to examine the role of selected socio-environmental factors in a larger series of cases and controls.

MATERIALS AND METHODS

Interview procedures

All cases and controls were interviewed between March 1966 and August 1968 by three instructed, experienced interviewers in the language and dialect of the interviewees. The questionnaire covered a variety of items, including social factors, medical history and exposure to selected substances by ingestion and inhalation. The answers were coded directly on the questionnaire and checked for consistency by one of us (KS).

The interviewers visited various clinics and hospital wards, according to a fixed schedule, and interviewed all of the cases and as many controls as time permitted, working systematically from bed to bed. Persons excluded from interview were patients who had been interviewed previously, patients who were too ill to be interviewed, patients absent from the wards for special examinations and patients who were unwilling to cooperate; there were very few in the last category.

Cases: The study comprised 379 Chinese patients with NPC in the clinics (outpatients) and wards (inpatients) of the Ear, Nose and Throat Department of the Outram Road General Hospital (now Singapore General Hospital) in whom the diagnosis of NPC had been confirmed by histological examination of the primary neoplasm.

Controls: Two groups of controls were used:

(1) Ear, Nose and Throat Department controls (ENTC), comprising 595 Chinese patients in the same clinics and wards as the NPC cases but with complaints other than NPC.

(2) Other hospital controls (OHC), comprising 1044 Chinese patients in the medical, surgical and orthopaedic (casualty) wards of the Outram Road and Thomson Road General Hospitals (now Toa Payoh Hospital) with diseases other than cancer or otorhinolaryngeal diseases. These two general hospitals were the only ones administered by the Singapore Ministry of Health during the period of this study. Only the former has an Ear, Nose and Throat Department.

All cases and controls were permanent residents of Singapore. Their distribution by age and sex is shown in Table 1. The controls, being hospital patients, may not be representative of the total Chinese population in Singapore; they were, however, comparable with the study group in as much as they represented groups of patients seeking treatment in government hospitals.

Cases and controls were not matched by socio-economic status. The great majority of NPC and ENTC were outpatients, whereas the majority of OHC were inpatients. Since most inpatients were non-paying and since outpatients may more often be persons from the upper income level, it was surmised that the ENTC group may contain relatively more persons from the higher socio-economic levels and the OHC group relatively more persons from the lower socio-economic levels than did the group of NPC patients. While these differences are not expected to be substantial, they should be considered in the interpretation of results.

Statistical procedures

Matching of controls by age and sex was not attempted because it was intended to use the controls for studies of other cancer sites which differ in these respects; differences are shown in Table 1. In addition, preliminary analysis revealed that the three interviewers showed significant heterogeneity in classifying some of the factors under study, despite prior efforts to promote uniformity of criteria

Table 1. Distribution of nasopharyngeal carcinoma cases and controls by age and sex

Age (yrs)	Cases		ENT controls		Other hospital controls	
	M	F	M	F	M	F
0- 9	0	0	0	0	1	0
10-19	4	1	21	22	32	7
20-29	21	5	65	41	82	23
30-39	54	25	94	62	113	51
40-49	76	32	56	70	138	64
50-59	73	37	45	52	179	107
60-69	29	9	27	30	140	46
70+	9	4	3	7	53	8
Total	266	113	311	284	738	306

ENT - Ear, Nose & Throat Department

and definition. Consequently, all comparisons reported below between the cases and each of the two control groups were adjusted for age, sex and interviewer. The method employed for obtaining the average relative risk and the summary corrected chi square with one degree of freedom was that of Mantel & Haenszel (1959).

RESULTS AND DISCUSSION

Results of analyses of 17 items in the questionnaire are summarized in Tables 2, 3, 4 and 5. The relative risks for NPC for each of the variables under investigation are shown separately with respect to the ENTC and the OHC groups.

Occupation

No single occupational group was shown to be at higher risk for NPC. In comparison with OHC, but not with ENTC (Table 2a), NPC cases comprised more persons of 'unknown' occupation and fewer workers in transport and communications. This finding (significant at the $P = 0.05$ level) probably reflects the bias towards a lower economic status in the OHC group.

Table 2. Social factors in the development of nasopharyngeal carcinoma (NPC)

	NPC patients compared with			
	ENT controls		Other hospital controls	
	Relative risk	χ^2	Relative risk	χ^2
(a) Occupation				
Professional and technical workers	0.721	0.484	1.429	0.743
Executive and managerial workers	(0.839)	0.000	(1.214)	0.000
Clerical workers	0.995	0.000	1.375	1.720
Sales workers	0.903	0.067	0.894	0.158
Agricultural workers and fishermen	0.770	0.222	0.574	3.034
Miners and quarrymen	(0.298)	0.241	(1.014)	0.000
Workers in transport and communications	0.797	0.328	0.537	5.329[a]
Craftsmen and labourers not classified elsewhere	1.281	1.827	0.954	0.056
Service, entertainment and recreation workers	1.197	0.624	0.982	0.000
Unknown	0.899	0.160	1.729	6.191[a]
(b) Level of education				
None, illiterate	1.339	2.110	0.934	0.130
None, literate	1.217	0.178	1.017	0.000
Primary school	0.871	0.661	0.771	3.298
Secondary school	0.914	0.106	1.557	5.450[a]
Other	(0.000)	0.000	(0.000)	0.001
College/University	0.739	0.182	3.379	3.853[a]
Unknown			(0.000)	0.000
(c) Language medium of education				
English	0.883	0.314	1.159	0.455
Chinese	0.874	0.549	0.988	0.000
Other	1.301	2.080	0.924	0.209

ENT - Ear, Nose & Throat Department

[a] $p < 0.05$

Values in parentheses are based on fewer than 5 NPC cases.

Several previous studies have indicated that there is no relationship between NPC and occupation (Ch'in & Szutu, 1940; Lin et al., 1973; Martin & Quan, 1951; Shanmugaratnam & Higginson, 1967). On the other hand, Andrews & Michaels (1968) reported the occurrence of NPC in three pilots of French, Finnish and British extraction, and Henderson et al. (1976) have reported positive associations with occupational exposures to fumes (2.0 ×), smoke (3.0 ×) and chemicals (2.4 ×). It is interesting to note that occupational exposures to nickel, chromium and radioactive materials have been associated with cancers of the nasal cavity, paranasal sinuses, larynx and lungs but not with nasopharyngeal cancer.

Education

Level of education (Table 2b) was investigated as a possible indicator of socio-economic status. A significantly higher relative risk was found for NPC patients with secondary and tertiary education when compared with OHC; however, this risk was marginally lower when the cases were compared with ENTC. These differences could again be due to bias in the composition of the control groups.

The language medium of education (Table 2c) was also included in the study, since persons who had attended Chinese medium schools could be expected to adhere more closely to certain customs that may be related to NPC. There were no significant differences between cases and either set of controls.

Nasal illnesses

A personal history of previous nasal illnesses during adult life (Table 3a) was associated with a significantly higher risk for NPC in those patients in comparison with both ENTC (2.8 ×) and OHC (40.2 ×);

Table 3. History of nasal illnesses in relation to the development of nasopharyngeal carcinoma (NPC)

	NPC patients compared with			
	ENT controls		Other hospital controls	
	Relative risk	χ^2	Relative risk	χ^2
(a) Personal history of nasal illnesses				
None	0.306	58.034[c]	0.022	614.988[c]
Yes, during childhood only	(0.476)	0.351	(0.881)	0.000
Yes, during adulthood only	2.756	45.326[c]	40.245	521.858[c]
Yes, throughout life	1.069	0.007	19.962	36.193[c]
Unknown	5.093	5.307[a]	4.296	8.074[b]
(b) Family history of nasal illnesses				
Yes	0.579	3.627	2.701	8.274[b]
No, or unknown	1.727	3.627	0.370	8.274

ENT - Ear, Nose & Throat Department

[a] $P < 0.05$ [b] $P < 0.01$ [c] $P < 0.001$

Values in parentheses are based on fewer than 5 NPC cases

in comparison with OHC, a higher risk (20.0 ×) was observed for NPC patients who had had illnesses during both childhood and adult life (all significant at P< 0.001). It is, of course, more than likely that the very nature of NPC may promote some bias in memory. However, the findings may also suggest that the environmental agent(s) responsible for NPC predispose to other nasal illnesses or, alternatively, that some non-malignant nasal or nasopharyngeal illness may predispose the nasopharyngeal mucosa to the action of environmental carcinogens. A positive relationship with previous nasal symptoms was also recorded by Lin et al. (1973) and Henderson et al. (1976).

A family history of nasal illnesses (Table 3b) was associated with a higher risk (8.3 ×) for NPC patients when compared with OHC and with a lower risk (0.6 ×) in comparison with ENTC. While these differences may be due, at least in part, to bias in memory due to the nature of their present illnesses, the possibility remains that a family history of some form of nasal illness may be associated with a higher risk for both NPC patients and ENTC, since the latter group included patients with various nasal allergies.

Use of Chinese medicines

The customary use of Chinese medicines in treating illnesses of various sorts (Table 4a) was associated with an elevated risk (1.5 ×, significant at P = 0.05) when compared with OHC. The use of Chinese medicines specifically for the nose and throat was associated with much higher risks for NPC patient's when compared with both ENTC and OHC (Table 4b). The risk differentials followed the same patterns as for

Table 4. Types of medicines used in relation to the development of nasopharyngeal carcinoma (NPC)

	NPC patients compared with			
	ENT controls		Other hospital controls	
	Relative risk	χ^2	Relative risk	χ^2
(a) Type of medicines usually used				
Chinese	1.261	1.380	1.470	5.478[a]
Other	0.793	1.380	0.680	5.478
(b) Use of Chinese medicines for nose and throat				
No	0.476	19.094[c]	0.110	165.201[c]
Yes, during childhood only	(0.834)	0.000	(0.703)	0.059
Yes, during adulthood only	2.033	15.715[c]	19.599	181.111[c]
Yes, throughout life	1.074	0.000	3.491	7.881[b]
Unknown	4.161	3.956[a]	1.629	0.674

ENT - Ear, Nose & Throat Department

[a] P < 0.05 [b] P < 0.01 [c] P < 0.001

Values in parentheses are based on fewer than 5 NPC cases.

personal history of nasal illnesses (Table 3a) and may to a large extent be due to use of such medicines after the development of cancer. They are applied directly, sometimes by inhaling or blowing powdered preparations into the nasal passages. Lin et al. (1973) also found a higher use of herbal drugs and nasal balms and oils among NPC patients. The chemistry and biological effects of such medicines should be investigated further.

Ingested substances

The use of soya sauce more than twice daily was associated with a significantly higher risk in NPC patients (1.5 ×, significant at P = 0.01) when compared with OHC (Table 5a). However, the absence of a clear dose-response pattern or of significant differences in comparison with ENTC raise the possibility of bias. The occasional consumption of Chinese tea (once daily) was associated with a reduced risk for NPC (0.7 ×) when compared with OHC, but the fluctuating dose-response pattern suggests that this difference is spurious (Table 5b). No relationship between NPC and the drinking of Chinese tea was observed by Lin et al. (1973) or Henderson et al. (1976).

There were no significant differences in risk of NPC with respect to the use of various so-called cooling drinks (Table 5c) or to the consumption of alcohol (Table 5d).

Cigarettes

Persons who had smoked cigarettes for 10 years or more had a higher risk for NPC when compared with ENTC, but there was no significant difference when compared with OHC. The pattern of distribution in Tables 6a and 6b suggests that the risk differential with ENTC, although highly significant, arose from the presence of more non-smokers and fewer smokers of long duration in the ENTC group rather than from any positive relationship between NPC and cigarette smoking. Lin et al. (1973) found that persons who smoked more than 20 cigarettes per day had more than twice the risk for NPC than those who had never smoked; they found no significant difference with past smokers and light smokers. However, other investigators (Henderson et al., 1976; Martin & Blady, 1940; Shanmugaratnam & Higginson, 1967; Simmons & Ariel, 1949) have failed to find any positive relationship between NPC and cigarette smoking. The fact that the remarkable geographical distribution of NPC bears no relationship to patterns of cigarette consumption or to the incidence of lung cancer indicates that it is most unlikely that cigarette smoking is an important causal factor.

Cooking fuels

The relative risk for NPC was significantly less in users of gas (0.6 ×) and significantly more in users of firewood (1.7 ×) when compared with ENTC (Table 6c). No significant differences were observed when compared with OHC. It is possible that the difference arose from the greater use of gas and lesser use of firewood by ENTC,

Table 5. Ingested substances in relation to the development of nasopharyngeal carcinoma (NPC)

	NPC patients compared with			
	ENT controls		Other hospital controls	
	Relative risk	χ^2	Relative risk	χ^2
(a) Soya sauce				
< Once daily	0.618	1.825	0.786	0.394
Once daily	1.694	1.641	1.085	0.020
Twice daily	0.837	1.007	0.790	2.986
> Twice daily	1.314	1.689	1.532	6.730[b]
Unknown	0.973	0.000	0.754	0.133
(b) Chinese tea				
< Once monthly	0.930	0.101	1.052	0.039
< Once daily	0.934	0.114	0.742	3.902[a]
Daily	1.166	0.568	1.279	3.042
Unknown	1.060	0.000	1.099	0.000
(c) 'Cooling' drinks				
Never or unknown	0.920	0.197	0.884	0.518
< Once weekly	0.896	0.364	1.034	0.012
Weekly or more	1.283	1.663	1.087	0.298
(d) Alcohol				
Never	0.895	0.537	0.792	2.777
< Once monthly	1.030	0.020	1.342	2.843
< Once weekly	0.803	0.330	0.889	0.119
< Once daily	1.176	0.249	0.959	0.043
Daily	1.497	1.882	1.345	2.023
Unknown	0.786	0.242	0.903	0.055

ENT - Ear, Nose & Throat Department

[a] $P < 0.05$ [b] $P < 0.01$

since this group may include more persons of a higher socio-economic and educational level (Table 2b). It is also relevant that there have been marked changes in the use of cooking fuels in Singapore during the last 20 years. Although the question referred to the main type of fuel used over a period of more than 10 years, there may have been differences in interpretation by responders.

Table 6. Inhaled substances in relation to the development of nasopharyngeal carcinoma (NPC)

	NPC patients compared with			
	ENT controls		Other hospital controls	
	Relative risk	χ^2	Relative risk	χ^2
(a) Cigarettes - duration				
Never	0.659	5.609[a]	1.052	0.091
< 1 year	(3.895)	1.385	(1.972)	0.375
1-4 years	0.620	1.369	0.802	0.146
5-9 years	0.560	2.645	0.814	0.235
10+ years	1.840	11.171[c]	0.929	0.198
Unknown	2.825	2.005	1.888	1.459
(b) Cigarettes - frequency				
Never or unknown	0.704	3.887[a]	1.113	0.486
1-10 per day	1.141	0.237	1.004	0.000
11-20 per day	1.146	0.239	0.981	0.000
> 20 per day	1.291	1.566	0.896	0.504
(c) Cooking fuels				
Gas	0.585	9.414[b]	0.904	0.289
Electricity	1.048	0.000	1.280	0.814
Charcoal	0.691	2.715	0.754	1.661
Firewood	1.713	7.474[b]	0.866	0.773
Kerosene	1.260	1.996	1.246	2.279
Other			(1.728)	0.000
Unknown	1.142	0.133	1.125	0.061
(d) Incense - duration				
Never	0.942	0.028	1.310	2.165
Yes, during childhood only	0.582	1.785	0.594	1.981
Yes, during adulthood only	(0.329)	0.680	(0.302)	0.871
Yes, throughout life	1.239	1.205	0.962	0.061
Unknown	1.245	0.000	1.455	0.047
(e) Incense - frequency				
Never	0.784	1.249	1.275	1.830
< Once weekly	0.895	0.372	0.930	0.184
Weekly or more	1.272	2.335	1.048	0.032
Unknown	0.971	0.000	0.530	2.898
(f) Anti-mosquito coils				
Yes	1.418	5.852[a]	1.320	4.116[a]
No or unknown	0.705	5.852	0.758	4.116

ENT - Ear, Nose & Throat Department

[a] $P < 0.05$ [b] $P < 0.01$ [c] $P < 0.001$

Values in parentheses are based on fewer than 5 NPC cases.

Incense

There was no difference in the use of incense between cases and either set of controls (Tables 6d and 6e). Negative results in this regard were also obtained by Lin et al. (1973); however, Sturton et al. (1966) found that in comparison with other cancer patients, NPC cases included more persons exposed to burning incense (this observation was only true for males below the age of 50 [P = 0.05] and not for males over the age of 50 or for females).

Anti-mosquito coils

Exposure to fumes from burning anti-mosquito coils was associated with higher risks for NPC when compared with both ENTC (1.4 ×) and OHC (1.3 ×), both significant at P = 0.05 (Table 6f). Further investigations are needed to confirm this association and to study the effects of smoky atmospheres in general.

COMMENTS

Housing conditions were not included in our study since it was difficult to obtain comparable information on the basis of hospital interviews. Lin et al. (1973) reported that persons working under poorly ventilated conditions have an NPC risk more than twice that in persons without this experience. The hypothesis that the use of salted fish and braised or dried vegetables may be etiologically involved in NPC (Ho, 1972a, b) was also not included in this study. Henderson et al. (1976) found no relationship with current use of salted fish; however, in view of the finding of nitrosamines in both of these items, they should be investigated in future studies.

The large number of comparisons resulting from the responses of NPC patients for each of the 77 variables comprising the 17 items investigated in this study and those of each of two groups of controls may have produced some positive results simply because statistically significant differences may be expected in 5% of comparisons on the basis of chance alone. It must also be remembered that the NPC cases and the control groups might have been subject to different degrees of selection by socio-economic status: as explained above, there is a possibility that one of the control groups (ENTC) may have comprised relatively more persons at the higher socio-economic level and that the other (OHC) may have comprised relatively more persons at the lower socio-economic level. It is important that this possible source of bias be kept in mind in evaluating the biological significance of the observed differences. For these reasons, differences with respect to only one of the control groups are not likely to be important unless they were of a high order of statistical significance (say, P = 0.01) and also showed a clear, sequential dose-response pattern.

SUMMARY

A total of 379 Singapore Chinese patients with NPC were interviewed by use of a questionnaire covering the following items: occupation, level of education, language medium of education, personal and family history of nasal illnesses, types of medicines used, use of Chinese medicines for the nose and throat, use of soya sauce, Chinese tea, cooling drinks and alcohol, cigarette smoking (number and duration), cooking fuels and use of incense (frequency and duration) and of anti-mosquito coils. The same questionnaire was given to two groups of controls: 595 patients with diseases of the ear, nose and throat other than NPC and 1 044 patients with diseases other than cancer or otorhinolaryngeal disease. NPC patients differed significantly from both groups of controls in that they showed stronger associations with personal history of nasal illnesses, family history of nasal illnesses, use of Chinese medicines for the nose and throat and exposure to smoke from anti-mosquito coils.

ACKNOWLEDGEMENTS

The cases and controls used in this investigation were provided by the heads of the respective hospital units. The interviewers were Miss H.C. Ng, Miss C. Wong and Mrs Y.S. Wong. Mrs W.K. Quah, Mrs C.L. Yap, Miss L.W. Quek and Miss S.K. Tan provided secretarial assistance. This investigation was supported in part by Public Health Service Research Grant No. CA 08448 from the National Cancer Institute, USA.

REFERENCES

Andrews, P.A.J. & Michaels, L. (1968) Aviator's cancer. *Lancet, ii*, 85, 640

Buell, P. (1965) Nasopharynx cancer in Chinese of California. *Brit. J. Cancer, 19*, 459-470

Buell, P. (1974) The effect of migration on the risk of nasopharyngeal cancer among Chinese. *Cancer Res., 34*, 1189-1191

Ch'in, K.Y. & Szutu, C. (1940) Lymphoepithelioma, a pathological study of 97 cases. *Chin. med. J., Suppl III*, 94-119

Clifford, P. & Beecher, J.L. (1964) Nasopharyngeal cancer in Kenya: clinical and environmental aspects. *Brit. J. Cancer, 18*, 25-43

Cooper, R.L. & Campbell, J.M. (1955) The etiology of respiratory tract cancer in the South African Bantu, II. Chemical identification of carcinogens. *Brit. J. Cancer, 9*, 533-538

Fong, Y.Y. & Chan, W.C. (1973) Bacterial production of di-methyl nitrosamine in salted fish. *Nature (Lond.), 243*, 421-422

Fong, Y.Y. & Walsh, E.O. (1971) Carcinogenic nitrosamines in Cantonese salt dried fish. *Lancet, ii*, 1032

Henderson, B.E., Louie, E.R.N., Jing, J.S.H., Buell, P. & Gardner, M.B. (1976) Risk factors associated with nasopharyngeal carcinoma. *New Engl. J. Med., 295*, 1101-1106

Henle, W., Henle, G., Ho, H.C., Burtin, P., Cachin, Y., Clifford, P., de Schryver, A., de-Thé, G., Diehl, V. & Klein, G. (1970) Antibodies to Epstein-Barr virus in nasopharyngeal carcinoma, other head and neck neoplasms and control groups. *J. nat. Cancer Inst., 44*, 225-231

Ho, H.C. (1967) *Nasopharyngeal carcinoma in Hong Kong*. In: Muir, C.S. & Shanmugaratnam, K., eds, *Cancer of the Nasopharynx (UICC Monograph Series No. 1)* Copenhagen, Munksgaard, pp. 58-63

Ho, H.C. (1972a) *Current knowledge of the epidemiology of nasopharyngeal carcinoma - a review*. In: Biggs, P.M., de-Thé, G. & Payne, L.N., eds, *Oncogenesis and Herpesviruses (IARC Scientific Publications No. 2)*, Lyon, pp. 357-366

Ho, J.H.C. (1972b) Nasopharyngeal carcinoma (NPC). *Advanc. Cancer Res., 15*, 57-92

Hou-Jensen, K. (1964) On the occurrence of post nasal space tumours in Kenya. *Brit. J. Cancer, 18*, 58-68

Klein, G., Geering, G., Old, L.J., Henle, G., Henle, W. & Clifford, P. (1970) Comparison of the anti-EBV titer and the EBV-associated membrane reactive and precipitating antibody levels in the sera of Burkitt lymphoma and nasopharyngeal carcinoma patients and controls. *Int. J. Cancer, 5*, 185-194

Lin, T.M., Chen, K.P., Lin, C.C., Hsu, M.M., Tu, S.M., Chiang, T.C., Jung, P.F. & Hirayama, T. (1973) Retrospective study on nasopharyngeal carcinoma. *J. nat. Cancer Inst., 51*, 1403-1408

Mantel, N. & Haenszel, W. (1959) Statistical aspects of the analysis of data from retrospective studies of disease. *J. nat. Cancer Inst., 22*, 719-748

Martin, H.E. & Blady, J.V. (1940) Cancer of nasopharynx. *Arch. Otolaryngol. (Chicago), 32*, 696-727

Martin, H. & Quan, S. (1951) The racial incidence (Chinese) of nasopharyngeal cancer. *Ann. Otolaryngol. (St. Louis)*, *60*, 168-174

Schoental, R. & Gibbard, S. (1967) Carcinogens in Chinese incense smoke. *Nature (Lond.)*, *216*, 612

Shanmugaratnam, K. (1967) *Nasopharyngeal carcinoma in Asia.* In: Shivas, A.A., ed, *Racial and Geographical Factors in Tumour Incidence (University of Edinburgh Press Monograph 2)*, Edinburgh, pp. 169-188

Shanmugaratnam, K. (1971) Studies on the etiology of nasopharyngeal carcinoma. *Int. Rev. exp. Path.*, *10*, 361-413

Shanmugaratnam, K. & Higginson, J. (1967) *Aetiology of nasopharyngeal cancer: report on a retrospective survey in Singapore.* In: Muir, C.S. & Shanmugaratnam, K., eds, *Cancer of the Nasopharynx (UICC Monograph Series No. 1)*, Copenhagen, Munksgaard, pp. 130-134

Simmons, M.W. & Ariel, I.M. (1949) Carcinoma of nasopharynx: report of 150 cases. *Surg. Gynec. Obstet.*, *88*, 763-775

Simons, M.J., Wee, G.B., Day, N.E., Morris, P.J., Shanmugaratnam, K. & de-Thé, G.B. (1974) Immunogenetic aspects of nasopharyngeal carcinoma. I. Differences in HL-A antigen profiles between patients and control groups. *Int. J. Cancer*, *13*, 122-134

Simons, M.J., Wee, G.B., Goh, E.H., Chan, S.H., Shanmugaratnam, K., Day, N.E. & de-Thé, G.B. (1976) Immunogenetic aspects of nasopharyngeal carcinoma. IV. Increased risk in Chinese of nasopharyngeal carcinoma associated with a Chinese-related HLA profile (A_2, Singapore 2). *J. nat. Cancer Inst.*, *57*, 977-980

Sturton, S.D., Wen, H.C. & Sturton, O.G. (1966) Etiology of cancer of the nasopharynx. *Cancer*, *19*, 1666-1669

Wolf, H., zur Hausen, H. & Becker, V. (1973) EB viral genomes in epithelial nasopharyngeal carcinoma cells. *Nature (Lond.)*, *244*, 245-247

Zippin, C., Tekewa, I.S., Bragg, K.U., Watson, D.A. & Linden, G. (1962) Studies on heredity and environment in cancer of the nasopharynx. *J. nat. Cancer Inst.*, *29*, 483-490

zur Hausen, H., Schulte-Holthausen, H., Klein, G., Henle, W., Henle, G., Clifford, P. & Santesson, B. (1970) EBV DNA in biopsies of Burkitt tumours and anaplastic carcinomas of the nasopharynx. *Nature (Lond.)*, *228*, 1056-1058

ENVIRONMENTAL FACTORS IN THE ETIOLOGY OF NASOPHARYNGEAL CARCINOMA: REPORT ON A CASE-CONTROL STUDY IN HONG KONG

A. GESER, N. CHARNAY, N.E. DAY & G. DE-THE

International Agency for Research on Cancer,
Lyon, France

H.C. HO

Department of Radiology and Oncology,
Queen Elizabeth Hospital,
Wylie Road,
Kowloon, Hong Kong

INTRODUCTION

The outstanding feature of the epidemiology of nasopharyngeal carcinoma (NPC) is that a high incidence is confined to Cantonese and several other South Chinese populations (Ho, 1967). Furthermore, Cantonese immigrants seem to bring their high incidence with them wherever they go: to Singapore (Shanmugaratnam, 1973), to Taiwan (Lin et al., 1971) or to the US (Buell, 1965; King & Haenszel, 1973; Zippin et al., 1962). The restriction of high risk to South Chinese populations suggests that genetically determined susceptibility plays an important role in the etiology of NPC. This impression has recently been reinforced by the finding that an HLA antigen profile is associated with a high risk for nasopharyngeal carcinoma (Simons et al., 1974, 1976).

That environmental factors may nevertheless be significant in the causation of NPC is indicated by studies on Chinese immigrants to the US (King & Haenszel, 1973), which disclosed that the mortality of NPC was lower in Chinese who were born in the US than in those born in China.

Many environmental factors have been proposed as possible risk factors in NPC, and some of these propositions have been supported by findings from controlled studies. Shanmugaratnam & Higginson (1967) compared the environments of NPC patients and those of other cancer and non-cancer patients in Singapore and found that the drinking of Chinese tea and education in the Chinese language medium were positively associated with NPC. However, the associations were weak, and the authors concluded that there was no basis for postulating a causal relationship.

Lin et al. (1973) compared the environments of NPC patients with those of neighbourhood controls in Taiwan and found that the smoking of cigarettes and working in poorly ventilated places were strongly associated with NPC. They also found positive associations with previous diseases of the nose, the use of nasal balms and marital status.

In a case-control study of NPC patients in California, Henderson et al. (1976) found that both previous diseases of the ear, nose or throat and occupational exposure to fumes, smoke and chemicals increased the risk for NPC.

Armstrong & Kutty[1] compared the 'self-specific' environment of NPC patients and controls in Malaysia and found that NPC is associated with lower socio-economic status, traditional lifestyle, a diet with less meat and fruit and possibly with levels of occupational air pollution.

The associations of some of the environmental factors described above with NPC risk were supported by several studies, others by only one. We report here the results of a further case-control study, carried out in Hong Kong, in the search for environmental factors in the causation of NPC.

MATERIALS AND METHODS

The aim of the retrospective study reported here was to compare NPC patients and controls to determine whether people who contract NPC have lived in a peculiar environment or have experienced anything different from their fellow citizens. The study was carried out by interviewing NPC patients and suitably selected controls (see below) with regard to experiences and exposures that have been incriminated in the etiology of NPC in the past (see de-Thé et al., 1976).

Since the recollections of patients (those with NPC as well as control patients) may be influenced by traumatic experiences during their illness, other adult members of each household were also interviewed regarding socio-economic conditions, religious practices and dietary habits in the household. In addition, a comparison was made

---

[1] Unpublished data

of weaning habits practised by mothers in the NPC and in the control families to see whether there was anything peculiar in the diet fed to the children in NPC families during this vulnerable period.

Environmental factors

The following factors, which have been implicated in the causation of NPC, were investigated in the interviews:

Demography: age, sex and marital status; place of origin, place of birth and length of residence

Socio-economic status: monthly income by individual and by family; number of domestic possessions of value; level of education; occupational status; religious habits

Dietary habits: consumption of cereals, meats, fish (including salt fish), vegetables, fats, dairy products and others; consumption of spices and condiments; preference for specific traditional Chinese dishes; preference for tinned foods

Drinking and smoking habits: consumption of tea, coffee, alcoholic drinks and soft drinks; smoking of cigarettes, cigars or pipes

Health and hygiene: previous illness, especially diseases of the ear, nose and throat; action taken in case of illness; choice of western or local practitioner or drugs; brushing of teeth; deaths in the family from cancer in general and from NPC in particular

Exposure to air pollution: domestic (from kitchen fires or incense burning); occupational

Weaning habits: length of time breast-fed; age of child at weaning; type of food given during and after weaning

Methods of analysis

The analysis of the present data consisted essentially of contrasting the NPC patients and their households with the control patients and their households in terms of frequency of exposure to environmental factors covered by the study.

Three types of comparison were made:

(1) NPC patients with controls 'proper', i.e., age- and sex-matched hospital controls paired with the NPC patients

(2) Households of NPC patients with those of control patients; here, the household is the unit, and the comparison units are paired as above

(3) Breast-feeding habits in households with an NPC case and in households without; here no pairing is involved.

Study population

The *NPC patients* were those hospitalized at the Department of Radiotherapy and Oncology, Queen Elizabeth Hospital, Hong Kong, between

January 1973 and February 1974; 150 NPC patients were selected (by rotation) for interviewing from a total of about 350 NPC admissions during this period. Nearly all NPC cases in Hong Kong are seen at this Department; the patients included in the study are thus representative of all NPC cases in Hong Kong.

Two sets of controls were used:

(1) *Hospital controls*: For each NPC patient a control patient was selected from the wards of the Queen Elizabeth Hospital. These controls were matched for sex and age, allowing for a variance of plus or minus five years. The intention was to use patients with other cancers hospitalized at the Queen Elizabeth Hospital at the time of the study, but it turned out to be difficult to find enough cancer patients to match NPC patients aged from 25-35 years; nine patients with thyreotoxicosis were therefore selected to supplement the controls. The numbers of controls in the various diagnostic groups were as follows:

Diagnosis	Sex	Number of controls
Lung cancer	M	34
	F	9
Cancer of mouth and	M	29
upper respiratory tract	F	13
Cancer of the digestive	M	15
tract	F	3
Other diseases, including	M	27
9 thyreotoxicoses	F	20
Total		150

It was realized that the use of lung cancer patients as controls would invalidate the comparison of smoking habits in NPC patients and controls, but since lung cancer patients constituted a major category of those available for matching with NPC patients, they were accepted into the study.

(2) *Household controls*: In each household (NPC as well as control), a special questionnaire was filled in during an interview with the senior woman of the household regarding socio-economic conditions, religious practices and dietary habits in the house.

Comparability of NPC patients and controls

The comparability of NPC patients and controls was assessed with respect to age and sex composition as well as place of origin in China.

This was carried out for the patients themselves (Table 1) as well as for the members of their households (Table 2).

Table 1. Age and sex distribution of patients with nasopharyngeal carcinoma (NPC) and control patients

Age (yrs)	Males			Females		
	NPC	Controls	Total	NPC	Controls	Total
15-19	1	1	2	0	0	0
20-24	1	3	4	2	2	4
25-29	3	1	4	0	1	1
30-34	7	4	11	4	2	6
35-39	7	4	11	5	2	7
40-44	15	15	30	7	6	13
45-49	20	14	34	8	14	22
50-54	15	22	37	10	6	16
55-59	15	11	26	3	5	8
60-64	13	20	33	2	2	4
65+	8	10	18	4	5	9
Total	105	105	210	45	45	90

The NPC families had a slight excess in the younger age groups (0-9 years for males and for females), with a corresponding shortage in the 20-29 year age group. This difference is small, but some difference in the lifestyle of the family groups might arise from the fact that the members of the NPC households are slightly younger than those of the control households.

Place of origin: Practically all families now living in Hong Kong migrated from some part of China in the past, the majority after the Second World War. The members of both NPC and non-NPC households (including the patients themselves) were questioned about their place of origin. The replies (Table 3) show that slightly more control families originated from provinces other than Kwangtung but that 96% of NPC families and 92% of non-NPC families came from that area.

Table 4 shows from where within Kwangtung the families originated. In both groups, most came from Canton and Hong Kong; however, 36.7% of the control families came from neighbouring areas (Sze Yop, Chiu Chau or Hakka), whereas only 24.7% of the NPC families did so. This

Table 2. Age and sex distribution of members of families of nasopharyngeal carcinoma (NPC) patients and control families

Age (yrs)	Males			Females		
	NPC families	Control families	Total	NPC families	Control families	Total
0- 4	24 (9.9)[a]	21 (8.3)	45	21 (7.2)	9 (3.1)	30
5- 9	30 (12.3)	25 (9.9)	55	39 (13.3)	26 (8.9)	65
10-14	46 (18.9)	41 (16.3)	87	47 (16.0)	47 (16.0)	94
15-19	48 (19.7)	46 (18.2)	94	41 (14.0)	50 (17.1)	91
20-29	45 (18.5)	67 (26.6)	112	41 (14.0)	64 (21.8)	105
30-39	10 (4.1)	15 (5.9)	25	20 (6.8)	16 (5.5)	36
40-49	14 (5.8)	9 (3.6)	23	29 (9.9)	29 (9.9)	58
50+	26 (10.7)	28 (11.1)	54	55 (18.8)	52 (17.7)	107
Total	243	252	495	293	293	586

[a] Figures in parentheses denote the percentage of the final total number of families.

Table 3. Chinese province of origin of members of families of nasopharyngeal carcinoma (NPC) patients and control families

Family	Kwangtung	Fukkien	Other	Total
NPC	515	5	15	536
Control	495	7	38	540
Total	1010	12	54	1076

Table 4. Town of origin in Kwangtung province of members of families of nasopharyngeal carcinoma (NPC) patients and control families

Family	Hong Kong	Canton	Sze Yap	Chiu Chau	Hakka	Elsewhere	Not classified	Total
NPC	18	307	91	34	2	43	20	515
Control	19	241	120	51	10	41	13	495
Total	37	548	211	85	12	84	33	1010

difference should be kept in mind when interpreting the findings, since lifestyle is partly determined by place of origin.

RESULTS

The replies of NPC patients and controls, or of their respective households, were first compared in terms of frequency. All items which occurred with significantly different frequency (simple chi-square test) are listed in Table 5 (for individuals) and Table 6 (for households). These tables also show the level of significance, the direction of the difference and the relative risk associated therewith.

Table 5. Factors associated with different frequency in nasopharyngeal carcinoma (NPC) patients and controls, with level of significance and relative risk

Factor	Frequency in		Level of significance P	Relative risk and 95% confidence interval
	NPC patients (%)	control patients (%)		
Socio-economic condition: belonging to the four lowest occupational classes (among those employed just prior to illness)	76/92 (82.6)	45/75 (60.0)	< 0.01	3.17 1.56 - 6.44
Religious affiliation: Buddhist or ancestor worshiper	111/150 (74.0)	86/150 (57.3)	< 0.01	2.12 1.30 - 3.45
Health: illness of ear after age of 15 years	38/144 (26.4)	17/150 (11.3)	< 0.01	2.80 1.50 - 5.25
illness of nose after age of 15 years	43/150 (28.7)	9/150 (6.0)	< 0.001	6.30 2.94 - 13.40

From this analysis the following differences emerged:

Socio-economic conditions

Neither the level of income nor the number of substantial possessions differed between households of NPC patients and controls. There were more NPC patients than controls in the four lowest occupational levels; this difference is significant ($P < 0.01$) and is associated with a relative risk of 3.17 (see Table 5).

Religious practices

More NPC patients than controls adhered to Buddhism and ancestor worship ($P < 0.01$; relative risk = 2.1). Ancestral altars and altars for door gods were kept more often in NPC households than in control households; the relative risks for the two kinds of altar are 2.1 and 2.2, respectively.

The habit of burning incense was more frequent in NPC households (65%) than in control households (54%), but this difference was not significant ($P = 0.08$).

Diet

Of the sixty different food items included in the questionnaire, the following were found to be consumed with different frequencies in NPC and non-NPC households (see also Table 6):

Table 6. Factors associated with different frequency in households (HH) of nasopharyngeal carcinoma (NPC) patients and of controls, with level of significance and relative risk

Factor	Frequency in NPC HH (%)	Frequency in Control HH (%)	Significance of difference P	Relative risk (95% confidence interval)
Religious habits:				
ancestral altar	42/148 (28.4)	24/149 (16.1)	< 0.05	2.06 (1.17-3.63)
altar for door god	38/148 (25.7)	20/149 (13.4)	< 0.001	2.23 (1.23-4.05)
burning of incense	96/148 (64.9)	81/149 (54.4)	= 0.08[a]	
Dietary habits:				
bread eaten often	74/147 (50.3)	103/147 (70.0)	< 0.01	0.43 (0.27-0.70)
tinned food eaten often	10/147 (6.8)	23/147 (15.6)	< 0.02	0.39 (0.18-0.86)
tinned food with fish	14/93 (15.1)	31/112 (27.7)	< 0.05	0.46 (0.23-0.94
Use of spices:				
fennel	3/143 (2.1)	16/141 (11.3)	< 0.01	0.17 (0.05-0.59)
mustard paste	31/144 (21.5)	55/143 (38.5)	< 0.001	0.44 (0.26-0.74)
chilli sauce	29/144 (20.1)	55/144 (38.2)	< 0.001	0.41 (0.24-0.69)
Chinese wine	59/145 (40.7)	79/144 (54.9)	< 0.02	0.56 (0.35-0.90)

[a] Not significant

Bread: Bread was consumed more often in the households of controls ($P < 0.001$), and the relative risk was 0.43.

Tinned food: Tinned foods of all kinds, and especially those containing fish, were consumed more frequently in control than in NPC households.

Spices: Among spices, shrimp oil, fennel, mustard sauce and chilli paste were used less frequently in NPC households than in those of controls. The use of Chinese wine as a flavouring in various dishes was also less frequent in NPC households.

Drinking habits

The drinking habits of the two groups did not differ with respect either to alcoholic or to non-alcoholic beverages. In particular, the proportion of tea drinkers was similar in NPC patients (84.5%) and controls (77.3%). There was no tendency for the NPC patients to drink tea at a higher temperature or to drink more cups per day. Only with respect to the kind of tea did the two groups differ significantly: the NPC patients more rarely (35.2%) consumed green tea than the controls (48.7%) ($P < 0.05$; relative risk = 0.57). The suggestion in earlier case-control studies (Shanmugaratnam & Higginson, 1967) that NPC patients have an excess of tea drinking was thus not confirmed.

Smoking habits

Cigar and pipe smoking were equally frequent among NPC patients and controls. The frequency and duration of cigarette smoking in NPC patients and controls are presented separately for each diagnostic group of controls in Table 7. Among the male NPC patients matched to lung cancer patients the proportion of cigarette smokers was slightly lower (76%) than in the controls (88%), but the number of years smoked and the average number of cigarettes per day were similar in these two groups.

Table 7. Amount of cigarette smoking in nasopharyngeal carcinoma (NPC) patients and their matched controls by diagnostic group of controls and by sex

Diagnosis of controls	Sex	Total no./Proportion of smokers		Average years of cigarette smoking[a]		Average no. of cigarettes smoked per day[a]	
		Controls	NPC	Controls	NPC	Controls	NPC
Lung cancer	M	34/88%	34/76%	26	27	21	21
	F	9/33%	9/22%	30	32	9	18
Cancer of mouth and upper respiratory tract	M	29/83%	29/79%	28	28	22	21
	F	13/46%	13/62%	25	24	12	12
Cancer of digestive tract	M	15/87%	15/67%	25	18	24	17
	F	3/0%	3/67%	-	40	-	23
Other diseases	M	27/78%	27/67%	23	24	25	20
	F	20/10%	20/15%	20	24	33	8
All	M	105/84%	105/73%	26	26	23	20
	F	45/24%	45/33%	25	26	16	13

[a] Among cigarette smokers

For the three other diagnostic groups of controls shown in Table 7 there was a higher proportion of cigarette smokers in male controls than in NPC patients. The number of females in each subgroup was too small to show any pattern. On the whole, both male NPC patients and controls appear to belong to a population of heavy cigarette smokers: approximately 80% had smoked an average of 20 cigarettes per day for nearly 25 years.

In order to determine whether there were more heavy cigarette smokers among lung cancer patients than in other groups of patients, the average number of cigarettes smoked per day was compared (for males) in NPC patients and in controls by diagnostic group of controls (Table 8). Among the controls with lung cancer, 65% were heavy smokers (20 cigarettes or more per day) *versus* 53% among their matched NPC patients. This excess of heavy smokers among controls was found in all four subgroups and was most pronounced in the group in which the controls had 'other diseases': here 63% of the controls and only 30% of the NPC patients were heavy smokers.

Table 8. Number of cigarettes smoked per day by male nasopharyngeal carcinoma (NPC) patients and controls, by diagnostic category of controls

	Lung cancer	Matched NPC cases	Mouth & upper respiratory tract cancer	Matched NPC cases	Digestive tract cancer	Matched NPC cases	Other diseases	Matched NPC cases	Total Controls	NPC cases
Non-smokers	4	8	5	6	2	5	6	9	17	28
1-9 per day	0	1	3	1	1	0	2	1	6	3
10-19 per day	5	6	3	10	1	4	1	6	10	26
20-29 per day	16	14	9	7	3	5	10	4	28	30
30- per day	6	4	7	4	4	0	7	4	24	12
Unknown amount	3	1	2	1	4	1	1	3	10	6
Total smokers	30	26	24	23	13	10	21	18	88	77
Total	34	34	29	29	15	15	27	27	105	105

Since the controls used in the present study included patients with cancers known to be associated with cigarette smoking, the study cannot throw any light on the question of whether there is an association between NPC and smoking.

Previous illness

A history of illness of the ear, nose or throat before the age of 15 years was equally frequent in NPC patients and controls. After this age, both ear and nose troubles were more frequent in the NPC patients, the relative risks being 2.8 and 6.3, respectively (see Table 5). The main ailments were otitis media, in the case of ear trouble, and bleeding, in the case of nose complaints. The frequency of illness of the throat after 15 years of age was not significantly different in NPC patients (19.5%) as compared to control patients (14.0%) (P = 0.26).

Weaning habits

A total of 108 mothers in the NPC households and 103 in the control households were interviewed regarding weaning habits. The only significant difference found in the type of food given to the babies during and after weaning was that in the NPC households 75% of the mothers claimed to have given their babies salted fish after weaning *versus* 53.4% of those among controls (P< 0.01; relative risk = 2.6).

Multivariate analysis

The next step in the analysis was to investigate whether any of the factors described above played an independent role or whether they were all indicators to a greater or lesser extent of traditional Chinese life style.

The variables considered were:

(1) the adherence to traditional Chinese lifestyle, such as keeping of altars in the house and avoiding new food habits, such as eating bread and tinned food;

(2) the use of Chinese spices; and

(3) the feeding of salted fish to babies being weaned from the breast.

Of the many variables that could have been used to express adherence to traditional lifestyle, 11 were chosen for an initial analysis: bread; frequency of use of tinned food; ancestral altars; Buddhist altars; kitchen god altars; door god altars; land god altars; burning of incense; burning of candles; where do you go for medical treatment (Chinese or not)? did you ever have a medical check-up? Others were excluded because they were either very rare or very common, or because they appeared to be almost identical to one or more of the other variables, or because alone they seemed unrelated to risk for NPC. Of these 11 variables, three, the use of bread, ancestral altars and Buddhist altars, discriminated as well between cases and controls as did the full set of 11.

Six dietary items were selected for inclusion in the analysis: oyster soy; vinegar; xanthozylon seeds; flavour essence; mustard paste; and Chinese wine. When included with the three traditional lifestyle variables, a significant improvement in fit was obtained. However, only one of the six dietary variables, rare use of Chinese wine, had a significant regression coefficient. This single dietary variable, plus the three lifestyle variables, gave as good a discrimination between cases and controls as the nine variables together.

On the basis of these four variables, an index of 'traditional lifestyle' was computed for each individual NPC case and control from the formula:

$$\text{Index} = -\text{frequency of wine drinking} - \text{frequency of bread consumption} + 0.9 \times \text{ancestral altars} + 0.7 \times \text{Buddhist altars}$$

Each NPC case and control was classified according to the level of the index, as shown in Table 9. There are clearly more NPC cases than controls with high index values, and the relative risk for NPC between high and low values is 6.5 ($P < 0.0001$).

Table 9. Relationship between traditional life style and risk for nasopharyngeal carcinoma

	Index of traditional lifestyle		
	Low	Medium	High
Cases	25	42	31
Controls	42	39	8

Table 10 shows the joint factors of consumption of salted fish during weaning and the index of traditional lifestyle. The effect of the use of salted fish clearly remains after correcting for traditional lifestyle. The apparent reversal of the effect in the most traditional group is not significant. This means that consumption of salted fish during weaning affects the risk of contracting NPC and is independent of the effect of a traditional lifestyle.

Table 10. Joint effect of traditional lifestyle and consumption of salted fish during weaning on risk for nasopharyngeal carcinoma (NPC)

Household	Index of traditional lifestyle					
	Low		Medium		High	
	Consumption of salted fish during weaning					
	-	+	-	+	-	+
Control	18	24	21	18	1	7
NPC	7	18	10	32	8	23

Overall relative risk = 2.22; 95% confidence interval = 4.46;
χ^2 for heterogeneity = 3.76 on 2 degrees of freedom, not significant

DISCUSSION

Retrospective studies such as the present case-control study harbour an unavoidable source of bias, derived from the fact that the patients have gone through a traumatic experience, in this case that of having cancer in the nasopharynx, whereas the comparison groups have not. This difference may influence the individuals' recollection of earlier exposures and may create a difference in replies obtained in interviews. Another bias which is easier to counteract is interviewer bias derived from the fact that the interviewer knows who is an NPC patient and who is not. The risk of these biases and the general vagueness of human recollections about what happened in a somewhat distant past may reduce the validity of results obtained in a case-control study and make it imperative that they should be corroborated by findings in other studies before they are accepted.

The results of two published and one unpublished case-control studies of NPC patients, together with the results of the present study, are summarized in Table 11, which lists environmental factors found to be significantly associated (positively or negatively) with NPC and also gives the relative risk attached to each of these factors. No one factor was found to be associated with NPC in all four studies. Only one factor was found to be positively associated in three studies, *viz*, a history of nasal symptoms, which carried relative risks of 2.1 in Taiwan, 4.9 in California and 6.3 in Hong Kong. *A priori* it would seem possible that a disease of the nose might predispose to cancer of the nasopharynx. A closer scrutiny of the data in the present study reveals, however, that it is illness close to the age of onset of NPC that is most strongly related to the tumour. This indicates that the nasal symptoms reported by the NPC patients may be early symptoms of NPC and not the cause of it.

Exposure to air pollution was found to be positively associated with NPC in two studies: in Taiwan, poor ventilation at work increased the risk 2.6 times, and in California occupational exposure to smoke carried a relative risk of 7.5. In Malaysia, on the other hand, people who spent more than average time in zones with heavy air pollution had a reduced relative risk (0.9).

That air pollution at work did not emerge as a risk factor in the present study in Hong Kong may be due to the fact that we asked only about the type of occupation and not about the kind of work actually done or the amount of air pollution at the place of work. The evidence in favour of industrial air pollution as a risk factor in NPC seems consistent with the higher risk of NPC in males and may be worthwhile pursuing in future studies, in spite of the somewhat equivocal results from the available retrospective studies.

In two studies the consumption of chilli was found to be negatively associated with NPC: in Hong Kong, the use of chilli sauce carried a relative risk of 0.4, and in Malaysia the use of raw chilli carried a

Table 11. Factors found to be associated with the risk of contracting nasopharyngeal carcinoma (NPC) in case-control studies from four different countries

Reference, place, period	Factors associated with NPC	Relative risk (RR) and P values
Lin et al. (1971), Taiwan, 1969-71	Smoking of cigarettes	20-29 cigarettes RR = 2.93; P<0.01 ⩾ 30 cigarettes RR = 3.13; P<0.001
	Use of herbal drugs	occasionally RR=1.68 frequently RR=3.51
	Use of nasal balms or oils	occasionally RR=1.34 frequently RR=2.76; P<0.001
	History of nasal symptoms	Paranasal sinusitis RR=2.05
	Conditions at work	Poor ventilation RR=2.55; P<0.05
This study, Hong Kong, 1973-74	Level of occupation	From lowest levels RR=3.2; P<0.01
	History of otorhinolaryngeal illness	In ear after age 15 yrs RR=2.8; P<0.01 In nose after age 15 yrs RR=6.3; P<0.001
	Religious practices	Buddhist or ancestor worshipping RR=2.1; P<0.01 Ancestral altar in house RR=2.1; P<0.05 Altar for door god in house RR=2.2; P<0.01
	Dietary habits in the household	Bread eaten often RR=0.43; P<0.001 Tinned food eaten often RR=0.39; P<0.02 Consumption of tinned fish RR=0.46; P<0.05
	Weaning habits	Salted fish after weaning RR=2.6; P<0.01
	Use of spices	Fennel RR=0.17; P<0.01 Mustard paste RR=0.44; P<0.001 Chilli sauce RR=0.41; P<0.001 Chinese wine RR=0.56; P<0.02
Henderson et al. (1976), Los Angeles county, California, USA, 1971-74	History of otorhinolaryngeal illness	Ear and nose only RR=4.9
	Beverage	Wine RR=0.7 (95% confidence limits 0.4-1.1) Tea RR=0.5 (95% confidence limits 0.3-1.0)
	Occupational exposure	To fumes for more than 10 yrs RR=1.7 To smoke for more than 10 yrs RR=7.5 To chemicals for more than 10 yrs RR=2.7 (all P< 0.05)
Armstrong & Kutty (unpublished), Selangar, Malaysia, 1973-74	Dietary habits in the family	Eating of rice RR=0.5; P⩽0.01 Eating of bread RR=0.7; P⩽0.05 Eating of beef RR=0.3; P⩽0.05 Eating of fresh fruit RR=0.5; P⩽0.05 Eating of sliced raw chilli RR=0.6; P⩽0.05 Drinking of milk RR=0.6; P⩽0.05
	Length of time spent in special environment (men only)	Industrial work place RR=1.9; P⩽0.01 Squatter housing RR=3.6; P⩽0.01 Old low-cost housing RR=3.5; P⩽0.01 New low-cost housing RR=1.2; P⩽0.01 Time in office RR=0.5; P⩽0.01 Time in street, shopping RR=0.3; P⩽0.01 Time in heavy air pollution RR=0.7; P⩽0.01
	Possessions in the family	Car RR=0.5; P⩽0.05 Electric fan RR=0.3; P⩽0.01 Refrigerator RR=0.4; P⩽0.01 Television set RR=0.4; P⩽0.01

risk of 0.6. According to present concepts of oncology, it is difficult to see how the use of chilli in any form could possibly protect against cancer in the nasopharynx, and, although the interviewing in the NPC patients was meant to explore conditions prevailing before the onset of the tumour, it is quite possible that the reported low consumption of chilli in NPC patients may reflect abstention from this highly irritating spice during the early and yet unrecognized stages of the illness.

Eating of bread was found to be negatively correlated with NPC in two studies: the relative risks were 0.4 in Hong Kong and 0.7 in Malaysia. Again, it is not likely that the consumption of bread, as such, could protect against NPC, and it seems more plausible that a low intake of bread is a feature of a more traditional lifestyle in Chinese communities and that it is the traditional way of life which for some reason or another is associated with a high risk for NPC.

A multivariate analysis of the data obtained in the present study showed that close adherence to a traditional Cantonese lifestyle increased the risk of contracting NPC by a factor of 6.5 and that low consumption of bread was the most powerful expression of traditionalism of all the factors included in the study.

The present finding that the feeding of salted fish to babies during weaning increases the risk for NPC has not been investigated in other studies, and this possibility clearly needs to be followed up.

SUMMARY

A case-control study was undertaken of Cantonese NPC patients hospitalized in the Queen Elizabeth Hospital, Hong Kong. One age- and sex-matched control was selected for each NPC case from hospitalized patients with cancers other than NPC. A total of 150 NPC patients and 150 controls were interviewed in order to compare the two groups with respect to socio-economic status, dietary habits and health status.

In addition to the individual patients and controls, healthy members of their respective households were also interviewed, in order to obtain information not influenced by the experience of having cancer. Weaning habits were compared in the households of NPC patients and those of controls by asking women who had ever breast fed a child about food supplements they had given to the baby during, and immediately after, weaning.

The following factors were found to be positively associated with NPC:

(1) belonging to the four lowest occupational classes;

(2) practising Buddhism or ancestor worship and having religious altars in the house; and

(3) having a history of previous illnesses of the ear or nose after the age of 15 years.

The following factors were found to be negatively associated with NPC:

(1) eating of bread;

(2) eating of tinned food; and

(3) use of spices.

The study of weaning habits disclosed that salted fish was given to babies just after weaning more often in households with an NPC case than in control households.

A multivariate analysis showed that traditional lifestyle and the consumption of salted fish during weaning are independent risk factors for NPC. This analysis also revealed that two or three of the many expressions of a traditional lifestyle included in the study could account for the total increase in NPC risk associated with this way of life, although it is quite possible that other, as yet unidentified, factors are just as important.

ACKNOWLEDGEMENT

This work was performed in part under contract no. N01 CP 4-3296 within the Virus Cancer Program of the National Cancer Institute, USA.

REFERENCES

Buell, P. (1965) Nasopharyngeal cancer in Chinese of California. *Brit. J. Cancer, 19*, 459-470

de-Thé, G., Ho, J.H.C. & Muir, C. (1976) *Nasopharyngeal carcinoma.* In: Evans, A.S., ed., *Viral Infections of Humans*, New York, Plenum, pp. 539-563

Henderson, B.E., Louie, E., Jing, J.S.H., Buell, P. & Gardner, M.B. (1976) Risk factors associated with nasopharyngeal carcinoma. *New Engl. J. Med., 295*, 1101-1106

Ho, H.C. (1967) *Nasopharyngeal carcinoma in Hong Kong.* In: Muir, C.S. & Shanmugaratnam, K., eds, *Cancer of the Nasopharynx* (*UICC Monograph Series No. 1*), Copenhagen, Munksgaard, pp. 58-63

King, H. & Haenszel, K. (1973) Cancer mortality among foreign and native born Chinese in the United States. *J. chron. Dis., 26*, 623-646

Lin, T.M., Hsu, M.M., Cheng, K.P., Chiang, T.C., Jung, P.F. & Hirayama, T. (1971) Morbidity and mortality of cancer of the nasopharynx in Taiwan. *Gann Monogr.*, *10*, 137-144

Lin, T.M., Chen, K.P., Lin, C.C., Hsu, M.M., Chiang, T.C., Jung, P.F. & Hirayama, T. (1973) Retrospective study on nasopharyngeal carcinoma. *J. nat. Cancer Inst.*, *51*, 1403-1408

Shanmugaratnam, K. & Higginson, J. (1967) *Aetiology of nasopharyngeal carcinoma: report on a retrospective survey in Singapore.* In: Muir, C.S. & Shanmugaratnam, K., eds, *Cancer of the Nasopharynx* (*UICC Monograph Series No. 1*), Copenhagen, Munksgaard, pp. 130-137

Shanmugaratnam, K. (1973) Cancer in Singapore - ethnic and dialect group variations in cancer incidence. *Singapore med. J.*, *14*, 68-81

Simons, M.J., Wee, G.B., Day, N.E., de-Thé, G., Morris, P.J. & Shanmugaratnam, K. (1974) Immunogenetic aspects of nasopharyngeal carcinoma. I. Differences in HLA antigens profiles between patients and comparison groups. *Int. J. Cancer*, *13*, 122-134

Simons, M.J., Wee, G.B., Goh, E.H., Chan, S.H., Shanmugaratnam, K., Day, N.E. & de-Thé, G. (1976) Immunogenetic aspects of nasopharyngeal carcinoma. IV. Increased risk in Chinese for nasopharyngeal carcinoma associated with a Chinese related HLA profile (A2, Sin-2). *J. nat. Cancer Inst.*, *57*, 977-980

Zippin, C., Tekawa, I.S., Bragg, K.U., Watson, D.A. & Linden, G. (1962) Studies on heredity and environment in cancer of the nasopharynx. *J. nat. Cancer Inst.*, *29*, 483-490

ENVIRONMENTAL BACKGROUNDS OF YOUNG CHINESE NASOPHARYNGEAL CARCINOMA PATIENTS

E.N. ANDERSON, Jr

Department of Anthropology,
University of California,
Riverside, Ca. 92502, USA

M.L. ANDERSON

Kaiser Hospital,
Fontana, Ca., USA

H.C. HO

Medical and Health Department
Institute of Radiology and Oncology,
Queen Elizabeth Hospital,
Kowloon, Hong Kong

INTRODUCTION

Nasopharyngeal carcinoma (NPC) afflicts Chinese far more frequently than other racial groups, and, among Chinese, the disease occurs most frequently in those originating from the southern province, Kwangtung (Guangdong) (Ho, 1967, 1972). Among these, a group, known as 'boat people' (mostly Tankas), who have been living and working in boats along the south China coast for centuries, have a significantly higher incidence rate of NPC than do Hong Kong Chinese land-dwellers, the majority of whom are also from Kwangtung (Ho, 1967, 1971). As early as 1921, Todd (1921) reported 103 cases of cervical adenopathy from the Kung Yee Medical College and Hospital in Canton, the capital of Kwangtung, and commented on the high frequency of cancer of the neck glands. We now know that most of the cases he saw must have been NPC.

Thus, this cancer is not a product of our modern environment but is probably connected with some traditional environmental factor(s).

For this reason, we undertook a study of the environmental backgrounds of young Chinese NPC patients in Hong Kong. We chose young patients because their mothers or other elder relatives were more likely to be available to give information about the patients' environments during infancy and early childhood; such information is often not obtainable for older patients. Furthermore, events of a shorter past are easier to recall.

Another important reason for studying the early environments of Chinese NPC patients is that, from an analysis of the age-specific incidence rates in this group, Ho (1975) speculated that the early steep rise in rates from 20-24 years of age could be due to exposure to carcinogenic agents in early life, since clinical manifestation of these carcinomas usually requires a latent period of 20 years or more.

MATERIALS AND METHODS

The Medical and Health Department Institute of Radiology and Oncology, based at Queen Elizabeth Hospital, Kowloon, and Queen Mary Hospital, Hong Kong Island, treats about 90% of all NPC patients diagnosed in Hong Kong and has detailed records of all cases. Its files revealed 31 patients diagnosed when they were less than 25 years of age and known to be still alive. Three could not be located, two had apparently left Hong Kong, and two were too ill to be interviewed. Of the remaining 24, all but two were interviewed with their families; the two exceptions were interviewed only briefly in hospital and refused further contact. The other 22 and their families proved to be extremely cooperative and helpful. Sixteen subjects were interviewed in their homes, preferably those of their parents when the subjects had left home because of marriage, and six insisted on meeting us in restaurants, for reasons of convenience or because the family did not want to hear about the disease. Most of the interviews were carried out in the presence of several persons, typically including most of the close family members; one exception was an orphan who had no close relatives in Hong Kong.

An interview lasted from two to four hours. It followed a set pattern but was not standardized and did not involve a questionnaire. It was felt that such less obviously formal interviewing would permit more detailed and probing enquiry, especially with regard to follow up of items of interest. A questionnaire covering the same material would have been formidably long, daunting the most cooperative respondent. Leading questions were scrupulously avoided. Observations about the patient's home environment were, when possible, integrated into the questions. Attempts were always made to induce a respondent to add more detail, but pressure was not applied to obtain an answer to an obviously touchy or painful question.

The rules of interviewing were: (1) to have a pre-planned schedule of questions; (2) during interviewing, to subdivide the questions progressively, especially with regard to food and medicines; (3) to follow up all interesting or exceptional responses with further questioning, until the subject could not be more specific; and (4) never to push too hard. If a matter proved to be too painful to discuss or if the respondent claimed to be unable to remember something, it was dropped; however, if at all possible, the issue was returned to later from another angle. This was done in order to cross-check certain key areas of interest, the importance of which cannot be over-emphasized. Here it is often useful to have two or three interviewers, each of whom reformulates the question; subjects often classify things in different ways.

The interviews began by taking background data: age, birth date and place, residential and occupational history (in full detail), education, family size and patient's position among the family members with whom he lives. Food habits were covered in the following order: person who cooks; fuel used; and food items consumed - meats, seafoods, starches, salt, sugar, cooking oils, drinks, spices, bean products, vegetables and fruits. Then, child rearing practices, especially foods given the subject in infancy, were discussed with the mother, or with another older relative when the mother was deceased or in mainland China. Medicines used, traditional Chinese or western, led to questions about past illnesses, an area in which less cooperation was obtained. Environment other than food was then covered: cleaning materials used in the home, smoke and soot in the home and surroundings, occupational exposure to chemicals, pollution, etc., housing conditions, changes in local conditions. Finally, questions were posed concerning the subject's recreational activities, feelings of well-being, attitudes toward life, perception of any dramatic changes or crucial events during life, and his/her interest in a possible follow-up interview, to which the 22 cooperating subjects agreed.

RESULTS

Of the 24 patients interviewed, 14 were male and 10 female; this ratio is lower than the 2.3 sex incidence ratio for the 0-24 age group in the Hong Kong Chinese population for the period 1970-1974 (Ho[1]). Seventeen were Cantonese, two Hakkas, two Chiuchows (Teochews) and three Cantonese-speaking boat people ('Tanka'), two of whom were sisters. The boat people were thus over-represented, since they constitute less than 1.3% of the Hong Kong population, according to the 1971 census (Hong Kong Government Census and Statistics Department[1]). Twenty of the patients interviewed were born in Hong Kong (11 in Kowloon, three in the city of Victoria on Hong Kong Island and two on Cheung Chow Island) and the remaining four in mainland China. Seventeen lived in urban

---

[1] Unpublished data

Kowloon, where the majority of the population resides, three in Victoria, two in the New Territories and two on boats.

Four of the 24 subjects had a family history of NPC: the mother of one patient and a grandmother of another had NPC, and both of two 'Tanka' sisters had the disease. These latter were the two patients who refused detailed interviewing.

Most of the subjects came from relatively poor backgrounds: the parents of most had been farmers, fishermen or poor urban labourers. Thus, in their early childhood about 17 of the subjects had received diets and, more importantly, medical care that was limited by family poverty. Only five had middle-class backgrounds, their parents being owners of a small family workshop, business workers or, in one case, a civil servant. All of the families felt that vegetables and fruits were bad for babies, whilst meat and fish were good, and the children had been fed accordingly. Only three of the subjects smoked cigarettes, in moderation, and seven drank small amounts of alcohol. None of the families used folk medicine or food therapy to any significant extent.

In addition to the three boat people who lived away from all sources of air pollution, several of the subjects spent varying amounts of time on farms in rural environments. The rest of the sample were distributed widely through urban Hong Kong and Kowloon, where the air outside and in the older buildings is close and highly polluted; however, the NPC patients interviewed had not been more highly exposed than the rest of the population. Occupational exposure to air contaminants was experienced by seven of the subjects, who worked in textile factories; however, about half of the Hong Kong industrial workforce is so employed, and textile factory workers elsewhere do not have a high risk for NPC.

Cantonese cooking methods often include rapid stir-frying with the attendant liberation of large clouds of hot food vapours; however, in the families in our sample, food was more frequently boiled or steamed. Furthermore, the subjects themselves had not normally assisted in cooking. The kitchens seen or described were not usually poorly ventilated or close to living quarters: many of them were quite separate from the living quarters, located outside the house on verandahs. Ho (1967) has pointed out that the boat people do their cooking in the open and yet have the highest incidence rates for NPC. In addition, the cooking is done by females, yet they have an age-standardized male:female incidence ratio of 3.1:1, compared with 2.48:1 for the whole Hong Kong population for the period 1969-1973 (Ho[1]).

Ho (1972) has discounted the relevance of the burning of Buddhist incense in NPC. Three of the families interviewed in our study were Christian and had never burnt it in or near their homes; only four of the rest had done so. These findings indicate that inhalants are probably not associated with NPC.

---

[1] Unpublished data

In obtaining information about food we were helped by the fact that the subjects were young and their families could thus remember what they had eaten from infancy on. In addition, the subjects had not had time to have contact with many foods; among other reasons, eating out in restaurants and tea-houses is, like smoking, something of an older person's privilege. Many of the subjects were not old enough to have eaten anything but small snacks away from home, and others had just begun to do so. Many of the subjects came from very poor or very remote rural backgrounds and thus had not been exposed to rare, unusual or expensive foods.

Pork was the meat eaten commonly by all subjects; beef and other meats were eaten only rarely. Pork is usually eaten fresh but is also marinated and roasted and sold precooked as *cha siu*; not all patients had eaten this in childhood, but all had eaten it sometime in their lives. Pork is also made into sausages (*laap cheung*, literally, 'cured intestines'), with Chinese liquor, salt and water; and it is sliced thickly and made into bacon (*laap yuk* or 'cured meat') by salting and sun-drying. Everyone had eaten these preparations, especially the former, which is a standard Cantonese food in cold weather. Both are considered to be too greasy to eat in warm weather, but many patients ate small pieces every day in winter.

Fish was the main seafood eaten and formed the chief source of animal protein, far ahead of meat. People of inland origin had eaten more freshwater fish (mostly species of carp) as children than boat people, who had eaten almost none. All currently ate a great deal of fresh marine fish, and most always had. All, without exception, had eaten salted fish and had received it as one of their first solid foods. The first solid food of the average Hong Kong baby is soft rice (rice cooked with a great deal of water until it is mushy) containing fish, either fresh (usually) or salted (often). Some of those who had rarely eaten salted fish had often eaten dried squid, which is cured in a similar way. Other seafoods were rarely or never eaten; dried shrimps, oysters and other shellfish were completely avoided by some families.

It is safe to say that all subjects had eaten most south Chinese vegetables (various cabbage greens, such flavourings as ginger, onion and native Chinese onion-like alliums, and many roots and tubers) and the common fruits (oranges, pears, apples, grapes, bananas, mandarin oranges). On the other hand, most had never eaten, except perhaps occasionally, exotic vegetables, rare fruits or spices. The typical Chinese spices such as star anise and five-spice powder were virtually never used by most of the families. Most subjects disliked and avoided spicy foods; many had never eaten strong spices.

Tea is considered to be bad for children and is not usually given to them in Cantonese homes. Fifteen of the 22 subjects who were fully interviewed reported that they drank only boiled water during childhood, except for a very little milk and fruit juice.

With regard to bean products, all subjects regularly consumed soya sauce and bean curd in amounts normal for Hong Kong residents. All had eaten *tau si*, a black fermented product made of salted soya beans. Not all had eaten the other soya bean products, e.g., *min si jeung* (flour and soya bean sauce) and *fu yu* (fermented, pickled bean curd), about which we asked in particular.

We asked separately and in some detail about infant feeding. Seven subjects were never breast-fed. Otherwise, all of the subjects shared a common and characteristic history: first solid food consisted of soft rice cooked with fish, fresh or salted, or sometimes with minced meat, including offal, or with such flavourings as thin soup, peanut oil or honey dates (jujubes preserved in honey). No significant quantities of fruit or vegetables were given. Babies who were not breast-fed were usually fed rice paste and little or nothing else. These diets, in all 22 cases, would have been inadequate in vitamin C and probably in the B vitamins, notably B_6, B_{12} and folic acid. The lack of vitamin C would have been very severe in those who were not breast-fed, and it is incredible that they survived.

Fifteen were notably choosy in their food habits and disliked most strongly flavoured foods. Twelve listed bland vegetables among their favourite foods and listed none that were strongly flavoured; only four liked curried or spicy foods. The six subjects whom we took to restaurants for interviews selected only the very blandest foods, notably, vegetable soup.

Twelve subjects had histories of poor health, as reported by their parents and other family members, and in several cases the mother stressed that this child had always been the weakest, most sickly and thinnest of the family, with the poorest appetite. We believe that many of the remaining ten families were reticent and that the patients from these families may also have been in poor health; cross-checking in two cases showed that although the mother reported that the child had always been in good health, he had actually been quite sickly.

DISCUSSION

The following factors were common to all of the NPC patients studied:

(1) All subjects had eaten pork, including cured sausages, most available vegetables and fruits, marine fish (fresh and salted), rice, bread, noodles, ginger, soya sauce, bean curd and fermented black beans.

(2) No other foods were eaten in significant quantities by all of the patients.

(3) No other environmental factors were shared even by most subjects.

(4) Most of the patients had a history of poor health, inactivity, strong food prejudices, a preference for relatively bland foods and poor infant nutrition.

In view of the prevalence of the latter factors, we formulated a very rough index of each subject's personality as expressed in the interview. Setting the behaviour of the 'average' adolescent or young Chinese Hong Kong resident at zero, we laid out a scale from 0 to 5, on the basis of our assessment of how withdrawn, tense, anxious and frail-seeming the subject was. Stage 5 applied to persons so severely withdrawn and anxious as to be unable to function normally; one such subject was among those interviewed and was clearly in serious need of professional psychiatric help. Stages in between were laid out on the basis of the subjects' responses and appearance. We observed and assessed willingness to talk and answer questions fully and to volunteer information, rather than to answer as briefly as possible, degree of activity and fondness of sports and outings, range of prejudices about foods and personal descriptions of tiredness, worry and tension. The stages in which the 22 subjects were classified were: one subject, 0; four, 1; six, 2; seven, 3; four, 4; and one, 5.

Obviously, this assessment must be very subjective; however, it is unlikely that we would have been totally mistaken about an entire group of people. The same phenomena were also noted by our field assistant and, often, by the subjects' families. Many of the latter commented on how different the subject had been from his siblings or on the fact that the subject had not changed since childhood in these regards.

Such reports indicate that not all of these traits arose as a result of the development of NPC; although the shattering physical and psychological effects of NPC - believed by our subjects to be almost certainly fatal - may account for many of the psychological traits observed, a number of them cannot be explained in this way.

These findings permit one of the following hypotheses: (a) chronic ill health can produce the personality type observed and render the person more susceptible to NPC; (b) this personality type, by itself, predisposes to NPC; (c) the personality type is mainly an effect of NPC. Further work is required to test which, if any, of these hypotheses is valid.

It is improbable that any of the fresh foods eaten by all patients are suspect: pork, ginger, vegetables and both freshwater and marine fish are eaten throughout eastern Asia - not only these foods in general, but the specific species and varieties involved. Soya sauce is also employed widely in this area, and the Cantonese do not consume more than others. The soya sauces used by our subjects came from many sources, ruling out the possibility that one particular kind was suspect.

The remaining foods eaten by all subjects were all wet-salted, slightly fermented (or spoiled), cured protein products: *laap cheung*, salted fish, *tau si* and dried squid. Salted fish was the most commonly eaten and was fed to babies; the other items were not fed to the very young. Huang et al. (1977) (using combined gas chromatography-high-resolution mass spectrometry, with a detection limit of 1 μg/kg) found *N*-nitrosodimethylamine (NDMA) at levels of 1-35 μg/kg of raw material in several samples of Cantonese salted fish, but none in *laap cheung*.

Nitrosamines are known to be potent carcinogens in laboratory animals, but whether the NDMA or other agents present in salted fish play a part in the genesis of NPC remains to be proven. Our subjects' consumption of salted foods, including salted fish, was more or less average by Hong Kong standards. Although many boat people eat salted fish every day, no such persons were among the 22 interviewed (which, however, included only one boat family); the motives for eating salted fish among most of the families were fundamentally economic or a desire for variety.

Our findings are consistent with the hypothesis of Ho (1975) that NPC has a multifactorial etiology: in southern Chinese, the consumption of salted fish and lack of vitamin C, especially in early life, are possible environmental factors, in addition to others, such as a genetic predisposition and Epstein-Barr virus. We would like to add that sickly, withdrawn children are probably more susceptible to NPC than others.

SUMMARY

Twenty-four Chinese NPC patients under 25 years of age at the time of diagnosis were interviewed. The interviews were carried out in the presence of their families in 22 cases and concentrated on the environmental background of the subject's infancy and early childhood. An analysis of the results eliminated household inhalants, aerial contaminants, medicines, food therapy, spices, fresh foods and soya sauce as likely factors in carcinogenesis. The only remaining foods eaten by all subjects and worthy of consideration were *laap cheung*, salted fish and *tau si*. Salted fish was the most commonly eaten and the only one fed to babies. In childhood, the subjects had rarely or never been fed vegetables or fruits. Most had, since childhood, been characteristically sickly, inactive, withdrawn and choosy about their food. It would appear that consumption of salted fish and vitamin C-deficiency in early childhood are important environmental factors and that a certain personality type may be associated with an increased risk.

ACKNOWLEDGEMENTS

This work was supported by IARC/CRA and financed by contract number N01 CP 43296 with the National Cancer Institute, USA. We are grateful to Mrs P. Liu for typing this manuscript.

REFERENCES

Ho, H.C. (1967) *Nasopharyngeal carcinoma in Hong Kong.* In: Muir, C.S. & Shanmugaratnam, K., eds, *Cancer of the Nasopharynx (UICC Monograph Series No. 1)*, Copenhagen, Munksgaard, pp. 58-63

Ho, H.C. (1971) Incidence of nasopharyngeal cancer in Hong Kong. *UICC Bull. Cancer, 9*, 5

Ho, J.H.C. (1972) Nasopharyngeal carcinoma (NPC). *Advanc. Cancer Res., 15*, 57-92

Ho, H.C. (1975) Epidemiology of nasopharyngeal carcinoma. *J. roy. Coll. Surg. (Edinb.), 20*, 223-235

Huang, D.P., Gough, T.A., Webb, K.S. & Ho, H.C. (1977) Volatile nitrosamines in some traditional southern Chinese food products. *Brit. J. Cancer* (in press)

Todd, P.J. (1921) Some practical points in the surgical treatment of cervical tumours. *Chin. med. J., 35*, 21-25

EPIDEMIOLOGY OF MALIGNANT TUMOURS OF THE NASOPHARYNX IN FRANCE: RETROSPECTIVE AND PROSPECTIVE STUDIES

J. BRUGERE & D. POINT

Head and Neck Unit,
Medical Section,
Fondation Curie,
Paris, France

H. SANCHO-GARNIER

Department of Statistical Medical Research,
Institut Gustave Roussy,
Villejuif, France

G. SCHWAAB

Head and Neck Department,
Institut Gustave Roussy,
Villejuif, France

Nasopharyngeal cancer (NPC) is very uncommon in France: this location represents only 3% of all malignant tumours of the upper digestive and respiratory tracts treated in the Institut Gustave Roussy (Villejuif) and Fondation Curie (Paris). We have made a retrospective study of two series of patients treated in these centres for malignant tumours of the nasopharynx, comprising 355 cases from the Institut Gustave Roussy (1959-1974) and 286 from the Fondation Curie (1951-1976).

PATHOLOGICAL DISTRIBUTION

In adults, carcinomas represent 80% of malignancies of the nasopharynx and malignant lymphomas, 16% (Table 1). In children (Table 2), three types of cancer of the nasopharynx have been observed:

malignant lymphomas, embryonal sarcomas and epidermoid carcinomas. At the Head and Neck and Pediatrics Departments of the Institut Gustave Roussy, 54 malignant nasopharyngeal tumours were seen in children under 15 years of age between 1959-1973.

Table 1. Malignant tumours of the nasopharynx seen in adults at the Institut Gustave Roussy (IGR) and the Fondation Curie (FC)

	No. of patients			
	IGR	FC	Total	Percent
Carcinoma	296	213	609	80
Malignant lymphoma	44	61	105	16
Miscellaneous	15	12	27	4
Total	355	286	641	100

Table 2. Malignant tumours of the nasopharynx seen in children at the Head and Neck and Pediatrics Departments of the Institut Gustave Roussy between 1952-1973

Malignant lymphoma	20
Embryonal sarcoma	17
Epidermoid carcinoma	17
Total	54

This was found to be the main and almost the only location of epidermoid carcinomas in children. In adults, 50% of epidermoid carcinomas of the nasopharynx seen in the two centres are of the undifferentiated type, and 21% are lymphoepitheliomas of the Regaud-Schmincke type (Table 3). No correlation was observed between geographic origin of the patient and pathological type of tumour.

SEX AND AGE DISTRIBUTION

Of the NPC in these two series, 74% occurred in males. The sex ratio for 509 cases was 3:1.

Table 3. Carcinomas of the nasopharynx seen in adults at the Institut Gustave Roussy (IGR)[a] and the Fondation Curie (FC)

	No. of patients			
	IGR	FC	Total	Percent
Squamous-cell carcinoma	78	70	148	29
Undifferentiated carcinoma	160	94	254	50
Lymphoepithelioma	58	49	107	21
Total	296	213	509	100

[a] Data reported by Brugère et al., 1975

NPC occurs at all ages, with peaks observed at about 55 years in males and 45 years in females. Thirty percent of cases occurred in patients under 39 years of age (Table 4).

Table 4. Carcinomas of the nasopharynx in adults: age distribution of 509 cases

Age	M	F	Total	Percent
15-19	17	7	24	5
20-29	33	10	43	8
30-39	59	27	86	17
40-49	77	31	108	21
50-59	118	30	148	29
60-69	58	16	74	14
70-79	16	9	25	5
80-89	1	0	1	-
Total	379	130	509	

DISTRIBUTION BY GEOGRAPHIC ORIGIN

Patients native to France represent less than 50% of the cases of NPC followed in the two institutions: as a result of agreements between these centres and with other countries that refer patients, 38% of cases seen at the Institut Gustave Roussy and 59% of those seen at the Fondation Curie are French natives. For the same reasons, Arabs native to North Africa represent 30% of cases at the Institut Gustave Roussy and 11% at the Fondation Curie. Further cases of NPC originate in other countries bordering the Mediterranean Sea, especially Italy, Portugal, Spain, Romania and Greece. The remaining cases come from the West Indies, Central Europe and North Vietnam (Table 5).

Table 5. Carcinomas of the nasopharynx seen at the Institut Gustave Roussy (IGR) and the Fondation Curie (FC): geographic origin of patients.

	IGR	FC	Sub-total	Percent of total
France	112	126	238	47
North Africa (Arabs)	88	24	112	22
North Africa (Europeans)	20	20	40	8
Other Western European countries . .	29	27	56	11
West Indies	21	2	23	-
Central Europe	14	7	21	-
Vietnam	10	4	14	-
Miscellaneous	2	3	5	-
Total	296	213	509	

It is interesting to note that 8% of the cases observed in the two centres occurred in Europeans born of parents who had lived for one, two or three generations in North Africa. This group, which lives in an area with an intermediate rate of risk for NPC, was first suspected in 1969 and may be of interest for a comprehensive approach to the illness. However, it is often difficult to determine geographic origin in a retrospective study: generally, no details are available regarding parents, travels and durations of stay in different countries.

LIMITS OF THE RETROSPECTIVE STUDY

With regard to occupation and use of tobacco and/or of alcohol, the available data are incomplete and often reflect only preconceived ideas of doctors about the origin of this disease. Thus, in 213 files examined at the Fondation Curie, occupation was given in 78%, use of tobacco in 43% and use of alcohol in only 24%.

The low reporting of use of alcohol and tobacco may be explained by the fact that it is currently taught that these factors are not correlated with NPC.

Information about occupation can seldom be used, because it is incompletely registered: exposures are not specified, duration of working life is not given, and past occupations of retired patients are not specified. For example, only small numbers of workers and farmers are indicated as suffering from NPC (Table 6), although these categories have a high risk of other cancers of the upper digestive and respiratory tracts.

Table 6. Carcinomas of the nasopharynx seen in a retrospective study at the Fondation Curie: distribution by occupation

Occupation	No. of cases
Manual workers	60
Office workers	81
Farmers	9
No occupation	16
Occupation unknown	47

THE PROSPECTIVE STUDY

A prospective study of nasopharyngeal tumours and malignant tumours of the nasal and paranasal sinuses was carried out in the Institut Gustave Roussy between 1975 and 1976. Sixteen institutes, oncological centres, university head and neck departments and private radiotherapists agreed to make available to us data on their patients by completing forms specifying age, sex, geographic origin, place of birth of patient and relatives, successive residences, travels and stays in endemic regions, occupations and occupational exposures, previous diseases or neoplasias, social and economic levels, use of tobacco, alcohol, tea, coffee, dried meats and fish, previous radiations or traumas and diseases and neoplasias in relatives. In addition, a second, very complete form describes initial status of the disease, pathological report, treatment given and results.

The same forms were used for other cancers of the upper digestive and respiratory tracts, especially cancers of the nasal and paranasal sinuses that share certain features with NPC. A control group consisted of patients with other cancers seen in the same head and neck departments during the same period and of outpatients who had no evidence of malignant disease.

In addition, biopsy specimens of nasopharyngeal tissue and sera were sent to the International Agency for Research on Cancer, and, when possible, sera were obtained after treatment. To date, we have collected 188 NPC files in this prospective study; 55 come from three centres in Athens, Milan and Tunis, whose cases of NPC serve as a control group, and 133 come from 16 French centres or institutions.

The preliminary data obtained from this enquiry are as follows:

(1) Of the 133 malignant nasopharyngeal tumours, only 43 NPC and 11 other malignancies of the nasopharynx occurred in the group of French-born natives. Assuming that other head and neck departments of general hospitals and other private radiotherapists see the same ethnic distribution in new cases of NPC, the annual rate in France is probably 100-150 new cases, i.e., a yearly rate of 0.3 per 100,000.

The other patients with NPC treated in France come from North Africa (especially Algeria), Italy, Portugal, Spain and the West Indies.

(2) The correlation between geographic origin and pathological classification (Table 7) shows that well-differentiated carcinomas and malignant lymphomas occur mostly in Western European patients, whereas undifferentiated carcinomas and lymphoepitheliomas have no significant pattern of distribution.

Table 7. NPC prospective study: geographic origin

Pathology	% of patients		
	North Africa (Arabs)	Western Europe	Other countries
Well-differentiated carcinoma	5	79	16
Undifferentiated carcinoma	32	57	11
Lymphoepithelioma	38	35	27
Malignant lymphoma	7	86	7

(3) At the present stage of this study, no obvious correlation can be made between NPC and place of birth or travels and stays in different countries, e.g., for European patients in North Africa.

(4) The sex ratio (Table 8) for lymphoepitheliomas and undifferentiated carcinomas is as expected (3:1 to 2:1), but that for well-differentiated carcinomas (20:1) is closer to that seen for other carcinomas of the upper digestive and respiratory tracts. This is the first trend we have observed that seems to set apart the well-differentiated carcinomas from other NPCs.

Table 8. NPC prospective study: sex ratio

Pathology	Sex ratio
Well-differentiated carcinoma	20:1
Undifferentiated carcinoma	3:1
Lymphoepithelioma	2:1
Malignant lymphoma	1:1
Other cancers of the upper digestive and respiratory tracts	12:1
No tumour	1:1

(5) The correlation between patient's age and pathological classification (Table 9) shows that lymphoepitheliomas occur at the lowest age, and well-differentiated carcinomas occur at roughly the same age as do the other carcinomas of the upper digestive and respiratory tracts.

Table 9. NPC prospective study: age

Pathology	Age (yrs)
Well-differentiated carcinoma	53 ± 7
Undifferentiated carcinoma	45 ± 8
Lymphoepithelioma	35 ± 8
Malignant lymphoma	60 ± 7
Other cancers of the upper digestive and respiratory tracts	57 ± 7

(6) It has not been possible to make a correlation with occupation, due to the small number of cases.

(7) The percentage of heavy drinkers (40g alcohol a day or more) is approximately the same in the three groups of patients with nasopharyngeal malignancies and much lower than for other carcinomas of the upper digestive and respiratory tracts (Table 10).

(8) With regard to the consumption of tobacco (Table 11), patients with epidermoid carcinomas were found to smoke twice as much as patients with lymphoepitheliomas.

The main objectives of this prospective study are better to estimate the extent of NPC in France, to detect the geographic origins of patients and to discriminate clinical features according to pathological types. A European committee of pathologists is working on the cases comprising this study.

Table 10. NPC prospective study : use of alcohol

Pathology	% of patients consuming	
	0-40g/day	40-80g/day
Epidermoid carcinoma	67	33
Lymphoepithelioma	73	27
Malignant lymphoma	73	27

Table 11. NPC prospective study: use of tobacco

Pathology	% of patients consuming	
	0-10g/day	20-40g/day
Epidermoid carcinoma	44	56
Lymphoepithelioma	73	27
Malignant lymphoma	45	55

Some of the data collected to date are not relevant, but we hope in the coming months to examine about 200 other cases treated during the same period, thanks to the cooperation of other ear, nose and throat units and radiotherapists. This study has therefore not yet been terminated, since we hope in the near future to increase its value by further data.

SUMMARY

Certain epidemiological conclusions have been drawn from a retrospective study of 509 cases of NPC treated in France. NPC was found to represent 3% of cancers of the upper digestive and respiratory tracts and 80% of nasopharyngeal malignancies in adults; 30% are squamous-cell carcinomas. The sex ratio was found to be 3:1. Less than 50% of cases occur in natives of France.

A prospective study initiated by the Institut Gustave Roussy lead to the collection of data on 133 new cases of NPC treated in France in 1975 and 1976. The annual rate of NPC in France is about 0.3/100,000. A number of factors set apart well-differentiated epidermoid carcinomas from other forms of NPC: sex ratio (20:1), age of patients, geographic origin and the use of tobacco were similar to those seen in cases of epidermoid carcinomas of the upper digestive and respiratory tracts.

ACKNOWLEDGEMENT

The prospective study at the Institut Gustave Roussy was supported by grant no. 73-A-5 from that Institute.

REFERENCE

Brugère, J., Eschwege, F., Schwaab, G., Micheau, C. & Cachin, Y. (1975) Les carcinomes du naso-pharynx (cavum): aspects cliniques et évolutifs. *Bull. Cancer (Paris)*, *62*, 319-330

DISCUSSION OF RISK FACTORS FOR NASOPHARYNGEAL CARCINOMA

B.E. HENDERSON & E. LOUIE

Department of Community and Family Medicine,
University of Southern California,
School of Medicine,
Los Angeles, Ca., USA

Previous epidemiological studies of nasopharyngeal carcinoma (NPC) have been largely descriptive and, although of considerable value in demonstrating the existence of certain high-risk populations, have necessarily provided only limited information about suspected risk factors (Clifford, 1970; Ho, 1972a; Muir, 1971). The high rates among southern Chinese both in China and abroad and the intermediate rates among populations admixed with Chinese have suggested a strong genetic control over expression of the disease. However, even if such racially determined genetic susceptibility exists, other evidence suggests that an environmental trigger must be present. Chinese migrants to Hawaii and California show a decreasing rate of NPC in succeeding generations (Buell, 1974; Zippin et al., 1962); and there is an increased rate of NPC among low-risk racial groups born and raised in high-risk areas, such as California whites born in southeast Asia and Jews born in Asia or North Africa (Buell, 1973; Muir, 1971).

The search for this environmental trigger has stimulated the studies reviewed at this symposium (Geser et al.[1]; Henderson et al., 1976; Hirayama[2]; Shanmugaratnam et al.[3]). It is the purpose of this paper to review those presentations and to compare them with other analytical studies. Two series of NPC cases have been published in the English literature (Lin et al., 1973; Shanmugaratnam & Higginson, 1967). The most recent case-control study of NPC, carried out in Kwangtung Province, People's Republic of China (Hu & Huang, 1972) was originally published

[1] See p. 213

[2] See p. 167

[3] See p. 199

in Chinese but has been partly abstracted into English and was reviewed by Wen (1974). One additional study is to be published in the near future (Armstrong et al., 1978).

A comparison of risk ratios for selected factors from the above studies is given in Table 1. There are, of course, limitations to comparisons of data from studies conducted in several geographical areas: the method of case and control selection varied within each area. Nevertheless, all of these studies have focused on populations derived from southern China, and most were conducted during the years 1964-1974.

The high risk of NPC among Chinese from Kwangtung province has been verified repeatedly. Interestingly, Henderson et al. (1976) also reported a higher risk for other foreign-born populations and particularly for Mexican-Americans. 'Never-married' status has been a risk factor in the majority of studies, as has lower socioeconomic status. Both Geser et al.[1] and Armstrong et al. (1978) have suggested that a more traditional way of life is linked with a lower socio-economic status. The relationship between traditional life style, as defined by Geser et al.[1] (frequency of wine drinking, frequency of bread consumption + 0.9 × ancestral altars + 0.7 × Buddhist altars), and risk for NPC was quite strong ($RR = 6.5$, $P < 0.0002$).

A prior history of ear and nose disease and of the use of traditional Chinese medication for nasal symptoms (balms or oils) has been a relatively consistent finding, when studied. Geser et al.[1] noted that a history of illness of the ear, nose and throat was equally frequent in cases and controls under 15 years of age, the excess risk being confined to adult life. Similar findings were noted by Shanmugaratnam et al.[2]. It is difficult to be certain whether the presence of disease of the nose and ear (if it is indeed increased in patients at risk for NPC and not due to recall bias) is a predisposing risk factor or whether it is secondary to the same common etiological agent(s). In our study (Henderson et al., 1976) we also collected data on prior hospitalization for disease of the nose; we found that, although the frequency was low (1% in controls), there was a positive association with risk for NPC (relative risk = 4.4).

The consumption of many foods and beverages has also been extensively studied, with largely negative results. Chinese tea was associated with NPC in studies in Singapore and Hong Kong but not in those in Malaysia and California. Consumption of alcohol has not regularly been associated with risk for NPC, in contrast to cancers elsewhere in the pharynx. Use of Cantonese salted fish is discussed below.

---

1 See p. 213

2 See p. 199

Table 1. Risk ratios for selected factors in case-control studies of nasopharyngeal carcinoma

Population studied	Reference	Year of study	Number of cases/controls	Source of controls	Risk factors: Place of origin	Marital status (never married)	Low/high socio-economic class	Prior history of ENT disease	Ever use of nasal balms or oils	Exposure to smoke: Occupational	Exposure to smoke: Other	Exposure to smoke: Ever use of cigarettes	Use of food and drink: Chinese tea	Use of food and drink: Salted fish	Use of food and drink: Alcohol
Chinese (Singapore)	Shanmugaratnam & Higginson (1967)	1961-1962	63/63	Hospital	Kwangtung *vs* other China 1.4	1.1	1.8	NA[a]	Balms 1.3 Oils 0.7	No association[b]	Incense 1.0 Opium 0.8	0.7	2.2	NA	No association[b]
Chinese (Kwangtung Province)	Hu & Huang (1972) (abstracted in English by Wen, 1974)	1964-1965	304/238	Hospital & clinic	Kwangtung *vs* other China 5.4	1.4	1.2	1.5	NA	Chef experience 2.7	Wood for cooking 1.5	1.4 (>1 pk 1.8)	NA	NA	1.3
Chinese (Singapore)	Shanmugaratnam et al. (this symposium)	1966-1968	379/1639	ENT Clinic & hospital		NA	0.8-1.0	Nose 20.0 FHNS[c] 2.7	3.5	No association[b]	Wood for cooking 0.9 Incense 1.0 Anti-mosquito coils 1.3	1.0 (>10 yrs 0.9)	1.3	NA	1.3
Chinese & Taiwanese (Taiwan)	Lin et al. (1973)	1969-1970	343/1017	Neighborhood	China *vs* Taiwan ~ 3.0	1.9	NA	2.1	2.8	Poor ventilation 2.6	NA	(>30 cig/day) 3.1	NA	NA	No association[b]
Chinese (Hong Kong)	Geser et al. (this symposium)	1973-1974	150/150	Other cancer cases	Kwangtung *vs* other China 2.1	No association[b]	3.2	Ear 2.8 Nose 6.3	NA	No association[b]	Cooking fuel - no association[b] Incense 1.6	NC[d]	1.6	No association[b] except at weaning 2.6	No association[b]
Chinese, Whites & others (California, USA)	Henderson et al. (1976)	1971-1974	156/267	Hospital & clinic	Foreign-born 1.4	NA	NA	Ear 1.9 Nose 2.1	NA	Fumes 2.0 Smoke 3.0 Smoke for >10 yrs 7.5	NA	1.0 (>40 cig/day) Males - 0.8	0.5	2.1 (Chinese only)	Beer 1.0 Wine 0.7 Liquor 1.2
Chinese (Malaysia)	Armstrong et al. (1978)	1973-1974	60/150	Random population sample	Cantonese *vs* other 1.5	1.3	2.1	NA	NA	Industrial workplace (males) 1.9 Petrol, oil 2.2 Wood dust 1.2	Charcoal/wood for cooking 2.1 Incense 1.3	0.9	0.5	0.8	NA

[a] NA = Data not available

[b] Details of data and relative risk calculations not presented - no statistical association found

[c] FHNS = Family history of nasal symptoms

[d] NC = Type of controls invalidates direct comparison of smoking data.

Exposure to smoke has been a suggested risk factor for NPC ever since Dobson (1924) first noticed the heavy exposure to smoke from wood and charcoal fires used for indoor cooking in the chimney-less houses of south China. Two of the studies listed in Table 1 (Armstrong et al., 1978; Hu & Huang, 1972) reported a positive association with use of fossil fuels for cooking, whereas Shanmugaratnam et al.[1] did not. In addition, Djojopranoto & Soesilowati (1967), who studied 53 Indonesian and Chinese NPC cases and compared them with 53 other ear, nose and throat disease controls in Indonesia, reported that 'the only significant difference was a greater use of wood fires for cooking by nasopharyngeal cancer patients'.

Other sources of inhaled smoke, including incense and anti-mosquito coils, have also been extensively investigated. Generally, when positive associations have been found the risk ratios are low (see Shanmugaratnam et al.[1]). Potential exposure to inhaled carcinogens has also been studied in occupational settings. Hu & Huang (1972) reported that experience of working as a chef at any time during life was a significant risk factor (relative risk = 2.7) for NPC and suggested that this was due to exposure to cooking fires and fumes. Other studies have not found people in specific occupations to be at risk. However, Lin et al. (1973) found a strong association (relative risk = 2.6) with working 'in a place with poor ventilation'. Armstrong et al. (1978) found an association between exposure to an industrial workplace (relative risk = 1.9) and to petrol and oil (relative risk = 2.2) and wood dust (relative risk = 1.2) and risk for NPC. Henderson et al. (1976) reported a significant positive association between occupational exposure to smoke and fumes and risk for NPC in both Chinese and non-Chinese patients; the relative risk was 7.5 for more than 10 years of smoke exposure. Geser et al.[2] found no positive association with exposure to potential inhaled carcinogens, except for incense; however, more than one half of the 'controls' had cancers of the lung, mouth or upper respiratory tract, which might overmatch for common etiological mechanisms such as smoke inhalation.

Use of cigarettes has generally not been associated with risk for NPC, although excessive cigarette smoking (more than 1 pack/day) carried an increased risk in the studies of Hu & Huang (1972) and Lin et al. (1973). The high risk (relative risk= 3.1) for heavy smokers found by Lin et al. (1973) is not consistent with results of other studies and may be due to methodological bias (Louie et al., 1977). Cigarette smoking has not been widespread among rural Chinese until relatively recently.

It would seem, therefore, that at least one potential cause of nasopharyngeal carcinoma would be inhalation of carcinogens (Table 2).

---

1 See p. 199

2 See p. 213

Table 2. Evidence in support of two hypotheses of NPC etiology

Inhaled carcinogens	Salted fish
1. Traditional life style	1. Traditional life style
2. Chimney-less houses of south China	2. Correlates with NPC rates in China
3. Exposure to fossil fuels	3. High risk of 'boat' people
4. Industrial exposure to smoke or poor ventilation at home	4. Associated with weaning in Hong Kong
5. Similarity in pathogenesis to other respiratory cancers	5. Significant association with frequency of use (California)
6. Known carcinogenicity of soot in man	6. Known carcinogenicity of nitrosamines
7. Pulmonary tumours with chimney soot and polycyclic aromatic hydrocarbons	7. Nasal cavity tumours in rats fed raw salted fish

For whites, contact with such carcinogens might occur primarily at the workplace, whereas, for foreign-born people, exposure could occur primarily during childhood in the home environment. The existence of disease of the ear and nose may alter the normal air currents of the nasal cavity in such a way as to produce stasis and chronic irritation in localized areas of the nasopharynx (Proetz, 1953). In these circumstances, the potential of even weak carcinogenic substances may be enhanced.

The hypothesis that inhaled carcinogens are the important risk factor in nasopharyngeal carcinoma is also consistent with knowledge of the cause of other respiratory carcinomas, e.g., cigarette smoking and cancer of the lung, hypopharynx and oropharynx and larynx (Doll et al., 1970; USDHEW, 1971). The site of action of inhaled carcinogens must depend on particle size and route of inhalation as well as on local tissue factors. Inefficient combustion of fossil fuels, such as occurs in indoor cooking on a wood fire, characteristically yields large particles (median diameter, 5-10 μm), which are trapped by the ciliated epithelium of the upper respiratory tract, including the nasopharynx (Willeke & Whitby, 1975).

Soot from wood and charcoal fires was originally shown to be carcinogenic to the scrotal skin of chimney sweeps by Pott (1775). Experimental data has confirmed the carcinogenic potential of soot (Passey, 1922).

Two major objections to the hypothesis that NPC is caused by carcinogens in inhaled smoke have been raised by Ho (1972b). Women, who are more heavily exposed to cooking fires, have lower risks for NPC than men. Equally important, Ho demonstrated that the 'fisher "boat" people who spend most of their lives in their boats and cooked their food in the open air', have high rates of NPC. In collaboration with Ho we have recently confirmed this high rate among Hong Kong boat people.

Searching for an alternative explanation of the high risk for NPC in southern Chinese, Ho has proposed exposure to Cantonese salted marine fish (Table 2). The ungutted fish has been found to contain appreciable quantities of *N*-nitrosodimethylamine (Fong & Chan, 1973; Fong & Walsh, 1971). Salted fish are a traditional food for southern Chinese but apparently not for northern Chinese, who are at low risk for NPC. Ho (1972b) has suggested that the 'boat' people eat larger quantities of salted fish, because they prefer to sell fresh-caught fish to provide their major source of income.

Exposure to nitrosamines or other possible carcinogens in salted fish could come from cooking, inhalation of fumes during eating, or by ingestion. This latter exposure would necessitate that the carcinogen become blood borne and then focus actively uniquely on the nasopharynx. The role of exposure to salted fish was not included in the first four studies listed in Table 1. Geser et al.[1] and Armstrong et al. (1978) found that current use of salted fish was similar in cases and controls; Henderson et al. (1976) reported that there was no significant difference in current use of salted fish. The latter statement was based on the summary relative risk of 2.1, which was not significantly different from 1.0 (95% confidence limits, 0.60-6.28, $P = 0.18$); however, in reanalysing this data by frequency of consumption of salted fish (Table 3), a significant positive association was found: the chi-square for trend was 5.27, $P = 0.02$. Geser et al.[1] did find a positive association between exposure to salted fish during the weaning period and risk for NPC (relative risk = 2.6).

Huang et al.[2] detected volatile *N*-nitrosodimethylamine in Cantonese salted fish. Equally important is the report of Huang et al.[3] that four of ten female WA albino rats developed carcinoma of the nasal cavity when fed a diet of Cantonese salted fish. No nasal tumors were detected when rats were fed *N*-nitrosodimethylamine; however, Druckrey et al. (1967) did produce nasal cavity carcinoma in rats by artificial inhalation of *N*-nitrosodimethylamine. Interestingly, subcutaneous administration of *N*-nitrosodiethylamine produced nasal

---

[1] See p. 213

[2] See p. 309

[3] See p. 315

Table 3. Frequency of current use of salted fish among Chinese cases and controls in California

Frequency of current use of salted fish	Cases	Controls	RR[a]
More than once a week	24	21	3.1
Weekly	13	17	2.1
At least monthly	30	52	1.6
Never	7	19	1.0

[a] Risk ratio compared to 1.0 for 'never use'

cavity tumours in European hamsters (Mohr et al., 1972); however, this *N*-nitrosamine was not detected as a volatile by-product of Cantonese salted fish (Huang et al.[1]).

Thus, there is experimental evidence to support J. Ho's (1975) contention that exposure, by inhalation or ingestion, to *N*-nitrosamines in Cantonese salted fish is a major risk factor for NPC. As yet, this hypothesis does not satisfactorily explain the male excess of NPC.

Another approach to unravelling the etiology of NPC in Chinese has been reported by Anderson et al.[2]. A search for childhood exposure to environmental factors was made among 22 patients with NPC in Hong Kong diagnosed before age 25. Most of the patients 'come from relatively poor backgrounds' and only three smoked cigarettes. The 'kitchens seen or described were not usually poorly ventialted'; however, when these patients were children the primary fuel used for cooking was wood or charcoal in 19 cases. All currently ate fresh fish and 'without exception had eaten salted fish and had received it as one of their first solid foods'.

In summary, two basic hypotheses have been advanced for the etiology of NPC. Although inhalation of smoke (as in certain occupations) may be one explanation for the occasional NPC case seen in industrialized countries, solid evidence to support this mechanism for the risk for NPC in southern Chinese is lacking. Exposure, by inhalation or ingestion, to *N*-nitrosamines or allied compounds in Cantonese salted fish has gained considerable support as a causative factor from recent epidemiological and experimental studies. Further, careful study of dietary patterns, especially during childhood, of southern Chinese are needed.

---

[1] See p. 309

[2] See p. 231

ACKNOWLEDGEMENT

This work was supported by grants IR13-CA-21549 and P01-CA-17054.

REFERENCES

Armstrong, R.W., Kutty, M.K. & Armstrong, M.J. (1978) Self-specific environments associated with nasopharyngeal carcinoma in Selangor, Malaysia. *Soc. Sci. Med.* (in press)

Buell, P. (1973) Race and place in the etiology of nasopharyngeal cancer: a study based on California death certificates. *Int. J. Cancer, 11*, 268-272

Buell, P. (1974) The effect of migration on the risk of nasopharyngeal cancer among Chinese. *Cancer Res., 34*, 1189-1191

Clifford, P. (1970) A review on the epidemiology of nasopharyngeal carcinoma. *Int. J. Cancer, 5*, 287-309

Dobson, W.C. (1924) Cervical lymphosarcoma (letter to editor). *Chin. med. J., 38*, 386

Doll, R., Morgan, L.G. & Speizer, F.E. (1970) Cancers of the lung and nasal sinuses in nickel workers. *Br. J. Cancer, 24*, 623-632

Djojopranoto, M. & Soesilowati (1967) *Nasopharyngeal cancer in East Java (Indonesia).* In: Muir, C.S. & Shanmugaratnam, K.S., eds, *Cancer of the Nasopharynx (UICC Monograph Series* Vol. 1*)*, Copenhagen, Munksgaard, pp. 43-46

Druckrey, H., Preussmann, R., Ivankovic, S. & Schmähl, D. (1967) Organotrope carcinogene Wirkungen bei 65 verschiedenen *N*-nitroso-Verbindungen an BD-Ratten. *Z. Krebsforsch., 69*, 103-201

Fong, Y.Y. & Chan, W.C. (1973) Dimethylnitrosamine in Chinese marine salt fish. *Food Cosmet. Toxicol., 11*, 841-845

Fong, Y.Y. & Walsh, E.O. (1971) Carcinogenic nitrosamines in Cantonese salt-dried fish. *Lancet, ii*, 1032

Henderson, B.E., Louie, E., Jing, J.S., Buell, P. & Gardner, M.B. (1976) Risk factors associated with nasopharyngeal carcinoma. *New Engl. J. Med., 295*, 1101-1106

Ho, H.C. (1972a) *Current knowledge of the epidemiology of nasopharyngeal carcinoma - a review.* In: Biggs, P.M., de-Thé, G. & Payne, L.N., eds, *Oncogenesis and Herpesviruses*, Lyon, International Agency for Research on Cancer (*IARC Scientific Publications No. 2*), pp. 357-366

Ho, H.C. (1972b) Nasopharyngeal carcinoma (NPC). *Adv. Cancer Res., 15*, 57-92

Ho, H.C. (1975) Epidemiology of nasopharyngeal carcinoma. *J. R. Coll. Surg. (Edinb.), 20*, 223-225

Hu, M.S. & Huang, H.L. (1972) Retrospective study on the etiological factors of nasopharyngeal carcinoma. *New Med. (Canton), 12*, 10 (in Chinese)

Lin, T.M., Chen, K.P., Lin, C.C., Hsu, M.M., Tu, S.M., Chiang, T.C., Jung, P.F. & Hirayama, T. (1973) Retrospective study on nasopharyngeal carcinoma. *J. natl Cancer Inst., 51*, 1403-1408

Louie, E., Henderson, B.E., Buell, P., Jing, J.S., Menck, H.R. & Pike, M.P. (1977) Selected observations on the epidemiology of pharyngeal cancers. *Natl Cancer Inst. Monogr., No. 47*

Mohr, U., Althoff, J. & Page, N. (1972) Tumors of the respiratory system induced in the common European hamster by *N*-diethylnitrosamine. *J. natl Cancer Inst., 49*, 595-597

Muir, C.S. (1971) Nasopharyngeal carcinoma in non-Chinese populations with special reference to Southeast Asia and Africa. *Int. J. Cancer, 8*, 351-363

Passey, R.D. (1922) Experimental soot cancer. *Br. med. J., ii*, 1112

Pott, P. (1775) *Cancer scroti.* In: *Chirurgical Observations*, London, Howes, Clarke & Collins, p. 63

Proetz, A.W. (1953) Respiratory air currents and their clinical aspects. *J. Laryngol. Otol., 67*, 1-17

Shanmugaratnam, K. & Higginson, J. (1967) *Aetiology of nasopharyngeal cancer: report on a retrospective survey in Singapore.* In: Muir, C.S. & Shanmugaratnam, K., eds, *Cancer of the Nasopharynx* (*UICC Monograph Series* Vol. 1), Copenhagen, Munksgaard, pp. 130-134

USDHEW (US Department of Health, Education and Welfare, Public Health Service, Health Services and Mental Health Administration) (1971) *The Health Consequences of Smoking. A report to the Surgeon General*, Washington DC, US Government Printing Office

Wen, C.P. (1974) *China Medicine As We Saw It*, J.R. Quinn, ed., Washington DC, John E. Fogarty International Center for Advanced Study in the Health Sciences, US Department of Health, Education and Welfare, Public Health Service, National Institutes of Health, pp. 289-344

Willeke, K. & Whitby, K.T. (1975) Atmospheric aerosols: size, distribution, interpretation. *J. Air Pollut. Control Assoc.*, *25*, 529-534

Zippin, C., Tekawa, I.S., Bragg, K.U., Watson, D.A. & Linden, G. (1962) Studies on heredity and environment in cancer of the nasopharynx. *J. natl Cancer Inst.*, *29*, 483-490

ETIOLOGY OF NASOPHARYNGEAL CARCINOMA – GENETIC AND CHEMICAL FACTORS

HLA FREQUENCIES IN CANCER: A THIRD STUDY

S.T. PERDUE & P.I. TERASAKI

Department of Surgery,
School of Medicine,
University of California,
Los Angeles, Ca 90024, USA

M.R. MICKEY

Department of Biomathematics,
University of California,
Los Angeles, Ca 90024, USA

In two previous studies, we reported that most cancers have at best a weak association with HLA (Takasugi et al., 1973; Terasaki et al., 1977). Because the strong linkage disequilibria between various HLA loci correspond to high associations between specificities in random populations, we might expect linkages between the HLA region and disease susceptibility genes to appear as associations in population studies of HLA-associated diseases. A certain number of conflicting reports with regard to antigen associations with cancer can be expected due to the problem of sampling variations alone. In this study, a third, independent group of patients was analysed and compared with earlier groups. A follow-up 'disease' haplotype analysis, using a second group of patients selected independently of those in our first haplotype study (Terasaki & Mickey, 1975), was also performed.

MATERIALS AND METHODS

For the phenotype study, 526 patients and 629 controls were selected from Caucasian persons HLA-typed in this laboratory between September 1975 and February 1977. All persons were unrelated to each other; controls were primarily normal blood donors from Los Angeles and Bethesda. Groups for the haplotype analysis included persons HLA-typed in this laboratory between September 1974 and December 1976, and they were carefully selected to eliminate any overlap in patients or controls from the previous haplotype study (Terasaki & Mickey, 1975). They comprised 711 patients with six types of cancer; 549 normal donors served as controls; all were Caucasians.

The standard microcytotoxicity test was used for HLA typing. At least three antisera were used for each of the 25 specificities listed in Table 1. Phenotype analysis was done using a chi-square computation. Haplotype analysis to compute disease-associated haplotype frequencies was performed using formulae described previously (Terasaki & Mickey, 1975).

Patients were categorized by the description of their disease submitted by the physician at the time their blood sample was received. Comparisons of analyses were made for diseases that occurred in two or three of the studies.

RESULTS

A total of seven cancer categories were studied for the phenotype analysis. Significant deviations were found for 12 antigens at the P= 0.05 level; however, only the elevated level of A29 in acute myeloid leukaemia (AML) patients remained significant when P values were corrected for the number of antigens tested (Table 1). The antigen frequencies in general are remarkably stable compared with those in earlier studies. The largest differences in the control groups were a 4-5% decrease in AW30 and BW35; both of these antigens are still being clarified, and their definitions and assignments may have varied in our laboratory. The elevated BW35 frequencies in patients with breast cancer, lung cancer and lymphoma should be viewed with caution considering the variation in the normal controls.

Table 1. Frequencies of HLA antigens in patients with various types of cancer

	N	A 1	A 2	A 3	A 9	A 10	A 11	A 28	A 29	AW 30	AW 32	B 5	B 7	B 8	B 12	B 13	B 14	B 18	B 27	BW 15	BW 16	BW 17	BW 21	BW 22	BW 35	BW 40
Controls	629	29	48	23	19	16	12	10	6	5	7	10	25	22	25	5	9	10	8	10	11	9	5	6	17	11
Patients																										
ALL	81	23	51	27	27[a]	18	16	4	4	4	6	6	28	16	31	6	6	9	14	9	12	4	11[a]	1	22	11
AML	92	21	41	16	28[a]	15	14	10	17[b]	6	5	6	18	12[a]	21	0	11	10	6	14	15	6	5	11	20	21[a]
Breast cancer	87	31	41	17	24	13	13	13	9	6	11	9	20	23	24	6	8	11	7	15	6	7	3	2	26[a]	15
Hodgkin's disease	51	18	51	22	33	27	10	10	4	6	6	8	25	10	22	2	8	10	12	12	24	4	2	4	25	14
Lung cancer	124	31	52	23	23	14	10	4	5	6	6	10	19	24	22	7	9	13	9	10	14	11	6	2	16	8
Lymphoma	54	39	48	15	20	15	6	15	6	17[a]	11	17	22	13	22	15[a]	20[a]	6	9	7	6	7	4	7	15	9
Ovarian cancer	37	30	43	16	22	11	22	8	3	14	3	14	22	22	24	14[a]	0	8	11	22[a]	14	3	8	5	16	5

ALL - acute lymphocytic leukaemia

AML - acute myeloid leukaemia

[a] P≤ 0.05

[b] P≤ 0.002

Levels of several antigens were consistently high in all studies of particular diseases (Table 2). A2 and B27 were elevated in patients with acute lymphocytic leukaemia (ALL), A29 and BW22 were high in AML

Table 2. Trends in HLA specificities in patients with various types of cancers compared with those in controls (P≤ 0.05 in at least one study)

Cancer	Antigen	Antigen frequency								
		1976-1977 study			1973-1975 study[a]			1970-1972 study[b]		
		Patients No.	%	Controls[c] %	Patients No.	%	Controls[d] %	Patients No.	%	Controls[e] %
ALL	A2	81	51	48	215	56[f]	47	NA		
	A9		27[f]	19		19	21			
	B27		14	8		11[f]	7			
	BW21		11[f]	5		3	6			
AML	A9	92	28[f]	19	151	20	21	NA		
	A29		17[g]	6		9	6			
	AW32		5	7		12[f]	7			
	B8		12[f]	22		22	21			
	BW22		11	6		9[f]	4			
	BW40		21[f]	11		12	12			
Breast cancer	A1	87	31	29	377	26	31	384	32[f]	27
	BW35		26[f]	17		25	21		20	22
Hodgkin's disease	B5	51	8	10	101	11	11	321	17[f]	11
	B7		25	25		25	23		19[f]	25
	B18		10	10		12	7		14[f]	9
Lung cancer	BW35	124	16	17	180	17	21	250	16[f]	22
Lymphoma	A29	54	6	6	100	14[f]	6	51	12	7
	AW30		17[f]	5		12	10		8	10
	B13		15[f]	5		2	5		6	4
	B14		20[f]	9		12	10		12	7
	BW35		15	17		23	21		35[f]	22
Ovarian cancer	B12	37	24	25	74	14[f]	24	69	14	24
	B13		14[f]	5		0	5		1	4
	BW15		22[f]	10		5	10		9	3

[a], [b] Previously reported (Takasugi et al., 1973; Terasaki et al., 1977)

[c] N= 629 [d] N= 1536 [e] N= 906

[f] 0.002< P≤ 0.05 , without correction for number of antigens

[g] P≤ 0.002

ALL - acute lymphocytic leukaemia

AML - acute myeloid leukaemia

NA - not available

patients, and B14 was somewhat elevated in lymphoma patients. The frequency of A29 in lymphoma patients, which was increased in the earlier studies, was the same as that of controls in this study.

Certain antigen-disease associations are inconsistent from one study to another and may reflect random sample variations (Table 2). Such associations include BW21 in ALL, AW32 in AML, B13 and AW30 in lymphoma and A1 in breast cancer patients. The inconsistent results obtained in patients with ovarian cancer, compared with those of the first two studies, may be due to the relatively small number (37) of patients tested. Possible associations of Hodgkin's disease with B5, B7 and B18 that were indicated in the 1973 study were not confirmed in either subsequent study.

Patients with AML showed elevated levels of BW40 and decreased levels of B8 in this study. Those with either ALL or AML have increased frequencies of A9, whereas these frequencies were normal in the earlier study. It should be noted that this extra A9 is entirely in the AW24 component for both types of leukaemia.

Haplotype analysis was done for six cancer categories. Those frequencies of disease haplotypes that were significantly different from in controls in either this or the 1975 study are shown in Table 3.

Several results were similar in both studies, even though the differences may have been statistically significant in only one. These include considerable increases for A3-B8 in ALL and for A11-B13 in breast cancer patients, as well as a virtual absence of A2-B5 in AML patients. All of the individual antigens of these haplotypes occur with normal frequency in the corresponding disease.

Other haplotypes that were significantly different from those in controls in one study were at least numerically so in the other; i.e., A9-BW22, A11-B5 and A2-BW40 in AML and A1-B8 in lymphoma patients. The remaining results were inconsistent in the two studies, emphasizing the fact that large numbers of patients are needed in order to obtain meaningful haplotype analyses.

DISCUSSION

This study confirms the finding that there are no strong associations between HLA-A and -B locus antigens and the types of cancers studied; however, some consistent results indicate that there may, in fact, be some linkage between HLA and cancer.

One problem that causes inconsistent results among different studies may be variations in patient populations, i.e., two given samples may be drawn from different subpopulations of a disease group. Several studies, for example, have reported an increase in A2 in ALL patients (Rogentine et al., 1972; Sanderson et al., 1973; Walford et al., 1970); others have not found this difference (Dickson, 1975; Klouda et al., 1974; Thorsby et al., 1971). Klouda et al. (1974)

Table 3. HLA disease haplotypes significantly different in patients with various cancers from those in controls ($P \leq 0.05$ in at least one study)

Cancer	Haplotype	Disease haplotype freq./1000					
		1977 study			1975 study		
		Patients		Controls[a]	Patients		Controls[b]
		No. tested	Hapl. freq.	Hapl. freq.	No. tested	Hapl. freq.	Hapl. freq.
ALL	1- 8	181	60	72	103	0[d]	89
	3- 8		46[d]	1		33	8
	3- 7		52	55		0[d]	62
	1-17		0[d]	22		25	20
AML	1- 8	134	80	72	75	0[d]	89
	9[c]-22		7	3		63[d]	2
	2- 5		0[d]	28		0	22
	11- 5		59[d]	7		9	3
	2-40		100[d]	26		32	24
Breast cancer	11-13	110	23	0	512	11[d]	0
	28-12		0	6		24[d]	8
Lung cancer	1- 7	173	16	18	179	63[d]	12
Lymphoma	1- 8	63	67	72	87	0[d]	89
Ovarian cancer	9[c]-35	50	9	19	108	57[d]	15

[a] N= 549

[b] N= 1500

[c] AW24 was used in place of A9 for the 1977 study.

[d] $P \leq 0.05$

ALL - acute lymphocytic leukaemia

AML - acute myeloid leukaemia

found different antigen profiles in newly diagnosed ALL patients and in those who survived longer, and they postulate that both A9 and B27 may be associated with increased survival time. B27 was elevated in ALL patients in our study, and A9 (specifically AW 24) was also increased; we showed only a small numerical increase in the frequency of A2 in these patients. Dickson (1975) found a significantly raised A9 frequency in patients with leukaemia, particularly in those with the myeloid types; our results showed the same trend.

Some investigators have reported an increase in the haplotypes A1-B8 and A2-B12 in ALL patients (Thorsby et al., 1971). Our haplotype analysis of 181 ALL patients showed no deviation in disease haplotype frequency for either A1-B8 or A2-B12 compared to that in normal controls.

It appears that it is necessary to exercise caution in carrying out population studies of possible associations of HLA and cancer. This is particularly evident in the case of haplotype analysis in which the use of small numbers of patients may give meaningless results because of the many variables involved.

SUMMARY

Frequencies of 25 HLA antigens in 526 Caucasian patients were compared to those in 629 healthy controls who were HLA-typed between September 1975 and February 1977. Haplotypes were compared for 711 patients and 549 controls typed between September 1974 and December 1976. Frequency deviations were found in those with ALL, AML, breast cancer, lymphoma and ovarian cancer, but only the increase in A29 in AML patients was statistically significant when corrected for the number of specificities. Interesting associations, when compared with earlier studies, include elevation of AW24 in both ALL and AML patients and increased B27 in ALL patients. Significant haplotype differences were increased A3-B8 and absence of A1-BW17 in ALL patients and increased A11-B5 and A2-BW40 as well as absence of A2-B5 in AML patients.

ACKNOWLEDGEMENT

This work was supported by Public Health Service Contract N01-CP43211 within the Virus Cancer Program of the Division of Cancer Cause and Prevention, National Cancer Institute, USA.

REFERENCES

Dickson, A. (1975) A raised incidence of HL-A2 plus HL-A9 and other anomalies of the HL-A antigens of patients with leukemia. *Acta Haematol.*, *54*, 143-151

Klouda, P.T., Lawler, S.D., Till, M.M. & Hardisty, R.M. (1974) Acute lymphoblastic leukemia and HL-A: a prospective study. *Tissue Antigens*, *4*, 262-265

Rogentine, G.N., Yankee, R.A., Gart, J.J., Nam, J. & Trapani, R.J. (1972) HLA antigens and disease: acute lymphocytic leukemia. *J. clin. Invest.*, *51*, 2420-2428

Sanderson, A.R., Mahon, G.H., Jaffe, N. & Das, L. (1973) Incidence of HL-A antigens in acute lymphocytic leukemia. *Transplantation*, *16*, 672-674

Takasugi, M., Terasaki, P.I., Henderson, G., Mickey, M.R., Menk, H. & Thompson, R.W. (1973) HLA antigens in solid tumors. *Cancer Res.*, *33*, 648-650

Terasaki, P.I. & Mickey, M.R. (1975) HL-A haplotypes of 32 diseases. *Transplant. Rev.*, *22*, 105-119

Terasaki, P.I., Perdue, S.T. & Mickey, M.R. (1977) *HLA frequencies in cancer: a second study*. In: Mulvihill, J.J., ed., *Genetics of Human Cancer*, New York, Raven Press, pp. 321-327

Thorsby, E., Engeset, A. & Lie, S.O. (1971) HL-A antigens and susceptibility to diseases: a study of patients with acute lymphoblastic leukemia, Hodgkin's disease, and childhood asthma. *Tissue Antigens*, *1*, 147-152

Walford, R.L., Finkelstein, S., Neerhout, R., Konrad, P. & Shanbrom, E. (1970) Acute childhood leukemia in relation to the HL-A human transplantation genes. *Nature (Lond.)*, *225*, 461-462

NASOPHARYNGEAL CARCINOMA AND HISTOCOMPATIBILITY ANTIGENS

M.J. SIMONS & S.H. CHAN

Immunology Research and Training Centre, University of Singapore

S. DARMALINGAM

Department of Radiology, University of Kuala Lumpur, Kuala Lumpur, Malaysia

G.B. WEE & K. SHANMUGARATNAM

Department of Pathology, University of Singapore

U. PRASAD

Ear, Nose and Throat Department, University of Kuala Lumpur, Kuala Lumpur, Malaysia

E.H. GOH

Ear, Nose and Throat Department, Singapore General Hospital

H. BETUEL

Centre de Transfusion Sanguine de Lyon, Beynost, France

J.H.C. HO & J.C.W. CHAU

Medical and Health Department Institute of Radiology, Queen Elizabeth Hospital, Kowloon, Hong Kong

N.E. DAY & G. DE-THE

International Agency for Research on Cancer, Lyon, France

INTRODUCTION

The purpose of this paper is to enlarge on the results already published concerning the relationship between nasopharyngeal carcinoma (NPC) and histocompatibility antigens. Previous papers (Simons et al., 1974, 1975, 1976) have described an association among Chinese between risk for NPC and the HLA antigens A2 and B-Sin 2. A further paper (Betuel et al., 1975) described the HLA profile of Tunisian NPC patients. In previous papers, NPC patients were classified by ethnic group and, among Chinese, by dialect group but were otherwise treated as homogeneous. Studies relating HLA antigens to risk for other malignancies have clearly shown that both susceptibility and survival can be modified by HLA type (Rogentine et al., 1973, 1977). In this paper, the differential effects of HLA antigen type on susceptibility and survival status, the interaction with age and some preliminary results with regard to other ethnic groups will be considered.

MATERIALS AND METHODS

Lymphocyte separation and HLA typing were performed as described earlier (Simons et al., 1976). The cases consist of histologically confirmed cases of NPC who were typed since the discovery of the B-locus antigen Sin 2. The analysis in this paper is confined to 141 cases from whom a blood sample was obtained within two months of diagnosis, i.e., newly diagnosed patients, and to 39 patients from whom blood was taken more than five years after diagnosis, i.e., long-term survivors. Control samples consisted of cord blood obtained from 238 women at the main Singapore maternity hospital.

RESULTS

Chinese subjects

Susceptibility. The effect of HLA genes on disease susceptibility can best be studied in newly diagnosed cases, thus avoiding varying times of survival. The hypothesis of an increased risk for the joint occurrence of A2 and B-Sin 2 was proposed on the basis of data from patients other than those in the present series; thus, in examining the effect of these two antigens, one-sided uncorrected significance levels are appropriate. For other antigens, nominal significance levels need correction for the number of comparisons.

Table 1 gives the antigen and gene frequencies for the HLA loci A and B in the NPC cases and in the controls. For locus A antigens, the excess of A2 among NPC cases is less than that found previously, a reflection probably of the improved survival associated with A2 (see below). The highly significant deficit of A11 among HLA cases is more striking than observed previously; this finding is related to the excess of BW17, since there is a high negative disequilibrium (Δ) value between these two antigens among NPC cases.

For locus B antigens, the relative risk associated with B-Sin 2 is slightly less than observed previously but still highly significant. Of great interest is the emergence of a new association, the very clear increase in risk associated with BW17. Among the NPC patients, but not among the controls, there is an apparent negative association between BW17 and B-Sin 2 (Table 2); that is, among NPC cases there is a deficit of individuals lacking both BW17 and B-Sin 2 and no

Table 1. Frequency of HLA locus A and B antigens among newly diagnosed Chinese nasopharyngeal carcinoma (NPC) patients and among healthy Chinese controls

Antigen	NPC patients n= 141			Controls n= 238			
	Number	Antigen frequency (%)	Gene frequency	Number	Antigen frequency (%)	Gene frequency	Significance
A1	1	0.7	0.004	0	0	0	
A2	86	61.0	0.376	126	52.9	0.314	χ^2 = 2.33[a] P = 0.064
A3	1	0.7	0.004	1	0.4	0.002	NS
A9	47	33.3	0.183	65	27.3	0.147	NS
A10	13	9.2	0.047	12	5.0	0.026	NS
A11	57	40.4	0.228	144	60.5	0.372	χ^2 = 14.3 P = 0.004[b]
A28	0	0	0	1	0.4	0.002	NS
A29	1	0.7	0.004	3	1.3	0.006	NS
AW19	22	15.6	0.081	49	20.6	0.109	NS
Blank	52	36.9	0.073	73	30.7	0.022	NS
B5	19	13.5	0.070	30	12.6	0.065	NS
B7	1	0.7	0.004	4	1.7	0.008	NS
B8	1	0.7	0.004	1	0.4	0.002	NS
B12	2	1.4	0.007	8	3.4	0.017	NS
B13	19	13.5	0.070	48	20.2	0.107	NS
B14	0	0	0	0	0	0	NS
B18	1	0.7	0.004	4	1.7	0.008	NS
B27	4	2.8	0.014	17	7.1	0.036	NS
BW15	26	18.4	0.097	53	22.3	0.118	NS
BW16	14	9.9	0.051	26	10.9	0.056	NS
BW17	40	28.4	0.154	34	14.3	0.074	χ^2 = 11.1 P = 0.02[b]
BW21	0	0	0	0	0	0	NS
BW22	9	6.4	0.032	29	12.2	0.063	NS
BW35	8	5.7	0.029	12	5.0	0.026	NS
BW37	2	1.4	0.007	1	0.4	0.002	NS
BW40	53	37.6	0.210	98	41.2	0.233	NS
B-Sin 2	48	34.0	0.188	54	22.7	0.121	χ^2 = 5.80 P = 0.008[a]
Blank	37	26.2		58	24.4		

[a] One-sided
[b] Two-sided, corrected for 26 antigens
NS - not significant

Relative risk for A2 = 1.39
" " " A11 = 0.44
" " " B-Sin 2 = 1.76
" " " BW17 = 2.38

Table 2. Joint occurrence of BW17 and B-Sin 2 among newly diagnosed nasopharyngeal carcinoma (NPC) patients and controls

	NPC patients BW17					Controls BW17			
		+	-	Total			+	-	Total
B-Sin 2	+	7	41	48	B-Sin 2	+	7	47	54
	-	33	60	93		-	27	157	184
	Total	40	101	141		Total	34	204	238

$\chi^2 = 6.81$ $P < 0.01$

Odds ratio = 3.22^{-1}

$\chi^2 = 0.10$

Odds ratio = 1.16^{-1}

corresponding increase in individuals carrying both antigens. The much greater disequilibrium among NPC cases than among controls is further evidence that both antigens play a role in determining the risk for NPC.

Table 3 gives the number of individuals with either BW17 or B-Sin 2 among NPC cases and among controls. Notwithstanding the number of possible ways in which one can choose a pair of antigens, i.e., 325, a value of 19.8 for a χ^2 on 1 degree of freedom is highly significant.

Table 3. Occurrence of either BW17 or B-Sin 2 among newly diagnosed nasopharyngeal carcinoma (NPC) cases and among controls

	BW17 or B-Sin 2	Neither BW17 nor B-Sin 2	Total
NPC patients	81	60	141
Controls	81	157	238
Total	162	217	379

χ^2= 19.8 P= 0.00001 Relative risk = 2.62

The joint occurrence of A2 and B-Sin 2 among the newly diagnosed NPC patients and controls is shown in Table 4. The difference between the two groups is highly significant, indicating clearly that the A2 B-Sin 2 phenotype increases susceptibility for the disease and is not a factor that primarily affects survival.

Table 4. Joint occurrence of A2 and B-Sin 2 among newly diagnosed nasopharyngeal carcinoma (NPC) cases and controls

	Joint occurrence of A2 and B-Sin 2	One or both of A2 and B-Sin 2 lacking	Total
NPC patients	41	100	141
Controls	41	197	238
Total	82	297	379

χ^2= 7.33 P= 0.0034 (one-sided) Relative risk = 1.97

Table 5 gives the disequilibrium (Δ) values, as obtained from phenotype frequencies (Mattiuz et al., 1970), for locus A and B antigens in the normal Chinese population and among NPC cases. Clearly, A2-B-Sin 2 and AW19-BW17 stand out as the antigen pairs in greatest disequilibrium. There is also considerable disequilibrium between BW17 and a locus A blank. Since the latter includes locus A homozygotes, a clearer picture is obtained by considering haplotypes obtained from family studies. Table 6 gives the joint occurrence of BW17, AW19 and A blank on 134 haplotypes obtained from 34 families of NPC patients (in some families full haplotyping was impossible, in others a second wife and her children were included). The association

Table 5a HLA antigen phenotypes and delta values in total normal Chinese (n= 238)

Locus B antigen (no. pos. in brackets)	Locus A antigens (no. positive in brackets)									
	A1(0)	A2(126)	A3 (1)	A9 (65)	A10 (12)	A11 (144)	A28 (2)	A29 (3)	AW19 (49)	Blank (74)
B5 (30)	0	16[a] 0.0004[b]	0	11 0.007	2 0.0011	20 0.007	1 0.002	0	7 0.002	3
B7 (4)	0	2 - 0.0004	0	0	0	2 - 0.0014	0	3 0.006	0	1
B8 (1)	0	1 0.001	0	0	0	0	1 0.002	0	0	0
B12 (8)	0	5 - 0.002	0	1 - 0.003	0	3 - 0.006	0	0	1 - 0.002	6
B13 (48)	0	22 - 0.012	0	16 0.008	2 - 0.0011	33 0.015	0	0	11 0.003	12
B14 (0)	0	0	0	0	0	0	0	0	0	0
B18 (4)	0	1 - 0.004	0	3 0.005	0	2 - 0.001	0	0	1 0.0004	1
B27 (17)	0	6 - 0.01	0	8 0.009	0	11 0.003	0	0	3 - 0.007	6
BW15 (53)	0	30 0.007	0	15 0.002	1 - 0.004	32 0.0003	0	1 0.001	11 - 0.0002	16
BW16 (26)	0	15 0.004	0	6 - 0.003	0	16 0.001	1 0.002	0	4 - 0.003	10
BW17 (34)	0	16 - 0.007	0	5 - 0.01	0	16 - 0.017	0	0	16 0.023	15
BW21 (0)	0	0	0	0	0	0	0	0	0	0
BW22 (29)	0	12 0.011	0	10 0.006	1 - 0.001	20 0.009	0	0	9 0.008	6
BW35 (12)	0	6 - 0.001	0	5 0.004	1 0.001	7 - 0.001	0	0	2 - 0.001	3
BW37 (1)	0	0	0	0	0	1 0.001	0	0	0	1
BW40 (98)	0	49 0.012	0	32 0.017	5 0.002	59 - 0.001	0	1 - 0.001	16 - 0.013	34
Sin 2 (54)	0	41 0.042	1 0.002	7 - 0.022	4 0.003	29 - 0.014	1 0.002	1 0.001	5 - 0.017	19
Blank (57)	0	30	1	11	8	37	0	0	12	15

[a] Number of subjects

[b] Delta value

Table 5b. HLA antigen phenotypes and delta values in total Chinese NPC patients (n= 141)

Locus B antigen (no. pos. in brackets)	Locus A antigens (no. positive in brackets)									
	A1 (1)	A2 (86)	A3 (1)	A9 (47)	A10 (14)	A11 (57)	A28 (0)	A29 (0)	AW19 (23)	Blank (53)
B5 (19)	0	14[a] 0.015[b]	1 0.003	9 0.012	2 0.001	8 0.002	0	0	0	4
B7 (1)	0	1 0.002	0	0	0	1 0.003	0	0	0	0
B8 (1)	0	1 0.002	0	0	1 0.003	0	0	0	0	0
B12 (2)	0	1 - 0.001	0	0	0	1 0.001	0	0	1 0.003	1
B13 (19)	0	7 - 0.029	0	7 0.003	1 - 0.004	10 0.011	0	0	4 0.004	9
B14 (0)	0	0	0	0	0	0	0	0	0	0
B18 (1)	0	1 0.002	0	1 0.003	0	0	0	0	0	0
B27 (4)	0	0	0	1 - 0.002	2 0.006	3 0.006	0	0	2 0.005	0
BW15 (26)	0	18 0.013	0	7 - 0.008	2 - 0.002	17 0.032	0	0	0	8
BW16 (14)	0	12 0.02	0	5 0.002	0	3 - 0.013	0	0	3 0.003	5
BW17 (40)	0	15 - 0.067	0	12 - 0.007	3 - 0.004	9 - 0.04	0	0	17 0.048	24
BW21 (0)	0	0	0	0	0	0	0	0	0	0
BW22 (9)	0	5 - 0.003	0	4 0.005	0	1 - 0.013	0	0	1 - 0.002	7
BW35 (8)	0	5 0.001	0	6 0.015	0	3 - 0.001	0	0	0	2
BW37 (2)	0	1 0.001	0	0	0	2 0.006	0	0	0	1
BW40 (53)	1 0.003	29 - 0.025	0	18 0.002	7 0.008	23 0.009	0	0	6 - 0.011	22
Sin 2 (48)	0	41 0.076	0	14 - 0.011	4 - 0.004	17 - 0.014	0	0	5 - 0.012	15
Blank (35)	1	21	1	10		16	0	0	7	8

[a] Number of subjects
[b] Delta value

Table 6. Occurrence on the same haplotype of BW17 with either AW19 or a locus A blank in 34 families of nasopharyngeal carcinoma patients

	BW17		
	+	-	Total
AW19	4	4	8
A blank	5	1	6
Other locus A antigen	1	119	120
Total	10	124	134

of BW17 with A blank, and to a lesser extent with AW19, is very strong. Table 7 compares the occurrence of BW17 with A blank in NPC patients and controls.

Table 7. Joint occurrence of BW17 and either AW19 or A blank among nasopharyngeal carcinoma (NPC) patients and controls

	Joint occurrence of BW17 and either AW19 or A blank		
	+	-	Total
NPC patients	36	105	141
Controls	26	212	238
Total	62	317	379

$\chi^2 = 13.8$ P= 0.0002 Relative risk = 2.80

Survival. In order to assess the effect that HLA antigens may have on survival after diagnosis, newly diagnosed cases are compared with cases who have survived at least five years after diagnosis. No account is taken of clinical stage at diagnosis, since this is clearly independent of HLA type and thus cannot act as a confounding factor.

Table 8 compares the frequency of BW17 between the two groups: BW17 clearly indicates a poor prognosis; B-Sin 2 has a lower frequency in the five-year survival group, but the effect is less marked and does not reach statistical significance.

Table 8. Frequency of BW17 among newly diagnosed nasopharyngeal carcinoma (NPC) patients and those surviving five years after diagnosis

NPC patients	BW17		
	+	-	Total
Newly diagnosed	40	101	141
5-year survivors	3	36	39
Total	43	137	180

$\chi^2 = 6.09$ (with Yates' correction) P= 0.014

Table 9 shows the effect on survival of A2 when it occurs without BW17 or B-Sin 2. The improved survival among those with A2 is evident.

Table 9. Frequency of A2 in the absence of B-Sin 2 or BW17 among newly diagnosed nasopharyngeal carcinoma (NPC) patients and among those surviving five years after diagnosis

NPC patients	A2 (in the absence of BW17 and Sin 2)		
	+	-	Total
Newly diagnosed	34	107	141
5-year survivors	17	22	39
Total	51	129	180

$\chi^2 = 5.71$ P= 0.017

Age. In newly diagnosed cases under 30 years of age, there is a lower frequency of the joint occurrence of A2 and B-Sin 2 than in older age groups and a higher frequency of A blank and BW17. There is, curiously, also a relative excess of B-Sin 2 occurring without A2 (Table 10).

Table 10. Occurrence of A2 with B-Sin 2 among nasopharyngeal carcinoma patients, by age

Age group	B-Sin 2 without A2	B-Sin 2 with A2	Total
Less than 30 years	3	1	4
30 years or more	4	40	44
Total	7	41	48

P= 0.008 (Fisher's exact test)

Malays

There are considerable differences at the A locus between NPC cases and controls (Table 11): the largest difference is in the size of the blank, which remains highly significant after correction for the number of comparisons. None of the locus B antigens show an association with NPC. There is also a deficit of the AW19 complex among the Malay NPC cases, which does not, however, achieve statistical significance after correction for the number of antigens.

Table 11. Frequency of locus A antigens among Malay nasopharyngeal carcinoma (NPC) patients and among Malay controls

	NPC patients n= 34			Controls n= 106			
	No.	Antigen frequency (%)	Gene frequency	No.	Antigen frequency (%)	Gene frequency	χ^2
A1	1	2.9	0.015	8	7.5	0.030	
A2	6	17.6	0.093	36	34.0	0.187	3.26
A3	3	8.8	0.045	3	2.8	0.014	
A9	22	64.7	0.406	61	57.5	0.348	
A10	2	5.9	0.030	16	15.1	0.079	
A11	12	35.3	0.196	29	27.4	0.148	
A28	0	0	0	1	0.9	0.005	
AW19	2	5.9	0.030	29	27.4	0.148	5.69
Blank	21	61.8	0.185[a]	29	27.4	0.041[a]	13.27

[a] by subtraction from 1

Significance level for blank = 0.00028 (nominal)
= 0.0073 (corrected for 26 antigens)

Relative risk = 4.29

DISCUSSION

The results presented above demonstrate that HLA antigens play a role in determining both susceptibility for NPC and survival after diagnosis.

The distribution of both locus A and locus B antigens is very significantly different in newly diagnosed NPC patients as compared to the normal population. Even though fewer numbers of cases were available for comparison, significant differences also emerged between long-term survivors and newly diagnosed cases.

Evidently, for the purpose of establishing disease associations with the HLA system, survival and susceptibility must be very sharply distinguished. Little weight can be given to studies in which the survival status of the patients in the different disease groups is not taken into account. In previous studies in the present series, the mixing of long-term survivors with newly diagnosed cases had obscured the BW17 association with susceptibility, and, as happened with acute lymphocytic leukaemia, confounded survival and susceptibility in the association with A2.

Among the Chinese, there are two locus B antigens, B-Sin 2 and BW17, that are associated with susceptibility, as for juvenile diabetes (B8 and BW15). However, unlike juvenile diabetes, the joint occurrence of the two antigens does not appear further to increase the risk. A possible interpretation of this result would be that a single dominant disease susceptibility gene is in disequilibrium with both B-Sin 2 and BW17. Dominance would imply that among NPC cases only one haplotype would normally carry the DS gene, and thus the frequency of only one of the two locus B antigens would be increased. In very simple terms, if the gene frequency of locus B alleles on a chromosome carrying the DS gene is given by q_1, q_2, ..., and the gene frequency of locus B alleles in the general population is p_1, p_2, ..., then if NPC cases have one haplotype carrying the DS gene and the other haplotype distributed as in the normal population, the frequency of antigen i among NPC cases is given by

$$p_i + q_i - p_i q_i,$$

and the frequency of joint occurrence of i and j is given by

$$p_i q_j + p_j q_i.$$

Substitution of the values for p from Table 1 gives values of q for B-Sin 2 of 0.250 and for BW17 of 0.227. The corresponding gene frequencies in the normal population are 0.121 and 0.074. The frequency of joint occurrence of B-Sin 2 and BW17 is then 0.046, giving an expected number in Table 2 of 6.49, as compared to 7 observed. The model clearly gives an adequate description of the negative association between the two antigens.

Both BW17 and B-Sin 2 occur in significant disequilibrium with first locus antigens, and, in fact, among the antigens which occur with appreciable frequency, the two largest Δ values correspond to the pairs A2-B Sin 2 and AW19-BW17. It seems likely that the AW19-BW17 disequilibrium is associated with the A blank-BW17 disequilibrium. That is to say, the A locus blank probably corresponds to a specificity of the cross-reacting AW19 complex, for which typing sera were not included in the trays. Sera against AW29, AW30, AW31 and AW32, but not against AW33 were included; and anti-serum against AW34, formerly Malay 2, was also not included.

An attempt to equate the blank not identifiable with our present panel of sera is planned in a future series. The excess of a locus A blank among Malay NPC patients is of considerable interest. Firstly, it extends the role of HLA antigen in NPC to a non-Chinese population (although the Malays are certainly Chinese-related). Secondly, corresponding to the excess of the blank, there is a deficit of the AW19 complex as defined by the sera used. It thus seems likely that the A blank associated with BW17 among Chinese is the same A blank as found in excess among Malay NPC patients and forms part of the AW19 group. Clearly, however, insufficient numbers of Malay patients have been typed, no distinction has been made with respect to survival status, there has been insufficient precision in typing the AW19 complex and Malay 2, or AW34, needs to be included. Further comments are unwarranted until a study has been performed to fill these deficiencies.

Extension of the HLA-NPC association to a completely non-Chinese-related population is suggested by initial observations from Melbourne (Simons & Mathews[1]), where a very high frequency of A3 was found in a small series. This observation requires confirmation in a larger study.

SUMMARY

New data are presented concerning the relationship between NPC and HLA antigens among Chinese. When attention is confined to newly diagnosed cases, it can be shown that, apart from the increased risk associated with the joint occurrence of A2 and B-Sin 2, there is also an increased risk associated with BW17 and a decrease in risk associated with A11. Among long-term survivors, however, BW17 is appreciably decreased, whereas A2 in the absence of B-Sin 2 or BW17 is increased. Among Malays, a non-Chinese group, there is an excess among NPC patients of a locus A blank, a blank which is probably associated with the AW19 complex.

REFERENCES

Betuel, H., Cammoun, M., Colombani, J., Day, N.E., Ellouz, R. & de-Thé, G. (1975) The relationship between nasopharyngeal carcinoma and the HL-A system among Tunisians. *Int. J. Cancer, 16*, 249-254

Mattiuz, P.L., Ihde, D., Piazza, A., Ceppellini, R. & Bodmer, W.F. (1970) *New approaches to the population: genetic and segregation analysis of the HL-A system.* In: Terasaki, P.I., ed., *Histocompatibility Testing*, Copenhagen, Munksgaard, pp. 193-205

---

[1] Personal communication

Rogentine, G.N. Trapani, R.J., Yaulice, R.A. & Henderson, E.S. (1973) HLA antigens and acute lymphocytic leukaemia: the nature of the HL-A2 association. *Tissue Antigens, 3*, 470-476

Rogentine, G.N., Jr, Dellon, A.L. & Chretien, P.B. (1977) *Prolonged disease-free-survival in bronchogenic carcinoma associated with HLA AW19 and B5: a follow-up.* In: Dausset, J. & Svejgaard, A., eds, *First International Symposium on HLA and Disease, Paris*, Copenhagen, Munksgaard (in press)

Simons, M.J., Wee, G.B., Day, N.E., Morris, P.J., Shanmugaratnam, K. & de-Thé, G. (1974) Immunogenetic aspects of nasopharyngeal carcinoma. I. Differences in HL-A antigen profiles between patients and comparison groups. *Int. J. Cancer, 13*, 122-134

Simons, M.J., Wee, G.B., Day, N.E., Chan, S.H., Shanmugaratnam, K. & de-Thé, G.B. (1975) Probable identification of an HL-A second-locus antigen associated with a high risk of nasopharyngeal carcinoma. *Lancet, i*, 142-143

Simons, M.J., Wee, G.B., Goh, E.H., Chan, S.H., Shanmugaratnam, K., Day, N.E. & de-Thé, G. (1976) Immunogenetic aspects of nasopharyngeal carcinoma. IV. Increased risk in Chinese of nasopharyngeal carcinoma associated with a Chinese-related HLA profile (A2, Singapore 2). *J. nat. Cancer Inst., 57*, 977-980

GENETIC COMPONENTS IN SUSCEPTIBILITY TO NASOPHARYNGEAL CARCINOMA

R.L. KIRK, N.M. BLAKE & S. SERJEANTSON

The John Curtin School of Medical Research, Canberra, Australia

M.J. SIMONS & S.H. CHAN

WHO Immunology Research and Training Centre, Singapore

INTRODUCTION

The increased incidence of nasopharyngeal carcinoma (NPC) among Chinese has been well documented (Shanmugaratnam, 1971; Shanmugaratnam & Wee, 1973) and suggests that genetic susceptibility to etiological factors or genetic inability to control the established disease may contribute to the observed epidemiological pattern. During the last few years Simons and his colleagues have presented evidence in support of this possibility (Simons & Day, 1975; Simons et al., 1974, 1975, 1976). They have focussed attention on the histocompatibility system and have shown that the combination of HLA A2-HLA B Sin 2 is significantly increased in NPC patients, the association being stronger in more severe cases, judged by shorter survival time, and in those over the age of 30 years[1]. The same workers have postulated that this association may be due to linkage disequilibrium with a specific disease susceptibility or immune-response gene at or near the HLA-D locus (Simons et al., 1976).

To explore further the possibility that genetic susceptibility may be involved in the increased frequency of NPC among Chinese we have carried out a survey of 25 red-cell enzyme and five serum protein systems in both affected and normal Chinese living in Singapore.

---

[1] See p. 271

One of the red-cell enzyme systems, glyoxalase (GLO), and one of the serum protein systems, properdin factor B (Bf), are controlled by genes closely linked to the HLA system on chromosome 6. The other enzyme and serum protein systems, in those cases in which information is available, are controlled by genes on other chromosomes: they may serve, therefore, as indicators of possible involvement of other parts of the genome in susceptibility to NPC.

MATERIALS AND METHODS

Chinese patients in Singapore suspected to be suffering from NPC were classified as NPC-positive when confirmed by histological examination or as NPC-negative. Some NPC-negative persons were confirmed histologically as NPC-positive after varying periods of time ; the NPC-negative patients are thus not a satisfactory control group. In the present investigation a control series was assembled from two other sources: a small group, comprising a total of 30 persons, consisted of non-affected spouses of patients; the remaining controls were non-related members of families included in a survey of Chinese living in a large Singapore housing development. They were all non-NPC cases and were representative of Chinese of low and medium income levels.

Cells and serum (or plasma) were separated immediately after collection of venipuncture blood samples, and portions were frozen for subsequent typing. Samples were transported to Canberra at dry-ice temperature, and red-cell enzyme and serum protein systems were studied using methods described previously (Malcolm et al., 1972; Woodfield et al., 1974).

RESULTS

Because of known differences in incidence of NPC among Chinese speaking different dialects (Shanmugaratnam & Wee, 1973), we have restricted our study, both of patients and controls, to those persons for whom dialect information was available. The method of selecting controls was such that the distribution of dialect groups was different particularly with regard to the percentage of Hokkien. The distribution of persons classified as NPC-negative was more similar to that of the NPC-positives (Table 1). As noted below, for certain comparisons the distribution of controls was adjusted to that of the NPC-positive series by using weighting factors for the five dialect groups considered, Cantonese, Hokkien, Teochew, Hakka/Khek and Hainanese.

The distribution of phenotypes and the gene frequencies derived from them in 11 of the systems that showed variation are given in Table 2. The gene frequencies of the controls are based on a dialect-standardized sample, in order to make them directly comparable

Table 1. Numbers of nasopharyngeal carcinoma (NPC) patients and controls sampled, by dialect

	No. of NPC +ve (%)	No. of NPC -ve (%)	No. of controls (%)
Cantonese	61 (26.64)	49 (27.84)	74 (30.83)
Hokkien	81 (35.37)	70 (39.77)	60 (25.00)
Teochew	43 (18.78)	36 (20.45)	51 (21.25)
Khek/Hakka	26 (11.35)	8 (4.55)	22 (9.17)
Hainanese	18 (7.86)	13 (7.39)	33 (13.75)
Total	229	176	240

to the NPC-positives. Variation was also noted in several other systems, particularly glucose 6-phosphate dehydrogenase (G6PD), for which 11 of 202 patients, but only 1 of 138 NPC-negatives and 0 of 194 controls, were classified as B-negative. Since many of the samples, particularly those from patients, had been stored for several months before testing, we do not place great confidence in these results. Future investigations should aim at testing for G6PD activity in fresh material; more careful evaluation of the system is needed, especially in view of the postulated protective effect against cancer of the B-negative phenotype (Beaconsfield & Rainsbury, 1968; Beaconsfield et al., 1965). It is of interest to note that our evidence suggests the opposite: that patients have a significantly higher frequency of the B-negative phenotype than do the controls.

Several other variants were detected in 18 systems not included in Table 2: among the patients, there were two persons with malate dehydrogenase, one with glutamate-oxaloacetate transaminase and phosphohexose isomerase variants, and 12 with some change in peptidase D. A similar frequency of these sporadic variants was found among the NPC-negative and control groups.

Single locus analysis

Four systems in Table 2 show differences of 4% or more between the frequencies of genes among patients compared with those among controls standardized for dialect. In six of 11 comparisons, the

Table 2. Phenotypes and gene frequencies for variable genetic marker systems in nasopharyngeal carcinoma (NPC) patients and two groups of controls

System	NPC +ve			NPC -ve			Controls (standardized for dialect)		
	No.	%	Gene frequency	No.	%	Gene frequency	No.	%	Gene frequency
Haemoglobin (Hb) A	223	99.11	Hb^A .9956	170	99.42	Hb^A .9971	194	100.0	Hb^A 1.0000
AE	2	0.89	Hb^E .0044	1	0.48	Hb^E .0029	0	0.00	Hb^E 0.0000
Phosphoglucomutase (PGM) (1)									
1-1	127	56.44	PGM_1^1 .7400	93	54.70	PGM_1^1 .7441	122	51.26	PGM_1^1 .7192
2-1	78	34.67	PGM_1^2 .2556	65	38.24	PGM_1^2 .2471	96	40.34	PGM_1^2 .2748
2-2	18	8.00	.0044	9	5.29	.0088	16	6.72	.0070
6-1	1	0.44	PGM_1^X	2	1.18	PGM_1^X	2	0.84	PGM_1^X
6-2	0	0.00		1	0.59		0	0.00	
Others[a]	1	0.44		0	0.00		2	0.84	
Acid phosphatase (P)									
A	16	6.99	p^a .2729	16	9.09	p^a .2500	12	5.00	p^a .2220
AB	93	40.61	p^b .7271	56	31.82	p^b .7500	86	35.83	p^b .7780
B	120	52.40		104	59.09		142	59.17	
6-Phosphogluconate dehydrogenase (PGD)									
A	212	92.58	PGD^A .9629	157	89.71	PGD^A .9486	200	83.33	PGD^A .9189
AC	17	7.42	PGD^C .0371	18	10.29	PGD^C .0514	39	16.25	PGD^C .0772
AR	0	0.00		0	0.00		1	0.42	PGD^R .0029
Adenosine deaminase (ADA) 1-1	171	85.07	ADA^1 .9154	145	85.80	ADA^1 .9260	25	89.29	ADA^1 .9464
2-1	26	12.94	ADA^2 .0846	23	13.61	ADA^2 .0740	3	10.71	ADA^2 .0536
2-2	4	1.99		1	0.59		0	0.00	
Glutamate-pyruvate transaminase (GPT) 1-1	63	30.29	GPT^1 .5072	35	24.31	GPT^1 .4757	54	23.58	GPT^1 .5082
2-1	85	40.86	GPT^2 .4928	67	46.53	GPT^2 .5208	115	50.22	GPT^2 .4828
2-2	60	28.85		41	28.47	.0035	55	24.02	.0090
Others	-	-		1	0.69	GPT^6	5	2.18	GPT^6
Esterase D (Es D)									
1-1	79	38.53	EsD^1 .6341	40	36.04	EsD^1 .6261	87	37.18	EsD^1 .6119
2-1	102	49.76	EsD^2 .3659	59	53.15	EsD^2 .3739	109	46.58	EsD^2 .3881
2-2	24	11.71		12	10.81		38	16.24	
Glyoxalase (GLO)									
1-1	2	1.19	GLO^1 .1607	1	1.06	GLO^1 .1789	5	3.01	GLO^1 .1815
2-1	50	29.76	GLO^2 .8393	32	33.68	GLO^2 .8211	43	25.90	GLO^2 .8185
2-2	116	69.05		62	65.26		118	71.08	
Properdin factor B (Bf) S	134	86.45	Bf^S .9290	66	89.19	Bf^S .9459	119	85.61	Bf^S .9059
FS	20	12.90	Bf^F .0710	8	10.81	Bf^F .0541	14	10.07	Bf^F .0941
F	1	0.65		0	0.00		6	4.32	
Haptoglobin (Hp) 1-1	24	11.21	Hp^1 .3113	16	11.43	Hp^1 .3107	26	12.44	Hp^1 .3545
2-1	84	39.25	Hp^2 .6887	55	39.29	Hp^2 .6893	89	42.58	Hp^2 .6455
2-2	104	48.60		69	49.29		90	43.06	
'0'	2	0.93		0	0.00		4	1.91	
Transferrin (Tf) C	200	93.46	Tf^C .9386	134	95.71	Tf^C .9786	204	97.61	Tf^C .9888
CD	13	6.07	Tf^D .0570	6	4.29	Tf^D .0214	5	2.39	Tf^D .0112
BC	1	0.47	Tf^B .0044	0	0.00		0	0.00	

[a] Other rare PGM(1) alleles have been combined with the 6 allele as PGM_1^X.

NPC-negative group had gene frequencies intermediate between those of patients and controls; of the other five comparisons, in two the gene frequencies of NPC-positives and NPC-negatives was almost identical, and in three the gene frequencies of the NPC-negatives were more divergent from the controls than were those of the patients.

For two systems, 6-phosphogluconate dehydrogenase (PGD) and transferrin, significant differences in gene frequencies were observed between NPC-positives and standardized controls, with a probability of less than 1%; a third system, red-cell acid phosphatase, approached significance ($\chi^2_{(1)} = 3.3$), but as noted below, the dialect groups were heterogeneous for the difference in acid phosphatase gene frequencies.

It is of interest to consider whether the gene frequencies of our control series were representative of those of the Chinese population in Singapore. In a previous investigation (Blake et al., 1973), we tested 378 Chinese blood donors for several red-cell enzyme systems. Four of these are among the 11 systems shown in Table 2, and the relevant data are reproduced in Table 3: there were no significant differences between the gene frequencies of the blood donors and those of our controls. We have no information about the dialect groups of the blood donors, so that gene frequencies could not be standardized for this variable; however, if NPC-positives are compared with the non-standardized blood donors, the difference in gene frequencies is now significant for red-cell acid phosphatase ($\chi^2_{(1)} = 5.74$; $P = 0.02$), and the difference in gene frequency for PGD is still significant ($\chi^2_{(1)} = 5,74$; $P = 0.02$).

In view of these differences in gene frequency, red-cell acid phosphatase and PGD merit more detailed analysis. Accordingly, in Table 4 the frequencies of the $\underline{p}^a$ and $\underline{PGD}^A$ alleles are given for the main linguistic groups; Hakka, Khek and Hainanese have been combined because of the relatively small numbers of persons in each. The $\underline{p}^a$ allele has a higher frequency among patients in each linguistic group, except for the Cantonese; $\underline{PGD}^A$ has a higher frequency among patients in all of the linguistic groups. It is not clear whether the reversal in $\underline{p}^a$ frequency for the Cantonese is due to an unusually high value of $\underline{p}^a$ among the Cantonese controls or to a low value of $\underline{p}^a$ among the Cantonese NPC-positives. In neither system are the differences in gene frequency between dialect groups significant.

Effects of age

The HLA data suggest a difference between individuals who contract the disease early and older patients (Simons et al.[1]). We therefore tabulated our genetic marker data for the NPC-positive and NPC-negative series by two age categories. It was not possible to make a meaningful breakdown for the controls: they consisted of parents in a study of families, so that there will have been a bias towards

---

[1] See p. 271

Table 3. Phenotypes and gene frequencies of Singapore blood donors[a]

System		No	%	Gene frequency	
Haemoglobin (Hb)	A	376	99.47	$\underline{Hb}^A$	.9974
	AE	2	0.53	$\underline{Hb}^E$	.0026
Phosphoglucomutase (PGM) (1)	1-1	204	53.97	$\underline{PGM}_1^1$	.7315
	2-1	143	37.83	$\underline{PGM}_1^2$	.2632
	2-2	27	7.14		.0053
	6-1	2	0.53	$\underline{PGM}_1^X$	
	6-2	2	0.53		
	Others	0	0.00		
Acid phosphatase (p)	A	24	6.35	$\underline{p}^a$	.2143
	AB	114	30.16	$\underline{p}^b$	.7857
	B	240	63.49		
6-Phosphogluconate dehydrogenase (PGD)	A	327	86.51	$\underline{PGD}^A$	.9325
	AC	50	13.23	$\underline{PGD}^C$	.0661
	Others	1	0.26	$\underline{PGD}^X$	.0013

[a] From Blake et al., 1973

Table 4. Frequencies of the acid phosphatase ($\underline{p}^a$) and 6-phosphogluconate dehydrogenase ($\underline{PGD}^A$) alleles in nasopharyngeal carcinoma (NPC) patients and controls from various dialect groups in Singapore

Dialect group	NPC +ve Frequency			Controls Frequency		
	No. tested	$\underline{p}^a$	$\underline{PGD}^A$	No. tested	$\underline{p}^a$	$\underline{PGD}^A$
Cantonese	61	0.2459	0.9508	74	0.2635	0.9189
Hokkien	81	0.2531	0.9630	60	0.2083	0.9250
Teochew	43	0.3605	0.9767	51	0.2059	0.9216
Hakka/Khek/ Hainanese	44	0.2614	0.9659	55	0.2273	0.9000

older persons. The data for those persons whose age was recorded are given in Table 5. Because of the relatively small number of persons below the age of 30, gene frequencies were calculated only for those aged 30 and over.

Table 5. Distribution of phenotypes in younger and older nasopharyngeal carcinoma (NPC) +ve and NPC-ve patients in Singapore (Rare phenotypes have been shown as additions to heterozygote 2-1's)

			Less than 30 years		30 years and over			
System	NPC	Phenotype	No.	%	No.	%	Gene frequencies	
Haemoglobin (Hb)	+ve	A	33	97.06	190	99.48	Hh^A	.9974
		AE	1	2.94	1	0.52	HB^E	.0026
	-ve	A	42	100.00	128	99.22	HB^A	.9961
		AE	0	0.00	1	0.78	Hb^E	.0039
Phosphoglucomutase (PGM)	+ve	1-1	19	55.88	108	56.54	PGM^1	.7382
		2-1	13 + 1	41.18	66	34.55	PGM^{Others}	.2618
		2-2	1	2.94	17	8.90		
	-ve	1-1	26	61.90	67	52.34	PGM^1	.7344
		2-1	14	33.33	51 + 3	42.19	PGM^{Others}	.2656
		2-2	2	4.76	7	5.47		
Acid phosphatase (P)	+ve	A	4	11.76	12	6.15	p^a	.2744
		AB	10	29.41	83	42.56	p^b	.7256
		B	20	58.82	100	51.29		
	-ve	A	1	2.33	15	11.28	p^a	.2744
		AB	13	30.23	43	32.33	p^b	.7256
		B	29	67.44	75	56.39		
6-Phosphogluconate dehydrogenase (PGD)	+ve	A	29	87.88	183	93.37	PGD^A	.9668
		AC	4	12.12	13	6.63	PGD^C	.0332
	-ve	A	39	90.70	118	89.39	PGD^A	.9470
		AC	4	9.30	14	10.61	PGD^C	.0530
Adenosine deaminase (ADA)	+ve	1-1	27	90.00	144	84.21	ADA^1	.9094
		2-1	3	10.00	23	13.45	ADA^2	.0906
		2-2	0	0.00	4	2.34		
	-ve	1-1	34	80.95	111	87.40	ADA^1	.9331
		2-1	8	19.05	15	11.81	ADA^2	.0669
		2-2	0.	0.00	1	0.79		
Glutamate-pyrurate transaminase (GPT)	+ve	1-1	9	29.03	54	30.51	GPT^1	.5085
		2-1	13	41.94	72	40.68	GPT^2	.4915
		2-2	9	29.03	51	28.81		
	-ve	1-1	6	16.67	29	26.61	GPT^1	.5183
		2-1	13 + 1	38.89	54 + 1	50.46	GPT^2	.4817
		2-2	16	44.44	25	22.94		
Esterase D (Es D)	+ve	1-1	13	41.94	66	37.93	EsD^1	.6264
		2-1	16	51.61	86	49.43	EsD^2	.3736
		2-2	2	6.45	22	12.64		
	-ve	1-1	12	46.15	28	32.94	EsD^1	.6118
		2-1	11	42.31	48	56.47	EsD^2	.3882
		2-2	3	11.54	9	10.59		
Glyxolase (GLO)	+ve	1-1	0	0.00	2	1.38	GLO^1	.1586
		2-1	7	38.89	42	28.97	GLO^2	.8414
		2-2	11	61.11	101	69.66		
	-ve	1-1	0	0.00	1	1.41	GLO^1	.1620
		2-1	8	42.11	21	29.58	GLO^2	.8380
		2-2	11	57.89	49	69.01		
Properdin factor B (Bf)	+ve	S	13	86.67	119	87.50	Bf^S	.9338
		FS	2	13.33	16	11.76	Bf^F	.0662
		F	0	0.00	1	0.74		
	-ve	S	8	88.89	54	88.52	Bf^S	.9426
		FS	1	11.11	7	11.48	Bf^F	.0574
		F	0	0.00	0	0.00		
Haptoglobin (Hp)	+ve	1-1	3	11.11	21	11.35	Hp^1	.3162
		2-1	9	33.33	75	40.54	Hp^2	.6838
		2-2	15	55.56	89	48.11		
	-ve	1-1	2	5.88	14	13.21	Hp^1	.3208
		2-1	15	44.12	40	37.74	Hp^2	.6792
		2-2	17	50.00	52	49.06		
Transferrin (Tf)	+ve	C	25	92.59	175	93.58	Tf^C	.9652
		CD	2	7.41	11	5.88	Tf^D	.0348
		BC	0	0.00	1	0.53		
	-ve	C	32	94.12	102	96.23	Tf^C	.9811
		CD	2	5.88	4	3.77	Tf^D	.0189
		BC	0	0.00	0	0.00		

There were no significant differences in gene frequency between NPC-positive and NPC-negative cases for any of the 11 systems, nor when all age groups were combined. However, if the gene frequencies for the older patients (i.e., 30 years and over) are compared with those of the standardized controls, the discrepancies are slightly magnified for the acid phosphatase and PGD systems. What is of interest is that a larger proportion (24.4%) of the NPC-negative cases than of the NPC-positive cases (14.8%) were below age 30. Although there is no reason to believe that age affects the distribution of genes in our control population, if there is any genetic association with NPC, or with the disorders that bring the NPC-negatives to the attention of the clinician, then age is likely to be of importance. The differences for the NPC-positives in the present study are, however, slight, and a much larger series will be required to assess the heterogeneity that may result from age-incidence of the disease.

Chromosome 6 markers

Since a significant association has been demonstrated between NPC and the HLA antigens A2:Sin 2 (Simons et al., 1976), it could be expected that there is also an association with other genes closely linked to the HLA region on chromosome 6. The association between NPC and HLA is stronger with the HLA B locus than it is with the A locus and may be even higher with the postulated immune response locus in the HLA D region. The D locus is approximately midway between HLA B and the locus controlling GLO, and the properdin locus Bf is probably also in the region of HLA B (Weitkamp, 1976). If there is linkage disequilibrium between a postulated immune response (Ir) gene involved in NPC and other genes in the same region, then a shift in frequency of one or other allele at the GLO and Bf loci may occur.

It is apparent from Table 2 that there is a slight effect for both GLO and Bf, since the gene frequencies in both systems are approximately 2% different between NPC-positive cases and standardized controls; however, these differences are not significant ($\chi^2{}_{(1)}$= 0.51 and 1.03; P= 0.5 and 0.3, respectively). Furthermore, an examination of the combination of phenotypes in each person tested for both GLO and Bf showed no combination of alleles to be in excess of that expected by chance.

A multivariate approach

As indicated above, at least three of the systems given in Table 2 show significant differences in gene frequency between the NPC-positive patients and controls drawn from non-affected members of families of patients and from a normal sample of the Chinese population in Singapore. In addition, smaller differences that occur in other systems, although individually insignificant, may contribute to a genetic distinctiveness of the patient population.

As an approach to this problem, we applied the techniques of genetic distance analysis, used frequently to assess phylogenetic relationships. Several methods are available for such analysis, which, although based on different conceptual approaches, in practice give essentially the same hierarchical relationships between populations. We employed the distance measures developed by Morton (1969) and by Nei (1972).

Using the gene frequency data from Table 2, but excluding ADA because of the small number of controls tested, Nei's statistic generates distance matrices between the three populations as given in Table 6.

Table 6. Nei (1972) genetic distances between nasopharyngeal carcinoma (NPC)+ve, NPC-ve and control populations in Singapore (actual distance values x 10^4)

	Distance	±SD
NPC+ve - NPC-ve	5	2
NPC+ve - control	14	4
NPC-ve - control	9	3

All three distance values are significant at the conventional level, since they are more than twice their standard deviation. What is also of interest is that the NPC-negative patients are intermediate between the NPC-positive patients and the controls. An identical relationship is given by Morton's statistic, the NPC-negatives being almost midway between the NPC-positives and controls.

Since both NPC-positive and -negative patients are drawn from the Singapore population, it is of interest to examine how they relate to the main dialect groups. Using Morton's statistic, and again omitting ADA, the distance matrix can be reduced to two dimensions in an eigenvector diagram (Fig. 1): the NPC-positives are the most extreme population, with NPC-negatives intermediate to the four dialect groupings. It is important to emphasize that the number of controls in each dialect group is relatively small (see Table 5), and this undoubtedly contributes to the dispersion between the dialect groups on the eigenvector diagram. More important in the present context, however, is the distinctive genetic position of the NPC-positive patients.

DISCUSSION

The occurrence of diseases with markedly different prevalences in different localities poses a complex challenge to the medical scientist. At one extreme there are diseases in which there is an overwhelming contribution from a specific environmental factor, whilst at the other extreme it is possible to demonstrate the importance of an increased

FIG. 1. EIGENVECTOR DIAGRAM

Eigenvector diagram showing the genetic relationships of nasopharyngeal carcinoma (NPC)-positive and NPC-negative patients to normal controls in various dialect groups

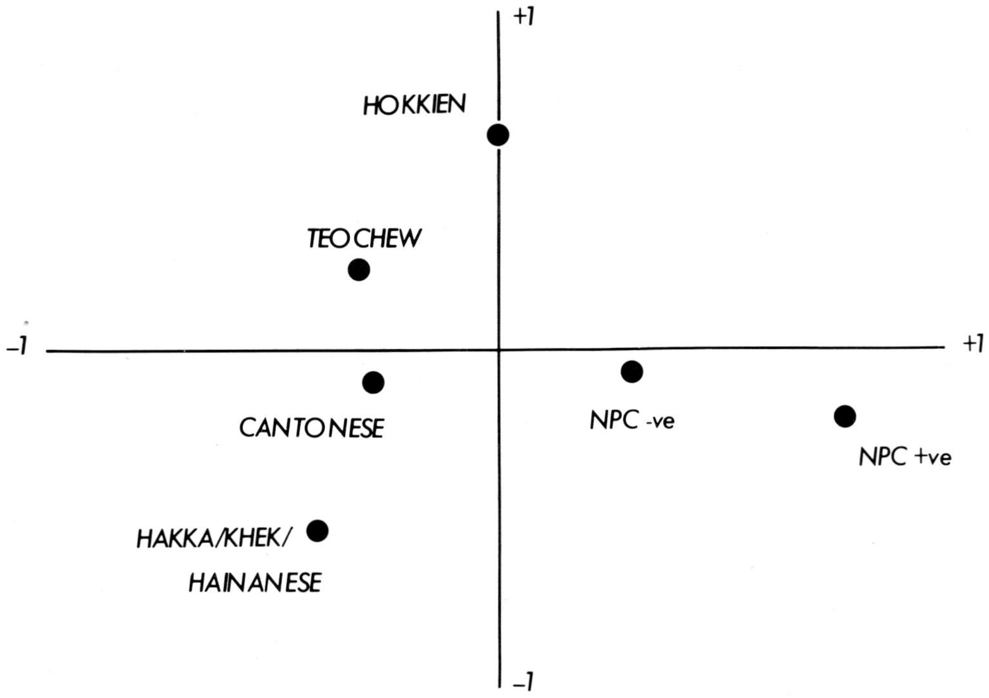

frequency of a single gene in particular populations. Many disorders, however, are likely to fall between these two extremes, and the analysis of the interaction between environmental factors and genetic constitution may be further complicated by imprecisions in nosological classification.

One approach to understanding the contribution of genetic factors to diseases has been through studies of their associations with specific genetic markers. In the past, many such studies have been opportunistic, making use of data or techniques readily available, such as blood grouping, for the genetic marker component. More recently, some of the significant associations that have been demonstrated, such as that between specific alleles of the α_1 anti-trypsin system and emphysema (Eriksson, 1965), have a plausible physiological basis, and it is probable that many more such meaningful associations will be demonstrated in the next few years.

Among those that are actively being studied at present, greatest attention is being given to the association of diseases with genes at the major histocompatibility (HLA) loci; for a review of such studies in relation to cancers at various sites, see Simons & Amiel (1977). Further impetus has been given to work of this kind by the possibility that Ir genes in man, corresponding to Ia genes in mice, are coded for by a region of chromosome 6 that is close to, or part of, the major histocompatibility region. A number of other genes are now known which are also coded for by regions of chromosome 6 close to the major histocompatibility region. Some of these gene products, such as complement components and Bf, may be directly involved in immune reactions, and particular alleles in these systems may be preferentially retained or lost in persons who develop active disease.

Many other sites on different chromosomes may also have genes that are involved in susceptibility to cancer, either by controlling enzymes which activate carcinogens, alter cell permeability or affect recognition sites for viruses on the cell surface or by replicating the virus within the cell as well as other parts of the total immune system. Examination of a broad range of genetic markers may be valuable, therefore, in indicating linkage disequilibria involving other chromosomes, or possibly even indicating direct physiological relationships between particular gene products and cell susceptibility or immune function.

In the present investigation, a comparison of gene frequencies in histologically confirmed cases of NPC with those in a carefully matched control population revealed that the patients were genetically distinct from normal Chinese. Of equal interest is that the analysis also showed that patients suspected to be suffering from NPC but histologically negative were intermediate in position between the positive cases and controls. This finding adds weight to the argument that there is a distinct genetic component in persons who are clinically and histologically suffering from NPC, since some, though not all, of the negative patients finally become histologically positive and should, therefore, have the same genetic traits as the other NPC-positives.

When the individual systems were examined, four of the 11 that showed variation in the present study had differences in gene frequency of 4% or more between NPC patients and controls. Two of these differences were significant - those for PGD and transferrin - and a third, red-cell acid phosphatase, though not significant in our own total data, is significantly different in NPC patients compared with Chinese blood donors in Singapore. On a dialect group basis, however, Cantonese show a reversal of the acid phosphatase relationship compared with that found in the other dialect groups: whether this is due to sampling problems or is a real phenomenon must be determined by further study.

It is not possible to describe the mechanism that gives rise to the genetic distinctiveness of NPC patients as a group. The distortion in gene frequencies at particular loci, such as that for PGD, could be due to linkage disequilibrium with some closely linked gene on chromosome 1 or to some direct involvement of PGD phenotypes in a metabolic process important for tumour cell growth or lymphocyte function. In the case of the transferrin polymorphism, one can speculate that there could be a relationship with viral invasion, since transferrin has antiviral activity (Martin & Jandl, 1959).

In broad terms, however, it appears that, whatever etiological factor or factors are responsible for conversion to the malignant state in NPC and which permit its establishment as a clinically and histologically recognizable entity, they operate on a selected portion of the total Chinese population, and this subpopulation is genetically distinct in its array of alleles at a number of loci of the total genome.

SUMMARY

A series of blood samples from more than 200 histologically confirmed Chinese patients with NPC in Singapore were typed for 25 genetically controlled red-cell enzyme and five serum protein systems. A comparable number of patients suspected of having NPC but histologically negative and a series of healthy unrelated Chinese were typed for the same systems.

The gene frequencies of NPC patients and controls differed by 4% or more in four of the 11 systems that showed variation; a further system, G6PD deficiency, also showed a significant difference between the two series but was excluded because of possible unreliability of the results from patients. Smaller differences existed in several other systems, including chromosome 6 markers closely linked to HLA.

An analysis of differences within dialect groups showed a consistent effect for PGD, but for red-cell acid phosphatase there was a reversal of the difference between patients and controls among the Cantonese. These results need a larger series to confirm their validity. A breakdown of patients into those 30 years of age or older and those under 30 slightly enhanced the differences in gene frequencies.

A multivariate analysis, using genetic distance statistics, showed a significant difference between NPC patients and controls, which is evident also when they are compared in the separate dialect groups. The histologically negative patients occupied an intermediate position.

The study indicates that etiological factors resulting in clinically and histologically confirmed NPC operate on a genetically distinct subpopulation of Chinese in Singapore.

ACKNOWLEDGEMENTS

This work was supported in part by a collaborative research agreement between the Unit of Biological Carcinogenesis of IARC and the IARC Research Centre, Department of Pathology at the University of Singapore, under Public Health Service Contract No. 1CP43296 within the Virus Cancer Program, National Cancer Institute, USA, and by the Jee Ah Chiou Fellowship in Cancer Research at the University of Singapore (to S.H.C.). In Australia, the costs of laboratory investigations were met by grants from the Australian National University. We acknowledge the valuable assistance of Mr Wee Guan Bok, Heng Swee Hiang and Nalini Srinivasan in Singapore in collecting and processing the samples. In Canberra, Mrs Kathy Sims, Ms Marjorie Coggan, Mrs Christine Hayes, Mrs Elizabeth Robertson, Mr Robert Taylor and Dr E.M. McDermid provided excellent assistance and advice at various stages of the project.

REFERENCES

Beaconsfield, P. & Rainsbury, R. (1968) G-6-PD deficiency and physiopathologic processes. *New Engl. J. Med.*, *278*, 914

Beaconsfield, P., Rainsbury, R. & Kalton, G. (1965) Glucose-6-phosphate dehydrogenase deficiency and incidence of cancer. *Oncologia*, *19*, 11-19

Blake, N.M., McDermid, E.M., Kirk, R.L., Ong, Y.W. & Simons, M.J. (1973) The distribution of red cell enzyme groups among Chinese and Malays in Singapore. *Singapore med. J.*, *14*, 1-8

Eriksson, S. (1965) Studies in alpha 1-antitrypsin deficiency. *Acta med. scand.*, *177*, Suppl. 432

Malcolm, L.A., Woodfield, D.G., Blake, N.M., Kirk, R.L. & McDermid, E. M. (1972) The distribution of blood, serum protein and enzyme groups on Manus Island (Admiralty Islands, New Guinea). *Human Heredity*, *22*, 305-322

Martin, C.M. & Jandl, J.H. (1959) Inhibition of virus multiplication by transferrin. *J. clin. Invest.*, *38*, 1024

Morton, N.E. (1969) Human population structure. *Ann. Rev. Genet.*, *3*, 53-74

Nei, M (1972) Genetic distance between populations. *Amer. Naturalist*, *106*, 283-292

Shanmugaratnam, K. (1971) Studies on the etiology of nasopharyngeal carcinoma. *Int. Rev. exp. Path.*, *10*, 361-413

Shanmugaratnam, K. & Wee, A. (1973) *Ethnic-dialect·group variations in cancer incidence in a Chinese population.* In: Doll, R. & Vodopija, I., eds, *Host Environment Interactions in the Etiology of Cancer in Man (IARC Scientific Publications No. 7)*, Lyon, pp. 67-82

Simons, M.J. & Amiel, J.L. (1977) *HLA and malignant diseases.* In: Dausset, J. & Svejgaard, A., eds, *First International Symposium on HLA and Disease, Paris, 1976*, Copenhagen, Munksgaard, (in press)

Simons, M.J. & Day, N.E. (1975) *HLA patterns and NPC.* In: Henderson, B., ed., *Proceedings of the Symposium on Epidemiology and Cancer Registries in the Pacific Basin, Hawaii, USA, 1975*, (in press)

Simons, M.J., Wee, G.B., Day, N.E., Morris, P.J., Shanmugaratnam, K. & de-Thé, G. (1974) Immunogenetic aspects of nasopharyngeal carcinoma. I. Differences in HL-A antigen profiles between patients and control groups. *Int. J. Cancer*, *13*, 122-134

Simons, M.J., Wee, G.B., Chan, S.H., Shanmugaratnam, K. & de-Thé, G. (1975) Probable identification of an HL-A second-locus antigen associated with a high risk of nasopharyngeal carcinoma. *Lancet*, *i*, 142-143

Simons, M.J., Wee, G.B., Goh, E.H., Chan, S.H., Shanmugaratnam, K., Day, N.E. & de-Thé, G. (1976) Immunogenetic aspects of nasopharyngeal carcinoma. IV. Increased risk in Chinese of nasopharyngeal carcinoma associated with a Chinese-related HLA profile (A2, Singapore 2). *J. nat. Cancer Inst.*, *57*, 977-980

Weitkamp, L.R. (1976) Linkage of GLO with HLA and Bf: effect of population and sex on recombination frequency. *Tissue Antigens*, *7*, 273-279

Woodfield, D.G., Scragg, R.F.R., Blake, N.M., Kirk, R.L. & McDermid, E.M. (1974) The distribution of blood, serum protein and enzyme groups among the Fuyuge speakers of the Goilala sub-district (Papua New Guinea). *Human Heredity, 24*, 507-519

CYTOGENETIC OBSERVATIONS ON THE MALIGNANT EPITHELIAL CELLS AND INFILTRATING LYMPHOCYTES OF NASOPHARYNGEAL CARCINOMA

J.E. JARVIS, S. FINERTY, M.A. EPSTEIN, P.A. TRUMPER & G. BALL

Department of Pathology,
University of Bristol Medical School,
University Walk,
Bristol BS8 1TD, UK

B.C. GIOVANELLA

Cancer Research Laboratory,
St Joseph Hospital,
Houston, Texas 77002, USA

INTRODUCTION

Nasopharyngeal carcinomas (NPC) consist of malignant squamous epithelial tumour cells with an invariable, moderate to heavy infiltration of non-malignant lymphoid cells (Gazzolo et al., 1972; Shanmugaratnam, 1971; Svoboda et al., 1967). NPC epithelial tumour cells carry the Epstein-Barr virus (EBV) genome (Huang et al., 1974; Klein et al., 1974; Wolf et al., 1973).

It has been known for some time that lymphoblastoid cell lines can be established from NPC biopsy samples cultured *in vitro* (de-Thé et al., 1970; Epstein et al., 1971), and this material is clearly suitable for cytogenetic analysis. Until recently it was not possible to obtain NPC epithelial tumour cells free of non-malignant infiltrating cells; however, it has now been shown that these infiltrating cells can be eliminated by passing NPC biopsy samples through athymic nude mice, in which only the malignant cells will grow (Klein et al., 1974).

Cells of EBV-carrying lymphoblastoid lines derived from non-malignant sources (blood from patients with infectious mononucleosis or from normal seropositive individuals, or lymphocytes from sero-negative donors which have been transformed *in vitro* by the virus) have been shown to differ in morphology, growth characteristics, and karyotype from those of lines derived from malignant EBV-containing lymphoblasts of Burkitt's lymphoma (BL) (Jarvis et al., 1974; Nilsson & Pontén, 1975; Zech et al., 1976). With regard to karyotype, BL-derived lines show a no. 14 chromosome abnormality (Manolov & Manolova, 1972) that is absent in EBV-carrying lines of non-malignant origin (Jarvis et al., 1974; Zech et al., 1976). It was therefore considered of interest to determine whether or not the no. 14 chromosome change was present in lymphoblastoid lines from NPC. It was also considered of interest to investigate the karyotype of the malignant epithelial cells of NPC and to look for any consistent pattern of chromosomal abnormalities or changes similar to those in the EBV-containing malignant cells of BL.

This paper describes cytogenetic studies on cultured lymphoblasts, and on NPC-derived squamous epithelial cells grown in nude mice.

MATERIALS AND METHODS

Lymphoblastoid cell lines

Seven NPC-derived cell lines were kindly supplie by Dr G.B. de-Thé, International Agency for Research on Cancer, Lyon, France; the designation and origin of the lines are shown in Table 1. The lines were established as described by de-Thé et al. (1970).

Cell culture

Cells were grown in Eagle's minimum essential medium with non-essential amino acids, 0.08% sodium bicarbonate, 10% fetal calf serum and 100 units per ml penicillin and streptomycin in stoppered conical flasks at 37°C.

Passage of tumour in nude mice

NPC biopsy material obtained in Nairobi, Kenya, was transplanted into outbred nude mice backcrossed with Swiss high-fertility strain breeders, as described elsewhere (Klein et al., 1974). The biopsy samples were obtained from the following patients: HW, female, aged 55, Unit no. 95410, secondary NPC cervical node; MM, male, aged 20, Unit no. 61764, recurrent NPC right orbit; JG, male, aged 51, Unit no. 81457, primary NPC; NM, female, aged 10/12, Unit no. 67480, secondary NPC cervical node; LOL, male, aged 55, Unit no. 107535, primary NPC. Mice were flown from Houston to Bristol for examination of chromosomes in the grafted NPC tumours.

Cytogenetic analysis

Chromosome spreads were prepared from the lymphoblastoid cell lines and stained by the banding technique described in earlier work (Jarvis et al., 1974).

To obtain epithelial tumour cells, tumour-bearing mice were given 4 μg per g bw Colcemid solution (CIBA laboratories, Horsham, Sussex, UK) intraperitoneally to induce *in vivo* spindle arrest (Visfeldt et al., 1972). The tumours were removed $3\frac{1}{2}$ hr later and were chopped finely in phosphate-buffered saline containing 0.125% trypsin (Wellcome Reagents Ltd, Beckenham, UK). The material in the trypsin was then rocked gently at 37°C for 30 min to give a cell suspension, after which the trypsin was inactivated by the addition of an equal volume of medium containing 20% fetal calf serum.

Dry metaphase spreads were prepared from the cell suspension and stained for banding in the same way as for the lymphoblastoid cell lines (Jarvis et al., 1974).

Examination of chromosomes

As many spreads as possible, up to a maximum of 25, were examined from each lymphoblastoid line (Table 1). Some difficulty was encountered in obtaining large numbers of satisfactory spreads of epithelial NPC tumour cells grown in nude mice; therefore, not more than 16 spreads of each NPC were examined (Table 2). All spreads examined were analysed for ploidy, chromosomal abnormalities and rearrangements, and the presence or absence of the no. 14 chromosome marker.

Preparation of material for electron microscopy

Fragments of tumours removed from mice were cut into 1 mm cubes in iced 4% glutaraldehyde; they were then post-fixed in osmium, dehydrated in graded ethanol solutions and embedded in epoxy resin. Sections were cut on a Porter-Blum microtome, contrast-stained with uranyl acetate and examined in a Phillips 201 electron microscope.

RESULTS

Electron microscopy of the tumours grown in nude mice confirmed the epithelial nature of the cells, which showed frequent desmosomes and cytoplasmic bundles of keratin fibrils.

Lymphoblastoid cells (Table 1)

Line LY26 was difficult to investigate since it consistently gave spreads of poor quality. Only seven spreads out of the large number examined were suitable for analysis.

The majority of the lines had a diploid cell population, and only two lines (LY26, LY38) were composed of tetraploid cells. With the exception of those in one line, most cells showed a normal karyotype; the chromosomal abnormalities and deletions present in rare cells did not follow a con istent pattern. All cells in the exceptional line (LY11) had a secondary constriction near the centromere of both no. 1 chromosomes.

Table 1. Cytogenetic analysis of cells from seven lymphoid lines derived from nasopharyngeal carcinomas

Designation	Sex	Origin	Mode	No. of spreads examined	Significant chromosomal abnormalities
LY11	M	Hong Kong	Diploid	15	Consistent secondary constriction near centromere of both no. 1
LY26	?	Hong Kong	Tetraploid	7	One spread had one abnormal no. 14 with an extra subterminal band
LY28	M	Hong Kong	Diploid	25	None
LY38	M	Hong Kong	Tetraploid	25	None
LY61	M	Hong Kong	Diploid	15	None
LY64	F	Hong Kong	Diploid	15	None
LY123	M	Morocco	Diploid	15	One spread had one abnormal no. 14 with an additional lightly-stained terminal region

In addition, one tetraploid spread in line LY26 showed an abnormal D14 chromosome that had an extra subterminal band; the other D14 chromosomes were normal. Another single spread, in the diploid LY123 line, contained a D14 chromosome with an additional lightly-stained region after the terminal band, again accompanied by a normal D14 chromosome. The no. 14 chromosomes in all other cells were normal.

Epithelial tumour cells (Table 2)

Chromosome spreads from JG were always unsatisfactory, and, although chromosome numbers could be counted, analysis was not possible. Two tumours, those from JG and MM, had near-diploid cell populations; the remainder contained hypo-tetraploid cells, apart from a single near-diploid cell in the tumour from NM.

Table 2. Cytogenetic analysis of epithelial tumour cells grown in nude mice from biopsy samples of five nasopharyngeal carcinomas from Kenya

Designation	Sex	No. of chromosomes per cell	No. of spreads examined	Chromosomal abnormalities
HW	F	60-66	15	Gross
MM	M	37-48	10	Minor
JG	M	36-44	5	Analysis not possible
NM	F	70-74 44	15 1	Gross Minor
LOL	M	56-66	12	Gross

Only minor chromosomal abnormalities were observed in the near-diploid cells from MM and in one from NM. The hypo-tetraploid spreads present in the tumours from HW, NM and LOL were complex with gross chromosomal abnormalities of uncertain origin. Major translocations were particularly frequent in cells from HW and LOL, but no consistent pattern of abnormality was shared by cells from the various different tumours. The no. 14 chromosomes were found to be normal in all spreads that could be analysed.

DISCUSSION

The characteristic abnormality in the no. 14 chromosome of BL cells both in biopsy samples and after culture (Manolov & Manolova, 1972) is clearly unrelated to EBV, since it has been shown to be lacking in EBV-carrying cells from other sources (Jarvis et al., 1974; Zech et al., 1976). It is now known that identical or somewhat similar abnormalities of the no. 14 chromosome are present in the cells of a variety of different lymphoid malignancies (Fukuhara et al., 1976; Prigogina & Fleischman, 1975; Wurster-Hill et al., 1973; Zech et al., 1976) and it would seem that no. 14 chromosomal abnormalities are often related to neoplastic changes in lymphoid cells *in vivo* in a relatively general way.

In view of this, and with the additional evidence from earlier work showing an absence of the marker in EBV-containing cells of non-malignant origin (Jarvis et al., 1974), it is not surprising that the cells of NPC-derived lymphoblastoid lines likewise lacked a consistent no. 14 chromosomal abnormality. The lymphocytes in NPC tumours have long been recognized as non-malignant infiltrating cells (Shanmugaratnam, 1971), and, although some are known to be T-cells (Klein, 1975; Yata et al., 1974), B-cells are also present. The latter, of course, include, in seropositive individuals, a minority that carry the EBV genome as a latent infection (see Epstein & Achong, 1977). If they are removed in NPC biopsy material and cultured, they give rise to virus-carrying lymphoblastoid lines (de-Thé et al., 1970; Epstein et al., 1971), as happens with such genome-containing cells from any other source.

Since no. 14 chromosomal abnormalities are associated with lymphoid malignancies, it is again not surprising that they have not been found in NPC epithelial tumour cells. These cells carry the EBV genome (Huang et al., 1974; Klein et al., 1974; Wolf et al., 1973) and are capable of supporting replication of the virus under certain conditions (Trumper et al., 1976); the absence of the chromosome marker thus provides confirmation that the no. 14 abnormality is not related to EBV.

The rare changes observed in no. 14 chromosomes of lymphoid cells (Table 1) are not considered to be significant, since they were found in only one cell of each of two lines and differed both from one another and from the more consistent abnormalities of lymphoid tumours

(Fukuhara et al., 1976; Prigogina & Fleischman, 1975; Wurster-Hill et al., 1973; Zech et al., 1976). They should perhaps be regarded as further examples of the general instability of no. 14 chromosomes in human lymphoid cells since, other such changes have been found from time to time in these cells after culture *in vitro* (Beatty-Desana et al., 1975; Hecht et al., 1975; Welch & Lee, 1975).

The chromosomal abnormalities in the epithelial cells were clearly more complex in the hypo-tetraploid than in the near-diploid tumours (Table 2), but it is obviously not possible to say for either group whether the abnormalities were present in the original material taken from the patient or whether they arose during passage in the nude mice. However, it seems likely that the gross changes found in the hypo-tetraploid cells arose during progression from diploidy to tetraploidy, since the single near-diploid cell from NM was less abnormal than were the NM hypo-tetraploid cells. In any event, the varied gross abnormalities found in the hypo-tetraploid cells from HW, NM and LOL presented no consistent pattern.

SUMMARY

Because of the presence of a No 14 chromosome marker abnormality in EB virus-carrying cells from African Burkitt's lymphoma (BL) but not from other origins, and the association of EB virus with nasopharyngeal carcinoma (NPC) as well as BL, both the malignant epithelial cells and the non-malignant lymphoid cells of NPC have been investigated cytogenetically.

Chromosome spreads from seven NPC-derived lymphoblastoid lines were examined after banding; five lines were diploid and two were tetraploid. No consistent no. 14 chromosome abnormalities were found. Apart from a secondary constriction near the centromere of both no. 1 chromosomes in all cells of one diploid line, no consistent significant abnormalities were seen.

Five NPC tumours, freed of infiltrating lymphoid cells by passage through nude mice, were similarly examined after spindle arrest *in vivo*. Two tumours were near-diploid, and three were hypo-tetraploid. Near-diploid cells had only minor chromosomal changes, but the hypo-tetraploid spreads from all tumours showed gross changes of uncertain origin, including frequent, major translocations. No. 14 chromosome marker changes were not seen, and there was no other consistent pattern of abnormality in tumour cells.

ACKNOWLEDGEMENTS

This work was assisted by the Cancer Research Campaign, London, UK, out of funds donated by the Bradbury Investment Company of Hong Kong and by the Stehlin Foundation for Cancer Research, Houston, Texas, USA. One of us (P.A.T.) is the recipient of a scholarship for training in research methods from the Medical Research Council, London, UK.

REFERENCES

Beatty-Desana, J.W., Hoggard, M.J. & Cooledge, J.W. (1975) Non-random occurrence of 7-14 translocations in human lymphocyte cultures. *Nature (Lond.)*, *255*, 242-243

de-Thé, G., Ho, H.C., Kwan, H.C., Desgranges, C. & Favre, M.C. (1970) Nasopharyngeal carcinoma. I. Types of cultures derived from tumour biopsies and non-tumourous tissues of Chinese patients with special reference to lymphoblastoid transformation. *Int. J. Cancer*, *6*, 189-206

Epstein, M.A. & Achong, B.G. (1977) Recent progress in EB virus research. *Ann. Rev. Microbiol.*, *31*, 421-445

Epstein, M.A., Achong, B.G. & Mansell, P.W.A. (1971) *A new virus in cultures of human nasopharyngeal carcinoma.* In: Nakahara, W., Nishioka, K., Hirayama, T. & Ito, Y., eds, *Recent Advances in Human Tumor Virology and Immunology*, Tokyo, University of Tokyo Press, pp. 163-171

Fukuhara, S., Shirakawa, S. & Uchino, H. (1976) Specific marker chromosome 14 in malignant lymphomas. *Nature (Lond.)*, *259*, 210-211

Gazzolo, L., de-Thé, G., Vuillaume, M. & Ho, H.C. (1972) Nasopharyngeal carcinoma. II. Ultrastructure of normal mucosa, tumor biopsies and subsequent epithelial growth *in vitro*. *J. nat. Cancer Inst.*, *48*, 73-86

Hecht, F., McCaw, B.K., Peakman, D. & Robinson, A. (1975) Non-random occurrence of 7-14 translocations in human lymphocyte cultures. *Nature (Lond.)*, *255*, 243-244

Huang, D.P., Ho, J.H., Henle, W. & Henle, G. (1974) Demonstration of Epstein-Barr virus-associated nuclear antigen in nasopharyngeal carcinoma cells from fresh biopsies. *Int. J. Cancer*, *14*, 580-588

Jarvis, J.E., Ball, G., Rickinson, A.B. & Epstein, M.A. (1974) Cytogenetic studies on human lymphoblastoid cell lines from Burkitt's lymphomas and other sources. *Int. J. Cancer, 14*, 716-721

Klein, G. (1975) *A summing-up.* In: de-Thé, G., Epstein, M.A. & zur Hausen, H., eds, *Oncogenesis and Herpesviruses II, Part 2 (IARC Scientific Publications No. 11)*, Lyon, pp. 365-397

Klein, G., Giovanella, B.C., Lindahl, T., Fialkow, P.J., Singh, S. & Stehlin, J.S. (1974) Direct evidence for the presence of Epstein-Barr virus DNA and nuclear antigen in malignant epithelial cells from patients with poorly differentiated carcinoma of the nasopharynx. *Proc. nat. Acad. Sci. (Wash.), 71*, 4737-4741

Manolov, G. & Manolova, Y. (1972) Marker band in one chromosome 14 from Burkitt lymphomas. *Nature (Lond.), 237*, 33-34

Nilsson, K. & Pontén, J. (1975) Classification and biological nature of established human hematopoietic cell lines. *Int. J. Cancer, 15*, 321-341

Prigogina, E.L. & Fleischman, E.W. (1975) Marker chromosome 14q+ in two non-Burkitt lymphomas. *Humangenetik, 30*, 109-112

Shanmugaratnam, K. (1971) Studies on the etiology of nasopharyngeal carcinoma. *Int. Rev. exp. Path., 10*, 361-413

Svoboda, D.J., Kirchner, F.R. & Shanmugaratnam, K. (1967) *The fine structure of nasopharyngeal carcinomas.* In: Muir, C.S. & Shanmugaratnam, K. eds, *Cancer of the Nasopharynx*, (*UICC Monograph Series No. 1*), Copenhagen, Munksgaard, pp. 163-171

Trumper, P.A., Epstein, M.A. & Giovanella, B.C. (1976) Activation *in vitro* by BUdR of a productive EB virus infection in the epithelial cells of nasopharyngeal carcinoma. *Int. J. Cancer, 17*, 578-587

Visfeldt, J., Poulsen, C.O. & Rygaard, J. (1972) Chromosome analyses of human tumours following heterotransplantation to the mouse mutant 'nude'. *Acta path. microbiol. scand., Section A, 80*, 169-176

Welch, J.P. & Lee, C.L.Y. (1975) Non-random occurrence of 7-14 translocations in human lymphocyte cultures. *Nature (Lond.), 255*, 241-242

Wolf, H., zur Hausen, H. & Becker, V. (1973) EB viral genomes in epithelial nasopharyngeal carcinoma cells. *Nature (New Biol.), 244*, 245-247

Wurster-Hill, D.H., McIntyre, O.R., Cornwell, G.G. & Maurer, L.H. (1973) Marker chromosome 14 in multiple myeloma and plasma cell leukaemia. *Lancet, ii*, 1031

Yata, J., Desgranges, C., de-Thé, G., Mourali, N., Ellouz, R., Tachibana, T. & Brugère, J. (1974) Nasopharyngeal carcinoma. VII. B and T lymphocytes in the circulating blood and in tumour tissue. *Biomedicine, 21*, 244-250

Zech, L., Haglund, U., Nilsson, K. & Klein, G. (1976) Characteristic chromosomal abnormalities in biopsies and lymphoid cell lines from patients with Burkitt and non-Burkitt lymphomas. *Int. J. Cancer, 17*, 47-56

ANALYSIS FOR VOLATILE NITROSAMINES IN SALT-PRESERVED FOODSTUFFS TRADITIONALLY CONSUMED BY SOUTHERN CHINESE

D.P. HUANG & J.H.C. HO

*Medical and Health Department Institute of Radiology and Oncology,
Queen Elizabeth Hospital,
Kowloon, Hong Kong*

T.A. GOUGH

*Department of Industry,
Laboratory of the Government Chemist,
London, UK*

INTRODUCTION

Epidemiological studies of nasopharyngeal carcinoma (NPC) by Ho (1971, 1972a, b, 1975) suggested that Cantonese salted fish and/or other salt-preserved food products traditionally consumed by southern Chinese may play a role in the development of this cancer, which has been known to be prevalent among southern Chinese for over half a century (Ho, 1975). Fong & Walsh (1971) reported the finding of volatile nitrosamines in Cantonese salted marine fish in the range of mg nitrosamine/kg of salted fish, using thin-layer chromatography after the method described by Sen et al. (1969).

Nitrosamines can induce malignant tumours in a wide variety of organs in many animal species. Several of the nitrosamines are known to induce squamous-cell carcinomas, adenocarcinomas and other tumours in the nasal cavities of experimental animals (Althoff et al., 1974; Cardesa et al., 1976; Herrold, 1970; Lijinsky et al., 1970; Mohr et al., 1972; Pelfrene & Garcia, 1976). In fact, virtually all organs of the animal body are susceptible to the carcinogenic action of at least one nitroso compound (Magee, 1968).

One of the unique features of nitrosamines is that they have an 'organotropic' carcinogenic effect (Lijinsky, 1977). In other words, carcinomas develop in the susceptible tissues, irrespective of the route of their administration to the animal. It seems likely that certain nitrosamines may be causally related to some human cancers.

We report here the results of analyses by a highly sensitive detection method for volatile nitrosamines, namely, combined gas chromatography and high-resolution mass spectrometry (GC-MS), of six types of salted fish and 10 other items of salted food products traditionally consumed by southern Chinese. The detection limit for each nitrosamine in the original raw food was 1 μg/kg.

MATERIALS AND METHODS

The following items were purchased in a market in Hong Kong: pork sausage, goose-liver sausage, salt-dried beans, soya bean paste, soy, shrimp paste, oyster sauce, soya bean curd, salt-dried egg yolk, fish sauce and six types of salted fish.

Samples of each of these foods were prepared as extracts according to the method described by Goodhead & Gough (1975) (Scheme 1). Two samples of each food, except two types of salted fish, were taken, and *N*-nitrosodimethylamine (NDMA) was added to one and *N*-nitrosodi-*n*-propylamine (NDPA) to the other, as internal standards. This was done in order to detect any NDPA and NDMA which may have been present naturally and, at the same time, to check the efficiencies of recovery of the nitrosamines. In samples of two of the types of salted fish, namely, anchovies and mixed fish heads, only NDPA was added.

After the extracts had been reduced to 2.5 ml in a Kuderna-Danish flask at 45°C, as shown in Scheme 1, the flask was cooled, 800 μl hexane added and evaporation continued until a volume of about 300 μl extract remained. This volume was measured accurately with a calibrated syringe, which was then used to transfer the sample into a septum-fitted vial for storage at 10°C in the dark, pending analysis by GC-MS.

The GC-MS system consisted of a Pye 104 chromatograph linked to an AEl MS 902 high-resolution mass spectrometer *via* a membrane separator (Gough & Webb, 1972). The chromatograph was fitted with a polar-packed column connected to a high-efficiency support coated open tubular (SCOT) column. A venting valve was placed between the two columns to prevent overload of the SCOT column by solvent and to minimize contamination of the mass spectrometer by extraneous material eluted from the columns. The mass spectrometer was operated at high resolution, and nitrosamines were detected by monitoring the parent ion of each nitrosamine at the appropriate retention time. The spectrometer was used in the peak-matching mode, which compares the mass of the nitrosamine with that of a suitable fragment ion of a fluorinated hydrocarbon.

SCHEME 1.

Determination of steam-volatile *N*-nitroso compounds in salt-preserved food products traditionally consumed by southern Chinese

500 gm salt-preserved food product

↓ + 500 ml water + 200 g NaCl
+ internal standard

steam distillation, collect 800 ml

↓ +160 g NaCl + 8 ml 10N H_2SO_4
Extract with 80 ml dichloromethane, 4 x

wash combined extracts with 140 ml 1.5 N NaOH,
dry over Na_2SO_4

↓

evaporate and reduce total volume to 2.5 ml in a
Kuderna-Danish flask at 45°C

↓

gas chromatography - mass spectrometry

Quantitative results were based on the mass spectrometric measurements, and the spectrometer was calibrated before and after sample analyses, using 1 and 10 µl/1 standard solutions of nitrosamines in hexane. The concentrations of nitrosamines in the original foodstuffs were calculated from the weight of food taken, the final volume of the extract and the efficiency of recovery of the nitrosamines, as determined in samples to which nitrosamines had been added.

All extracts were examined for the following nitrosamines: NDMA, *N*-nitrosodiethylamine, -dipropylamine, -dibutylamine, -piperidine and -pyrrolidine. The detection limit in the original raw food was 1 µg/kg for each nitrosamine, and the quantitative results have a precision of ± 20%.

RESULTS

Within the limits of detection, no volatile nitrosamine, other than those added as internal standards, was detected in any of the salted food products, except in four of the six types of salted fish; in these, NDMA was detected in the range of 1-35 μg/kg (Table 1).

Table 1. Occurrence of volatile nitrosamines in salted fish

Type of fish	No. of samples	Internal standard	Nitrosamine detected (μg/kg)
Anchovy	2	NDPA	NDMA (2, 35)
Croaker	1	NDPA	NDMA (8)
	2	NDMA	None
Red snapper	2	NDMA	None
	1	NDPA	None
	1	-	None
White herring	3	NDPA	NDMA (1, 1, 8)
	1	NDMA	None
Yellow croaker	2	NDPA	NDMA (7, 18)
	4	NDMA	None
Mixed fish heads	1	NDPA	None
	1	-	None

NDPA - *N*-nitrosodi-*n*-propylamine; NDMA - *N*-nitrosodimethylamine

DISCUSSION

For those samples of fish with which positive results were obtained, the levels are no higher than those encountered in cured meats consumed in Europe, where the incidence of NPC is low. Many possibilities could account for the difference in risk for NPC in these two population groups that consume foods containing NDMA. We are now investigating one of these - whether other carcinogens or procarcinogens could be formed as the result of cooking and as a result of interaction between nitrites and nitrates known to be present in the salted fish (Fong & Chan, 1973) and nitrosamine precursors in the stomach. We are also analysing the salted fish for non-volatile nitrosamines.

SUMMARY

Six types of salted fish and 10 other sorts of salted food products traditionally consumed by southern Chinese were analysed by GC-MS for the presence of volatile nitrosamines. The detection limit in the original raw food was 1 μg/kg for each nitrosamine. Only NDMA, in the range of 1-35 μg/kg, could be detected, in four of the six types of salted fish samples examined; and no nitrosamines were found in the other salted food products.

ACKNOWLEDGEMENTS

Thanks are rendered to the World Health Foundation (Hong Kong) and to The Hong Kong Anti-Cancer Society for financial assistance. The authors are also grateful to Mrs M. Ali for her technical assistance, to Mrs P. Liu for typing the manuscript and to Mr K.W. Leung for photographic assistance.

REFERENCES

Althoff, J., Mohr, U., Page, N. & Reznik, G. (1974) Carcinogenic effect of dibutylnitrosamine in European hamsters (*Cricetus cricetus*). *J. nat. Cancer Inst.*, *53*, 795-800

Cardesa, A., Pour, P., Haas, H., Althoff, J. & Mohr, U. (1976) Histogenesis of tumours from the nasal cavities induced by diethyl-nitrosamine. *Cancer*, *37*, 346-355

Fong, Y.Y. & Chan, W.C. (1973) Bacterial production of di-methyl nitrosamine in salted fish. *Nature (Lond.)*, *243*, 421-422

Fong, Y.Y. & Walsh, E.O. (1971) Carcinogenic nitrosamines in Cantonese salt-dried fish. *Lancet*, *ii*, 1032

Goodhead, K. & Gough, T.A. (1975) The reliability of a procedure for the determination of nitrosamines in food. *Fd Cosmet. Toxicol.*, *13*, 307-312

Gough, T.A. & Webb, K.S. (1972) The use of a molecular separator in the determination of trace constituents by combined gas chromatography and mass spectrometry. *J. Chromat.*, *64*, 201-210

Herrold, K. (1970) Upper respiratory tract tumours induced in Syrian hamsters by *N*-methyl-*N*-nitrosourea. *Amer. J. Cancer*, *6*, 223-233

Ho, J.H.C. (1971) *Genetic and environmental factors in nasopharyngeal carcinoma.* In: Nakahara, W., Nishioka, K., Hirayama, T. & Ito, Y., eds, *Recent Advances in Human Tumor Virology and Immunology*, Tokyo, University of Tokyo Press, pp. 275-295

Ho, J.H.C. (1972a) Nasopharyngeal carcinoma (NPC). *Advanc. Cancer Res.*, *15*, 57-92

Ho, H.C. (1972b) *Current knowledge of the epidemiology of nasopharyngeal carcinoma - a review.* In: Biggs, P.M., de-Thé, G. & Payne, L.N., eds, *Oncogenesis and Herpesviruses (IARC Scientific Publications No. 2)*, Lyon, pp. 357-366

Ho, H.C. (1975) Epidemiology of nasopharyngeal carcinoma. *J. roy. Coll. Surg. Edinb.*, *20*, 223-235

Lijinsky, W., Ferrero, A., Montesano, R. & Wenyon, C.E.M. (1970) Tumourogenicity of cyclic nitrosamines in Syrian golden hamster. *Z. Krebsforsch.*, *74*, 185-189

Lijinsky, W. (1977) How nitrosamines cause cancer. *New Scientist*, *73*, 216-217

Magee, P.N. (1968) Possible mechanism of carcinogenesis by *N*-nitroso compounds and alkylating agents. *Food Cosmet. Toxic.*, *6*, 572-573

Mohr, U., Althoff, J. & Page, N. (1972) European hamster as a model for respiratory carcinogenesis. *J. nat. Cancer Inst.*, *49*, 595-597

Pelfrene, A. & Garcia, H. (1976) Chemically induced esthesioneuroblastomas in rats. *Z. Krebsforsch.*, *86*, 113-119

Sen, N.P., Smith, D.C., Schwinghamer, L. & Marleau, J.J. (1969) Diethylnitrosamine and other *N*-nitrosamines in food. *J. Ass. off. analyt. Chem.*, *52*, 47

CARCINOMA OF THE NASAL AND PARANASAL REGIONS IN RATS FED CANTONESE SALTED MARINE FISH

D.P. HUANG & J.H.C. HO

Medical and Health Department
Institute of Radiology and Oncology,
Queen Elizabeth Hospital,
Kowloon, Hong Kong

D. SAW & T.B. TEOH

Medical and Health Department Institute of Pathology,
Sai Ying Pun Jockey Club Clinic,
Hong Kong

INTRODUCTION

Ho (1971) first suspected that Cantonese salted fish might be a possible etiological factor in the development of nasopharyngeal carcinoma (NPC) in Chinese populations, because it is commonly consumed by the southern Chinese, who have far higher rate of incidence of the disease than any other group. Furthermore, Ho (1975) pointed out that since NPC was already prevalent among the Chinese in Canton in the early nineteen twenties (Todd, 1921) and is among Chinese in Singapore (Shanmugaratnam & Muir, 1967), it is unlikely to be a product of the modern environment and that attention should be concentrated on traditional environmental factors. The fishing 'boat people' in Hong Kong, who live in boats and cook their food in the open, have a significantly higher incidence of NPC than do the land-dwellers, thus eliminating inhalants as a possible factor; in addition, the boat people consume relatively more salted fish.

Salted fish is fed to most southern Chinese as one of their first solid foods (Topley, 1973). Ho (1975) thinks that the early steep rise in the age-specific incidence rate of NPC in Chinese could be explained by exposure to an agent early in life. If this is so, salted fish is high on the list of suspects. It has been found by

Anderson et al.[1] to be the only non-fresh food fed to babies and to be the food eaten most commonly by 22 Hong Kong Chinese NPC patients diagnosed before the age of 25.

In the face of such persuasive epidemiological data, we proceeded to test the hypothesis in laboratory animals. At the same time, we looked for the presence of nitrosamines in some traditional southern Chinese food products; the results are reported elsewhere by Huang et al.[2]. The present report is concerned with the incidence and morphology of the tumours that developed in the nasal cavities and paranasal regions of experimental animals fed Cantonese salted fish as a part of their diet.

MATERIALS AND METHODS

Inbred WA albino rats, aged one month and weighing 150 g, and Syrian golden hamsters, also aged one month and weighing 100 g, were housed in plastic cages in groups of two, according to sex, and kept under standard conditions. They were supplied with a pelleted diet (Airport Animal Shelter, Animal Food and Bedding Division, Burlingams, Ca, USA) during the day; during the night, nightly for six months, animals were given a quantity of salted marine fish which had been steamed with water for 15 min in a closed container (30 g/rat and 20 g/hamster). Each animal generally consumed the whole amount; if not, a reduced amount of the pelleted diet was given the following morning.

Thereafter, the animals were given only the pelleted diet, but a soup prepared from salted fish heads replaced the drinking-water during the night for five consecutive nights per week; the animals were sacrificed after 1-2 years or when moribund. The soup was prepared in the following manner: 500 g of salted fish heads were added to 1 l of drinking-water and boiled for 1 hr in a covered container, giving a final volume of 500 ml of concentrated extract; this was diluted 1:5 with fresh drinking-water to give a sodium chloride concentration of 0.9 g/l. Twenty ml of this preparation were given to each animal. Fish heads were used, since, in practice, when the whole fish is not steamed (frequently on top of rice in a covered cooker), sometimes only the head is used to prepare a soup.

Twenty rats (10 males and 10 females) and 14 hamsters (8 males and 6 females) were given the above treatment, and 6 rats (3 males and 3 females) and equal numbers of hamsters served as controls.

Since *N*-nitrosodimethylamine (NDMA) has been detected in Cantonese salt-dried or salted marine fish (Fong & Chan, 1973; Fong & Walsh, 1971; Gough, 1974; Huang et al.[2]), NDMA

---

[1] See p. 231

[2] See p. 309

was added to the drinking-water of a second group of experimental animals comprising 15 rats (6 males and 9 females) and 18 hamsters (10 males and 8 females). Each animal was given 20 ml of a solution of 2.5 µl NDMA standard (Tokyo Kasei Kogyo Co. Ltd, Tokyo, Japan) in 100 ml drinking-water nightly for five consecutive nights per week, equivalent to a weekly intake of 2.5 mg. Six rats and 6 hamsters (3 males and 3 females in each group) served as controls.

A third group, comprising 14 rats and 12 hamsters, with an equal sex distribution, were administered 0.05 ml 1% (v/v) *N*-nitrosodiethylamine (NDEA) (0.5 mg) orally through a dropper once weekly. Six rats and 6 hamsters, with an equal sex distribution, served as controls. NDEA was included in the study as a positive control, since it is a known carcinogen of high potency, inducing nasal carcinomas in hamsters (Herrold, 1964; Mohr et al., 1972), rats (Thomas, 1965) and gerbils (Cardesa et al., 1976).

Sacrificed rats (no tumours were observed in hamsters) were sent for histopathological examination. Blocks taken from the heart, lungs, liver, spleen, kidney, trachea, oesophagus and stomach were fixed in 10% neutral phosphate-buffered formalin. Heads were fixed similarly, after removal of the skin and brain; after fixation, the whole head was decalcified in 8% formic acid for approximately three days, and six frontal (paracoronal) sections were taken at 5 mm intervals. The sections were further decalcified for another one to two days before being embedded in paraffin. Sections were stained routinely with haematoxylin and eosin; where tumours were found in the nasal and paranasal regions, the following, additional stains were used: periodic acid-Schiff (PAS), PAS after diastase treatment, alcian blue and Southgate's mucicarmine. Selected liver sections were also stained with PAS, PAS after diastase treatment and Gordon & Sweet's silver impregnation.

RESULTS

None of the control rats and none of the treated or control hamsters developed nasal or paranasal tumours. The following section refers, therefore, only to treated rats. The results are summarized in Table 1.

Rats administered salted fish

Of the ten males and ten females that received salted fish, four females developed carcinomas in the nasal or paranasal regions: two developed adenocarcinomas of the nasal cavity after 12 and 24 months, respectively (Figs 1 & 2), one developed an undifferentiated carcinoma in a paranasal sinus after 15 months (Fig. 3), and another showed a highly invasive squamous carcinoma in the upper posterior part of the right buccoalveolar sulcus after 24 months (Fig. 4). The two rats with nasal adenocarcinomas also developed a mammary adenocarcinoma and a nodular liver after 12 and 24 months' treatment, respectively.

Table 1. Development of carcinomas in the nasal or paranasal regions of WA albino rats treated with salted fish, *N*-nitrosodimethylamine (NDMA) or *N*-nitrosodiethylamine, (NDEA)

Treatment	Incidence	Treatment time (mths)	Site	Cell type	Origin
Salted fish	4/10 females	12	Nasal cavity	Adenocarcinoma	Unicentric
	0/10 males	24	Nasal cavities	Adenocarcinoma	Multicentric
		15	Paranasal sinus	Undifferentiated carcinoma	Unicentric
		24	Upper posterior buccoalveolar sulcus	Squamous carcinoma	Unicentric
NDMA	0/15	5-24	none	-	-
NDEA	2/7 females	12	Nasal cavity	Adenocarcinoma	Unicentric
	1/7 males	13	Nasal cavities	Adenocarcinoma	Multicentric
		15	Nasal cavities	Adenocarcinoma	Multicentric

One further rat killed after five months' treatment showed a slightly nodular, enlarged liver.

NDMA-treated rats

One of the 15 treated animals had an undifferentiated malignant growth about 3 cm in diameter involving one kidney after 10 months' treatment.

NDEA-treated rats

Of 14 treated animals, three developed nasal adenocarcinomas (Figs 5 & 6) and had large areas of hyperplasia in their livers. In another three rats, treated for 11½, 12 and 18 months, only enlarged, nodular livers were noted.

Histological findings

The nasal tumours that developed in the rats treated with salted fish and in those administered NDEA had very similar features, their microscopic appearances varying from those of well to moderately differentiated adenocarcinomas. The glandular structures were usually lined with single or multilayered, closely arranged cuboidal or tall columnar cells, with irregularly arranged nuclei exhibiting moderate hyperchromatism and pleomorphism (Figs 7 & 8). Heaping up of nuclei was seen in some areas; mitosis was rare. In one well-differentiated adenocarcinoma that developed in a rat given salted fish, prominent glandular and papillary formations as well as a few small solid areas of tumour cells were seen. The glandular and papillary processes were covered by compactly arranged, tall, columnar epithelial cells, with crowding or heaping of nuclei; abundant mucin was present in the cytoplasm and glandular lumen. The cells

FIG. 1. RAT NASAL TUMOUR INDUCED BY TREATMENT WITH SALTED FISH

Frontal section across the posterior part of the nasal cavities of a rat showing a nasal tumour (adenocarcinoma with some undifferentiated elements) on the left side, after 12 months' treatment with salted fish; H & E x5

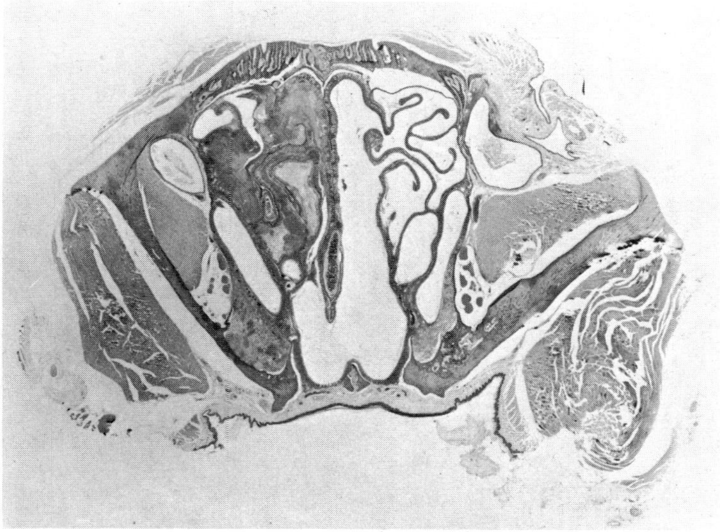

FIG. 2. RAT NASAL TUMOURS INDUCED BY TREATMENT WITH SALTED FISH

Frontal section of the posterior part of the nasal cavities of a rat showing tumours (adenocarcinomas) in both cavities, after 24 months' treatment with salted fish; H & E x 3.5

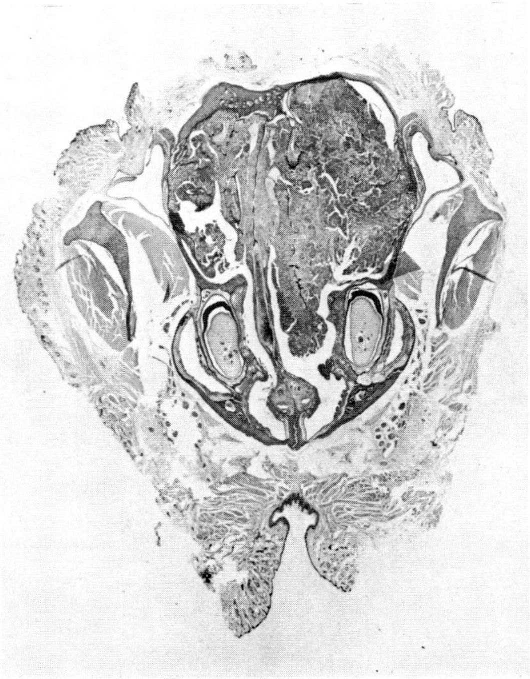

FIG. 3. TUMOUR IN RAT SINUS INDUCED BY TREATMENT WITH SALTED FISH

Frontal section of the maxillary sinuses of a rat showing a tumour (undifferentiated carcinoma) in the right sinus, after 15 months' treatment with salted fish; H & E x 4.5

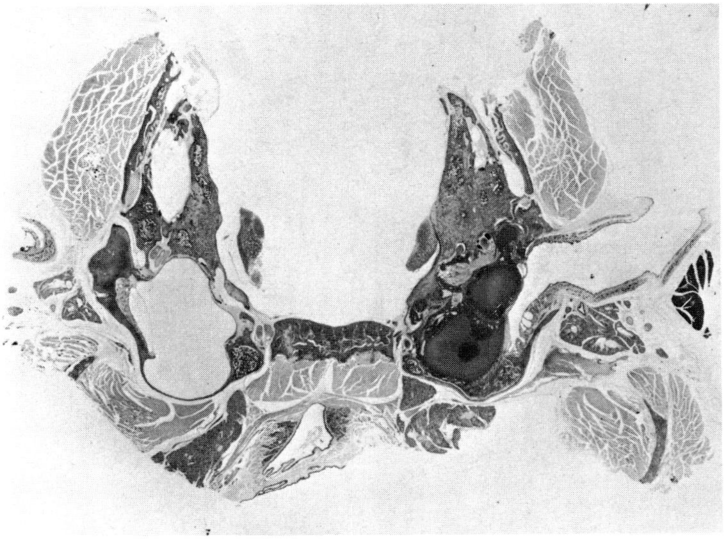

FIG. 4. ULCERATED GROWTH INDUCED BY TREATMENT WITH SALT FISH

Frontal section of ulcerated growth (arrow) in the buccoalveolar mucosa of a rat after 24 months' treatment with salted fish; H & E x 4.5

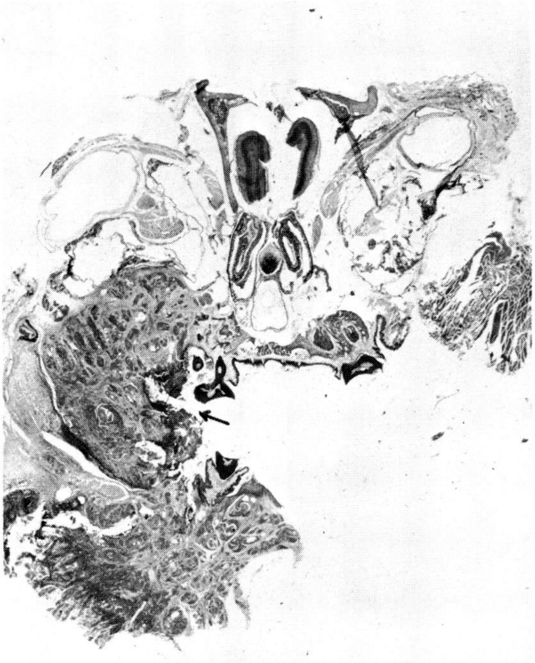

FIG. 5. MULTICENTRIC GROWTHS
INDUCED BY TREATMENT WITH *N*-NITROSODIETHYLAMINE

Frontal section of nasal cavities of a rat, showing multicentric growths (arrows) in the left cavity, after 13 months' treatment with *N*-nitrosodiethylamine; H & E x 5

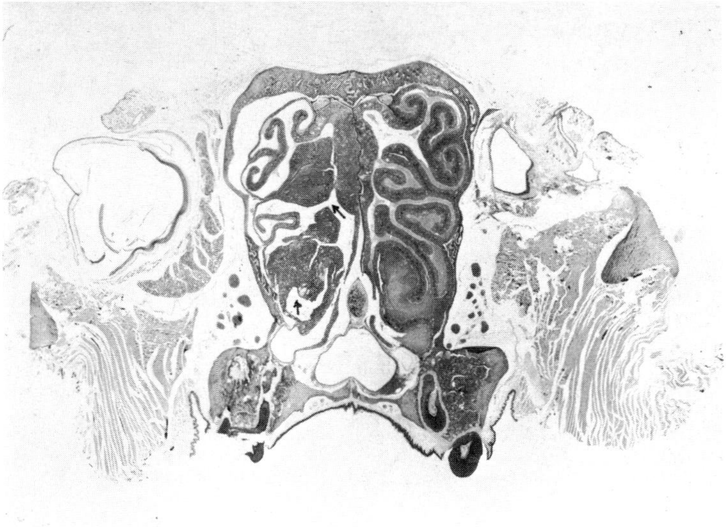

FIG. 6. MULTICENTRIC GROWTHS
INDUCED BY TREATMENT WITH *N*-NITROSODIETHYLAMINE

Frontal section of the nasal cavities of a rat showing multicentric growths (arrows) in both cavities, after 15 months' treatment with *N*-nitrosodiethylamine; H & E x 4.5

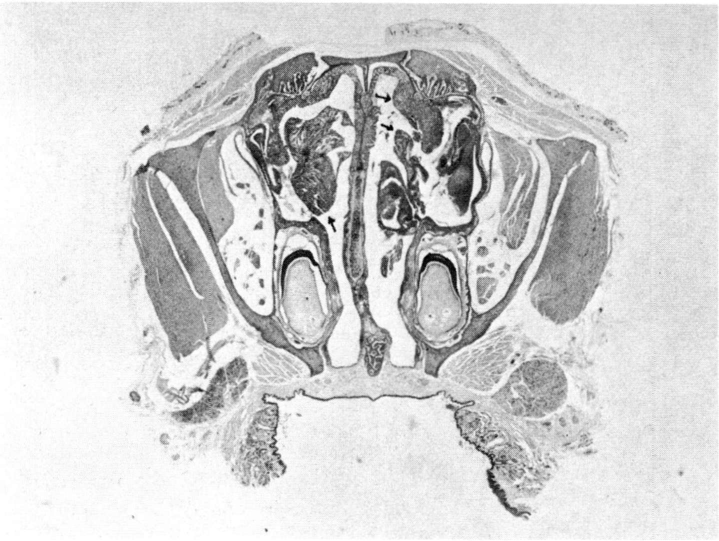

FIG. 7. RAT NASAL TUMOUR INDUCED BY TREATMENT WITH SALTED FISH

Higher magnification of tumour seen in Fig. 2, showing well-differentiated papillary adenocarcinoma cells; H & E x 150

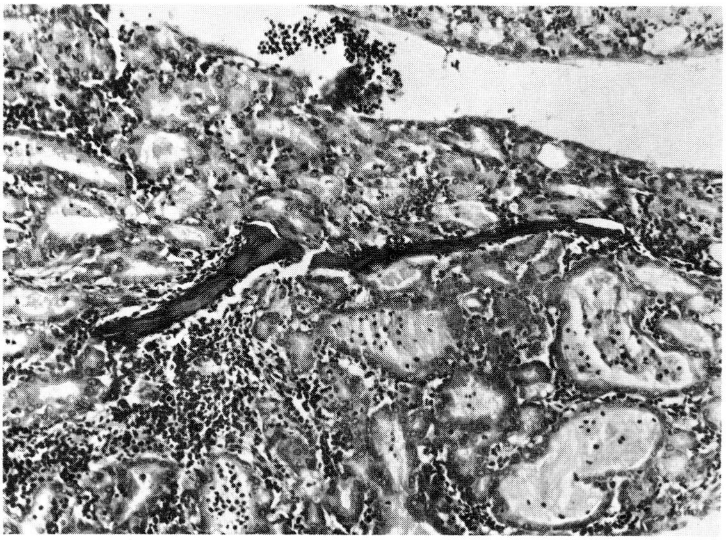

FIG. 8. RAT NASAL TUMOUR INDUCED BY TREATMENT WITH SALTED FISH

Another area of tumour seen in Fig. 2, showing irregular polygonal tumour cells with abundant mucinous cytoplasm displacing the nuclei to one side; H & E x 150

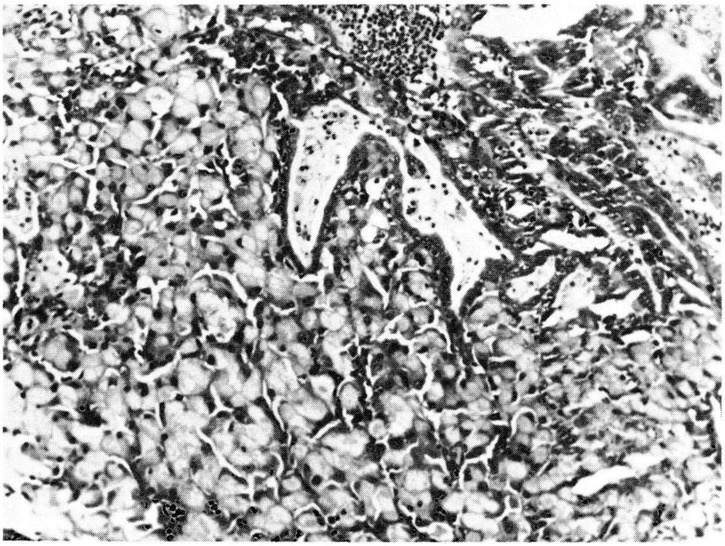

of the solid areas were moderately large and irregularly polygonal in shape; the nuclei were small, hyperchromatic and pushed to one side by the abundant mucinous cytoplasm. These closely resembled signet-ring cells (Fig. 9). Superior invasion of bone was seen in three of the five rats that developed nasal adenocarcinomas (Fig. 10).

FIG. 9. TUMOUR INDUCED BY *N*-NITROSODIETHYLAMINE

Higher magnification of tumour seen in Fig. 6, showing features of a well-differentiated adenocarcinoma; H & E x 150

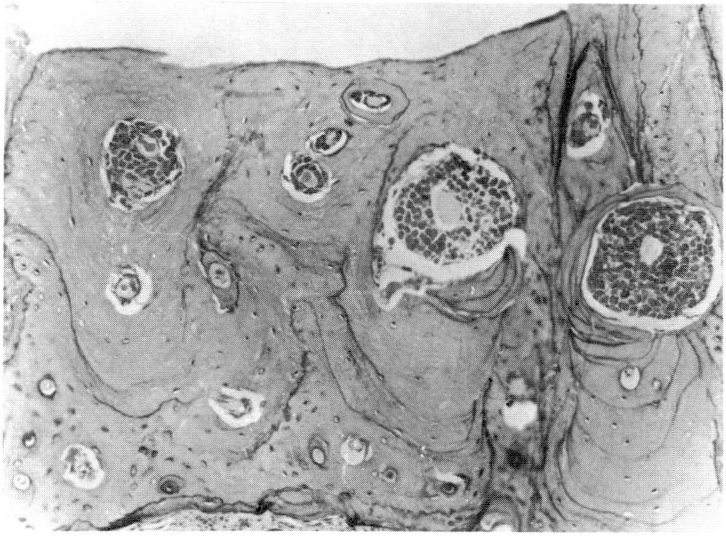

The growth in the right paranasal sinus of one rat given salted fish showed a relatively large area of central necrosis, surrounded by a compact zone of undifferentiated tumour cells with very scanty cytoplasm (Fig. 11). Scattered mucinous areas or droplets were seen among the tumour cells, and there was invasion of the adjacent bone in one area.

The ulcerated lesion in the upper posterior part of the bucco-alveolar sulcus of one rat given salted fish showed typical features of a well-differentiated squamous-cell carcinoma with abundant keratinization (Fig. 12). The growth infiltrated the adjoining soft tissue and the floor of the right paranasal sinus. The overlying epithelium lining the sinus cavity was intact.

The nodular lesions seen in the livers of rats treated with salted fish or NDEA exhibited changes varying from hyperplasia to neoplasia; varying degrees of bile-duct epithelial proliferation were also present in

FIG. 10. INVASION OF BONE FROM NASAL TUMOUR INDUCED BY TREATMENT WITH SALTED FISH

Invasion of bone by undifferentiated carcinoma cells from the nasal tumour seen in Fig. 1; H & E x 150

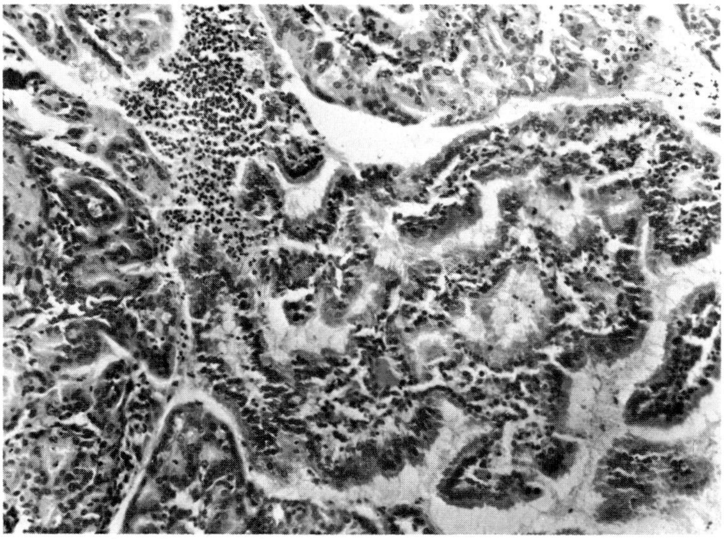

FIG. 11. UNDIFFERENTIATED CARCINOMA CELLS

Strands and masses of undifferentiated carcinoma cells in an area of the maxillary sinus tumour seen in Fig. 3; H & E x 260

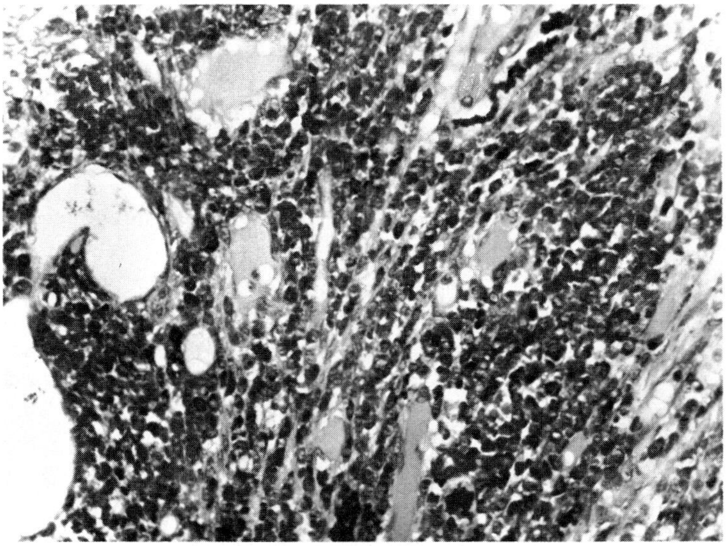

FIG. 12. WELL-DIFFERENTIATED SQUAMOUS CARCINOMA CELLS

Well-differentiated squamous carcinoma cells with keratin pearls, from tumour seen in Fig. 4; H & E x 250

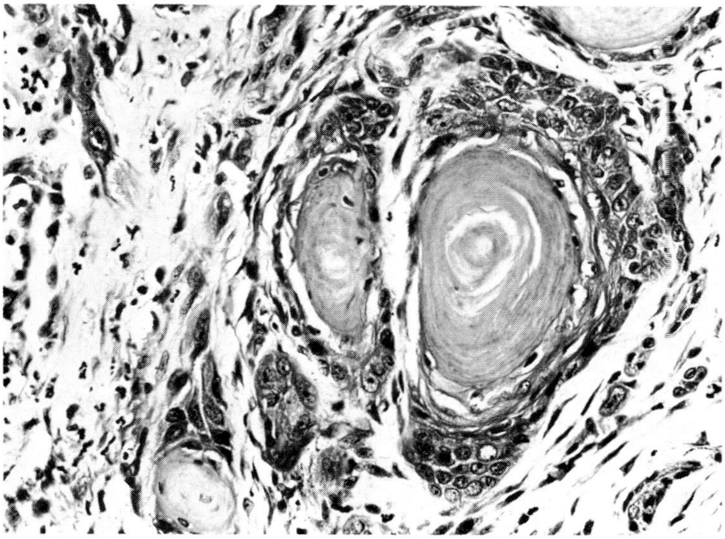

the parenchymal lesions. In the group of animals treated with salted fish, hyperplastic changes were seen in the liver and bile-duct epithelial cells of two rats. These features were more severe in the rat that developed a well-differentiated papillary adenocarcinoma in the nasal cavity after two years' treatment; many hyperplastic bile ducts were cystically dilated, with short, papillary infoldings projecting into the lumen. In the group of animals treated with NDEA, three rats that developed nasal adenocarcinomas also showed features of advanced hepatic hyperplasia; three other rats that developed liver lesions only exhibited changes characteristic of neoplasia. Lung metastases were observed in two of these animals after 12 and 18 months' treatment, respectively.

DISCUSSION

The development of carcinomas in four of 20 WA albino rats given salted fish in their diet from the age of one month, and in none of six controls, is unlikely to be coincidental. It certainly suggests that salted fish contains an unknown agent capable of inducing carcinomas in these rats systemically. The adenocarcinoma that developed in the breast of one rat and the squamous carcinoma seen in the buccoalveolar mucosa of another may be treated as isolated, coincidental findings; but the adenocarcinomas, one with multicentric origins, that developed in the nasal cavities of two rats and the undifferentiated carcinoma found in a paranasal sinus of another cannot be ignored.

The epithelial linings of the nasal and paranasal sinus cavities are both of the ciliated respiratory type and are continuous. It is likely, therefore, that the intracellular enzymes and metabolism of the cells in both cavities have much in common. The carcinomas that develop predominantly in this epithelium may result from a special susceptibility of this tissue to a hypothetical carcinogenic agent that occurs in salted fish.

Although the frequency of tumour induction, the site of the tumours induced and their histological type resemble those seen in NDEA-treated rats, NDEA has not been detected at the μg/kg level in several samples of salted fish analysed by Huang et al.[1]. On the other hand, although these authors found NDMA at levels of 1-35 μg/kg in salted fish, no nasal or paranasal tumours occurred in NDMA-treated animals in our study. Huang et al. detected no volatile nitrosamines other than NDMA in the salted fish samples analysed; however, they did not look for high-molecular weight, non-volatile nitrosamines.

Nitrosamines are suspected to be the carcinogenic agent involved because they are organotropic in their action, as is the agent causing tumours in rats given salted fish. Other chemical carcinogens or pro-carcinogens should not be overlooked, but it would seem logical next to look at non-volatile nitrosamines, and this project is already in hand.

SUMMARY

Cantonese salted fish is suspected on epidemiological grounds to be an etiological factor in human NPC. To determine whether this food contains a carcinogen which acts on the upper respiratory epithelial lining, WA albino rats and Syrian golden hamsters were given Cantonese salted fish in their diet for one to two years from the age of one month and examined for tumours in that area. Three of 20 treated rats, but no control rats and no treated or control hamsters, developed carcinomas (two adenocarcinomas and one undifferentiated) in the nasal or paranasal sinus cavities after 12 to 24 months' treatment. NDEA was given orally to a similar group of animals as a positive control, and NDMA, the only volatile nitrosamine detected

---
[1] See p. 309

in salted fish, was added to the drinking-water of a third group. Three of 14 NDEA-treated rats developed adenocarcinomas in the nasal cavities, but none of the other animals developed nasal or paranasal tumours. These findings lead us to suspect that salted fish may contain a carcinogen or procarcinogen that can act systematically on the epithelial cells of the nasal and paranasal cavities

ACKNOWLEDGEMENTS

Thanks are given to the World Health Foundation (Hong Kong) and The Hong Kong Anti-Cancer Society for financial assistance and to Mrs P. Liu for typing the manuscript.

REFERENCES

Cardesa, A., Pour, P., Haas, H., Althoff, J. & Mohr, U. (1976) Histogenesis of tumors from the nasal cavities induced by diethylnitrosamine. *Cancer, 37*, 346-355

Fong, Y.Y. & Chan, W.C. (1973) Bacterial production of di-methyl nitrosamine in salted fish. *Nature (Lond.), 243*, 421-422

Fong, Y.Y. & Walsh, E.O. (1971) Carcinogenic nitrosamines in Cantonese salt-dried fish. *Lancet, ii*, 1032

Gough, T.A. (1974) *Report of the Government Chemist*, London, HMSO, p. 45

Herrold, K. (1964) Induction of olfactory neuroepithelial tumors in Syrian hamsters by diethylnitrosamine. *Cancer, 17*, 114-121

Ho, H.C. (1971) Incidence of nasopharyngeal cancer in Hong Kong. *UICC Bull. Cancer, 9*, 5

Ho, H.C. (1975) Epidemiology of nasopharyngeal carcinoma. *J. roy. Coll. Surg. (Edinb.), 20*, 223-235

Mohr, U., Althoff, J. & Page, N. (1972) European hamster as a model for respiratory carcinogenesis. *J. nat. Cancer Inst., 49*, 595

Shanmugaratnam, K. & Muir, C.S. (1967) *Nasopharyngeal carcinoma, origin and structure.* In: Muir, C.S. & Shanmugaratnam, K., eds, *Cancer of the Nasopharynx*, Copenhagen, Munksgaard (*UICC Monograph Series No. 1*), pp. 153-162

Thomas, C. (1965) Durch nitrosamine experimentell erzeugte nasenhoehlentumoren bei der ratte. *V. Dtsch. Gesundh.-Path.*, *49*, 245-248

Todd, P.J. (1921) Some practical points in the surgical treatment of cervical tumours. *Chin. med. J.*, *35*, 21-25

Topley, M. (1973) In: Field, C.E. & Baber, F.M., eds, *Growing up in Hong Kong*, Hong Kong, Hong Kong University Press, p. 56

DISCUSSION SUMMARY

N.E. DAY

International Agency for Research on Cancer,
Lyon, France

The importance of identifying functional parameters related to HLA genotypes at high risk for nasopharyngeal carcinoma was stressed. Day reported that a range of serological activities (IgG and IgA antibodies against the Epstein-Barr viral capsid antigen, early antigen and nuclear antigen) against Epstein-Barr virus-related antigens had been determined in family members of nasopharyngeal carcinoma cases in Singapore, but a preliminary analysis had indicated no differences in serological profile between family members sharing two, one or no haplotypes with the nasopharyngeal carcinoma case. Ng pointed out that in Hong Kong IgA levels (against Epstein-Barr viral capsid and early antigen) appeared to be higher in family members of nasopharyngeal carcinoma cases than among the general population. There was some evidence that positive IgA levels could be a risk factor for this carcinoma.

Chan drew attention to results he had obtained on nasopharyngeal carcinoma patients in Singapore, where those that had the A2, B-Sin 2 phenotype had higher anti-Epstein-Barr virus early antigen titres and somewhat higher anti-viral capsid antigen titres. The combined genetic and serological profile was of some prognostic importance.

Simons commented on the elevated frequency of BW15 among the Japanese cases reported. In Singapore, several sera had shown cross-reactivity between BW15 and B-Sin 2. A high frequency of anti-nuclear antibody had also been found among the Japanese nasopharyngeal carcinoma cases.

Terasaki expressed surprise that the occurrence of B-Sin 2 in certain population groups was not related to incidence of nasopharyngeal carcinoma. He found significant linkage disequilibrium between A2 and B-Sin 2 among US Japanese and was surprised that a clear association with HLA was found only among Chinese. He proposed that a wider range of loci be investigated; a cline of incidence might be related to more general genetic susceptibility, involving several genes.

ETIOLOGY OF NASOPHARYNGEAL CARCINOMA – VIROLOGICAL FACTORS

EPSTEIN-BARR VIRUS – DISCOVERY, PROPERTIES AND RELATIONSHIP TO NASOPHARYNGEAL CARCINOMA

M.A. EPSTEIN

Department of Pathology,
University of Bristol Medical School,
University Walk,
Bristol BS8 1TD, UK

INTRODUCTION

As a result of careful clinical observation, Denis Burkitt came to realize that the various lymphoid tumours he was seeing so frequently in children in East Africa were merely different manifestations of a single, highly unusual and until then unrecognized malignant lymphoma (Burkitt, 1958). This tumour has rightly come to be known as Burkitt's lymphoma (BL), and where it is common in Africa it is commoner than all other tumours of childhood added together (Burkitt, 1963). After describing BL, Burkitt made a second and perhaps more important contribution when he showed that the distribution of the tumour in Africa is determined by temperature and rainfall (Burkitt, 1962a, b).

The great significance of BL immediately became apparent when Burkitt presented his findings for the first time outside Africa, in London in 1961. The fact that the incidence of the tumour could be influenced by climatic factors suggested that some biological agent, such as an oncogenic virus spread by a climate-dependent arthropod vector, was concerned in its causation.

DISCOVERY OF EPSTEIN-BARR VIRUS

In view of this possibility, it was decided to undertake an extensive investigation of African BL biopsy samples for the presence of viruses. The failure of direct virological tests on this material, the rationale for subsequent attempts to culture BL cells in order to test them after growth *in vitro* (Epstein et al., 1964a), and the way in which Epstein-Barr virus (EBV) was found in such cells by electron microscopy (Epstein et al., 1964b, 1965) have been described in several reviews (Epstein, 1970a, b, 1975; Epstein & Achong, 1970).

With the accumulation of epidemiological information (Haddow, 1964), the original hypothesis that an arthropod vector was spreading an oncogenic virus which might play a role in the causation of African BL (Burkitt, 1962a, b) required revision, and other mechanisms for a virus etiology have since emerged; it is now thought that the climate-dependence of this tumour involves holoendemic malaria as a cofactor (Burkitt, 1969). Thus, EBV continues to be of importance, is being studied on an increasing scale, and is widely regarded as a likely human tumour virus.

PROPERTIES OF EBV

Uniqueness

It was recognized from the outset on the basis of morphological examinations that EBV was clearly a herpes virus (Epstein et al., 1964b, 1965); yet the agent was evidently highly unusual in that it regularly failed to show activity in standard biological tests (Epstein et al., 1965). There was no surprise, therefore, when immunological investigations rapidly established that EBV was a new and distinct member of the herpes family (see Epstein & Achong, 1973).

Biochemistry

EBV is also unique at the biochemical level: it is now known that the virus genome consists of double-stranded DNA with a molecular weight of 10^8 Daltons (Becker & Weinberg, 1972; Pritchett et al., 1975), that this should be sufficient to code for over 100 proteins (Pritchett et al., 1976), and that the virus particle in fact contains at least 33 different structural polypeptides (Dolyniuk et al., 1976).

Biological behaviour

General: The general biology of EBV infection has recently been reviewed (Epstein & Achong, 1977). Briefly, EBV is transmitted horizontally and infects all human populations. Primary infection usually occurs during childhood, without symptoms, and is accompanied by seroconversion. The virus is then harboured for life as a productive infection in the oropharynx, with shedding of infectious virus in the buccal fluid, and as a non-productive latent infection of a few lymphocytes. If primary infection is delayed and acquired in young adult life, it is accompanied by infectious mononucleosis (IM) in 50% of cases. Delayed primary infection is related to affluence, and IM is therefore common in upper socio-economic classes. IM has long been known to be associated characteristically with kissing among young people, but it may, infrequently, accompany primary infection in children or in adults in later life.

The incidence of persons who shed infectious virus from the mouth varies in different populations and under different circumstances, but it is this source of virus which is responsible for natural primary infection by horizontal transmission. Only B lymphocytes have receptors for EBV; the small number of such cells that harbour the EBV genome as a latent infection provide the starting material for the lymphoblastoid cell lines which can be established *in vitro* from blood or lymph nodes of seropositive individuals (Epstein & Achong, 1977).

Transforming ability in vitro: It has been known for some time that cell lines cannot be established from B lymphocytes from normal seronegative donors (including B lymphocytes from fetal cord blood), unless EBV has been added to them *in vitro* (see Epstein & Achong, 1973, 1977). When this has been done, the virus enters the cells, EBV-determined nuclear antigen (EBNA) expression can be detected within 18 to 24 hours (Aya & Osato, 1974; Menezes et al., 1977; Wright et al., 1975), and the virus DNA is increased to 10 to 15 genome equivalents per cell. At about this time an event takes place which transforms the cell, induces cellular DNA synthesis (Gerber & Hoyer, 1971) and confers the power of continuous proliferation *in vitro*; the transformed lines which result maintain a steady load of 10 to 15 virus genome equivalents per cell irrespective of the number of cell generations through which they have passed (Thorley-Lawson & Strominger, 1976). Transformation *in vitro* by EBV seems to occur more readily with fetal cells than with adult cells from seronegative donors (Dalens et al., 1975; Gerber et al., 1976), and there is some difference in the behaviour of cell lines from these two sources (Gerber etal., 1976). It has been speculated that the transformation event may be related either to amplification of the virus genome load to 10 to 15 equivalents or to the linear integration into the host-cell genome of some of these EBV DNA molecules (Thorley-Lawson & Strominger, 1976).

But whatever the cause of transformation, there is much to be said for the view (Henle, 1968) that the changes brought about *in vitro* by EBV when it confers the power of unlimited proliferation on virus-free lymphocytes, resemble those of malignant transformation by known oncogenic animal viruses (see Epstein & Achong, 1973), even though inoculation experiments to prove this cannot, of course, be performed in man.

As mentioned above, continuous lymphoblastoid lines can also be established from B lymphocytes which harbour the virus *in vivo*, and there is growing evidence to suggest that the mechanism involved is different for cells already malignantly transformed *in vivo* as in BL, compared to that found with latently infected B lymphocytes from normal seropositive individuals or from patients with IM (Epstein & Achong, 1977; Rickinson et al., 1977).

Experimental carcinogenicity: EBV has been found to cause fatal malignant lymphoma when inoculated into owl monkeys or cotton-top marmosets (Epstein et al., 1973a, b, 1975; Shope et al., 1973), and a dose-dependent response has been observed with the second of these species (Deinhardt et al., 1975). In this connection it should be noted that marmoset lymphocytes infected and transformed into continuous lines by EBV in culture (Miller et al., 1972) grow into malignant tumours when inoculated into autologous hosts (Shope et al., 1973); so that, at least with marmoset cells, EBV does bring about true malignant transformation *in vitro*.

Strain differences

With EBV playing such widely different roles as etiological agent in IM, as transforming agent for human lymphocytes *in vitro*, as suspected human tumour virus in two widely differing malignancies and as harmless commensal in the great majority of normal human beings, efforts have been made to ascertain whether these different activities are associated with different strains of the virus.

At the present time, only one strain of virus that fails to conform to the standard has been found, and this, P3HR-1, emerged during cloning experiments (Hinuma etal., 1967). Although the P3HR-1 strain of EBV clearly lacks transforming ability (Miller etal., 1974), this is best regarded as a consequence of laboratory manipulation, since the parent virus, Jijoye, from which the P3HR-1 strain derives was fully transforming (Henle et al., 1967).

Apart from the P3HR-1 strain, the biochemical and antigenic similarities of all other EBV isolates from whatever source, do not suggest major strain differences (Gerber et al., 1976; Kawai et al., 1973; Kieff & Levine, 1974; Menezes et al., 1975; Miller et al., 1976; Nonoyama & Pagano, 1973; Pagano et al., 1976). However, strain heterogeneity is a possibility, and may perhaps be revealed in the future as more refined techniques become available.

RELATIONSHIP OF EBV TO NASOPHARYNGEAL CARCINOMA

The validity of the search for viruses associated with African BL has stood the test of time; since its discovery, EBV has been shown to have a remarkably close relationship with this tumour, and a recent review has discussed this in full (Epstein, 1977). In addition, an almost equally close relationship has emerged with another human malignancy, namely nasopharyngeal carcinoma (NPC). This tumour consists of poorly differentiated squamous epithelial malignant cells with a moderate to heavy infiltration of non-malignant lymphocytes (Gazzolo et al., 1972; Shanmugaratnam, 1971; Svoboda et al., 1967). NPC occurs rarely throughout the world, but has long been known to have its highest incidence among the southern Chinese in whom it is the commonest tumour in men and the second commonest in women (Shanmugaratnam, 1971). Areas with lower incidences (which are still remarkably high by comparison with those in the rest of the world) have been recognized in Kenya (Clifford, 1970) and in North Africa (Cammoun et al., 1974).

Seroepidemiology

The first hint of an association between EBV and NPC was provided by the demonstration (with immunodiffusion tests) of antibodies to the virus in sera from a substantial proportion of individuals with NPC (Old et al., 1966). Extensive seroepidemiological studies using immunofluorescence techniques have confirmed and amplified this. It is now known (Henle, 1971; Henle et al., 1970) that 100% of patients with NPC have antibodies to EBV capsid antigen (VCA), usually at high titre, in contrast to patients with carcinomas of the hypo- or oropharynx or with tumours of the nasopharynx other than carcinoma, who are either EBV antibody-negative or positive at low titre.

The pattern in NPC of antibody responses to other EBV-determined antigens (see Epstein & Achong, 1977) shows specific characteristics and variations that accompany clinical events in the course of the disease. Thus, although antibodies to all the antigens are raised, those directed against early antigen of the diffuse type (EA-D) (Epstein & Achong, 1977) predominate in a very unusual way (Henle et al., 1971), and there is an almost invariable and curious production of IgA antibodies to EBV VCA (Henle & Henle, 1976). Progress of NPC from early to later stages is accompanied by increases in all antibody levels; and successful treatment is characterized by loss of anti-EA-D and a gradual decline in the level of antibodies to VCA (Henle et al., 1973).

EBV in tumour cells

As with BL, so in NPC EBV particles have not been observed in tumour cells in biopsy samples (Gazzolo et al., 1972); this absence of virions parallels the situation with known animal oncogenic DNA viruses in relation to the tumours they cause. However, EBV DNA has been shown by nucleic acid hybridization to be present as multiple copies in all the squamous epithelial tumour cells of NPC (Wolf et al., 1973) and determines in the cells the expression of EBNA (Huang et al., 1974; Klein et al., 1974), again paralleling the behaviour of oncogenic DNA viruses, with EBNA perhaps corresponding to the nuclear T neoantigens.

It has already been mentioned that only B lymphocytes have so far been shown to have receptors for EBV, and the mode of entry of the virus into epithelial cells of the nasopharynx is not understood. There is some indication that there might be virus receptors on the malignant tumour cells of NPC (Glaser et al., 1976), so that their presence on the normal epithelial cells from which the tumour originates would not be surprising.

Alternatively, entry of the virus might result from the formation of intercellular bridges between EBV genome-containing lymphocytes and adjacent epithelial cells (Gazzolo et al., 1972), or by fusion of such cells during upper respiratory tract infection with syncytium-inducing banal viruses. Close contact between these cell types is known to occur in the postnasal space where the epithelium lies on cushions of lymphoid tissue (Shanmugaratnam, 1971), and some of the lymphoid cells must surely be of the B type and harbouring the EBV genome as a latent infection. Certainly, latently infected B cells are present in the nonmalignant lymphoid infiltration of NPC tumours, since, if they are removed in NPC biopsy material and cultured, they give rise to EBV-carrying lymphoblastoid lines (de-Thé et al., 1970; Epstein et al., 1971). In this connection it should be noted that many T cells are also known to be present in the infiltrate (Klein, 1975; Yata et al., 1974), and that, however they come to be infected, the EBV genome-containing malignant epithelial cells are fully capable of supporting replication of the virus, since they produce particles if activated under certain experimental conditions (Trumper et al., 1976).

DISCUSSION

Several features of the association of EBV with NPC are sufficiently unusual to call for comment. The fact that the virus genome and a virus-determined antigen (EBNA) have been found in the epithelial cells of NPCs from every part of the world (Desgranges et al., 1975; Huang et al., 1974; Klein et al., 1974; Wolf et al., 1973) suggests at the least a somewhat special relationship, and if EBNA really corresponds to a nuclear T-antigen, the parallel with known animal oncogenic DNA viruses must be borne in mind. There is evidence that NPC is a monoclonal disease (Fialkow, 1976; Fialkow et al., 1972), and the presence of EBV DNA in every tumour cell indicates that the original cell that underwent malignant transformation must in each case have been infected from the outset; i.e., EBV does not at a later stage infect tumour cells which happen to provide a suitable, accessible environment. Another argument against the possibility that infection is a casual passenger event is the characteristic antibody pattern seen in NPC, which changes with its progression or successful treatment (Henle & Henle, 1976; Henle et al., 1971, 1973).

The long-recognized high incidence of NPC in southern Chinese and related races of South East Asia (Clifford, 1970; Shanmugaratnam, 1971), and the moderately high incidence in parts of East and North Africa (Clifford, 1970; Cammoun et al., 1974), have indicated a genetically determined predisposition to NPC, the existence of which has recently been put on a firm basis by studies which have shown a three times greater risk of NPC associated with particular HL-A profiles in southern Chinese (Simons et al., 1974, 1975, 1976). There would also seem to be racial differences amongst NPC patients in the pattern of antibody responses to EBV antigens (de Schryver et al., 1974) and in the age at onset of the tumour (Clifford, 1970), but whether or not these differences have a truly genetic basis is not yet clear.

That environmental factors are also involved in the etiology of NPC is beyond doubt. Southern Chinese immigrants living in Australia and the US have the same high incidence of NPC as do the Chinese in

China, whereas their local-born descendants have a lower incidence, though nevertheless much higher than that in the surrounding Caucasian population (Clifford, 1970; Henderson, 1974). Furthermore, a definite risk factor has been demonstrated for members of low-risk racial groups born and raised in high-incidence regions (Henderson et al., 1976). However, despite extensive search, no specific environmental cofactors have so far been identified (Clifford, 1970; Shanmugaratnam, 1971).

Thus, the exact mechanisms in the causation of NPC remain obscure. A susceptible genetic constitution clearly plays a part, and some as yet unknown environmental cofactors are likewise important. In addition, EBV is regularly present in the tumour cells, has a relationship to them analogous to that of known oncogenic animal DNA viruses to the cells of the tumours they cause and is a virus capable of bringing about seeming malignant transformation of human cells *in vitro* and experimental tumour induction in sub-human primates. It looks, therefore, as if EBV plays some etiological role in NPC; but whether this is so and how it influences the undoubtedly complex interactions underlying the disease will be only emerge as a result of future investigations.

REFERENCES

Aya, T. & Osato, T. (1974) Early events in transformation of human cord leucocytes by Epstein-Barr virus: induction of DNA synthesis, mitosis, and the virus-associated nuclear antigen synthesis. *Int. J. Cancer, 13*, 341-347

Becker, Y. & Weinberg, A. (1972) *Molecular events in the biosynthesis of Epstein-Barr virus in Burkitt lymphoblasts.* In: Biggs, P.M., de-Thé, G. & Payne, L.N. eds, *Oncogenesis and Herpesviruses (IARC Scientific Publications No. 2)*, Lyon, pp. 326-335

Burkitt, D. (1958) A sarcoma involving the jaws in African children. *Brit. J. Surg., 46*, 218-223

Burkitt, D. (1962a) A children's cancer dependent on climatic factors. *Nature (Lond.), 194*, 232-234

Burkitt, D. (1962b) Determining the climatic limitations of a children's cancer common in Africa. *Brit. med. J., ii*, 1019-1023

Burkitt, D. (1963) A lymphoma syndrome in tropical Africa. *Int. Rev. exp. Path., 2*, 67-138

Burkitt, D.P. (1969) Etiology of Burkitt's lymphoma - an alternative hypothesis to a vectored virus. *J. nat. Cancer Inst., 42*, 19-28

Cammoun, M., Hoerner, G.V. & Mourali, N. (1974) Tumors of the nasopharynx in Tunisia: an anatomic and clinical study based on 143 cases. *Cancer, 33*, 184-192

Clifford, P. (1970) A review: on the epidemiology of nasopharyngeal carcinoma. *Int. J. Cancer, 5*, 287-309

Dalens, M., Zech, L. & Klein, G. (1975) Origin of lymphoid lines established from mixed cultures of cord-blood lymphocytes and explants from infectious mononucleosis, Burkitt lymphoma and healthy donors. *Int. J. Cancer, 16*, 1008-1014

Deinhardt, F., Falk, L., Wolfe, L.G., Paciga, J. & Johnson, D. (1975) *Response of marmosets to experimental infection with Epstein-Barr virus.* In: de-Thé, G., Epstein, M.A. & zur Hausen, H., eds, *Oncogenesis and Herpesviruses II, Part 2 (IARC Scientific Publications No. 11)*, Lyon, pp. 161-168

Desgranges, C., Wolf, H., de-Thé, G., Shanmugaratnam, K., Cammoun, N., Ellouz, R., Klein, G., Lennert, K., Muñoz, N. & zur Hausen, H. (1975) Nasopharyngeal carcinoma. X. Presence of Epstein-Barr genomes in separated epithelial cells of tumours in patients from Singapore, Tunisia and Kenya. *Int. J. Cancer, 16*, 7-15

de Schryver, A., Klein, G., Henle, W. & Henle, G. (1974) EB virus-associated antibodies in Caucasian patients with carcinoma of the nasopharynx and in long-term survivors after treatment. *Int. J. Cancer, 13*, 319-325

de-Thé, G., Ho, H.C., Kwan, H.C., Desgranges, C. & Favre, M.C. (1970) Nasopharyngeal carcinoma. I. Types of cultures derived from tumour biopsies and non-tumourous tissues of Chinese patients with special reference to lymphoblastoid transformation. *Int. J. Cancer, 6*, 189-206

Dolyniuk, M., Pritchett, R. & Kieff, E. (1976) Proteins of Epstein-Barr virus. I. Analysis of polypeptides of purified enveloped Epstein-Barr virus. *J. Virol., 17*, 935-949

Epstein, M.A. (1970a) Aspects of the EB virus. *Advanc. Cancer Res., 13*, 383-411

Epstein, M.A. (1970b) *Long-term tissue culture of Burkitt lymphoma cells.* In: Burkitt, D.P. & Wright, D.H., eds, *Burkitt's Lymphoma*, Edinburgh & London, E. & S. Livingstone, pp. 148-157

Epstein, M.A. (1975) Recent studies with EB virus. *Yale J. Biol. Med., 48*, 431-437

Epstein, M.A. (1977) *An assessment of the possible role of viruses in the aetiology of Burkitt's lymphoma.* In: Ito, Y., ed, *Viruses and Human Cancer*, Basel, Karger (in press)

Epstein, M.A. & Achong, B.G. (1970) *The EB virus.* In: Burkitt, D. P. & Wright, D.H., eds, *Burkitt's Lymphoma*, Edinburgh & London, E. & S. Livingstone, pp. 231-248

Epstein, M.A. & Achong, B.G. (1973) The EB virus. *Ann. Rev. Microbiol.*, *27*, 413-436

Epstein, M.A. & Achong, B.G. (1977) Recent progress in EB virus research. *Ann. Rev. Microbiol.*, *31*, 421-445

Epstein, M.A., Barr, Y.M. & Achong, B.G. (1964a) Avian tumor virus behavior as a guide in the investigation of a human neoplasm. *Nat. Cancer Inst. Monogr.*, *17*, 637-650

Epstein, M.A., Achong, B.G. & Barr, Y.M. (1964b) Virus particles in cultured lymphoblasts from Burkitt's lymphoma. *Lancet*, *i*, 702-703

Epstein, M.A., Henle, G., Achong, B.G. & Barr, Y.M. (1965) Morphological and biological studies on a virus in cultured lymphoblasts from Burkitt's lymphoma. *J. exp. Med.*, *121*, 761-770

Epstein, M.A., Achong, B.G. & Mansell, P.W.A. (1971) *A new virus in cultures of human nasopharyngeal carcinoma.* In: Nakahara, W., Nishioka, K., Hirayama, T. & Ito, Y., eds, *Recent Advances in Human Tumor Virology and Immunology*, Tokyo, University of Tokyo Press, pp. 163-171

Epstein, M.A., Rabin, H., Ball, G., Rickinson, A.B., Jarvis, J. & Meléndez, L.V. (1973a) Pilot experiments with EB virus in owl monkeys (*Aotus trivirgatus*). II. EB virus in a cell line from an animal with reticuloproliferative disease. *Int. J. Cancer*, *12*, 319-332

Epstein, M.A., Hunt, R.D. & Rabin, H. (1973b) Pilot experiments with EB virus in owl monkeys (*Aotus trivirgatus*). I. Reticuloproliferative disease in an inoculated animal. *Int. J. Cancer*, *12*, 309-318

Epstein, M.A., zur Hausen, H., Ball, G. & Rabin, H. (1975) Pilot experiments with EB virus in owl monkeys (*Aotus trivirgatus*). III. Serological and biochemical findings in an animal with reticuloproliferative disease. *Int. J. Cancer*, *15*, 17-22

Fialkow, P.J. (1976) Clonal origin of human tumors. *Biochim. biophys. Acta*, *458*, 283-321

Fialkow, P.J., Martin, G.M., Klein, G., Clifford, P. & Singh, S. (1972) Evidence for a clonal origin of head and neck tumors. *Int. J. Cancer*, *9*, 133-142

Gazzolo, L., de-Thé, G., Vuillaume, M. & Ho, H.C. (1972) Nasopharyngeal carcinoma. II. Ultrastructure of normal mucosa, tumor biopsies, and subsequent epithelial growth *in vitro*. *J. nat. Cancer Inst.*, *48*, 73-86

Gerber, P. & Hoyer, B.H. (1971) Induction of cellular DNA synthesis in human leucocytes by Epstein-Barr virus. *Nature (Lond.)*, *231*, 46-47

Gerber, P., Nkrumah, F.K., Pritchett, R. & Kieff, E. (1976) Comparative studies of Epstein-Barr virus strains from Ghana and the United States. *Int. J. Cancer, 17*, 71-81

Glaser, R., de-Thé, G., Lenoir, G. & Ho, J.H.C. (1976) Superinfection of epithelial nasopharyngeal carcinoma cells with Epstein-Barr virus. *Proc. nat. Acad. Sci. (Wash.), 73*, 960-963

Haddow, A.J. (1964) Age incidence in Burkitt's lymphoma syndrome. *E. Afr. med. J., 41*, 1-6

Henderson, B.E. (1974) Nasopharyngeal carcinoma: present status of knowledge. *Cancer Res., 34*, 1187-1188

Henderson, B.E., Louie, E., Jing, J.S., Buell, P. & Gardner, M.B. (1976) Risk factors associated with nasopharyngeal carcinoma. *New Engl. J. Med., 295*, 1101-1106

Henle, G., Henle, W. & Klein, G. (1971) Demonstration of two distinct components in the early antigen complex of Epstein-Barr virus-infected cells. *Int. J. Cancer, 8*, 272-282

Henle, W. (1968) Evidence for viruses in acute leukemia and Burkitt's tumor. *Cancer, 21*, 580-586

Henle, W. (1971) *Evidence for a relation of the Epstein-Barr virus to Burkitt's lymphoma and nasopharyngeal carcinoma.* In: Nakahara, W., Nishioka, K., Hirayama, T. & Ito, Y., eds, *Recent Advances in Human Tumor Virology and Immunology*, Tokyo, University of Tokyo Press, pp. 361-367

Henle, W. & Henle, G. (1976) Epstein-Barr virus-specific IgA serum antibodies as an outstanding feature of nasopharyngeal carcinoma. *Int. J. Cancer, 17*, 1-7

Henle, W., Diehl, V., Kohn, G., zur Hausen, H. & Henle, G. (1967) Herpes-type virus and chromosome marker in normal leukocytes after growth with irradiated Burkitt cells. *Science, 157*, 1064-1065

Henle, W., Henle, G., Ho, H.C., Burtin, P., Cachin, Y., Clifford, P., de Schryver, A., de-Thé, G., Diehl, V. & Klein, G. (1970) Antibodies to Epstein-Barr virus in nasopharyngeal carcinoma, other head and neck neoplasms, and control groups. *J. nat. Cancer Inst., 44*, 225-231

Henle, W., Ho, H.C., Henle, G. & Kwan, H.C. (1973) Antibodies to Epstein-Barr virus-related antigens in nasopharyngeal carcinoma. Comparison of active cases and long-term survivors. *J. nat. Cancer Inst., 51*, 361-369

Hinuma, Y., Konn, M., Yamaguchi, J., Wudarski, D.J., Blakeslee, J.R. & Grace, J.T. (1967) Immunofluorescence and herpes-type virus particles in the P3HR-1 Burkitt lymphoma cell line. *J. Virol., 1*, 1045-1051

Huang, D.P., Ho, J.H., Henle, W. & Henle, G. (1974) Demonstration of Epstein-Barr virus-associated nuclear antigen in nasopharyngeal carcinoma cells from fresh biopsies. *Int. J. Cancer*, *14*, 580-588

Kawai, Y., Nonoyama, H. & Pagano, J.S. (1973) Reassociation kinetics for Epstein-Barr virus DNA; nonhomology to mammalian DNA and homology of viral DNA in various diseases. *J. Virol.*, *12*, 1006-1012

Kieff, E. & Levine, J. (1974) Homology between Burkitt herpes viral DNA and DNA in continuous lymphoblastoid cells from patients with infectious mononucleosis. *Proc. nat. Acad. Sci. (Wash.)*, *71*, 355-358

Klein, G. (1975) *A summing-up*. In: de-Thé, G., Epstein, M.A. & zur Hausen, H., eds, *Oncogenesis and Herpesviruses II*, *Part 2* *(IARC Scientific Publications No. 11)*, Lyon, pp. 365-397

Klein, G., Giovanella, B.C., Lindahl, T., Fialkow, P.J., Singh, S. & Stehlin, J.S. (1974) Direct evidence for the presence of Epstein-Barr virus DNA and nuclear antigen in malignant epithelial cells from patients with poorly differentiated carcinoma of the nasopharynx. *Proc. nat. Acad. Sci. (Wash.)*, *71*, 4737-4741

Menezes, J., Leibold, W. & Klein, G. (1975) Biological differences between Epstein-Barr virus (EBV) strains with regard to lymphocyte transforming ability, superinfection and antigen induction. *Exp. Cell Res.*, *92*, 478-484

Menezes, J., Patel, P., Dussault, H. & Bourkas, A.E. (1977) Comparative studies on the induction of virus-associated nuclear antigen and early antigen by lymphocyte-transforming (B95-8) and non-transforming (P3HR-1) strains of Epstein-Barr virus, *Intervirology* (in press)

Miller, G., Shope, T., Lisco, H., Stitt, D. & Lipman, M. (1972) Epstein-Barr virus: transformation, cytopathic changes, and viral antigens in squirrel monkey and marmoset leukocytes. *Proc. nat. Acad. Sci. (Wash.)*, *69*, 383-387

Miller, G., Robinson, J., Heston, L. & Lipman, M. (1974) Differences between laboratory strains of Epstein-Barr virus based on immortalization, abortive infection, and interference. *Proc. nat. Acad. Sci. (Wash.)*, *71*, 4006-4010

Miller, G., Coope, D., Niederman, J. & Pagano, J. (1976) Biological properties and viral surface antigens of Burkitt lymphoma- and mononucleosis-derived strains of Epstein-Barr virus released from transformed marmoset cells. *J. Virol.*, *18*, 1071-1080

Nonoyama, M. & Pagano, J.S. (1973) Homology between Epstein-Barr virus DNA and viral DNA from Burkitt's lymphoma and nasopharyngeal carcinoma determined by DNA-DNA reassociation kinetics. *Nature (Lond.)*, *242*, 44-47

Old, L.J., Boyse, E.A., Oettgen, H.F., de Harven, E., Geering, G., Williamson, B. & Clifford, P. (1966) Precipitating antibody in human serum to an antigen present in cultured Burkitt's lymphoma cells. *Proc. nat. Acad. Sci. (Wash.)*, *56*, 1699-1704

Pagano, J.S., Huang, C-H. & Huang, Y-T. (1976) Epstein-Barr virus genome in infectious mononucleosis. *Nature (Lond.)*, *263*, 787-789

Pritchett, R.F., Hayward, S.D. & Kieff, E.D. (1975) DNA of Epstein-Barr virus. I. Comparative studies of the DNA of EBV from HR-1 and B95-8 cells. Size, structure and relatedness. *J. Virol.*, *15*, 556-584

Pritchett, R., Pedersen, M. & Kieff, E. (1976) Complexity of EBV homologous DNA in continuous lymphoblastoid cell lines. *Virology*, *74*, 227-231

Rickinson, A.B., Finerty, S. & Epstein, M.A. (1977) Comparative studies on adult donor lymphocytes infected by EB virus *in vivo* or *in vitro*: origin of transformed cells arising in co-cultures with foetal lymphocytes. *Int. J. Cancer*, *19*, 775-782

Shanmugaratnam, K. (1971) Studies on the etiology of nasopharyngeal carcinoma. *Int. Rev. exp. Path.*, *10*, 361-413

Shope, T., Dechairo, D. & Miller, G. (1973) Malignant lymphoma in cottontop marmosets after inoculation with Epstein-Barr virus. *Proc. nat. Acad. Sci. (Wash.)*, *70*, 2487-2491

Simons, M.J., Wee, G.B., Day, N.E., Morris, P.J., Shanmugaratnam, K. & de-Thé, G.B. (1974) Immunogenetic aspects of nasopharyngeal carcinoma. I. Differences in HL-A antigen profiles between patients and control groups. *Int. J. Cancer*, *13*, 122-134

Simons, M.J., Wee, G.B., Chan, S.H., Shanmugaratnam, K., Day, N.E. & de-Thé, G. (1975) *Immunogenetic aspects of nasopharyngeal carcinoma (NPC). III. HL-A type as a genetic marker of NPC predisposition to test the hypothesis that Epstein-Barr virus is an etiological factor in NPC.* In: de-Thé, G., Epstein, M.A. & zur Hausen, H., eds, *Oncogenesis and Herpesviruses II, Part 2 (IARC Scientific Publications No. 11)*, Lyon, pp. 249-258

Simons, M.J., Wee, G.B., Goh, E.H., Chan, S.H., Shanmugaratnam, K., Day, N.E. & de-Thé, G. (1976) Immunogenetic aspects of nasopharyngeal carcinoma. IV. Increased risk in Chinese of nasopharyngeal carcinoma associated with a Chinese-related HLA profile (A2, Singapore 2). *J. nat. Cancer Inst.*, *57*, 977-980

Svoboda, D.J., Kirchner, F.R. & Shanmugaratnam, K. (1967) *The fine structure of nasopharyngeal carcinomas.* In: Muir, C.S. & Shanmugaratnam, K. eds, *Cancer of the Nasopharynx (UICC Monograph Series No. 1)*, Copenhagen, Munksgaard, pp. 163-171

Thorley-Lawson, D. & Strominger, J.L. (1976) Transformation of human Lymphocytes by Epstein-Barr virus is inhibited by phosphonoacetic acid. *Nature (Lond.)*, *263*, 332-334

Trumper, P.A., Epstein, M.A. & Giovanella, B.C. (1976) Activation *in vitro* by BUdR of a productive EB virus infection in the epithelial cells of nasopharyngeal carcinoma. *Int. J. Cancer, 17*, 578-587

Wolf, H., zur Hausen, H. & Becker, V. (1973) EB viral genomes in epithelial nasopharyngeal carcinoma cells. *Nature (New Biol.), 244*, 245-247

Wright, J., Falk, L. & Deinhardt, F. (1975) *Appearance of Epstein-Barr virus nuclear antigen in human cordblood lymphocytes.* In: de-Thé, G., Epstein, M.A. & zur Hausen, H., eds, *Oncogenesis and Herpesviruses II, Part 1, (IARC Scientific Publications No. 11)*, Lyon, pp. 409-414

Yata, J., Desgranges, C., de-Thé, G., Mourali, N., Ellouz, R., Tachibana, T. & Brugère, J. (1974) Nasopharyngeal carcinoma. VII. B and T lymphocytes in the circulating blood and in tumour tissue. *Biomedicine, 21*, 244-250

THE ASSOCIATION BETWEEN UNDIFFERENTIATED NASOPHARYNGEAL CARCINOMA AND EPSTEIN-BARR VIRUS SHOWN BY CORRELATED NUCLEIC ACID HYBRIDIZATION AND HISTOPATHOLOGICAL STUDIES

M. ANDERSSON-ANVRET & G. KLEIN

Department of Tumor Biology,
Karolinska Institutet,
S104 01 Stockholm 60, Sweden

N. FORSBY

Department of Pathology,
Helsingborg Hospital,
Helsingborg, Sweden

W. HENLE

Children's Hospital of Philadelphia,
34th Street & Civic Center Blvd,
Philadelphia, Pa. 19104, USA

INTRODUCTION

The surface of the nasopharynx is lined with various types of epithelium (Ali, 1967). The histogenetic origin of nasopharyngeal carcinoma (NPC) is unclear, and several histopathological classifications have been proposed. Electron microscopic findings have lent support to the view that all types of NPC may be regarded as variants of squamous-cell carcinoma.

NPCs may be classified as squamous-cell carcinomas with various degrees of differentiation and as 'undifferentiated' carcinomas (Anvret-Andersson et al., 1977). Undifferentiated carcinomas occur most frequently.

A serological association between NPC and the Epstein-Barr virus (EBV) was discovered when Old and coworkers showed that NPC patients in the US had elevated antibody titres against an EBV-associated soluble antigen (Oettgen et al., 1967; Old et al., 1966). Later, it was shown that most NPC patients have highly elevated antibody titres against EBV-determined viral capsid (VCA) and membrane (MA) antigens (Henle et al., 1970; Lin et al., 1972; de Schryver et al., 1969). There was also an abnormally high frequency of antibodies against the EBV-determined early antigen (EA) complex, particularly the diffuse (D) component (Henle et al., 1971, 1973). A clear relationship was observed between the elevation of antibody titres against EBV-associated antigens and total tumour burden (Henle et al., 1970, 1973).

Patients with differentiated carcinomas of the nasopharynx showed no significant rise in anti-VCA, MA or EA titres, compared with controls (Henle et al., 1970; de Schryver et al., 1969). The same was true for carcinoma patients with head and neck tumours outside the postnasal space.

EBV DNA was detected in NPCs by nucleic acid hybridization (zur Hausen et al., 1970; Nonoyama et al., 1973). The viral genomes and the EBV-associated nuclear antigen, EBNA, were localized in the epithelial cells and not in the infiltrating lymphocytes as originally thought (Klein et al., 1974; Wolf et al., 1973, 1975).

Earlier reports dealing with the detection of EBV genomes in NPC biopsies indicated that while a substantial proportion of NPCs contained EBV DNA, a minority did not. No attempt was made, however, to type the EBV-DNA-positive and negative carcinomas histologically or to ensure that only biopsy material containing viable tumour tissue was used in the nucleic acid hybridization experiments.

The purpose of our study was to perform a parallel histological and nucleic acid hybridization test on each tumour. The biopsies were classified as (i) undifferentiated NPC; (ii) NPC with squamous differentiation; (iii) other types of nasopharyngeal tumours; and (iv) carcinomas of the head and neck regions outside the nasopharynx. In addition, the serum of each patient was tested for antibodies against VCA, EA(D) and EBNA. Representative biopsies were examined for the presence of EBNA-positive cells in smear preparations.

MATERIALS AND METHODS

Tumours

Biopsies were obtained in Nairobi from primary tumours of the nasopharynx or other regions of the head and neck. The biopsies were immersed in tissue culture medium and shipped to Stockholm in wet ice by a direct flight, reaching the laboratory within 24 hours. Upon arrival, the material was divided into two aliquots, one for nucleic acid hybridization and one for histopathological examination. Material from some biopsies was sent to Philadelphia, USA, for testing for EBNA, arriving there within 4-5 days' total transit time. Frozen sera were shipped to Philadelphia for EBV antibody tests.

Nucleic acid hybridization

EBV DNA was prepared by methods described elsewhere (Adams, 1975) and transcribed into ^{32}P-labelled EBV complementary RNA (cRNA), using *Escherichia coli* RNA polymerase and α-^{32}P-labelled cytosine triphosphate, as described previously (Lindahl et al., 1976).

Cellular DNA was prepared from the biopsies by standard procedures (Pettersson & Sambrook, 1973), and DNA-cRNA hybridization was performed as described by Lindahl et al. (1976). Briefly, 10 μg aliquots of cellular DNA were denatured and fixed to 13 mm nitrocellulose filters, according to the method of Gillespie & Spiegelman (1965). The filters, containing DNA, were incubated for 96 h at 45°C in 0.3 ml 0.9 M sodium chloride - 0.09 M sodium citrate, pH 7.5, containing 50% formamide, and supplemented with 1 ng ^{32}P-labelled EBV cRNA (1.5×10^8 cpm/μg). The filters were washed at 60°C, treated with RNAse and analysed for radioactivity. The DNA content of each filter was determined colorimetrically by the diphenylamine reaction. The data were used to correct the hybridization values to a DNA content of 10 μg/filter.

The average number of EBV genome equivalents per biopsy cell was calculated by comparison with a standard curve, obtained from filters that contained 10 μg cellular DNA from an EBV-DNA-negative human B-cell lymphoma line, U-698 M (Andersson & Lindahl, 1976) and small, known amounts (0.25-30 ng) of EBV DNA. The molecular weight of EBV DNA was taken to be 1×10^8 and that of human cellular DNA as 4×10^{12}. EBV-DNA-positive (Raji) and -negative (calf thymus or U-698 M) controls were included in each hybridization experiment. All determinations were performed at least in duplicate.

EBNA staining of biopsies

Fresh biopsy sections were cut into small fragments, and touch preparations were made from freshly cut surfaces on 6 x 30 mm coverslips, as described by Huang et al. (1974). The preparations were dried rapidly in front of a fan and then fixed in a precooled (-20°C) mixture of equal proportions of acetone and methanol for 3-5 min. The fixed smears were stained by the anti-complement immunofluorescence (ACIF) technique for EBNA-positive cells (Reedman & Klein, 1973). According to ACIF tests on EBNA-negative cells, the anti-EBNA-positive sera were free of antinuclear antibodies. Anti-EBNA-negative sera served as controls.

Antibody tests

All sera were titrated for antibodies against EBV-determined VCA, diffuse (D) and restricted (R) components of the EA complex and EBNA, using methods described previously (Henle & Henle, 1966; Henle et al., 1971; Reedman & Klein, 1973).

Histology

The part of the biopsy allocated for histological examination was fixed in buffered, neutral 10% formalin and embedded in paraffin. Sections were stained routinely with hematoxylin-eosin. If the diagnosis was doubtful, additional sections were stained for keratin, mucin, collagen or reticulin.

RESULTS

Most tumour biopsies studied were obtained from the postnasal space; the majority were classified as undifferentiated NPC. A few showed a certain degree of squamous differentiation, and some turned out to be other tumour types. Occasionally, metastatic biopsies were also studied. A few biopsies from head and neck tumours outside the nasopharynx were included in the study.

All biopsies were examined histologically. Tumours with extensive autolytic or necrotic changes were excluded. Biopsies that contained neither histologically recognizable tumour tissue nor detectable EBV DNA were also excluded.

Undifferentiated carcinomas of the nasopharynx

This group included all NPCs with no signs of squamous differentiation. Lymphoepitheliomas of the Schmincke and Regaud types (Capell, 1938; Ewing, 1929; Regaud, 1921; Schmincke, 1921) and transitional-cell carcinomas (Capell, 1938; Quick & Cutler, 1927) were entered into this category, together with a few carcinomas having spindle-cell, clear-cell, basaloid or pleomorphic appearances (Shanmugaratnam, 1972; Yeh, 1962). Occasionally, different areas of the same tumour showed cellular arrangements corresponding to different histological subtypes.

Table 1 is a summary of the data. The frequency of EBV-DNA-positive tumours is shown, with the mean numbers of EBV genome equivalents per cell and the geometric means of EBV antibody titres against VCA, EA (D) and EBNA. A more detailed tabulation of these results, listing individual patients, will be published elsewhere (Anvret-Andersson[1]).

All 51 biopsies derived from undifferentiated carcinomas of the nasopharynx were EBV-DNA-positive, with a mean EBV genome equivalent of 31.5 ± 3.3 viral genomes per cell. The range of EBV genome number copies among the different biopsies was very wide, between 2 and 137 viral genome equivalents per cell. This was conceivably due, at least in part, to the different proportions of viable tumour cells carrying EBV DNA, in comparison with non-viable tumour cells and with non-tumour cells without EBV DNA. The histopathological findings indicate a wide variation in the relative content of viable tumour tissue, but no attempt was made to quantitate this.

[1] Unpublished data

Table 1. Summary of EBV DNA and serological tests in the different histological categories examined

Histological diagnosis	No. of tumours examined	EBV-DNA-positive		Geometric mean EBV antibody titres against			
		No.	Mean no. of EBV genome equivalents per cell	VCA		EA (D)	EBNA
Undifferentiated carcinomas of the nasopharynx	51	51	31.5 ± 3.3		759 ± 88	141 ± 23	70 ± 9
Nasopharyngeal carcinomas with squamous-cell differentiation	4	2	(10, 2)	EBV-DNA-pos.	640	2/4 pos. (30)	20
				EBV-DNA-neg.	80	2/4 neg.	50
Other types of nasopharyngeal tumours[a]	7	1[b]	(30)	EBV-DNA-pos.	80	neg.	80
				EBV-DNA-neg.	71 ± 38	4/6 neg. 2/6 pos. (10, 40)	25 ± 6
Head and neck carcinomas outside the nasopharynx[c]	14	0	-		98 ± 25	12/14 neg. 2/14 pos. (10, 40)	19 ± 5

[a] Including cases of Burkitt's lymphoma, Hodgkin's disease, histiocytic lymphoma, lymphocytic lymphoma, mixed-cell type lymphoma and plasmocytoma

[b] Burkitt's lymphoma

[c] Carcinomas of the nose, maxilla, mandible, cheek, lip, tongue, palate, tonsil and parotis

Table 2 gives the results of an attempt to relate the mean number of EBV genome equivalents per cell in the undifferentiated NPCs to the anti-EBV serological picture. Twenty-two patients had VCA titres ranging between 1280 and 5120; their mean EBV genome equivalent number was 29 (range, 5-70 virus genomes per cell). Twenty-three patients had VCA titres between 320 and 640; their average EBV DNA copy number was 33, ranging between 2 and 137 EBV genome equivalents per cell. The remaining patients, who had lower VCA titres, are listed individually; their tumours contained relatively high numbers of EBV genome copies per cell. Thus, there is no correlation between the number of EBV genome equivalents and EBV antibody titres at the level of the individual patient; however, the EBV antibody titres of the undifferentiated carcinoma group were clearly much higher than those in the EBV-genome-negative tumour groups described below.

Nasopharyngeal carcinomas with squamous differentiation

This group included four NPCs with some signs of squamous differentiation, as indicated by the presence of polyhedral cells with distinct cell boundaries, 'intercellular bridges', pearls or keratinization. All four tumours in this category were poorly differentiated with only small foci of differentiation. One of the four contained 10, and another 2 EBV genome copies per cell, whereas the remaining two were EBV-DNA-negative.

Other types of nasopharyngeal tumours

Seven tumour biopsies, representing different types of malignant lymphomas, were included in this group. One biopsy contained 30 EBV genome equivalents per cell; histologically, it was shown to be a Burkitt's lymphoma. The remaining six were negative for EBV DNA.

Table 2. Summary of tests on undifferentiated nasopharyngeal carcinomas

No. of patients examined, or individual patient designation	Serum titres		No. of EBV genome equivalents per cell	
	VCA	EA (D)	No.	Mean
22	1280-5120	20-1280	5-70	29
23	320- 640	20- 320	2-137	33
M.M. 138339 PNS[a]	160	20	78	
cln[b]			62	
R.K. 17823 PNS	160	40	48	
K.M. 145010 PNS	160	20	26	
cln			76	
K.K. 167188 PNS	160	20	25	
cln			18	
K.K. 162628 PNS	160	10	3	
cln			25	
A.E. 121011 cln	80	20	19	

[a] Carcinoma of the postnasal space

[b] Cervical lymph node

The serological findings paralleled the positivity and negativity of the biopsies with respect to the presence of EBV genomes.

Head and neck carcinomas outside the nasopharynx

The 14 tumours included in this category were located in the regions indicated in footnote *c* of Table 1. They were all negative for EBV DNA, and two of the patients had antibodies against the EA (D) component. Eleven of the tumours were squamous-cell carcinomas, with various degrees of differentiation, ranging from high to poor. The remaining three comprised one adenocarcinoma and two adenoid cystic carcinomas.

EBNA tests on biopsy cells

These were performed on 15 tumours, including undifferentiated and differentiated NPCs and some non-nasopharyngeal head and neck carcinomas (Table 3). EBNA-positive cells were detected in 12 out of 18 EBV-DNA-positive biopsies; no EBNA-positive cells were found in six biopsies that had detectable EBV DNA or in three that had no EBV DNA. All six EBNA-negative but EBV-DNA-positive biopsies gave unsatisfactory touch preparations.

Table 3. Comparative EBV DNA and EBNA tests on biopsy specimens

Patient designation	Antibodies to			Tumour biopsy		Lymph node biopsy	
	VCA	EA (D)	EBNA	No. of EBV genomes per cell	EBNA	No. of EBV genomes per cell	EBNA
M.M. 138339	160	20	160	78	+		
M.K. 136453	1280	320	160	70	+		
K.S. 145037	5120	1280	40	61	+		
W.K. 78638	1280	160+	320	52	-		
K.M. 163859	1280	160	80	30	+		
K.M. 127225	1280	160	160	30	+	10	-
K.K. 167188	160	20	160	25	+	18	-
K.M. 153644	2560	320	40	25	+	28	-
G.I. 100999	1280	40	160	24	+		
B.O. 145838	640	160	40	15	-	11	+
J.N. 100070	640	40-80	20	10	+		
M.H. 135634	640	80-160	40	10	+	<1	-
N.A. 132943	320	320	160	7	-	11	+
K.E. 130849	80	<10	20	<1	-		
S.N. 163858	40	<10	40	<1	-		

DISCUSSION

The findings reported show unequivocally that all 51 undifferentiated NPCs tested were EBV-DNA-positive and showed correspondingly elevated anti-EBV antibody titres. The absence of undifferentiated NPCs that were EBV-DNA-negative was remarkable in view of the documented existence of rare EBV-negative Burkitt's lymphomas. It also suggests that the alleged EBV-negativity of a substantial fraction of previously reported

NPCs (e.g., Nonoyama et al., 1973) was spurious and must be attributed to a lack of parallel histological examination.

The present findings further emphasize the association between EBV and undifferentiated NPC. The consistent presence of the viral genome in a well-defined histological category and its equally consistent absence from other tumours is strongly suggestive of an etiological relationship, related to preneoplastic or neoplastic change.

SUMMARY

All of 51 undifferentiated carcinomas of the nasopharynx were EBV-DNA-positive and, in the few tests performed, EBNA-positive as well. Most of these patients also had high anti-EBV [VCA and EA (D)] antibody titres. Of four patients that had somewhat differentiated NPCs, two were EBV-DNA-positive with a corresponding serological picture, whereas two were negative with an EBV serology comparable to that of healthy donors. Of seven lymphomas localized in the nasopharynx, one was EBV-DNA-positive and corresponded histologically to Burkitt's lymphoma, whereas six others were EBV-DNA-negative. Fourteen head and neck carcinomas outside the nasopharynx were all EBV-DNA-negative. These results confirm the consistent and unique association of EBV DNA with undifferentiated carcinomas of the nasopharynx.

ACKNOWLEDGEMENTS

This work was supported by Contract No. N01 CP 33316 within the Virus Cancer Program of the National Cancer Institute, USA, by the Swedish Cancer Society and by the King Gustaf V Jubilee Fund.

REFERENCES

Adams, A. (1975) *Preparation of Epstein-Barr virus from P3HR-1 cells and isolation of the virus DNA.* In: Ablashi, D.V., Aaslestad, H.G. & de-Thé, G., eds, *Epstein-Barr Virus, Production, Concentration, and Purification,* Lyon, International Agency for Research on Cancer, pp. 129-146

Ali, M.Y. (1967) *Distribution and character of the squamous epithelium in the human nasopharynx.* In: Muir, C. & Shanmugaratnam, K., eds, *Cancer of the Nasopharynx*, Copenhagen, Munksgaard (*UICC Monograph Series* No. 1), pp. 138-146

Andersson, M. & Lindahl, T. (1976) Epstein-Barr virus DNA in human lymphoid cell lines: *in vitro* conversion. *Virology, 73*, 96-105

Anvret-Andersson, M., Forsby, N. & Klein, G. (1977) *Reassessment of the role of viruses associated with human neoplasia: nasopharyngeal carcinoma.* In: Ito, Y., ed., *Viruses and Human Cancers*, Basel, Karger (in press)

Capell, D.F. (1938) Pathology of nasopharyngeal tumours. *J. Laryngol. Otol., 53*, 558-580

de Schryver, A., Friberg, S., Jr., Klein, G., Henle, G., Henle, W., de-Thé, G., Clifford, P. & Ho, H.C. (1969) Epstein-Barr virus-associated antibody patterns in carcinoma of the postnasal space. *Clin. exp. Immunol., 5*, 443-459

Ewing, J. (1929) Lymphoepithelioma. *Amer. J. Pathol., 5*, 99-107

Gillespie, D. & Spiegelman, S. (1965) A quantitative assay for DNA-RNA hybrids with DNA immobilized on a membrane. *J. molec. Biol., 12*, 829-842

Henle, G. & Henle, W. (1966) Immunofluorescence in cells derived from Burkitt's lymphoma. *J. Bacteriol., 91*, 1248-1256

Henle, G., Henle, W. & Klein, G. (1971) Demonstration of two distinct components in the early antigen complex of Epstein-Barr virus-infected cells. *Int. J. Cancer, 8*, 272-282

Henle, W., Henle, G., Ho, H.C., Burtin, P., Cachin, Y., Clifford, P., de Schryver, A., de-Thé, G., Diehl, V. & Klein, G. (1970) Antibodies to Epstein-Barr virus in nasopharyngeal carcinoma, other head and neck neoplasms, and control groups. *J. nat. Cancer Inst., 44*, 225-231

Henle, W., Ho, H.C. & Kwan, H.C. (1973) Antibodies to Epstein-Barr virus-related antigens in nasopharyngeal carcinoma. Comparison of active cases with long-term survivors. *J. nat. Cancer Inst., 51*, 361-369

Huang, D.P., Ho, J.H.C., Henle, W. & Henle, G. (1974) Demonstration of Epstein-Barr virus-associated nuclear antigen in nasopharyngeal carcinoma cells from fresh biopsies. *Int. J. Cancer*, *14*, 580-588

Klein, G., Giovanella, B.C., Lindahl, T., Fialkow, P.J., Singh, S. & Stehlin, J. (1974) Direct evidence for the presence of Epstein-Barr virus DNA and nuclear antigen in malignant epithelial cells from patients with anaplastic carcinoma of the nasopharynx. *Proc. nat. Acad. Sci. (Wash.)*, *71*, 4737-4741

Lin, T.M., Yang, C.S., Ho, S.W., Chiou, J.F., Liu, C.H., Tu, S.M., Chen, K.P., Ito, Y.H., Kawamura, A. & Hirayama, T. (1972) Antibodies to herpes-type virus in nasopharyngeal carcinoma and control groups. *Cancer*, *29*, 603-609

Lindahl, T., Adams, A., Bjursell, G., Bornkamm, G.W., Kaschka-Dierich, C. & Jehn, U. (1976) Covalently closed circular duplex DNA of Epstein-Barr virus in a human lymphoid cell line. *J. molec. Biol.*, *102*, 511-530

Nonoyama, M., Huang, C.H., Pagano, J.S., Klein, G. & Singh, S. (1973) DNA of Epstein-Barr virus detected in tissue of Burkitt's lymphoma and nasopharyngeal carcinoma. *Proc. nat. Acad. Sci. (Wash.)*, *70*, 3265-3268

Oettgen, H.F., Aoki, T., Geering, G., Boyse, E.A. & Old, L.J. (1967) Definition of an antigenic system associated with Burkitt's lymphoma. *Cancer Res.*, *27*, 2532-2534

Old, L.J., Boyse, E.A., Oettgen, H.F., de Hawen, E., Geering, G., Williamson, B. & Clifford, P. (1966) Precipitating antibody in human serum to an antigen present in cultured Burkitt's lymphoma cells. *Proc. nat. Acad. Sci. (Wash.)*, *56*, 1699-1704

Pettersen, U. & Sambrook, J. (1973) Amount of viral DNA in the genome of cells transformed by adenovirus type 2. *J. molec. Biol.*, *73*, 125-130

Quick, D. & Cutler, M. (1927) Transitional cell epidermoid carcinoma; radiosensitive type of intra-oral tumor. *Surg. Gynecol. Obstet.*, *45*, 320-331

Reedman, B.M. & Klein, G. (1973) Cellular localization of an Epstein-Barr virus (EBV)-associated complement-fixing antigen in producer and non-producer lymphoblastoid cell lines. *Int. J. Cancer*, *11*, 499-520

Regaud, C. (1921) Discussion dans Reverchon, L. et Coutard, H. Lymphoepitheliome de l'hypopharynx traité par la roentgenthérapie. *Bull. Soc. franç. Otorhinolaryngol.*, *34*, 209-214

Schmincke, A. (1921) Über lymphoepitheliale Geschwülste. *Beitr. Path. Anat.*, *68*, 161-170

Shanmugaratnam, K. (1972) *The pathology of nasopharyngeal carcinoma. A review.* In: Biggs, P.M., de-Thé, G. & Payne, L.N., eds, *Oncogenesis and Herpesviruses*, Lyon (*IARC Scientific Publications No. 2*), pp. 239-248

Wolf, H., zur Hausen, H. & Becker, V. (1973) EB-viral genomes in epithelial nasopharyngeal carcinoma cells. *Nature-New Biol.*, *244*, 245-247

Wolf, H., zur Hausen, H., Klein, G., Becker, V., Henle, G. & Henle, W. (1975) Attempts to detect virus-specific DNA sequences in human tumours. III. Epstein-Barr viral DNA in non-lymphoid nasopharyngeal carcinoma cells. *Med. Microbiol. Immunol.*, *161*, 15-21

Yeh, S. (1962) A histological classification of carcinomas of the nasopharynx with a critical review as to the existence of lympho-epitheliomas. *Cancer*, *15*, 895-920

zur Hausen, H., Schulte-Holthausen, H., Klein, G., Henle, W., Henle, G., Clifford, P. & Santesson, L. (1970) EBV DNA in biopsies of Burkitt tumours and anaplastic carcinomas of the nasopharynx. *Nature (Lond.)*, *228*, 1056-1058

MORPHOLOGICAL TRANSFORMATION OF NASOPHARYNGEAL EPITHELIAL CELLS *IN VITRO* BY EPSTEIN-BARR VIRUS FROM B95-8 CELLS

D.P. HUANG & J.H.C. HO

Medical and Health Department Institute of Radiology and Oncology, Queen Elizabeth Hospital, Kowloon, Hong Kong

M.H. NG

Department of Microbiology, Pathology Building, University of Hong Kong, Queen Mary Hospital Compound, Hong Kong

INTRODUCTION

An association between nasopharyngeal carcinoma (NPC) and Epstein-Barr virus (EBV) was first suggested by the results of seroepidemiological studies (de Schryver et al., 1969; de-Thé et al., 1973; Henle & Henle, 1976; Henle et al., 1968, 1970a, b, 1971, 1973, 1976; Old et al., 1966, 1968; Reedman & Klein, 1973). It was confirmed subsequently by the demonstration of the persistence of EBV DNA and/or virus-determined nuclear antigens (EBNA) in NPC tumour cells (Desgranges et al., 1975; Huang et al., 1974; Klein et al., 1974; Nonoyama & Pagano, 1973; Nonoyama et al., 1973; Wolf et al., 1973, 1975; zur Hausen et al., 1970). Glaser et al. (1976) showed that the resident EBV genome in NPC cells could be activated by treatment with 5-iododeoxyuridine (IUDR) to synthesize EBV early antigens. Almost simultaneously, Trumper et al. (1976) treated NPC cells *in vitro* with 5-bromodeoxyuridine (BUDR) and observed a limited synthesis of what is believed to be EBV particles.

These findings appear largely to have satisfied the first two of Koch's three postulates, which are adopted conventionally to establish a causal relationship between an infectious agent and a given disease. The strict application of the third postulate is impossible in the case

FIG. 1. INFECTED NON-NEOPLASTIC NASOPHARYNX SPECIMEN

Infected non-neoplastic nasopharynx specimen outgrowth two weeks after culture, showing foci of cell piling and a disorientated cell distribution pattern. Giemsa x 80

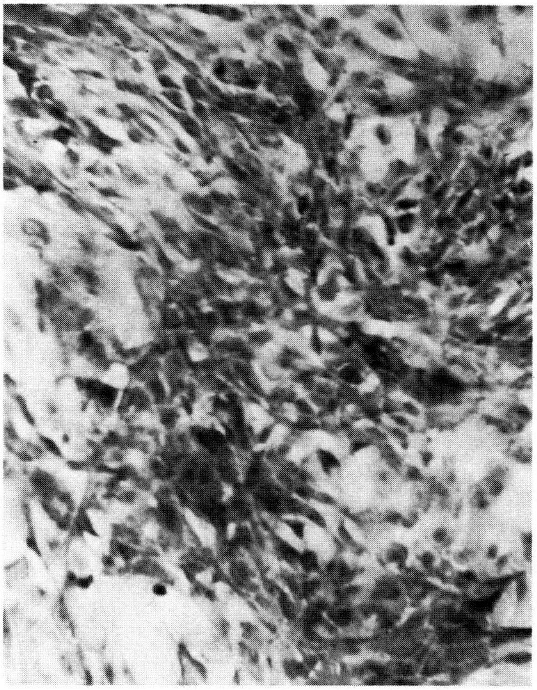

FIG. 2. UNINFECTED NON-NEOPLASTIC NASOPHARYNX SPECIMEN

Uninfected non-neoplastic nasopharynx specimen outgrowth two weeks after culture. The cells have a low nucleus:cytoplasm ratio and fine chromatin material in nuclei; mitosis is rare. Giemsa x 230

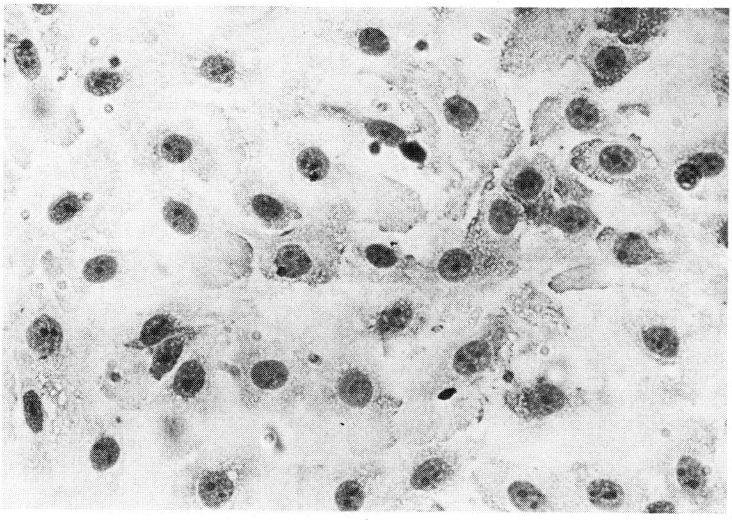

of NPC, since it would require the production of experimental NPC in man with this virus.

To circumvent this difficulty, we attempted to produce experimental tumours *in vitro* by infecting tissue fragments with EBV. We report here the preliminary findings of this study.

MATERIALS AND METHODS

Fresh biopsy specimens were obtained from non-neoplastic nasopharyngeal mucosa (NP) from patients examined either for exclusion of NPC or for exclusion of involvement of the nasopharynx by a tumour in an adjacent organ, from tonsillar mucosa of excised tonsils, from primary nasopharyngeal tumours and from primary lesions of the upper respiratory or alimentary tract other than NPC. All of the subjects were Chinese.

A portion of each of the biopsy specimens was submitted for routine histological examinations. Touch smear preparations from each specimen were fixed for EBNA staining before EBV infection. The remainder of the biopsy specimen was cut into approximately 2 mm fragments, washed with culture medium and treated with a B95-8 virus preparation for two hours at 37°C. The infected tissue fragments were then washed once with fresh medium and cultured on glass cover-slips in fresh growth medium (RPMI 1640, supplemented with 15% heat-inactivated fetal calf serum, Grand Island Biologicals, NY, USA, to which 100 units penicillin and 100 mg streptomycin per ml of medium were added). Cultures of uninfected tissue fragments were set up similarly as controls. Uninfected and infected tissue fragments were incubated in separate incubators at 37°C and provided with an atmosphere of 90% compressed air and 10% carbon dioxide. The tissue cultures were maintained by changing the medium twice weekly; observation of outgrowth was performed at the same time.

The B95-8 virus stock was prepared according to the method of Adams (1973) from the culture fluid of B95-8 cells and kept at -70°C for no more than four months. The infectivity of the virus preparation was assessed by its stimulatory effect on the rate of ^{3}H-thymidine incorporation by neonatal leucocytes. It was shown to affect neonatal leucocyte transformation at a maximum dilution of 1:50, with eventual formation of a number of cell lines. That this effect is virus-mediated was shown by its abolition when the infection of neonatal leucocytes was carried out in the presence of human sera with anti-EBV VCA reactivity, or when the leucocytes were treated overnight before infection and subsequently cultured with 100 standard units of human foreskin-cell interferon. The extent of stimulation was dependent on the concentration of infecting virus. A 1:50 dilution of this virus was used for infection of the tissue fragments; a single batch of virus preparation was used throughout

FIG. 3. INFECTED NON-NEOPLASTIC NASOPHARYNX SPECIMEN

Infected non-neoplastic nasopharynx specimen outgrowth two weeks after culture, showing marked cellular pleomorphism. Giemsa x 230

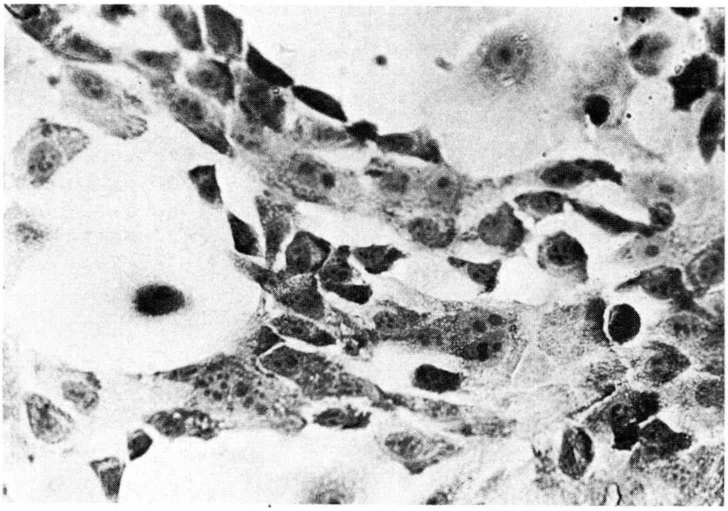

FIG. 4. INFECTED NON-NEOPLASTIC NASOPHARYNX SPECIMEN

Infected non-neoplastic nasopharynx specimen outgrowth two weeks after culture, with cells having an increased nucleus:cytoplasm ratio, many mitotic figures and coarse chromatin material. Giemsa x 230

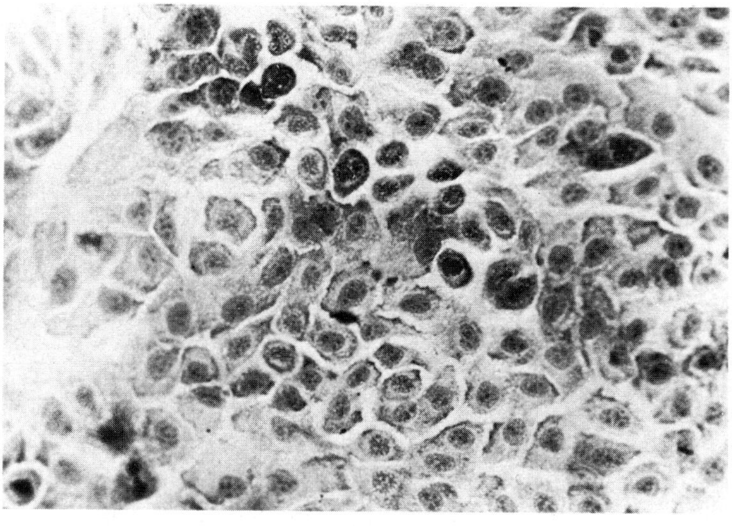

RESULTS

The diameters of outgrowth from six EBV-infected and six uninfected tissue fragments were measured and averaged on the 15th day after infection. The ratio of the average diameter of the infected fragment outgrowth to that of the uninfected fragment outgrowth was used as a measure of the effect of EBV infection; this ratio is referred to as the 'outgrowth ratio'. Table 1 summarizes the effects of infection with EBV on the different types of biopsy specimens.

As indicated by the outgrowth ratios for the short-term cultures, the NP biopsy specimens were highly susceptible to EBV infection, with 19 of the 20 biopsy specimens responding to the growth stimulatory effect of EBV infection. The biopsy specimens from the other sources responded at significantly lower frequencies: thus, only one of the nine tonsil specimens, two of the seven specimens from carcinomas of the upper respiratory and alimentary tracts and three of the 10 NPC specimens showed growth stimulation after infection with EBV.

Table 1. Growth of test and control tissue explants observed on the 15th day after infection with an Epstein-Barr virus preparation from B95-8 cell line

Tissue	No. of specimens[a]	Mean diameter of growth mm ± SD		Mean growth ratio infected:uninfected ± SD	p^b (*t test*)	No. with stimulation ≥1.8 / total	p^b (χ^2 test)
		Uninfected	Infected				
Non-neoplastic nasopharynx	20	12.25 ± 2.88	34.55 ± 14.75	2.83 ± 1.16		19 / 20	
Nasopharyngeal carcinoma	10	15.70 ± 3.23	20.30 ± 7.83	1.33 ± 0.50	<0.001	3 / 10	<0.001
Other tumours	7	14.00 ± 4.16	23.00 ± 13.84	1.65 ± 0.94[c]	<0.02	2 / 7	<0.005
Tonsil	9	23.78 ± 5.14	26.67 ± 7.35	1.14 ± 0.33	<0.001	1 / 9	<0.0005

[a] 6 uninfected and 6 B95-8 infected explants from each specimen were studied.
[b] All comparisons were with non-neoplastic nasopharynx explant.
[c] The large SD was due to the presence of 1 specimen with a growth ratio of 3.64; all the other specimens in the group had ratios of 1.0 and 2.0.

When comparing the effect of EBV on the various tissue fragments, we feel that the tonsil specimens are a better control for NP specimens than are NPC and other carcinomas, since tonsillar mucosa, like NP mucosa, overlies lymphoid tissue in Waldeyer's ring. Both are non-neoplastic epithelium, and both showed negative EBNA staining in touch smear preparations before EBV infection. The results shown in Table 1 indicate that NP tissue fragments are more susceptible to EBV infection than are tonsil tissue fragments.

FIG. 5. INFECTED NON-NEOPLASTIC NASOPHARYNX SPECIMEN

Infected non-neoplastic nasopharynx specimen outgrowth two weeks after culture, with cells having an increased nucleus:cytoplasm ratio, many mitotic figures, coarse chromatin material and vesicular nuclei. Giemsa x 230

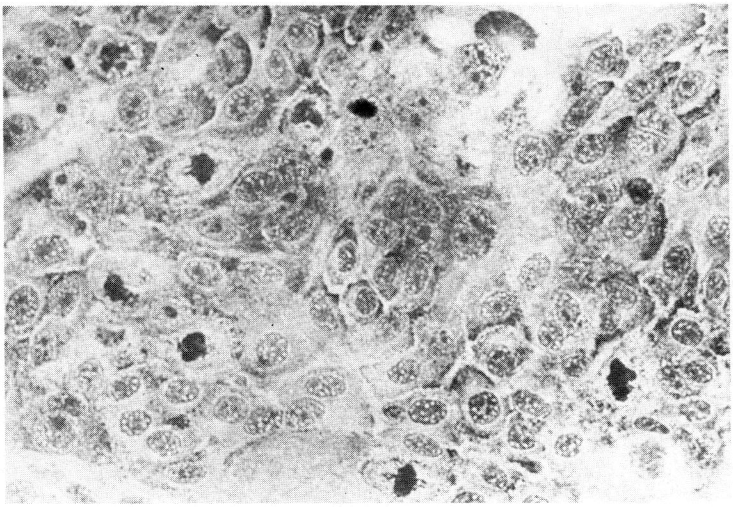

FIG. 6. INFECTED NON-NEOPLASTIC NASOPHARYNX SPECIMEN

Infected non-neoplastic nasopharynx specimen outgrowth two weeks after culture, showing a multi-nucleated giant cell with dense nuclear hyperchromasia in centre. Giemsa x 230

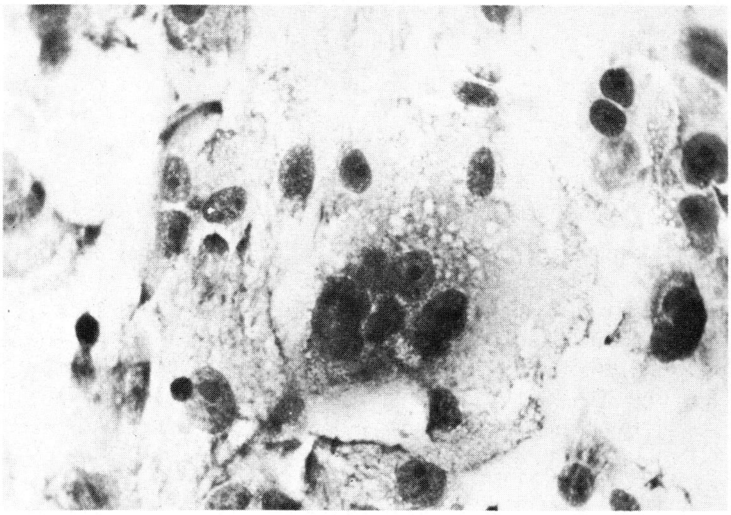

All of the NPC specimens, on the other hand, showed the presence of EBNA staining in touch smear preparations before EBV infection. The *in vitro* infection of these tissue fragments with B95-8 virus preparation differs from the infection of NP tissue fragments in that the former event is likely to represent superinfection; and the B95-8 virus preparation, as far as we are aware, has not been shown to affect superinfection.

From our preliminary tests it appears that some of the infected NP cells display EBNA, and this will be confirmed by including more positive and negative anti-EBNA sera in the EBNA test. We are also investigating whether NP mucosa is a unique target tissue for *in vitro* infection by EBV; this might be anticipated from the fact that NPC cells are the only non-lymphoid tumour cells that have so far been shown to harbour EB viral genomes.

We have also examined the morphology of the cells from the infected and uninfected NP outgrowths. After infection with the B95-8 virus preparations, the NP explants showed marked changes in growth characteristics and cellular morphology. The uninfected NP cells, on the other hand, grew slowly, spreading out in a mosaic pattern from the periphery of the tissue fragment, and showed signs of degeneration and detachment from the cover-slips about one month after explantation. In a light microscope at low power, it can be seen from the monolayer cell outgrowth that the uninfected NP cells have abundant cytoplasm and small nuclei. The infected NP explants, on the other hand, proliferated at a much higher rate, with foci of cell piling and a disorientated cell distribution pattern (Fig. 1). After the first week, the cells from the uninfected NP explants, when observed at high power, consisted predominantly of polyhedral cells of relatively uniform morphology, with a low nucleus:cytoplasm ratio, fine chromatin material and few mitotic figures (Fig. 2). In contrast, those from the infected NP explants showed marked cellular pleomorphism (Fig. 3), an increased nucleus:cytoplasm ratio, many mitotic figures and, sometimes, vesicular nuclei (Figs 4 & 5). There were also occasional multi-nucleated giant cells, and nuclear hyperchromasia was noted in many of the cells (Fig. 6).

DISCUSSION

Exposure of the normal nasopharyngeal mucosa in short-term culture to EBV prepared from B95-8 cells induced significant growth stimulation when compared with uninfected controls and with three other groups of biopsy specimens. In the infected NP outgrowth we also observed rapid cell proliferation, piling up of cells, formation of cell foci and changes in cell morphology.

All of these features indicate that these cells have undergone morphological transformation, but whether there is also a malignant transformation remains to be tested.

SUMMARY

Tissue fragments of fresh biopsy specimens from the non-neoplastic NP mucosa of 20 subjects, from the tumours of 10 NPC patients, from the mucosa of freshly removed tonsils from nine subjects and from the primary lesions of seven patients with malignancies of the upper respiratory or alimentary tract other than NPC were infected with EBV derived from B95-8 cells. A significantly higher frequency of growth stimulation and a greater mean growth ratio between infected and uninfected fragments from the same source were observed in the non-neoplastic NP mucosa specimens than in the others. In addition, the growth characteristics and the morphology of the cells in the infected non-neoplastic NP mucosal explants resembled those of transformed cells; but whether they possess malignant potential is being investigated.

ACKNOWLEDGEMENTS

Thanks are extended to the World Health Foundation (Hong Kong) and to The Hong Kong Anti-Cancer Society for financial assistance, to Mrs M. Ali for her technical assistance, to Mrs E. Seto for typing the manuscript and to Mr K.W. Leung for photographic assistance.

REFERENCES

Adams, A. (1973) Concentration of Epstein-Barr virus from cell culture fluids with polyethylene glycol. *J. gen. Virol.*, *20*, 391-394

de Schryver, A., Friberg, S., Jr, Klein, G., Henle, W., Henle, G., de-Thé, G., Clifford, P. & Ho, J.H.C. (1969) Epstein-Barr virus (EBV)-associated antibody patterns in carcinoma of the postnasal space. *Clin. exp. Immunol.*, *5*, 443-459

Desgranges, G., Wolf, H., de-Thé, G., Shanmugaratnam, K., Cammoun, N., Ellouz, R., Klein, G., Lennert, K., Muñoz, N. & zur Hausen, H. (1975) Nasopharyngeal carcinoma. X. Presence of Epstein-Barr genomes in separated epithelial cells of tumours in patients from Singapore, Tunisia and Kenya. *Int. J. Cancer*, *16*, 7-15

de-Thé, G., Sohier, R., Ho, J.H.C. & Freund, R., (1973) Nasopharyngeal carcinoma. IV. Evolution of complement-fixing antibodies during the course of the disease. *Int. J. Cancer, 12*, 368-377

Glaser, R., de-Thé, G., Lenoir, G. & Ho, J.H.C. (1976) Superinfection of epithelial nasopharyngeal carcinoma cells with Epstein-Barr virus. *Proc. nat. Acad. Sci. (Wash.), 73*, 960-963

Henle, G., Henle, W. & Diehl, V. (1968) Relation of Burkitt tumor associated herpes-type virus to infectious mononucleosis. *Proc. nat. Acad. Sci. (Wash.), 59*, 94-101

Henle, G., Henle, W., Zajac, B., Pearson, G., Waubke, R. & Scriba, M. (1970a) Differential reactivity of human sera with EBV-induced 'early antigens'. *Science, 169*, 188-190

Henle, G., Henle, W. & Klein, G. (1971) Demonstration of two distinct components in the early antigen complex of Epstein-Barr virus infected cells. *Int. J. Cancer, 8*, 272-282

Henle, G. & Henle, W. (1976) Epstein-Barr virus-specific IgA serum antibodies as an outstanding feature of nasopharyngeal carcinoma. *Int. J. Cancer, 17*, 1-7

Henle, W., Henle, G., Ho, H.C., Burtin, P., Cachin, Y., Clifford, P., de Schryver, A., de-Thé, G., Diehl, V. & Klein, G. (1970b) Antibodies to EB virus in nasopharyngeal carcinoma, other head and neck neoplasm and control groups. *J. nat. Cancer Inst., 44*, 225-231

Henle, W., Ho, J.H.C., Henle, G. & Kwan, H.C. (1973) Antibodies to Epstein-Barr virus-related antigens in nasopharyngeal carcinoma: comparison of active cases and long term survivors. *J. nat. Cancer Inst., 51*, 361-369

Huang, D.P., Ho, J.H.C., Henle, W. & Henle, G. (1974) Demonstration of Epstein-Barr virus-associated nuclear antigen in nasopharyngeal carcinoma cells from fresh biopsies. *Int. J. Cancer, 14*, 580-588

Klein, G., Giovanella, B., Lindahl, T., Fialkow, P.J., Singh, S. & Stehlin, J. (1974) Direct evidence for the presence of Epstein-Barr virus DNA and nuclear antigen in malignant epithelial cells from patients with anaplastic carcinoma of the nasopharynx. *Proc. nat. Acad. Sci. (Wash.), 71*, 4737-4741

Nonoyama, M., Huang, C.H., Pagano, J.S., Klein, G. & Singh, S. (1973) DNA of Epstein-Barr virus detected in tissue of Burkitt's lymphoma and nasopharyngeal carcinoma. *Proc. nat. Acad. Sci. (Wash.), 70*, 3265-3268

Nonoyama, M. & Pagano, J.S. (1973) Homology between Epstein-Barr virus DNA and viral DNA from Burkitt's lymphoma and nasopharyngeal carcinoma determined by DNA-DNA re-association kinetics. *Nature (Lond.), 224*, 44-47

Old, L.J., Boyse, E.A., Oettgen, H.F., De Harven, E., Geering, G., Williamson, B. & Clifford, P. (1966) Precipitating antibody in human serum to an antigen present in cultured Burkitt's lymphoma cells. *Proc. nat. Acad. Sci. (Wash.)*, *56*, 1699-1704

Old, L.J., Boyse, E.A., Geering, G. & Oettgen, H.F. (1968) Serologic approaches to study of cancer in animals and man. *Cancer Res.*, *28*, 1288-1299

Reedman, B.M. & Klein, G. (1973) Cellular localization of an Epstein-Barr virus (EBV) associated complement-fixing antigen in producer and non-producer lymphoblastoid cell lines. *Int. J. Cancer*, *11*, 499-520

Trumper, P.A., Epstein, M.A. & Giovanella, B.C. (1976) Activation *in vitro* by BUdR of a productive EB virus infection in the epithelial cells of nasopharyngeal carcinoma. *Int. J. Cancer*, *17*, 578-587

Wolf, H., zur Hausen, H. & Becker, V. (1973) EB viral genomes in epithelial nasopharyngeal carcinoma cells. *Nature (New Biol.)*, *244*, 245-247

Wolf, H., zur Hausen, H., Klein, G., Becker, V., Henle, G. & Henle, W. (1975) Attempts to detect virus-specific DNA sequences in human tumors. III. Epstein-Barr viral DNA in non-lymphoid nasopharyngeal carcinoma cells. *Med. Microbiol. Immunol.*, *161*, 15-21

zur Hausen, H., Schulte-Holthausen, H., Klein, G., Henle, W., Henle, G., Clifford, P. & Santesson, L. (1970) EB-virus DNA in biopsies of Burkitt tumors and anaplastic carcinomas of the nasopharynx. *Nature (Lond.)*, *228*, 1056-1058

EPSTEIN-BARR VIRUS-REGULATION STUDIES ON SOMATIC-CELL HYBRIDS DERIVED FROM THE FUSION OF BURKITT'S LYMPHOMA AND NASOPHARYNGEAL CARCINOMA CELLS WITH HUMAN OR MOUSE PARTNERS

G. KLEIN

Department of Tumor Biology,
Karolinska Institutet,
S 104 01 Stockholm 60, Sweden

INTRODUCTION

The relationships between the multiple Epstein-Barr virus (EBV) genomes carried in Burkitt's lymphoma (BL) and nasopharyngeal carcinoma (NPC) cells and the host cell are not well understood. In particular, it would be important to learn about the mechanisms that keep the viral genomes latent. More or less complete suppression of the viral cycle [the initiation of which is signalled by the appearance of early antigen (EA)] is a prerequisite for host-cell survival and proliferation. Since latency of multiple, complete genomes is the rule, both in the transformed (immortalized) lymphoid cell lines *in vitro* and in BLs and NPCs *in vivo*, and initiation of the viral cycle is the very rare exception, we must envisage the existence of finely poised and probably multiple regulation mechanisms, controlled by the viral and/or the cellular genome.

One of the few possible approaches towards the study of these regulations is somatic-cell hybridization. The purpose of the present report is to summarize briefly a variety of hybrid studies. Information has been obtained in relation not only to the regulation of the EBV cycle but also to a variety of markers on these cells.

CHROMOSOMAL PATTERNS AND EBV GENOME PERSISTENCE

These phenomena have been studied in two hybrid series (Spira et al., 1977). The first consists of four hybrid clones established by H. Harris by fusing the mouse ascites carcinoma cell, TA3Ha, and the BL cell, Daudi.

One of the four TA3Ha/Daudi clones was EBV DNA- and Epstein-Barr nuclear antigen (EBNA)-negative, and three were positive, at different levels. During serial passage, all three positive clones lost EBV DNA and EBNA in parallel. As in an earlier study on the A9/Daudi hybrid series (Klein et al., 1974b), the persistence of the EBV genome did not appear to depend on the presence of a large number of human chromosomes: EBV-carrying hybrids contained only a very small number of human chromosomes, and there was little further chromosome loss at the time the EBV genomes disappeared. In this particular series, loss of chromosome no. 21 was the most consistent feature that parallelled the loss of EBV; however, in view of the small size of the series, this could have been coincidental.

Another, very large series of hybrids was established and is presently being analysed in collaboration with Steplewski & Koprowski[1]. Over 200 hybrids were derived by the fusion of mouse or hamster fibroblasts with NPC biopsy cells. Interestingly, this series includes hybrids with a high average EBV DNA genome number per cell and 90-100% EBNA positivity. Even more surprisingly, several of the cloned hybrids appeared to maintain EBV in a much more stable fashion than the previously studied A9/Daudi or TA3Ha/Daudi hybrids.

Since NPC-derived, EBV-carrying epithelial cells have not yet been established in culture, it was important to know whether the EBV-carrying partner cell of the NPC biopsy/mouse fibroblast hybrid was the carcinoma cell itself or if it was an EBV-carrying lymphocyte. Further analysis showed that both events could occur. Critical evidence that it was the EBV-carrying carcinoma cell that participated was obtained by fusing a nude mouse-passaged, EBV-carrying NPC line, free of contaminating human lymphocytes (Klein et al., 1974a) with the mouse partner cell, IT-22. EBNA-positive hybrids were obtained, proving that it was possible to establish epithelial NPC/mouse hybrids. We have also found, however, that EBV-carrying non-epithelial cells could occasionally participate in fusion when a human biopsy was used as the partner. An EBV-carrying hybrid was derived by fusing a mouse fibroblast with a nasopharyngeally localized tumour that turned out on histological examination to be an EBV-negative lymphoma. Obviously, the EBV-carrying cell must have been a contaminating host cell, presumably a lymphocyte.

Chromosomal and isozyme tests performed by Steplewski & Koprowski[1] on the NPC/mouse fibroblast hybrids showed that several of them

---

[1] Unpublished data

contained only a very small number of chromosomes. The majority of the EBV-carrying hybrids contained either chromosome 20 or 21. However, some EBV-carrying hybrids lacked both 20 and 21, and one hybrid (BU-7) contained no detectable human chromosome; it was, nevertheless, 100% EBNA-positive and contained an average of 29 EBV DNA copies per cell, including both integrated and free circular forms (Falk et al.[1]). We saw no tendency for EBNA-negative sublines to segregate during continued propagation over five months: this raises the question of whether EBV genomes might have become inserted into the mouse genome, directly or through the vehicle of a small human chromosome piece.

None of the mouse/human hybrids in this or previous studies showed any spontaneous EBV production, nor were they inducible by iododeoxyuridine (IUDR) or by EBV (P3HR-1 strain) superinfection. In spite of this apparently complete extinction of all characteristics related to the EBV cycle in the interspecies hybrids, EBNA was fully expressed. In a combined, quantitative microfluorimetric and EBV DNA study, Ernberg et al. (1977) found a direct correlation between the number of EBV genome equivalents per cell and the amount of EBNA per nucleus in a variety of human EBV-carrying lines and in human/human hybrids. In more recent studies[1], EBV-carrying mouse/human hybrids showed the same correlation, confirming the autonomous expression of EBNA even in this, otherwise entirely nonpermissive, system.

EBNA is the only known function of the viral genome that is consistently expressed in all EBV DNA-carrying cells. It is a virally determined or virally changed chromosomal protein with strong DNA-binding properties (Baron et al., 1975; Lenoir et al., 1976; Luka et al., 1977; Ohno et al., 1977). Its autonomous expression suggests that it may play a regulatory role, perhaps at the transcription level. If it is instrumental in keeping the viral cycle suppressed, EBNA may be responsible not only for the prolonged latency but, indirectly or directly, for the transforming ('immortalizing') function of the viral genome.

In this connection, it may be relevant that *in vitro* conversion of the EBV-negative BL lines (e.g., Ramos or BJAB) to permanent carriers of EBV DNA and EBNA, by infection with either the B95-8 or the P3HR-1 strain of the virus, is accompanied by a series of biological changes similar to those that accompany the transformation of monolayer cultures by known, experimental oncogenic DNA (e.g., polyoma or SV40) or RNA (e.g., RSV) viruses. These changes include reduced capping of surface IgM concanavalin A, and other membrane receptors (Yefenof & Klein, 1974, 1976), increased agglutinability by concanavalin A (Yefenof et al., 1977), increased resistance to saturation conditions in culture, decreased dependence on serum concentration and independence of some dialysable serum factor(s) (Steinitz & Klein, 1977 a, b, c). In view of the fact that the same changes were found in a number of

[1] Unpublished data

independently EBV-converted sublines of both BJAB and Ramos, they are most likely due to the direct or indirect action of the viral genome. Since EBNA is the only known viral function expressed in the converted cells, its role in inducing them may be similar to the one that T antigens are believed to play in bringing about the pleiotropic cellular changes associated with SV40 or polyoma transformation.

REGULATION OF SPONTANEOUS EA AND VCA PRODUCTION

Spontaneous EBV-producer status, assessed by the appearance of EA and VCA in a small number of cells, was studied in two types of intraspecies hybrids. One was the hybrid between the EBV producer P3HR-1 line and the EBV-negative HeLa subline D-98, produced and studied by Glaser & Nonoyama (1974); the other was a hybrid between two EBV-carrying human BLs, one a low-level producer (Daudi), the other a non-producer (Raji) (Klein et al., 1976). While spontaneous production was extinguished in the lymphoma/nonlymphoma hybrid, it was maintained in the BL/BL hybrid. This correlates with the fact that other B-cell properties are extinguished in lymphoid/nonlymphoid hybrids but maintained in lymphoid/lymphoid hybrids (see 'surface markers' below).

Although hybrids between high-producer and non-producer BL lines have not yet been studied, the dominance of the producer status in BL/BL hybrids augurs well for the possibility of 'virus rescue' experiments.

INDUCTION OF EA BY IUDR AND BY P3HR-1 VIRUS SUPERINFECTION

A variety of patterns were observed with regard to EA induction by IUDR treatment or P3HR-1 virus superinfection, depending on the combination of partner cells (Klein et al., 1976, 1977a); Nyormoi et al., 1973). Within this variety, there was a good correlation in each hybrid between the EA induction responses following the two, very different EA-inducing treatments, compared to those in the parental cells, in spite of the different levels of response to the two treatments. This suggests that the same regulatory mechanisms control the responses of the cell to both. Suppressive and permissive hybrids have both been encountered, suggesting complex regulatory circuits in which the outcome is determined by the actual combinations of the target cells. Thus, the relatively limited EA inducibility of Raji dominated, both after fusion with the even less inducible Namalwa cell (Klein et al., 1977b; Nyormoi et al., 1973) (suggesting positive control) and also after fusion with the relatively more permissive Daudi cell (Klein et al., 1976) (suggesting negative control). Perhaps the most appropriate statement is that the Raji cell imposed its own level of inducibility on both partner cells.

Another interesting situation was encountered when Raji was fused with the EBV-negative BJAB cell (Klein et al., 1976). While BJAB itself responded with only minimal EA induction after P3HR-1 virus superinfection, the Raji/BJAB hybrid showed a higher EA inducibility than Raji, suggesting some kind of complementation between the participating genomes.

In this context, it is important to note that complementation phenomena have also been demonstrated between resident and superinfecting EBV genomes in relation to EA induction. Thus, Dalens & Adams (1977) found that EA induction by P3HR-1 virus in EBV genome-carrying Raji cells was much more resistant to ultraviolet radiation than was EA induction in the EBV-negative Ramos or BJAB lines. This can only be explained by assuming that the resident viral genome participates in EA induction. Another sort of evidence comes from the recent work of Fresen et al. (1977). While B95-8 virus transforms normal lymphocytes and induces EBNA in them and in the BJAB or Ramos line, it has so far failed to induce EA in Raji, BJAB or Ramos. In the experiments of Fresen et al., it did not induce EA in EBV-carrying convertants of BJAB and Ramos if they had been converted with the B95-8 virus but did so if they had been converted by P3HR-1 virus. This suggests complementation between the superinfecting B95-8 and resident P3HR-1 genome in EA induction. In a way, this is the mirror image of the complementation between the superinfecting P3HR-1 virus and the resident Raji-EBV genome in the experiments described above.

The fact that both the Raji/Daudi and the Raji/BJAB hybrids were either equally or more inducible to produce EA, both after exposure to IUDR and P3HR-1 virus superinfection, compared to Raji itself is interesting contrast to our recent finding (Shapiro et al.[1]) that the EA inducibility of Raji and Daudi cells by both IUDR and P3HR-1 virus decreases dramatically after tetraploidization. While the mechanism is obscure, it is apparent that duplication of the cell genome increases virus repression, whereas the complementation of viral and cellular genomes in a hybrid tends to do the opposite. This is also reflected at the level of EBV genomes: Andersson (1975) showed that the number of EBV DNA copies per cell is amplified, beyond simple addition, in the somatic hybrids Raji/Namalwa and Raji/BJAB, whereas in the tetraploid Raji cells it remained almost unchanged or showed only a slight increase (Shapiro et al.[1]).

Further studies on the suppressive controls that prevail in tetraploid cells, as contrasted to somatic hybrids, may reveal important new facts about the regulation of the EBV cycle.

SURFACE MARKERS

In all human/mouse hybrids so far studied, in which an EBV-carrying B-lymphoblast line was the human partner, all differentiated (B cell)

---

[1] Unpublished data

markers of the human partner cell, including surface immunoglobulin, Fc receptors, C3 receptors and EBV receptors, eclipsed completely.

In human/human hybrids, surface-marker expression depended on the lineage of the partners. In hybrids derived from the fusion of B-lymphoid lines with non-lymphoid partners, B-cell markers were also eclipsed. When two B-cell lines were fused, however, the situation was quite different (Klein et al., 1977a). Complement receptors, EBV receptors and Fc receptors showed a dominant expression, i.e., fusion of a line that had high receptor expression with a line that had negative or low receptor expression led to a hybrid that resembled the high expressor parent. HLA antigens and B-cell antigens were expressed in a codominant fashion.

An interesting situation was encountered in relation to β_2-microglobulin: the Daudi line lacks both β_2-microglobulin and HLA antigens; the Raji/Daudi hybrid was β_2-microglobulin-positive and showed the appearance of new HLA specificities, presumably the products of the 'silent' HLA genes of the Daudi cell that cannot be expressed in the absence of β_2-microglobulin.

ACKNOWLEDGEMENTS

This work was supported by Public Health Service Research Grant No. 5R01 CA 14054-04 and by the Swedish Cancer Society.

REFERENCES

Andersson, M. (1975) Amounts of Epstein-Barr virus DNA in somatic cell hybrids between Burkitt lymphoma-derived cell lines. *J. Virol.*, *16*, 1345-1347

Baron, D., Benz, W.C., Carmichael, G., Yocum, R.R. & Strominger, J.L. (1975) Assay and partial purification of Epstein-Barr virus nuclear antigen. In: *IARC Internal Technical Report 75/003, Epstein-Barr virus, production, concentration and purification.* Lyon, International Agency for Research on Cancer, pp. 257-262

Dalens, M. & Adams, A. (1977) Induction of Epstein-Barr virus associated early antigen in different lymphoid cell lines with ultraviolet irradiated P3HR-1 virus. *Virology* (in press)

Ernberg, I., Andersson-Anvret, M., Klein, G., Lundin, L. & Killander, D. (1977) Relationship between amount of Epstein-Barr virus-determined nuclear antigen per cell and number of EBV-DNA copies per cell. *Nature (Lond.)*, *266*, 269-270

Fresen, K.-O., Merkt, B., Bornkamm, G.W. & zur Hausen, H. (1977) Heterogeneity of Epstein-Barr virus originating from P3HR-1 cells. I. Studies on EBNA induction. *Int. J. Cancer*, *19*, 317-323

Glaser, R. & Nonoyama, M. (1974) Host cell regulation of Epstein-Barr virus. *J. Virol.*, *14*, 174-176

Klein, G., Giovanella, B.C., Lindahl, T., Fialkow, P.J., Singh, S. & Stehlin, J.S. (1974a) Direct evidence for the presence of Epstein-Barr virus DNA and nuclear antigen in malignant epithelial cells from patients with poorly differentiated carcinoma of the nasopharynx. *Proc. nat. Acad. Sci. (Wash.)*, *71*, 4737-4741

Klein, G., Wiener, F., Zech, L., zur Hausen, H. & Reedman, B. (1974b) Segregation of the EBV-determined nuclear antigen (EBNA) in somatic cell hybrids derived from the fusion of a mouse fibroblast and a human Burkitt lymphoma line. *Int. J. Cancer*, *14*, 54-64

Klein, G., Clements, G., Zeuthen, J. & Westman, A. (1976) Somatic cell hybrids between human lymphoma lines. II. Spontaneous and induced patterns of the Epstein-Barr virus (EBV) cycle. *Int. J. Cancer*, *17*, 715-724

Klein, G., Terasaki, P., Billing, R., Honig, R., Jondal, M., Rosén, A., Zeuthen, J. & Clements, G. (1977a) Somatic cell hybrids between human lymphoma lines. III. Surface markers. *Int. J. Cancer*, *19*, 66-76

Klein, G., Clements, G., Zeuthen, J. & Westman, A. (1977b) Spontaneous and induced patterns of the Epstein-Barr virus (EBV) cycle in a new set of somatic cell hybrids. *Cancer Let.*, *3*, 91-98

Lenoir, G., Berthelon, M.-C., Favre, M.-C. & de-Thé, G. (1976) Characterization of Epstein-Barr virus antigens. I. Biochemical analysis of the complement-fixing soluble antigen and relationship with Epstein-Barr virus-associated nuclear antigen. *J. Virol.*, *17*, 672-674

Luka, J., Siegert, W. & Klein, G. (1977) Solubilization of the Epstein-Barr virus determined nuclear antigen and its characterization as a DNA-binding protein. *J. Virol.*, *22*, 1-8

Nyormoi, O., Klein, G., Adams, A. & Dombos, L. (1973) Sensitivity to EBV superinfection and IUDR inducibility of hybrid cells formed between a sensitive and a relatively resistant Burkitt lymphoma cell line. *Int. J. Cancer*, *12*, 396-408

Ohno, S., Luka, J., Lindahl, T. & Klein, G. (1977) Identification of a purified complement fixing antigen as the Epstein-Barr virus-determined nuclear antigen (EBNA) by its binding to metaphase chromosomes. *Proc. nat. Acad. Sci. (Wash.), 74*, 1605-1609

Spira, J., Wiener, F., Andersson-Anvret, M., Povey, S. & Klein, G. (1977) Chromosome banding, isoenzyme analysis and determination of Epstein-Barr virus DNA content in human Burkitt lymphoma/mouse hybrids. *Int. J. Cancer* (in press)

Steinitz, M. & Klein, G. (1977a) Comparison between growth characteristics of an Epstein-Barr virus (EBV)-genome-negative lymphoma line and its EBV-converted subline *in vitro*. *Proc. nat. Acad. Sci. (Wash.), 72*, 3518-3520

Steinitz, M. & Klein, G. (1977b) Epstein-Barr virus (EBV)-induced change in the saturation sensitivity and serum dependence of established, EBV-negative lymphoma lines *in vitro*. *Virology, 70*, 570-573

Steinitz, M. & Klein, G. (1977c) Further studies on the differences in serum dependence in EBV negative lymphoma lines and their *in vitro* EBV converted, virus-genome carrying sublines. *Europ. J. Cancer* (in press)

Yefenof, E. & Klein, G. (1974) Antibody-induced redistribution of normal and tumor associated surface antigens. *Exp. Cell Res., 88*, 217-224

Yefenof, E. & Klein, G. (1976) Difference in antibody induced redistribution of membrane IgM in EBV-genome free and EBV positive human lymphoid cells. *Exp. Cell Res., 99* , 175-178

Yefenof, E., Klein, G., Ben Bassat, H. & Lundin, L. (1977) Differences in the Con A induced redistribution agglutination patterns of EBV genome free and EBV carrying human lymphoma lines. *Exp. Cell Res.* (in press)

EPSTEIN-BARR VIRUS-EPITHELIAL CELL INTERACTION AND ITS IMPLICATION IN THE ETIOLOGY OF NASOPHARYNGEAL CARCINOMA

G. LENOIR & G. DE-THE

International Agency for Research on Cancer, Lyon, France

The two major characteristics of nasopharyngeal carcinoma (NPC) are its genetic predisposition, as shown by ethnic, familial and histocompatibility studies, and its association with the Epstein-Barr virus (EBV), as testified by viral markers [viral DNA and EBV-determined nuclear antigen (EBNA)] that are consistently detected within epithelial tumour cells. These viral elements, which are also present *in vitro* in EBV-transformed lymphocytes and in Burkitt's tumour (BL) cells, seem to be indicators of the role of EBV in continued cell proliferation and of its oncogenic potential *in vivo*. However, the etiological role of EBV in NPC is still a matter of debate; the interaction of this virus with epithelial cells of the nasopharynx needs better to be understood. From a virological point of view, two major questions arise:

(1) How does the viral DNA become associated with epithelial carcinoma cells, since only B-type lymphocytes are at present known to have receptors for EBV?

(2) Is the expression of EBNA in the epithelial cells a marker of the malignant state; or, conversely, can EBNA-positive epithelial cells be found *in vivo* in the absence of a tumour?

A short recapitulation of the interaction of EBV with human B lymphocytes and its implication in the etiology of BL is necessary at this point (see also de-Thé & Lenoir, 1977). In the case of BL, the tumour cells are B lymphocytes, cells which are known to be the main targets of EBV. These tumour cells carry the EBV genome, express EBNA and can give rise to continuous lymphoblastoid cell lines after *in vitro* cultivation. In the case of infectious mononucleosis (IM), the EBNA-carrying lymphoblasts possess some of the characteristics of transformed cells, since they are able to grow *in vitro* as continuous cell lines. However, the *in vivo* proliferation of these cells is controlled by the 'immune surveillance' system of the organism and, in particular, by specific killer T lymphocytes (Svedmyr & Jondal, 1975).

EBNA-expressing lymphocytes can be detected in the absence of a tumour, in the peripheral blood (Klein et al., 1976) or in lymph nodes (Lenoir et al., 1977) of patients with severe IM during the acute phase of the disease. Thus, if EBNA-expressing lymphocytes can be found *in vivo* in the absence of malignancy, the direct interaction of EBV with lymphocytes, which results in EBNA-carrying lymphocytes, is not sufficient by itself to explain the development of the Burkitt's tumour. Other factors must be implicated, malarial infection, for example, which can act at two different levels, either by an action on the immune surveillance mechanism, allowing proliferation of the EBNA-carrying B lymphoblasts (although this would lead to the development of polyclonal tumours), or by increasing the neoplastic potential of the EBV-carrying lymphoblasts, resulting in a tumorous clone. The finding that BL tumours are uniclonal (Fialkow et al., 1970) and that the lymphoma cells exhibit a specific translocation involving the long arm of the no. 14 chromosome (Zech et al., 1976) - a genetic change that appears to be independent of the EBV infection - favours the latter hypothesis and, therefore, a multi-stage carcinogenic process at the cellular level in the development of BL.

What is the situation in the case of NPC? Laboratory studies on EBV-NPC epithelial cell interaction are difficult for two reasons:

(1) Only limited outgrowths of NPC epithelial tumour cells can be obtained from explant cultures, and these can be kept *in vitro* for only a few weeks, so that permanent lines cannot be established.

(2) Normal nasopharyngeal epithelial cells have only been found to be susceptible to EBV infection in tissue culture under exceptional conditions[1].

Three hypotheses can be proposed to explain how the viral DNA becomes associated with NPC cells and whether the presence of EBNA in the epithelial cell is a marker of the malignant state.

The first hypothesis (Fig. 1) suggests that the normal epithelial cell from the nasopharyngeal mucosa is permissive for EBV infection, i.e., the cell possesses EBV receptors and can replicate the virus. This would represent one site of production of the EBV detected in the saliva of sero-positive individuals. Transformation of such epithelial cells could result from direct interaction of the virus with this cell type. If this hypothesis were confirmed, the relationship of

---

[1] Desgranges & de-Thé, personal communication

FIG. 1. HYPOTHESIS 1

The normal epithelial cell is permissive for EBV infection.

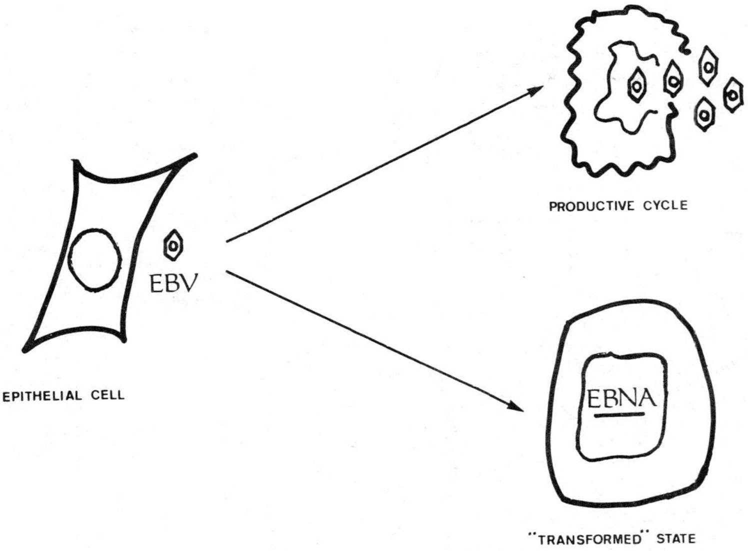

EBV with the epithelial cell would be similar to that known for B lymphocytes. However, the origin of the virus present in the saliva and throat-washings of most sero-positive individuals is still unknown. Furthermore, no-one has succeeded in infecting cells other than B lymphocytes with EBV: in reports of such studies (Al-Moslih et al., 1976; Huang et al.[1]), expression of EBV-related antigens was not proven satisfactorily.

The second hypothesis (Fig. 2) proposes that a malignant or pre-malignant change is required in the epithelial cells for them to become permissive for EBV infection. Two possibilities exist:

(1) The epithelial cell is already malignant when it is infected with EBV; the virus thus has no etiological role in the transformation process (passenger hypothesis).

(2) The epithelial cell is in a premalignant state when infected by the virus, which acts as a promoting factor for tumour development. The malignant transformation thus results from a multistage process at the cellular level, as has been proposed in the development of BL.

---

[1] See p. 359

FIG. 2. HYPOTHESIS 2

The normal epithelial cell is not permissive for EBV infection.
A malignant or premalignant change in the cell is required.

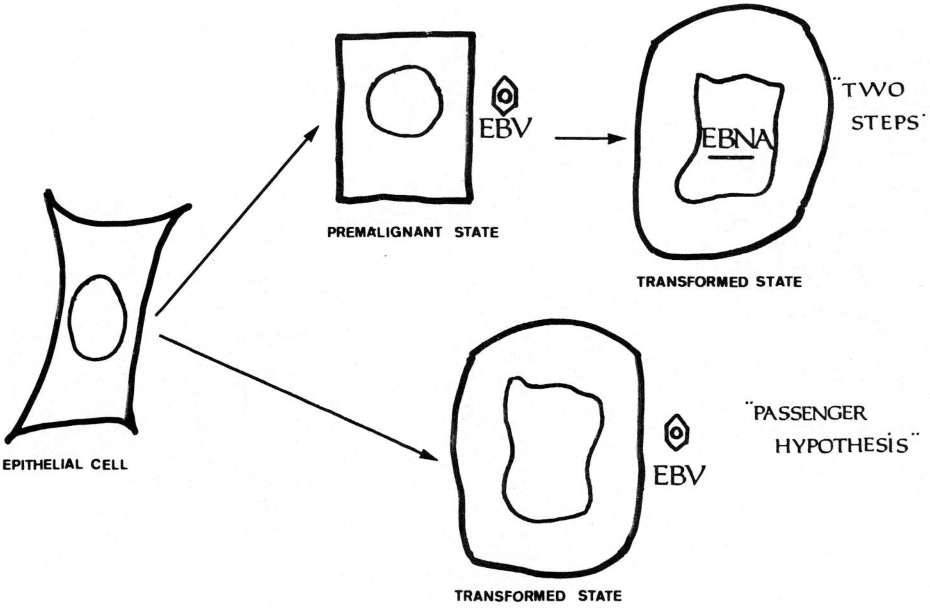

In either case, the influence of chemical carcinogens may be important: some of the data presented at this conference (see Huang et al.[1] with regard to rats fed salt-fish) should be kept in mind. However, the lack of an *in vitro* transformation assay makes testing of this hypothesis difficult. With regard to the passenger hypothesis, it would be interesting to see to what extent undifferentiated anaplastic carcinomas of the nasopharynx can be found that are free of EBV genomes, or if NPC can occur in EBV serologically negative individuals.

The third hypothesis (Fig. 3) implies that the epithelial cells have no receptors for EBV, but that infection results from a specific interaction of this cell with EBV-infected B lymphocytes, involving either a cell hybrid formation or a transfection process. Various observations may support this hypothesis:

---

[1] See p. 315

FIG. 3. HYPOTHESIS 3

The normal epithelial cell is not permissive for EBV infection. This occurs through either a transfection or a fusion process.

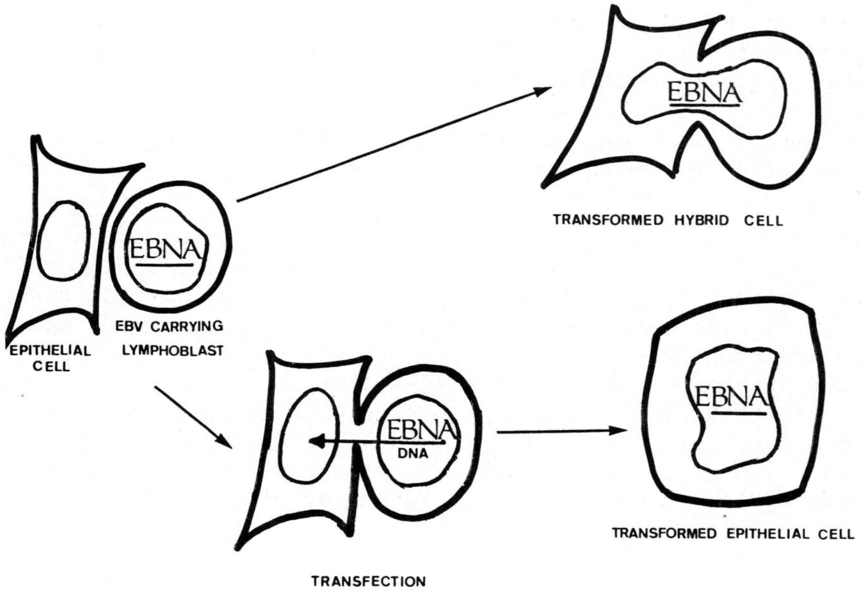

(1) NPC arises only in an anatomical region in which epithelial cells lie on a lymphocyte layer (the lymphoepithelium).

(2) In both normal and tumourous tissues of the nasopharynx, the lymphoid cells have been shown by electron microscopy to be closely associated with the epithelial cells, possibly by cytoplasmic bridges (Gazzolo et al., 1972).

(3) The nasopharyngeal region is also the site of replication of various myxoviruses, which are capable of cell fusion. Furthermore, a new human virus, characterized as the syncytial virus, was isolated from a NPC biopsy (Epstein et al., 1974). When NPC biopsies are cultured, polycaryons or tetraploid cells are found very frequently. Indirect evidence comes from the work of Glaser et al. (1977) on somatic hybrids of BL cells and of human epithelial cells, which shows that such hybrids are tumorigenic in nude mice, producing tumours with the histopathological features of undifferentiated anaplastic carcinoma.

Moreover, cell fusion has been shown to occur *in vivo* in an experimental mouse system (Wiener et al., 1972); this could provide the basis for a greatly increased genetic variation in the infected cell population.

The recent demonstration of the presence of neutralizing, EBV-specific IgA in throat-washings from NPC patients (Desgranges et al., 1977) and of the presence of the secretory piece of such IgA within malignant epithelial cells[1] raises the possibility that, in normal individuals, the virus, complexed with neutralizing IgA, can be trapped within the epithelial cells which produce the secretory piece. This emphasizes the need for defining whether secretion of anti-VCA IgA represents a risk factor in NPC development.

Finally, the demonstration by Glaser et al. (1976) and by Trumper et al. (1976) that viral genome present in epithelial cells of NPC is activated either by chemicals or by superinfection with the P3HR1 strain of EBV indicates that the tumour cells can replicate the virus and may possess EBV receptors. Unfortunately, this does not permit selection of one of the three hypotheses presented above; however, since it is possible that EBV viral particles could be rescued in this way, their biological activity could be tested directly to ascertain the differences between the NPC virus and EBV isolated from BL or IM (Kaschka-Dierich et al., 1976; Pagano et al., 1974).

SUMMARY

The etiological role of EBV in NPC is still a matter for debate. A major question is how the viral DNA becomes associated with the carcinoma cell, since only B lymphocytes are at present known to have receptors to EBV. The following hypotheses are proposed:

(1) The epithelial cells of the nasopharynx have EBV receptors *in vivo*; transformation of the epithelial cell thus results from a direct interaction between EBV and this cell type.

The epithelial cells of the nasopharynx are not permissive for EBV infection. In this case:

(2) Malignant or premalignant changes in the epithelial cells are required for EBV infection to take place. Thus, EBV may act either as a passive passenger or as an active promoter in NPC development.

---

[1] Desgranges, personal communication

Or, (3) infection of the epithelial cells results from a specific interaction (involving either transfection or hybrid formation) between an EBV-infected B lymphocyte and an epithelial cell within the nasopharynx. Here again, the virus may either be passive or act as an oncogenic factor.

Recent data are presented both for and against these hypotheses.

REFERENCES

Al-Moslih, M.I., White, R.J. & Dubes, G.R. (1976) Use of a transfection method to demonstrate a monolayer cell transforming agent from the EB3 line of Burkitt's lymphoma cells. *J. gen. Virol.*, *31*, 331-345

Desgranges, C., de-Thé, G., Ho, J.H.C. & Ellouz, R. (1977) Neutralizing EBV-specific IgA in throat washings of nasopharyngeal carcinoma (NPC) patients. *Int. J. Cancer*, *19*, 627-633

de-Thé, G. & Lenoir, G. (1977) *Comparative diagnosis of Epstein-Barr virus related diseases: infectious mononucleosis, Burkitt's lymphoma and nasopharyngeal carcinoma.* In: Kurstak, E. & Kurstak, C., eds, *Comparative Diagnosis of Viral Diseases*, Vol. 1, New York, Academic Press, pp. 195-240

Epstein, M.A., Achong, B.G. & Ball, G. (1974) Further observations on a human syncytial virus from a nasopharyngeal carcinoma. *J. nat. Cancer Inst.*, *53*, 681-688

Fialkow, P.J., Klein, G., Gartler, S.M. & Clifford, P. (1970) Clonal origin for individual Burkitt tumours. *Lancet*, *i*, 384-386

Gazzolo, L., de-Thé, G., Vuillaume, M. & Ho, J.H.C. (1972) Nasopharyngeal carcinoma. II. Ultrastructure of normal mucosa, tumor biopsies and subsequent epithelial growth *in vitro*. *J. nat. Cancer Inst.*, *48*, 73-86

Glaser, R., de-Thé, G., Lenoir, G. & Ho, J.H.C. (1976) Superinfection of epithelial nasopharyngeal carcinoma cells with Epstein-Barr virus. *Proc. nat. Acad. Sci. (Wash.)*, *73*, 960-963

Glaser, R., Ablashi, D.V., Nonoyama, M., Henle, W. & Easton, J. (1977) Enhanced oncogenic behavior of human and mouse cells after cellular hybridization with Burkitt tumor cells. *Proc. nat. Acad. Sci. (Wash.)*, *74*, 2574-2578

Kaschka-Dierich, C., Adams, A., Lindahl, T., Bornkamm, G., Bjursell, G., Klein, G., Giovanella, B.C. & Singh, S. (1976) Intracellular forms of Epstein-Barr virus DNA in human tumour cells *in vivo*. *Nature (Lond.)*, *260*, 302-306

Klein, G., Svedmyr, E., Jondal, M. & Person, P.O. (1976) EBV-determined nuclear antigen (EBNA) positive cells in the peripheral blood of infectious mononucleosis patients. *Int. J. Cancer*, *17*, 21-26

Lenoir, G., Virelizier, J.L., Griscelli, C. & de-Thé, G. (1977) *Epstein-Barr virus nuclear antigen (EBNA) positive cells in a lymph node of a child with severe primary EBV infection*. In: de-Thé, G., Henle, W. & Rapp, F., eds, *Oncogenesis and Herpes-viruses III*, Lyon, International Agency for Research on Cancer (*IARC Scientific Publications No. 24*) (in press)

Pagano, J.S., Huang, C.H., Klein, G., de-Thé, G., Shanmugaratnam, K. & Yang, C.S. (1974) *Homology of Epstein-Barr virus DNA in nasopharyngeal carcinoma from Kenya, Taiwan, Singapore and Tunisia*. In: de-Thé, G., Epstein, M.A. & zur Hausen, H., eds, *Oncogenesis and Herpesviruses II*, Lyon, International Agency for Research on Cancer (*IARC Scientific Publications No. 11*), pp. 179-190

Svedmyr, E. & Jondal, M. (1975) Cytotoxic effector cells specific for B cell lines transformed by Epstein-Barr virus are present in patients with infectious mononucleosis. *Proc. nat. Acad. Sci. (Wash.)*, *72*, 1622-1626

Trumper, P.A., Epstein, M.A. & Giovanella, B.C. (1976) Activation *in vitro* by BUdR of a productive EB virus infection in the epithelial cells of nasopharyngeal carcinoma. *Int. J. Cancer*, *17*, 578-587

Wiener, F., Fenyo, E.M., Klein, G. & Harris, H. (1972) Fusion of tumour cells with host cells. *Nature New Biol.*, *238*, 155-159

Zech, L., Haglund, U., Nilsson, K. & Klein, G. (1976) Characteristic chromosomal abnormalities in biopsies and lymphoid-cell lines from patients with Burkitt and non-Burkitt lymphomas. *Int. J. Cancer*, *17*, 47-56

EARLY AND LATE COMPONENTS OF EPSTEIN-BARR VIRUS-ASSOCIATED MEMBRANE ANTIGEN IN SUPERINFECTED DAUDI CELLS AND THEIR REACTIVITY WITH SERA FROM NASOPHARYNGEAL CARCINOMA PATIENTS

Y. HINUMA, T. SAIRENJI & M. MAEDA

Department of Microbiology,
Kumamoto University Medical School,
Kumamoto, Japan

Epstein-Barr virus (EBV)-determined membrane antigen (MA) was first demonstrated in Burkitt's lymphoma biopsy cells by membrane immunofluorescense (Klein et al., 1966). MA can be detected either on certain EBV-genome carrying lymphoid cell lines (Klein et al., 1972) or on non-producer lines experimentally superinfected with P3HR-1 strain EBV (Gergely et al., 1971; Pearson et al., 1971; Sairenji & Hinuma, 1975). MA appears at an early stage of the viral cycle and is apparently not influenced by DNA inhibitors (Dölken & Klein, 1976; Gergely et al., 1971; Sairenji & Hinuma, 1975). Ernberg et al. (1974) found that MA can be subdivided into two components, designated as early MA (EMA) and late MA (LMA), which differ with respect to their sensitivity to inhibitors of DNA synthesis and to their antigenicity. However, it was not known whether LMA was formed in EBV superinfected cells. The present investigation, in which an indirect membrane immunofluorescence technique was used, provides evidence that both EMA and LMA appear upon superinfection of Daudi cells. Furthermore, it is shown that sera from nasopharyngeal carcinoma (NPC) patients react with LMA to give a 'prozone' phenomenon.

When a culture of Daudi cells superinfected with P3HR-1 virus was treated with medium alone, high background levels of MA made it difficult to distinguish between passively adsorbed and newly synthesized MA. Addition to the culture of 0.1% trypsin 2 hr after infection removed most detectable MA from the cell surface and brought the background level down to that of uninfected cells, without disturbing *de novo* synthesis of MA, early antigen (EA) or viral capsid antigen (VCA).

The results were in agreement with our previous findings on superinfected NC37 (C-6 clone) cells (Sairenji & Hinuma, 1975) and with those of another report (Dölken & Klein, 1976) in which superinfected Raji cells were treated with papain. Important increases in the levels of MA, EA and VCA took place during the first 24 hr after infection; the frequencies of MA-, EA- and VCA-positive cells reached maximum levels (64%, 34% and 23%, respectively) 22 hr after infection.

Addition of 25 μg/ml puromycin at the time of virus infection completely inhibited MA, EA and VCA synthesis. In the presence of 20 μg/ml cytosine arabinoside (Ara-C), synthesis of both MA and VCA, but not of EA, was markedly inhibited. This suggests that the synthesis not only of VCA but also of MA, or a part of them, is dependent on DNA synthesis, which is blocked by Ara-C. Since it has been reported recently that phosphonoacetic acid specifically inhibits viral DNA synthesis in EBV-infected cells (Thorley-Lawson & Strominger, 1976; Yajima et al., 1976), the effect of disodium phosphonoacetate (PA) on the synthesis of MA, EA and VCA was also examined. No effect was observed on EA synthesis, even with 200 μg/ml of the drug; however, a dose-dependent inhibitory effect was observed on both MA and VCA synthesis. The presence of 200 μg/ml PA reduced the percentage of VCA-positive cells from 40% to 5%; with this dose 50% of MA-positive cells were still detectable. This effect of PA on MA synthesis was somewhat analogous to that in the experiments with Ara-C.

It was considered that if the Ara-C-sensitive component of MA in P3HR-1 virus superinfected Daudi cells is antigenically distinct from the Ara-C-insensitive component, a presumably polyvalent human serum could be differentially absorbed with the respective MA components. In absorption tests, the reactivity of the serum to the superinfected Daudi target cells was found to be greatly reduced by absorption with these cells *per se* but only slightly reduced by absorption with Ara-C-treated cells. In turn, the reactivity of the same serum to Ara-C-treated superinfected Daudi target cells was reduced more by absorption with these same cells than by absorption with non-treated superinfected cells. It was evident, however, that the superinfected Daudi cells possess the same antigen as do the Ara-C-treated cells, since the reactivity of the serum to the latter was to a certain extent reduced by absorption with the former. The results indicate that both of the two antigenically different components of MA, the Ara-C-sensitive and the Ara-C-insensitive antigens, occur on superinfected Daudi cells and that on the Ara-C-treated cells, only the Ara-C-insensitive component, and perhaps a small quantity of the Ara-C-sensitive component, occur.

One component of MA that is detectable in superinfected Daudi cells in the presence of Ara-C or PA is 'early' by definition because it appears without synthesis of viral DNA, which is blocked by these inhibitors (Gergely et al., 1971; Yajima et al., 1976). This antigen may correspond to the EMA synthesized in superinfected Raji cells in the presence of Ara-C (Ernberg et al., 1974). That another component of MA occurs on superinfected Daudi cells in the absence of DNA inhibitors was indicated by the marked reduction in the frequency of MA-positive cells in cultures treated with these inhibitors. This component may correspond to the LMA present in VCA-positive cells in producer cell lines (Ernberg et al., 1974).

On the basis of these findings, we attempted to determine the IgG immunoglobulin fraction antibody against the two components of MA in human sera. Two sera, one from a patient with NPC and another from a healthy adult, were titrated for antibody against LMA in superinfected Daudi cells by indirect membrane immunofluorescence. As shown in Figure 1, with the normal serum about 70% of cells were MA-positive in each dilution between 1:10 and 1:80, while further dilutions resulted in lower percentages. The serum from the NPC patient showed a different pattern: percentages of MA-positive cells obtained by reaction with either 1:10 or 1:20 dilutions of the serum were lower than those obtained with higher dilutions, 1:40, 1:80 and 1:160. This pattern resembles the prozone phenomenon seen in general antigen-antibody tests.

We therefore investigated whether the same phenomenon would occur in reactions of LMA with other NPC sera. Sera from five NPC patients and from five normal adults were tested for antibodies against LMA and EMA (Fig. 2). The prozone effect was observed in three out of five NPC sera with LMA but was not seen with EMA. None of the normal sera showed such an effect. It is not yet known why the prozone phenomenon was demonstrated in certain NPC sera and only in reaction with LMA. Further studies are required for confirmation of this phenomenon and for evaluation of its significance in relation to stages of NPC and other EBV-related diseases.

SUMMARY

Investigations were carried out on newly synthesized MA, VCA and EA in Daudi cells superinfected with the P3HR-1 strain of EBV and treated with trypsin to remove previously adsorbed MA-positive material from the cell surface. Synthesis of MA, VCA and EA was completely blocked by puromycin. A marked reduction in the frequency of MA-positive cells was observed in the infected cell cultures in the presence of either Ara-C or PA, but a fraction of the MA-positive cells was insensitive to the inhibitors. Differential absorption of an EBV antibody-positive human serum with Ara-C-treated or -untreated infected cells revealed two antigenically different components of MA: early (Ara-C-insensitive) and late (Ara-C-sensitive) MA. Three of five sera from patients with NPC, but none of five sera from normal adults, showed an apparent 'prozone' phenomenon in their reactivity against late but not early MA.

FIG. 1. REACTIVITY OF TWO HUMAN SERA

Reactivity of two human sera, one normal (VO-7) and one from a patient with nasopharyngeal carcinoma (NPC 32T), with late membrane antigen from superinfected Daudi cells; MA+ - membrane antigen-positive

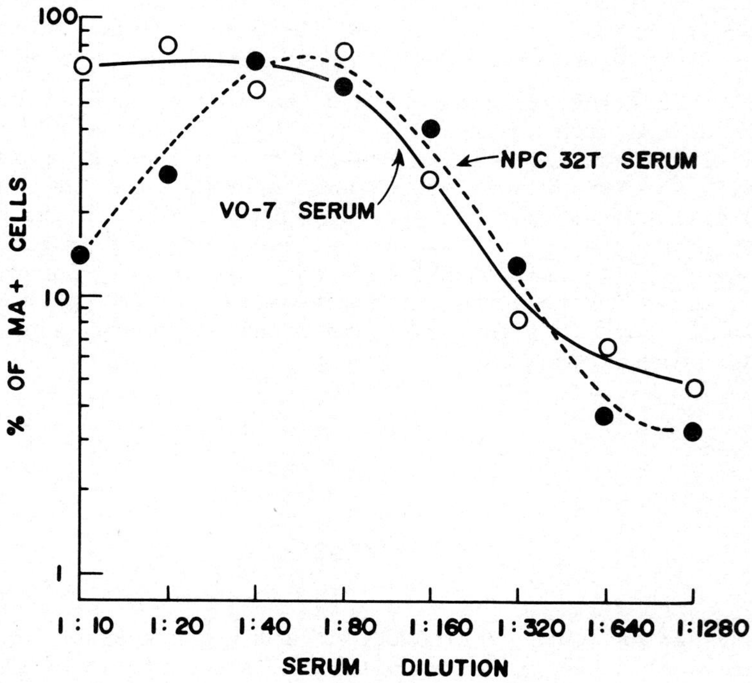

FIG. 2. REACTIVITY OF SERA

Reactivity of sera from normal adults (○) or from patients with nasopharyngeal carcinoma (NPC) (●) with late membrane antigen (LMA) and early membrane antigen (EMA) from superinfected Daudi cells.
MA+ - membrane antigen-positive

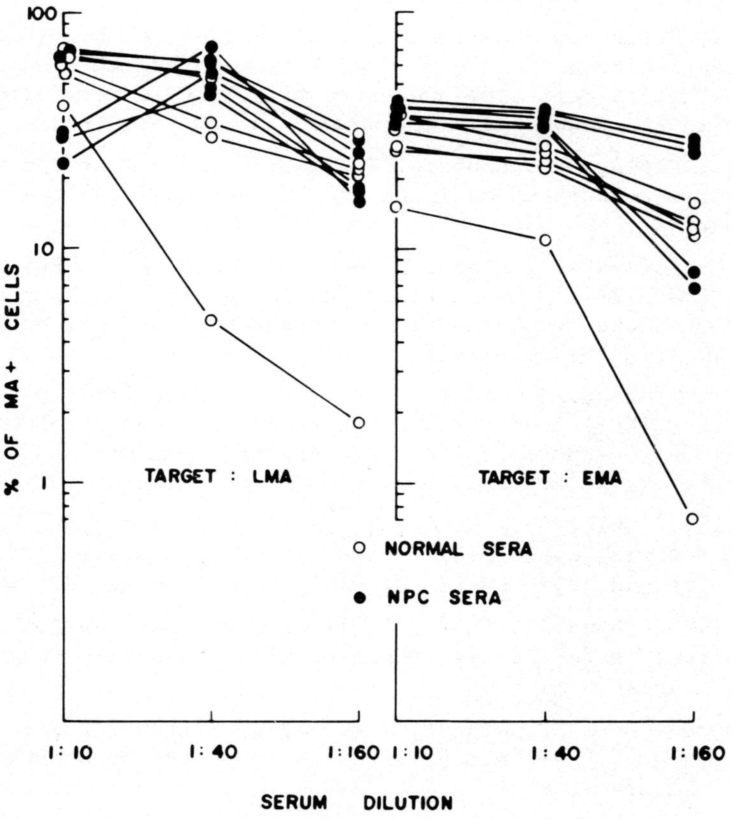

ACKNOWLEDGEMENT

This work was supported by a Grant-in-Aid for cancer research from the Ministry of Education, Science and Culture and the Ministry of Health and Welfare, Japan.

REFERENCES

Dölken, G. & Klein, G. (1976) Expression of Epstein-Barr-virus-associated membrane antigen in Raji cells superinfected with two different virus strains. *Virology*, *70*, 210-213

Ernberg, I., Klein, G., Kourilsky, F.M. & Silvestre, D. (1974) Differentiation between early and late membrane antigen on human lymphoblastoid cell lines infected with Epstein-Barr virus. I. Immunofluorescence. *J. nat. Cancer Inst.*, *53*, 61-65

Gergely, L., Klein, G. & Ernberg, I. (1971) Appearance of Epstein-Barr virus-associated antigens in infected Raji cells. *Virology*, *45*, 10-21

Klein, G., Clifford, P., Klein, E. & Stjernswärd, J. (1966) Search for tumor-specific immune reactions in Burkitt lymphoma patients by the membrane immunofluorescence reaction. *Proc. nat. Acad. Sci. (Wash.)*, *55*, 1628-1635

Klein, G., Dombos, L. & Gothoskar, B. (1972) Sensitivity of Epstein-Barr virus (EBV) producer and non-producer human lymphoblastoid cell lines to superinfection with EB-virus. *Int. J. Cancer*, *10*, 44-57

Pearson, G.R., Henle, G. & Henle, W. (1971) Production of antigens associated with Epstein-Barr virus in experimentally infected lymphoblastoid cell lines. *J. nat. Cancer Inst.*, *46*, 1243-1250

Sairenji, T. & Hinuma, Y. (1975) Ultraviolet inactivation of Epstein-Barr virus: effect on synthesis of virus-associated antigens. *Int. J. Cancer*, *16*, 1-6

Thorley-Lawson, D. & Strominger, J.L. (1976) Transformation of human lymphocytes by Epstein-Barr virus is inhibited by phosphonoacetic acid. *Nature (Lond.)*, *263*, 332-334

Yajima, Y., Tanaka, A. & Nonoyama, M. (1976) Inhibition of productive replication of Epstein-Barr virus DNA by phosphonoacetic acid. *Virology*, *71*, 352-354

HETEROGENEITY OF EPSTEIN-BARR VIRUS DERIVED FROM P3HR-1 CELLS

H. ZUR HAUSEN & K.-O. FRESEN

Institut für Virologie der Universität Freiburg,
Zentrum für Hygiene,
D-7800 Freiburg, Federal Republic of Germany

INTRODUCTION

Infection of cells of the human B lymphoma lines, BJAB and Ramos, with Epstein-Barr virus (EBV) derived from P3HR-1 and B95-8 cells results in conversion of the lymphoma cells to EBV-genome carriers after prolonged cultivation (Fresen & zur Hausen, 1976; Klein et al., 1975). Cells of such sublines express EBNA antigen (Reedman & Klein, 1973) but are usually negative for EB viral structural antigens, such as viral capsid antigen (VCA), or for the early antigen (EA) complex. Only P3HR-1 virus-converted cells reveal a small percentage (less than 0.01%) of EA- and VCA-positive cells (Fresen et al., 1977). The number of EBV-genome equivalents, as determined by nucleic acid hybridization, is low in cells of most of these lines, ranging between 1 and 5 genome copies per converted cell (Fresen et al., 1977).

In the course of these studies, different EBNA patterns were observed when EBNA-positive cells from P3HR-1 virus-converted lines were compared with those from B95-8 virus-converted cells (Fresen & zur Hausen, 1976; Fresen et al., 1977). Whereas B95-8 virus-converted cells revealed uniformly brilliant EBNA expression, the pattern in P3HR-1 virus-converted BJAB and Ramos cells was much more heterogeneous: apart from a few brilliantly stained nuclei, a faintly granular nuclear pattern predominated. These differences in EBNA expression were suggestive of heterogeneity in the infecting P3HR-1 virus, and further experiments were devised in order to study this possibility.

The results are summarized below; detailed experimental data are reported elsewhere (Fresen & zur Hausen[1]; Fresen et al., 1977; zur Hausen & Fresen, 1977).

RESULTS

Cloning experiments

Individual P3HR-1 virus-converted BJAB cells were isolated with a capillary tube and were placed into microplate wells containing a feeder layer of embryonic human fibroblasts. Cloning efficiency under these conditions was 30-40%. The results of these experiments are summarized in Figure 1.

FIG. 1. CLONING OF BJA-B1 CELLS CONVERTED TO EBNA EXPRESSION BY PRIOR INFECTION WITH EBV DERIVED FROM P3HR-1 CELLS

F (faintly granular), B (brilliant) and FB (heterogeneous, F and B) expression characterize the EBNA patterns observed. The empty circles indicate the segregation of EBNA-negative cells.

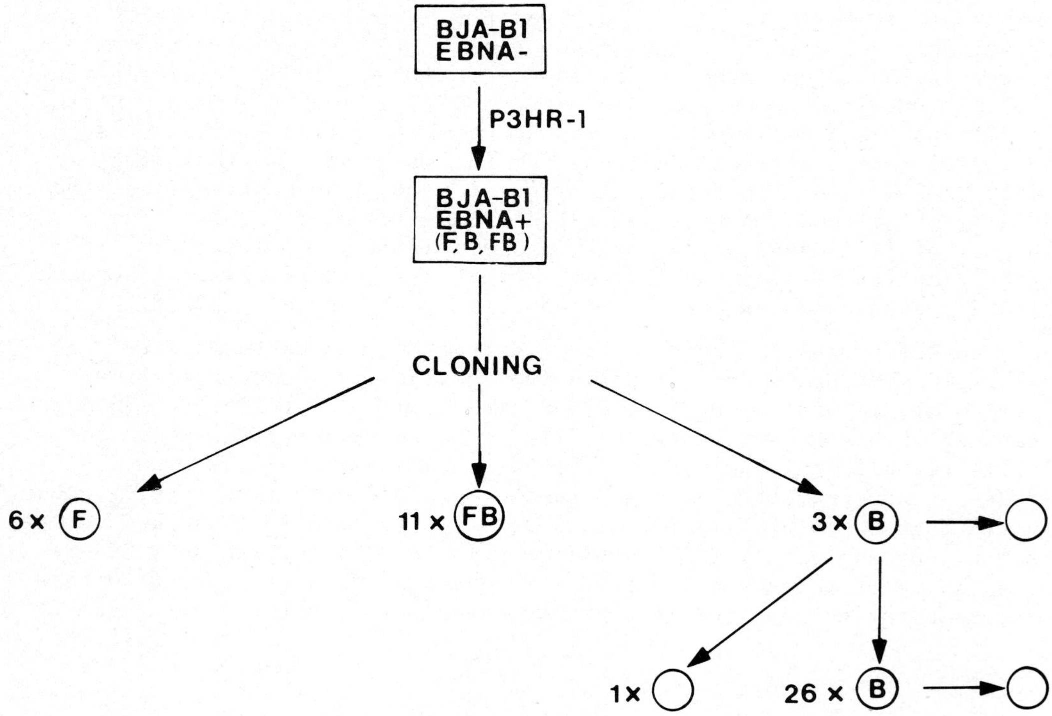

[1] Unpublished data

Twenty of these cloned sublines were analysed for EBNA expression: 11 showed the heterogeneous pattern of the parental converted line; six clones were obtained in which almost 100% of the cells exhibited only the faintly granular EBNA pattern; and in three clones, the cells showed brilliant EBNA expression, although 20-40% of the cells were EBNA-negative.

Subcloning of one of the lines showing brilliant EBNA expression (B1) resulted in 27 subclones. Except for one of these all revealed the same EBNA pattern as the parental clone: 30-80% were brilliantly EBNA-positive, and a corresponding percentage were EBNA-negative. The exceptional subclone (B1-28) showed no detectable EBNA expression. The data indicate that in these subclones brilliant EBNA expression accompanies segregation of EBNA-negative cells.

Nucleic acid hybridization

The EBV DNA content of EBV-converted lines and sublines was determined by reassociation kinetics (Fresen et al., 1977). Ramos and BJAB cells converted by B95-8 virus contained only a small number of EBV-genome copies, ranging between 1 and 2 genome equivalents per cell. In contrast, cells of the P3HR-1 virus-converted BJAB lines, and their clones and subclones, contained multiple EBV-genome copies per cell, ranging between 10 and 35 equivalents per cell. These data must be viewed with some reservation, however, about 0.01% of the P3HR-1 virus-converted cells synthesized EA and VCA. The P3HR-1 virus-converted Ramos cells contained only 1-2 genome equivalents.

No evidence for the presence of viral DNA was found in the B1-28 subclone that was negative for EBNA expression. These data indicate that the segregation of EBNA-negative cells in the clones showing brilliant EBNA expression is due to loss of viral DNA.

Induction of early antigens

EA was induced in BJAB and Ramos cells, as well as in their converted sublines, the faintly granular EBNA-expressing BJA-HRIK clone A 5, the brilliantly EBNA-expressing clone B 1-19 and the EBNA-negative subclone B 1-28 and in Raji cells by infecting them with EBV from P3HR-1 and B95-8 cells (zur Hausen & Fresen, 1977).

Under these conditions, EA induction by P3HR-1 virus increased by an average of 14-fold in cells containing EBV genome when compared with EBV-negative lines: EBNA induction in the latter ranged from 0.15-0.4%, and EBNA-positive lines showed between 1.04 and 6.15% EA-positive cells.

B 95-8 virus, which, it was previously reported, did not induce EA in human lymphoblasts (Miller et al., 1975), induced EA only in P3HR-1 virus-converted cells and, to a small extent, in Raji cells. EA induction was particularly significant in the A 5 clone (faintly granular EBNA expression), whereas cells of the brilliantly EBNA-expressing B 1-19 clone did not show increased EA synthesis. B 95-8 virus-converted cells were not induced to EA production by B 95-8 virus.

The kinetics of EA induction were investigated after infection of EBV genome-positive and -negative cells with various dilutions of P3HR-1 virus. EA induction was found to be directly proportional to the dilution of the infecting virus in EBV-genome-positive cells; and in EBV-genome-free cells, EA induction was reduced by the square of the dilution factor, thus following second-order kinetics. These data indicate that resident genomes complement superinfecting genomes in inducing EA and that two different populations of genomes present in P3HR-1 virus isolates are required for EA induction after infection of B lymphoblasts.

DISCUSSION

Infection of BJAB and Ramos cells with EBV of different origins leads to conversion of these cells to EBV-genome carriers. This system permits a first biological approach to the analysis of possible heterogeneities of EB viral preparations after cloning of the converted cells (Fresen & zur Hausen, 1976). After infection of these cells with P3HR-1 virus and subsequent cloning, two patterns of EBNA expression were observed: some clones uniformly revealed a faintly granular pattern, and another group of clones expressed brilliant EBNA staining. The latter group segregated varying percentages of EBNA-negative cells (Fresen et al., 1977). This suggests a labile association of viral DNA with the host-cell genome and emphasizes the intracellular heterogeneity of the P3HR-1 virus.

In nucleic acid hybridization experiments, EBNA expression was strictly correlated with the presence of EBV DNA. We were unable to correlate the intensity of EBNA fluorescence with the number of genome copies. Cells converted by B95-8 virus revealed brilliant EBNA expression, despite the presence of only 1-2 EBV genome copies per cell (Fresen et al., 1977). A subclone of EBNA-negative cells from P3HR-1 virus-converted BJAB cells contained no detectable concentrations of EBV DNA. The segregation of EBNA-negative cells apparently results from loss of viral DNA.

The heterogeneity of EBV genomes in P3HR-1 cells was underlined by studies of EA induction. The presence of EBV genomes substantially enhanced EA induction, when compared with EA induction of EBV-negative cells infected under the same conditions. Infection of the converted clones with B95-8 virus resulted in EA induction only in cells of the faintly granular EBNA-expressing A 5 clone and in those of the non-cloned parental line (BJA-HR 1 K). No EA induction was observed in the brilliantly EBNA expressing clone B1-19. A small but significant EA induction was shown in Raji cells after B95-8 virus infection. These data suggested a specific interaction of B95-8 viral DNA with one subpopulation of EBV molecules of the P3HR-1 virus mixture.

Complementation of EA induction following superinfection was clearly demonstrated by studying the kinetics of this induction after infecting EBNA-positive and EBNA-negative cells with various dilutions of the

P3HR-1 virus. EA induction in genome-positive cells followed first-order kinetics, but in EBNA-negative cells a reduction occurred according to second-order kinetics. This finding implies that P3HR-1 cells contain two populations of complementary genomes.

It remains to be established whether the observed heterogeneity of P3HR-1 virus also occurs in cells of other lines that contain EBV. Preliminary data suggest that cells of at least two additional lines contain heterogeneous EBV populations. The existence of complementary EB viral molecules in cells from human tumours could help to explain open questions concerning the pathogenesis of EBV-associated diseases.

SUMMARY

Infection of cells of the EBV-free human B-lymphoma lines BJAB and Ramos resulted in conversion of these cells to EBV-genome carriers expressing EBNA. EBV isolates from P3HR-1 cells induced a heterogeneous EBNA pattern: both a faintly granular pattern and brilliant EBNA-expression were observed. The two types of EBNA-expressing cells could be separated upon cloning. Brilliantly EBNA-expressing cells always segregated varying percentages of EBNA-negative cells. An EBNA-negative subclone derived from these cells was devoid of detectable EBV DNA. Nucleic acid hybridization experiments failed to reveal a correlation between the intensity of EBNA expression and the number of EBV genome equivalents per cell. EBV genome-containing cells had an average of 14-fold more cells showing EA synthesis after superinfection by P3HR-1 virus, when compared with EBNA-negative cells infected under identical conditions. Studies on the kinetics of EA induction in EBNA-positive and EBNA-negative cells indicate that complementation is required for the induction of EA after superinfection.

ACKNOWLEDGEMENTS

The excellent technical assistance of Mrs G. Menzel and Mrs M. Zeissler is gratefully appreciated. This work was supported by the Deutsche Forschungsgemeinschaft (SFB 118, Erlangen: 'Methodenforschung zur Früherkennung des Krebses').

REFERENCES

Fresen, K.O. & zur Hausen, H. (1976) Establishment of EBNA-expressing cell lines by infection of Epstein-Barr virus (EBV)-genome-negative human lymphoma cells with different EBV strains. *Int. J. Cancer, 17*, 161-166

Fresen, K.O., Merkt, B., Bornkamm, G.W. & zur Hausen, H. (1977) Heterogeneity of Epstein-Barr virus originating from P3HR-1 cells. I. Studies on EBNA induction. *Int. J. Cancer, 19*, 317-323

Klein, G., Giovanella, B., Westman, A., Stehling, J.S. & Mumford, D. (1975) An EBV-genome-negative cell line established from an American Burkitt lymphoma; receptor characteristics, EBV infectability and permanent conversion into EBV-positive sublines by *in vitro* infection. *Intervirology, 5*, 319-334

Miller, G., Robinson, J., Heston, L. & Lipman, M. (1975) *Differences between laboratory strains of Epstein-Barr virus based on immortalization, abortive infection and interference.* In: de-Thé, G., Epstein, M.A. & zur Hausen, H., eds, *Oncogenesis and Herpesviruses, II, Part 1 (IARC Scientific Publications No. 11)*, Lyon, pp. 395-408

Reedman, B.M. & Klein, G. (1973) Cellular localization of an Epstein-Barr virus-associated complement-fixing antigen in producer and non-producer lymphoblastoid cell lines. *Int. J. Cancer, 11*, 499-520

zur Hausen, H. & Fresen, K.O. (1977) Heterogeneity of Epstein-Barr virus. II. Induction of early antigens (EA) by complementation. *Virology* (in press)

EXPRESSION OF LATENT EPSTEIN-BARR VIRUS GENOMES IN HUMAN EPITHELIAL/BURKITT'S LYMPHOBLASTOID HYBRID CELLS

M. NONOYAMA & A. TANAKA

Laboratory of Molecular Virology,
Life Sciences Biomedical Research Institute, Inc.,
St. Petersburg, Fla 33710, USA

R. GLASER

Department of Microbiology and Special Cancer Research Center,
The Milton S. Hershey Medical Center,
Pennsylvania State University,
Hershey, Pa 17033, USA

Epstein-Barr virus (EBV) is suspected of inducing nasopharyngeal carcinoma (NPC) (zur Hausen et al., 1970), and epithelial cells from these tumours contain EBV genomes (Wolf et al., 1973). It has not, however, been possible to establish an NPC cell line, nor can any available monolayer cell line be infected with EBV. EBV infects only B lymphocytes from human and non-human primates *in vitro*; thus, hybrid cell lines obtained by fusion between monolayer cells and EBV genome-carrying B lymphocytes serve as a unique model system for studying the role of EBV genomes in carcinoma cells.

Raji cells were established from African Burkitt's lymphomas; they contained 50 EBV genomes per cell but were non-virus producing. HR-1 cells, also established from African Burkitt's lymphomas, were virus producing. Both Raji and HR-1 cells were successfully fused with D98 cells, a variant of HeLa cells, and the resulting hybrids have been maintained as monolayer cells in HAT selective medium for several years (Glaser & O'Neill, 1972). Each hybrid cell line, after being cloned in soft agar, contained EBV genomes in various amounts and was inducible for EBV antigens and virus particles by treatment with iododeoxyuridine (IUDR) (Glaser et al., 1973).

In Table 1, the pattern of IUDR induction of virus antigens is compared with virus DNA replication in each cell line. Cells were

Table 1. Early antigen (EA) and viral capsid antigen (VCA) formation, virus DNA replication and virus genome transcription in cells treated with IUDR

	Control				IUDR, 3 days on				IUDR, 3 days on and 3 days off			
Cell line	EA	VCA	Virus DNA replication	% Virus genome transcribed	EA	VCA	Virus DNA replication	% Virus genome transcribed	EA	VCA	Virus DNA replication	% Virus genome transcribed
Raji	-	-	-	25	+	-	-	30	+	-	-	50
D98/Raji	-	-	-	23	+	-	-	30	+	+	+	50
D98/HR-1	-	-	-	25	+	-	-	30	+	+	ND	50

ND - not determined

treated with 60 μg/ml IUDR for three days at 37°C and then maintained in normal medium for an additional three days. Viral capsid antigen (VCA) and early antigen (EA) were detected by indirect immunofluorescence tests,and virus DNA replication was examined by cRNA hybridization. All of the cell lines, Raji, D98/Raji and D98/HR-1, showed EA immediately after treatment with IUDR. No VCA was detected at that time but was obtained in hybrid, but not in Raji, cells three days after they were transferred to normal medium. Virus DNA replication was also inhibited in Raji cells. The data indicate that only the early functions of EBV genomes were expressed in Raji cells after IUDR induction; virus DNA replication and VCA formation were inhibited, possibly by a cellular control mechanism of Raji cells which disappeared after hybridization with D98 cells (Glaser & Nonoyama, 1974).

DNA-RNA hybridization kinetic studies were conducted on the above system to determine the extent of virus genome transcription in each cell line under the various conditions. Highly labelled virus DNA (3×10^6 cpm/μg) was obtained by superinfection of Raji cells with HR-1 EBV in the presence of H^3-thymidine (Tanaka et al., 1976) and was mixed with a large excess of cellular RNA. The mixture was then denatured and reannealed at 66°C. The amount of DNA-RNA hybrid was determined by S-1 nuclease, a single-stranded, specific nuclease. Self-hybridization of H^3-DNA at the end of the reaction was approximately 20% in each sample, and the value was corrected for the DNA-RNA hybridization kinetics. Percent transcription of virus DNA (α) and the fraction (a) of virus mRNA in total cellular RNA used were calculated from the equation of $D/D_o = \alpha(1 - e^{kaR_ot})$ (Frenkel & Roizman, 1972), where D_o and D are the total and hybridized amounts of virus DNA, respectively, k is a kinetic constant, R_o is total RNA used in the reaction, and t is time required for the hybridization.

Figure 1 is a typical graphical presentation of DNA-RNA hybridization kinetics for virus-specific mRNA in Raji cells either treated or not with IUDR. Untreated Raji cells already contained some virus-specific mRNA, which was transcribed from 25% of total virus DNA. The amount of virus mRNA increased slightly after three days' treatment with IUDR, but the obvious induction of virus genome transcription occurred only after transfer to fresh medium, where transcription of virus DNA reached 50%, indicating that the entire virus genome was transcribed.

FIG. 1. TRANSCRIPTION OF EBV GENOMES IN RAJI CELLS

RNA obtained from Raji cells was reacted with H^3-EBV DNA as described in the text; the amount of DNA-RNA hybrid was measured by S-1 nuclease, and the percentage was plotted, by use of a computer, against total RNA used in the reaction (R_o) x time required for the hybridization (t).

△: RNA from untreated cells

◇: RNA from cells treated with IUDR

⬡: RNA from cells treated with IUDR, followed by incubation in fresh medium

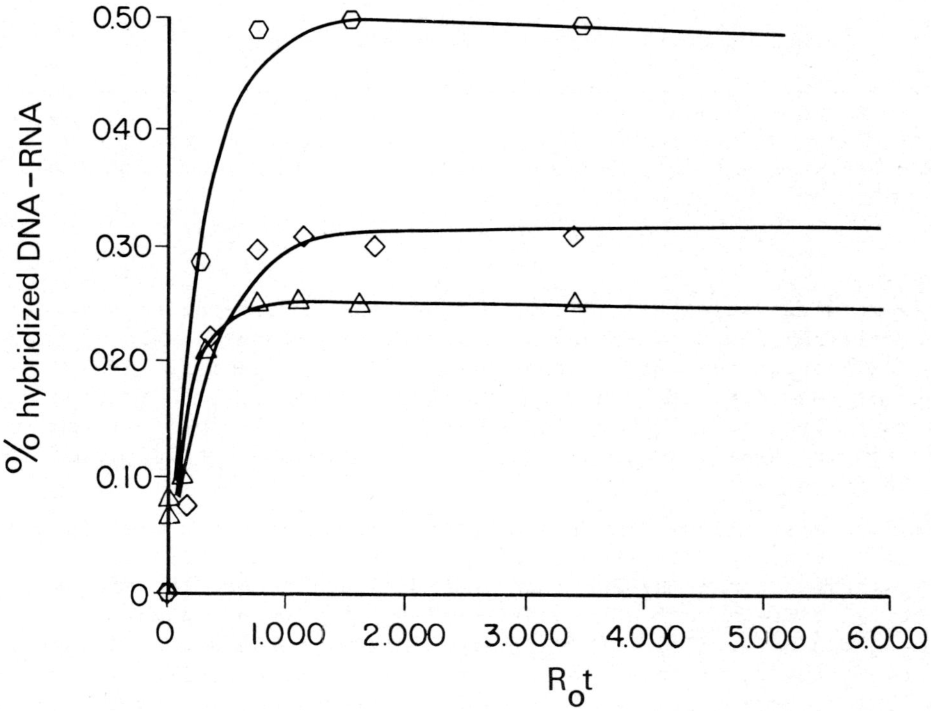

Similar results were obtained in D98/Raji and D98/HR-1 cells, with and without IUDR treatment (Table 2). Latent virus genomes were transcribed in every cell line at the level of 25%, and treatment with IUDR slightly increased the transcription level. When the treated cells were transferred to fresh medium, all of the virus genes were transcribed.

Table 2. Correlation between number of EBV genomes per cell and amount of virus RNA in the cells

Cell line	IUDR	n^a	Ratio		Genomes/cell[b]
Raji	none	5.30×10^{-3}	1	1	50
	3 days on	2.64×10^{-3}	0.50		
	on and off	2.82×10^{-3}	0.53		
D98/Raji	none	1.50×10^{-3}	1	0.28	17
	3 days on	9.10×10^{-4}	0.60		
	on and off	8.80×10^{-4}	0.59		
D98/HR-1	none	7.45×10^{-4}	1	0.14	7
	3 days on	6.30×10^{-4}	0.80		
	on and off	4.06×10^{-3}	5.40		

[a] n (= ka) was shown from the equation, $D/Do = \alpha (1-e^{kaR_o t})$ (Frenkel & Roizman, 1972).

[b] The number of genome equivalents per cell was obtained by cRNA hybridization, as described by Nonoyama & Pagano (1971).

The results indicate that latent virus DNA is controlled similarly in the original lymphocytes and in the hybrid cells and that treatment with IUDR induces complete transcription of virus genomes. The absence of VCA formation and virus DNA replication in IUDR-treated Raji cells must, therefore, be attributed to a post-transcriptional control present in the cells; this effect was eliminated by hybridization with D98 cells.

Table 2 also allows comparison of the amount of virus mRNA in the cells and the number of virus genomes per cell. The total amounts of virus mRNA found in D98/Raji and D98/HR-1 cells were 28% and 14%, respectively, of those found in Raji cells, whereas the number of virus genomes per cell in D98/Raji and D98/HR-1 cells were 34% and 14%, respectively, of those in Raji cells (50 genomes/cell). The linear relationship between the amount of virus-specific RNA and the number of virus genomes per cell suggests that every copy of the latent virus genomes may participate in the transcription of virus mRNA.

SUMMARY

Expression of latent Epstein-Barr virus genomes in somatic-cell hybrids of Burkitt's lymphoblastoid cells has been studied. Treatment of the hybrid cells, D98/Raji and D98/HR-1, with IUDR induced the formation of EA and VCA and replication of virus DNA, whereas the same treatment of Raji cells induced only the formation of EA. The patterns of transcription of virus genomes in these three cell lines were, however, very similar: 25% without treatment with IUDR, 30% immediately after the treatment and 50% (entire genome transcription) three days after being transferred to fresh medium. The amount of virus RNA in the cells, calculated from DNA-RNA hybridization kinetics, was proportional to the number of virus genomes per cell, suggesting that every copy of virus DNA in these cells is actively transcribed.

ACKNOWLEDGEMENTS

We thank Dr B. Roizman, who let us use his computer for the calculation of DNA-RNA hybridization kinetics, and Mr T. Bibb, Ms M. Whitman and Ms J. Gorodecki for their technical assistance. This work was supported by grants CA 21665-01 and CA 15038 from the National Institutes of Health, USA, and by contracts NO 1 CP 53516 and NO 1 CP 33250 within the Virus Cancer Program of the National Cancer Institute, USA.

REFERENCES

Frenkel, N. & Roizman, B. (1972) Ribonucleic acid synthesis in cells infected with herpes simplex virus: controls of transcription and of RNA abundance. *Proc. nat. Acad. Sci. (Wash.)*, *69*, 2654-2658

Glaser, R. & Nonoyama, M. (1974) Host cell regulation of induction of Epstein-Barr virus. *J. Virol.*, *14*, 174-176

Glaser, R., Nonoyama, M., Decker, B. & Rapp, F. (1973) Synthesis of Epstein-Barr virus antigens and DNA in activated Burkitt somatic cell hybrids. *Virology, 55*, 62-69

Glaser, R. & O'Neill, F.J. (1972) Hybridization of Burkitt lymphoblastoid cells. *Science, 176*, 1245-1247

Nonoyama, M. & Pagano, J.S. (1971) Detection of Epstein-Barr viral genome in non-productive cells. *Nature (New Biol.), 233*, 103-106

Tanaka, A., Miyagi, M., Yajima, Y. & Nonoyama, M. (1976) Improved production of Epstein-Barr virus DNA for nucleic acid hybridization studies. *Virology, 74*, 81-85

Wolf, H., zur Hausen, H. & Becker, V. (1973) EB viral genomes in epithelial nasopharyngeal carcinoma cells. *Nature (New Biol.), 244*, 245-247

zur Hausen, H., Schulte-Holtehausen, H., Klein, G., Henle, W., Henle, G., Clifford P. & Samtessen, L. (1970) EBV DNA in biopsies of Burkitt tumors and anaplastic carcinomas of the nasopharynx. *Nature (Lond.), 228*, 1056-1058

DETECTION AND QUANTITATION OF ADENOVIRUS TYPE 12 TRANSFORMING DNA SEGMENTS AND THEIR APPLICATION IN ETIOLOGICAL STUDIES OF HUMAN NEOPLASIA

K. FUJINAGA, S. YANO, S. OJIMA & Y. SAWADA

Department of Molecular Biology,
Cancer Research Institute Sapporo Medical College,
Sapporo 060, Japan

INTRODUCTION

The oncogenic capacity of DNA viruses lies in a small region of the viral genome, the transforming segment, and cells can be transformed by this segment when it is isolated from the viral DNA molecule (Graham et al., 1974; Shiroki et al., 1977; Yano et al., 1977a). Cell lines transformed by DNA tumour viruses often contain only a part of the viral genome, the portion including the transforming segment; yet they can synthesize virus-specific mRNA and virus-specific proteins (Flint et al., 1976; Fujinaga & Green, 1966; Fujinaga et al., 1974; Levinson & Levine, 1977; Levinson et al., 1976; Ortin & Doerfler, 1975; Ortin et al., 1976; Sambrook et al., 1974). This indicates that the isolated DNA segment with oncogenic capacity can provide an appropriate and sensitive probe for detecting viral genomes in tumour cells. Detection of the transforming segment in cellular DNA is thus important in investigations of the viral etiology of tumours, including human cancers. In this communication, we discuss a method for the detection and quantitation of the transforming DNA sequence of adenovirus type 12 (Ad 12) and its significance in etiological studies of human neoplasia.

ISOLATION AND PURIFICATION OF Ad 12 TRANSFORMING DNA SEGMENTS

Restriction endonucleases *Eco*RI (EndoR·*Eco*RI) and *Hin*dIII (EndoR·*Hin*dIII) cleave the Ad 12 DNA molecule into six (A∿F) and 16 (A∿O) specific fragments, respectively; cleavage maps have been made of the Ad 12 DNA molecule after exposure to these enzymes (Mulder et al., 1974; Ortin et al., 1976; Yano & Fujinaga[1]; Yano et al., 1977a). Yano et al. (1977a) and Shiroki et al. (1977) have located the transforming gene(s) at the left-hand end of the molecule, in the *Eco*RI-C and in the *Hin*dIII-G regions.

Ad 12 DNA was digested with *Eco*RI or *Hin*dIII, and the *Eco*RI-C or the *Hin*dIII-G fragment was separated from other DNA fragments by electrophoresis on 1.4% agarose gel and eluted electrophoretically (Yano et al., 1977b). The *Eco*RI-C or the *Hin*dIII-G fragment was further purified by extraction with phenol and chloroform-isoamylalcohol, as described previously (Yano et al., 1977b). Preparations of *Eco*RI-C (16% of the viral genome) and *Hin*dIII-G (7.2% of the viral genome) thus obtained showed transforming ability in a clonal rat embryo cell line, 3Y1, and several transformed cell lines were established by these DNA fragments (Shiroki et al., 1977; Yano et al., 1977a). In the experiments described below, the *Eco*RI-C and *Hin*dIII-G fragments thus isolated, purified and identified as transforming segments were used to detect and quantitate Ad 12 transforming genes in tumour and transformed cells.

DETECTION AND QUANTITATION OF VIRAL DNA SEQUENCES IN RAT CELL LINES TRANSFORMED BY *Eco*RI-C OR *Hin*dIII-G FRAGMENTS OF Ad 12 DNA

Rat cell lines transformed by the *Eco*RI-C (CY-1) or the *Hin*dIII-G fragment (GY-1) synthesize T antigen and induce tumours in rats (Shiroki et al., 1977). Viral DNA sequences were also shown to be present in these cells (Shiroki et al., 1977; Yano et al., 1977a). DNA from CY-1 and GY-1 cells was prepared by the phenol-chloroform-isoamylalcohol method, as described elsewhere (Fujinaga et al., 1973) and was further purified by Sephadex G-50 column chromatography. DNA-DNA reassociation of ^{32}P-labelled *Eco*RI fragments of Ad 12 DNA was carried out in the presence or absence of unlabelled cellular DNA isolated from transformed rat cells.

As shown in Figure 1, cellular DNA from CY-1 cells accelerated reassociation of the *Eco*RI-C fragment only; no acceleration was observed in the reassociation reactions of any of the other five *Eco*RI fragments (Fig. 2), indicating that these fragments do not occur in CY-1 cells (less than a half copy per haploid cell DNA quantity, if any). That only part of the *Eco*RI-C sequence is present in CY-1 cells was suggested by the fact that the reassociation reaction of ^{32}P-labelled *Eco*RI-C fragments in the presence of CY-1 cell DNA (see plot in Fig. 1) deviates from linearity (Fujinaga et al., 1974).

[1] Unpublished data

FIG. 1. REASSOCIATION OF ^{32}P-LABELLED *Eco*RI FRAGMENTS (A-F) OF ADENOVIRUS TYPE 12 (Ad 12) DNA IN THE PRESENCE OF CALF THYMUS DNA AND CY-1 CELLULAR DNA

^{32}P-labelled Ad 12 DNA (3.27×10^5 cpm/μg) was cleaved with *Eco*RI, and the resulting six DNA fragments were separated and purified as described in the text. Each reaction mixture contained 212 μg/ml of either calf thymus DNA (●) or CY-1 cellular DNA (○) and labelled probes of fragment A (3.36×10^{-3} μg/ml), fragment B (2.80×10^{-3}μg/ml), fragment C (2.50×10^{-3} μg/ml), fragment D (2.01×10^{-3} μg/ml), fragment E 2.44×10^{-3} μg/ml) or fragment F (2.50×10^{-3} μg/ml). Reassociation reactions were carried out at 68°C in 0.4 M phosphate buffer at pH 6.8, and DNA was quantitated by batch elution from hydroxyapatite (Yano et al., 1977a).

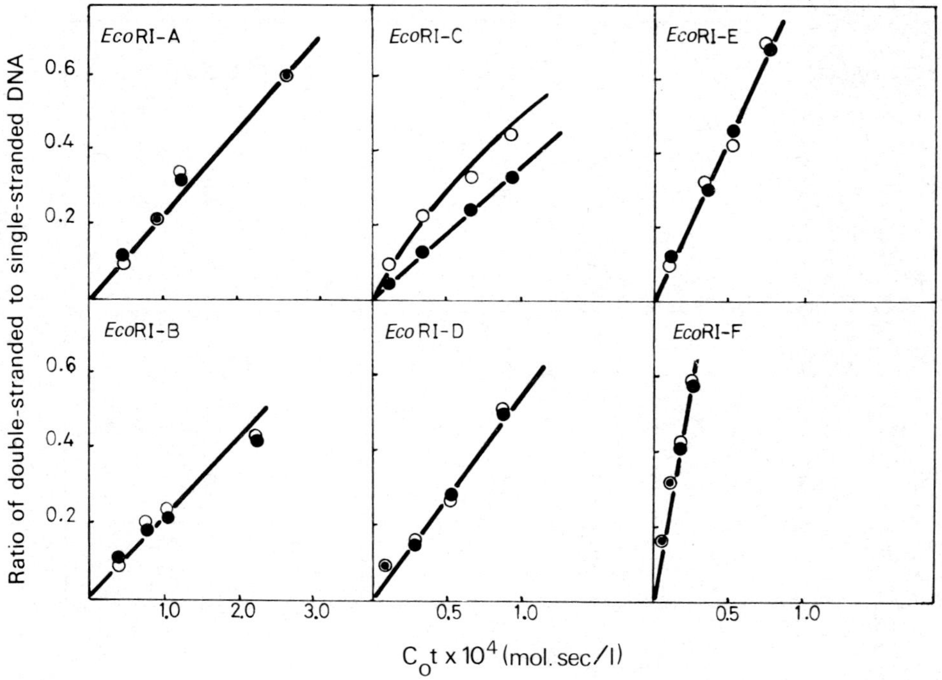

A further, detailed analysis of viral DNA sequences in CY-1 cells was performed, using smaller-sized fragments as probes (Yano et al., 1977a). CY-1 cellular DNA increased the reassociation rate of ^{32}P-labelled *Hin*dIII-G and *Hin*dIII-I in the *Eco*RI-C fragment. Reassociation kinetics showed the presence of most, if not all, of the entire *Hin*dIII-G sequence, with 1.69 copies per haploid cell DNA quantity; on the other hand, only a part of the *Hin*dIII-I fragment was indicated in these cells. A portion of

FIG. 2. REASSOCIATION OF ^{32}P-LABELLED *Hin*dIII-G FRAGMENT OF ADENOVIRUS TYPE 12 DNA IN THE PRESENCE OF DNA OF VARIOUS ORIGINS

Reassociation of ^{32}P-labelled *Hin*dIII-G fragment (3.96×10^5 cpm/μg, 2.75×10^{-3} μg/ml) of adenovirus type 12 DNA in the presence of calf thymus DNA and DNA from either W-3, Raji, P3HR-1, NC37, acute myelogenous leukaemic cells (AML) or normal human spleen (NHS). Five hundred microliters of reaction mixture (0.4 M sodium phosphate, pH 6.8) contained 267 μg/ml calf thymus DNA (●) or DNA from various cell lines or tissues (○), each sheared sonically and heat denatured. Reassociation was carried out at 68°C and stopped after various periods. Single- and double-stranded DNA was quantitated by batch elution from hydroxyapatite (Yano & Fujinaga, unpublished data).

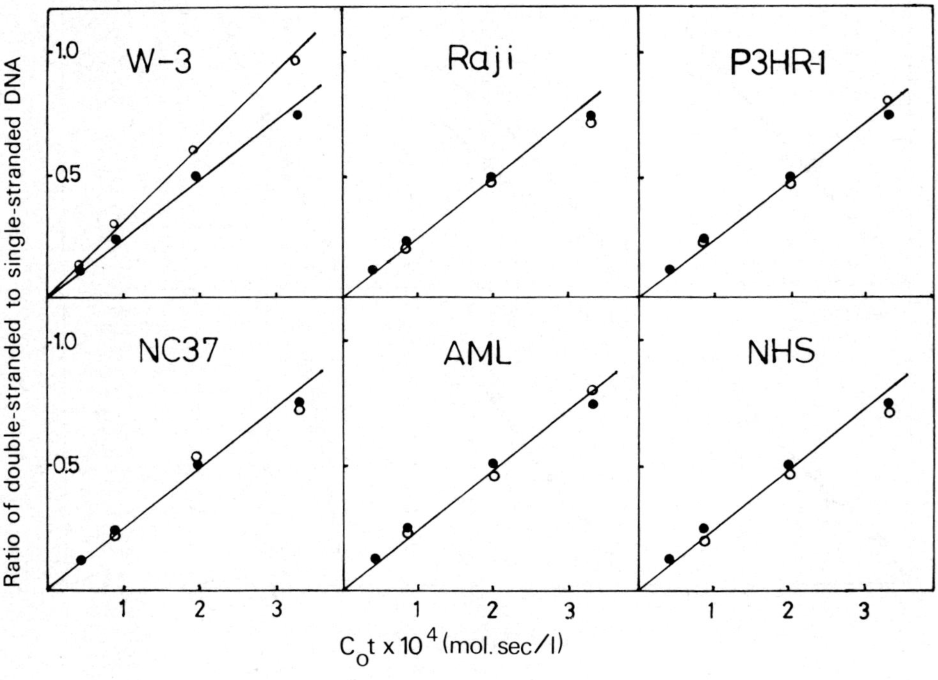

the *Hin*dIII-G sequence was demonstrated in DNA from GY-1 cells, 3Y-1 cells transformed by the *Hin*dIII-G fragment of Ad 12 DNA, using ^{32}P-labelled

*Hin*dIII-G fragments as the probe (Shiroki et al., 1977). The sequence of *Hin*dIII-I, the fragment mapped adjacent to *Hin*dIII-G, was absent from the cell (less than one half copy per haploid cell DNA quantity).

We do not yet know whether all of the viral DNA sequences in these cells are present at a single and specific site in cellular DNA in the form of a tandem array. Further studies are now in progress.

ABSENCE OF Ad 12 TRANSFORMING GENE(S) IN CERTAIN HUMAN NEOPLASIAS

The experiments described above show that transforming gene(s) of Ad 12 exist in the *Hin*dIII-G fragment of the viral DNA molecule, which represents only 7.2% of the left end of the molecule. Moreover, all of the cell lines transformed by Ad 12 virion or by Ad 12 DNA fragments contain this portion of the viral DNA molecule (Green et al., 1976; Yano & Fujinaga[1]; Yano et al., 1977). This indicates that the *Hin*dIII-G fragment of Ad 12 DNA that contains transforming gene(s) will, when isolated, provide one of the most appropriate probes for investigating the Ad 12 viral etiology of tumours.

The ^{32}P-labelled *Hin*dIII-G fragment of Ad 12 DNA was isolated and purified from viral DNA, labelled *in vivo* as described previously, and used to detect Ad 12 transforming gene(s) by DNA-DNA reassociation techniques. As shown in Figure 2 and in Table 1, the Ad 12 transforming gene sequence was readily detected in Ad 12 transformed rat cells (W-3) by an acceleration of the reassociation rate of the *Hin*dIII-G fragment. No such sequence was found in Burkitt's lymphoma cell lines (Raji and P3HR-1), in KB cells, in cells from patients with acute myelogenous leukaemia and in normal cells (NC37) and tissues (normal human spleen, hamster embryo, AKR mouse embryo, Fischer rat embryo). Using *Hin*dIII-G fragment nick-translated *in vitro* and labelled with α-^{32}P-dATP and α-^{32}P-dCTP as described by Green et al. (1976), no Ad 12 transforming gene sequence could be detected in Raji cells, in P3HR-1 cells, in normal human spleen or in cells from patients with chronic myelogenous leukaemia or monocytic leukaemia (Fig. 3, Table 2).

Since Ad 31 DNA has transforming DNA sequences homologous to those of Ad 12 DNA (Fujinaga et al., 1977), the absence of Ad 12 transforming genes from the DNA of the human tumour cells studied suggests that neither Ad 12 nor Ad 31 is a major cause of these human neoplasias. Recently, a similar analysis (Mackey et al., 1976), using the *Eco*RI-C fragment of Ad 12 DNA as a probe, provided evidence that Ad 12 plays no role in the etiology of human gastrointestinal tumours.

Tumour cells and cells transformed by DNA tumour viruses often contain only a part of the viral genome, the portion including the transforming gene(s), and its detection and quantitation in tumour cell DNA provides evidence for or against a possible etiological role of the

[1] Unpublished data

Table 1. Absence of *Hin*dIII-G fragment of adenovirus 12 (Ad 12) DNA in certain types of human neoplasia[a]

Cell line or tissue[b]	Increased rate factor	*Hin*dIII-G copies per haploid cell DNA quantity[c]
Raji	0.959	< 0.5
P3HR-1	1.021	< 0.5
NC37	0.959	< 0.5
Acute myelogenous leukaemic cells	0.968	< 0.5
Normal human spleen	0.968	< 0.5
KB	0.968	< 0.5
Hamster embryo	0.968	< 0.5
Mouse (AKR) embryo	0.979	< 0.5
Rat (Fischer) embryo	0.979	< 0.5
W-3[d]	1.191	2.1
Salmon sperm	1.000	-

[a] From Yano & Fujinaga, unpublished data

[b] Samples contained 266 μg/ml DNA and 2.32 ng/ml ^{32}P-labelled *Hin*dIII-G fragment of Ad 12 DNA isolated from viral DNA labelled *in vivo* as described in the legend to Figure 2

[c] Calculated from the increased rate factor, using values of 2.0×10^{12} daltons for the molecular weight of haploid cell DNA and 1.7×10^{6} daltons for the molecular weight of *Hin*dIII-G fragment

[d] Rat cells transformed by Ad 12

virus in a human neoplasia. In the case of the larger herpes viruses, including Epstein-Barr virus which has genomes weighing 10^{8} daltons, transforming gene(s) might represent only one percent or so of the whole viral genome; the approach described herein could thus provide a very powerful and important investigatory tool.

Table 2. Absence of *Hin*dIII-G fragment of adenovirus 12 (Ad 12) DNA in certain types of human neoplasia[a]

Expt	Cell line or tissue	DNA (mg/ml)	*Hin*dIII-G[b] (ng/ml)	Increased rate factor	*Hin*dIII-G copies per haploid cell DNA quantity[c]
1	P3HR-1	2.15	4.13	1.18	<0.5
	CML[d]	2.06	4.13	1.05	<0.5
	GY-1[e]	2.10	4.13	11.0	positive[f]
	Calf thymus	2.02	4.13	1.00	-
2	ML[g]	1.98	3.64	1.131	<0.5
	Raji	2.01	3.64	1.176	<0.5
	Normal human spleen	2.01	3.64	1.090	<0.5
	W-3[h]	2.05	3.64	2.246	2.7
	Calf thymus	2.02	3.64	1.000	-

[a] From Sawada & Fujinaga, unpublished data

[b] ^{32}P-labelled *Hin*dIII-G fragment of Ad 12 DNA prepared by *in vitro* nick-translation after purification as described in the legend to Figure 3

[c] Calculated from the increased rate factor, using values of 2.0 x 10^{-2} daltons for the molecular weight of haploid cell DNA and 1.7 x 10^6 daltons for the molecular weight of *Hin*dIII-G fragment

[d] Leukaemic cell DNA from a patient with chronic myelogenous leukaemia

[e] Rat cell line transformed by Ad 12 *Hin*dIII-G fragment

[f] Only a portion of the *Hin*dIII-G fragment was present; further, detailed analysis is required for an accurate estimation.

[g] Leukaemic cell DNA from a patient with monocytic leukemia

[h] Rat cells transformed by Ad 12

SUMMARY

The oncogenic capacity of the tumour virus lies in a small region of the viral genome, and tumour cells and cells transformed by DNA tumour viruses often contain only a part of the viral genome, the portion including the transforming gene(s). The detection and quantitation of these gene(s) in tumour cell DNA can provide evidence for or against a possible etiological role of the virus in human neoplasia. In this communication, the isolation, purification and identification of the transforming segment of Ad 12 are described.

FIG. 3. REASSOCIATION OF NICK-TRANSLATED ^{32}P-*Hin*dIII-G FRAGMENT OF ADENOVIRUS 12 DNA IN THE PRESENCE OF DNA OF VARIOUS ORIGINS

Reassociation of nick-translated ^{32}P-*Hin*dIII-G fragment of adenovirus 12 DNA in the presence of DNA from calf thymus, W-3, monocytic leukaemia cells, Raji or normal human spleen. Twenty microliters of reaction mixture (0.4 M sodium phosphate, pH 6.8) contained 3.64 ng/ml labelled nick-translated fragment (1.00×10^7 cpm/μg) and 2.0 mg/ml calf thymus DNA (●), W-3 (○), monocytic leukaemia cells (△), Raji (□) or normal human spleen (+). Reassociation was carried out at 68°C and stopped after various periods, followed by the batchwise quantitation of single- and double-stranded DNA on hydroxyapatite (Sawada & Fujinaga, unpublished data).

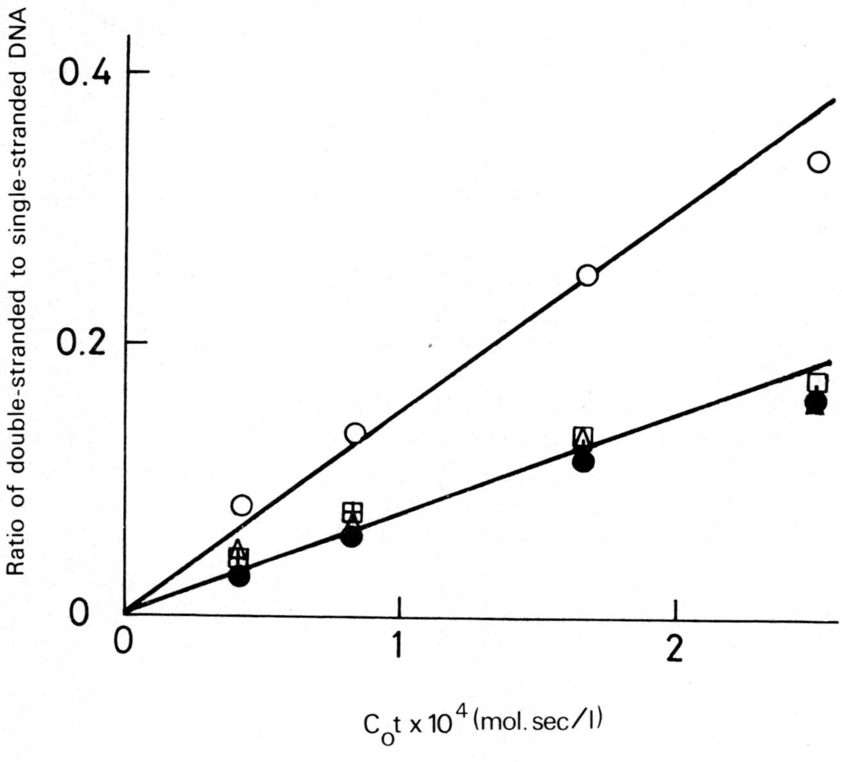

No detectable Ad 12 transforming gene sequence was found in cellular DNA from several types of human neoplasia, using labelled transforming DNA sequences, the *Hin*dIII-G fragment from labelled viral DNA or the nick-translated *Hin*dIII-G fragment as a probe.

ACKNOWLEDGEMENTS

We thank Dr T. Osato, Hokkaido University School of Medicine, for providing lymphoblastoid cell lines and Drs I. Urushizaki and K. Kikuchi, Sapporo Medical College, for providing clinical material. We also thank Dr Y. Ito, Faculty of Medicine, Kyoto University, for his critical reading of the manuscript. This work was supported in part by grants from the Ministry of Education, Science and Culture, Japan and from the Princess Takamatsu Fund for Cancer Research.

REFERENCES

Flint, S.J., Sambrook, J., Williams, J.F. & Sharp, P.A. (1976) Viral nucleic acid sequences in transformed cells. IV. A study of the sequences in transformed cells in four lines of adenovirus 5-transformed rodent cells using specific fragments of the viral genome. *Virology, 72*, 456-470

Fujinaga, K. & Green, M. (1966) The mechanism of viral carcinogenesis by DNA mammalian viruses: virus specific RNA in polysomes of adenovirus tumor and transformed cells. *Proc. nat. Acad. Sci. (Wash.), 55*, 1565-1574

Fujinaga, K., Rankin, A., Yamazaki, H., Sekikawa, K., Bragdon, J. & Green, M. (1973) RD-114 virus:analysis of viral gene sequences in feline and human cells by DNA-DNA reassociation kinetics and RNA-DNA hybridization. *Virology, 56*, 484-495

Fujinaga, K., Sekikawa, K., Yamazaki, H. & Green, M. (1974) Analysis of multiple viral genome fragments in adenovirus 7 transformed hamster cells. *Cold Spring Harbor Symp. Quant. Biol., 39*, 633-636

Fujinaga, K., Ojina, S., Yano, S. & Shinagawa, M. (1977) The transforming DNA sequence common to highly oncogenic human adenoviruses Type 12, 18 and 31. *Proc. Japan. Acad., 53* (in press)

Graham, F.L., Abrahams, P.J., Mulder, C., Heijnecker, H.L., Warnaar, S.O., de Vries, F.A.J., Fiers, W. & van der Eb, A.J. (1974) Studies on *in vitro* transformation by DNA and DNA fragments of human adenoviruses and simian virus 40. *Cold Spring Harbor Symp. Quant. Biol. 39*, 637-650

Green, M.R., Chinnadurai, G., Mackey, J.K. & Green, M. (1976) A unique pattern of integrated viral genes in hamster cells transformed by highly oncogenic human adenovirus 12. *Cell*, *7*, 419-428

Levinson, A.D., Levine, A.J., Anderson, S., Osborn, M., Rosenwirth, B. & Weber, K. (1976) The relationship between group C adenovirus T antigen and the adenovirus single-strand DNA binding protein. *Cell*, *7*, 575-584

Levinson, A.D. & Levine, A.J. (1977) The isolation and identification of the adenovirus group C tumor antigens. *Virology*, *76*, 1-11

Mackey, J.K., Rigden, P.M. & Green, M. (1976) Do highly oncogenic group A human adenoviruses cause human cancer? Analysis of human tumors for adenovirus 12 transforming DNA sequences. *Proc. nat. Acad. Sci. (Wash.)*, *73*, 4657-4661

Mulder, C., Sharp, P.A., Delius, H. & Pettersson, U. (1974) Specific fragmentation of DNA of adenovirus serotype 3, 5, 7 and 12 and adeno-simian virus 40 hybrid virus Ad2+ ND1 by restriction endonuclease *Eco*RI. *J. Virol.*, *14*, 68-77

Ortin, J. & Doerfler, W. (1975) Transcription of the genome of adenovirus type 12. I. Viral mRNA in abortively infected and transformed cells. *J. Virol.*, *15*, 27-35

Ortin, J., Scheiatmann, K.-H., Greenberg, R., Westpahl, M. & Doerfler, W. (1976) Transcription of the genome of adenovirus type 12. III. Maps of stable RNA from productively infected human cells and abortively infected and transformed hamster cells. *J. Virol.*, *20*, 355-372

Sambrook, J., Botchan, M., Gallimore, P., Ozane, B., Pettersson, U., Williams, J. & Sharp, P.A. (1974) Viral DNA sequences in cells transformed by simian virus 40, adenovirus type 2 and adenovirus type 5. *Cold Spring Harbor Symp. Quant. Biol.*, *39*, 615-632

Shiroki, K., Handa, H., Shimojo, H., Yano, S., Ojima, S. & Fujinaga, K. (1977) Establishment and characterization of rat cell lines transformed by restriction endonuclease fragment of adenovirus 12 DNA. *Virology*, *82* (in press)

Yano, S., Ojima, S., Fujinaga, K., Shiroki, K. & Shimojo, H. (1977a) Transformation of a rat cell line by the adenovirus type 12 DNA fragment. *Virology*, *82* (in press)

Yano, S., Tsuchida, N. & Fujinaga, K. (1977b) Analysis of DNA from adenovirus 12-transformed cells for virus-specific DNA sequences with viral DNA fragments cleaved with restriction endonuclease. *Gann*, *68*, 107-114

INTERACTION BETWEEN EPSTEIN-BARR VIRUS AND TYPE-C VIRUS IN HUMAN CELLS

T. OSATO, K. YAMAMOTO, T. MATSUO & T. AYA

Department of Virology,
Cancer Institute,
Hokkaido University School of Medicine,
Sapporo 060, Japan

F. MIZUNO

Department of Bacteriology,
Asahikawa Medical College,
Asahikawa 071-01, Japan

M. NONOYAMA

Life Sciences, Inc.,
St Petersburg, Fla 33710, USA

The oncogenic potential in man of Epstein-Barr virus (EBV) has been well established by observation of *in vitro* conversion of normal lymphocytes into lymphoblasts with infinite replicative capabilities (Miller, 1974).

The present paper concerns the significance of possible cofactor(s) that influence EBV oncogenesis, as shown by investigations of the interaction between EBV and type-C virus in human lymphoid cells, which confirm and extend our previous work (Osato et al., 1975b).

FVNC CELL LINE

The experimental system in which our interaction studies were carried out was a human lymphoid FVNC cell line, shown in Figure 1. The FVNC cell line was established in our laboratory several years ago

FIG. 1. FVNC CELLS OF LYMPHOID MORPHOLOGY
GIEMSA x 620

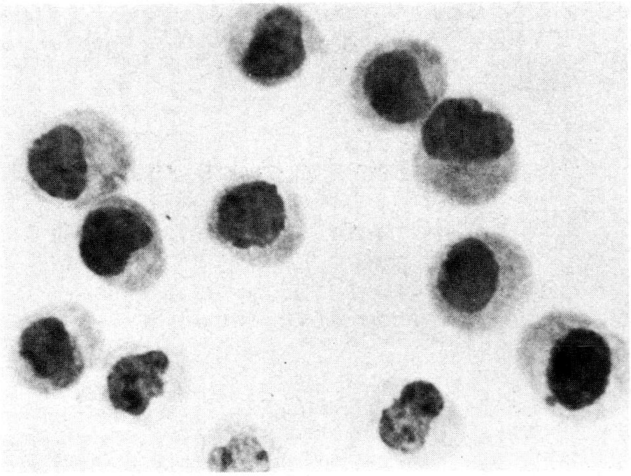

by exposing EBV genome-positive human lymphoid NC-37 cells to type-C Friend murine leukaemia virus (Osato et al., 1975a). As shown in Table 1 and Figure 2, the FVNC cells contained only one or two EBV genomes per cell, in contrast to NC-37 cells which had 80 copies;

Table 1. Occurrence of Epstein-Barr virus (EBV) genomes and Epstein-Barr virus nuclear antigen (EBNA) in FVNC and NC-37 cells

Cells	cpm/50 μg cell DNA[a]	No. of EBV genomes/cell	% EBNA-positive cells[b]
FVNC	103	$\leqslant$ 2	100
NC-37	3215	80	100

[a] cRNA-DNA hybridization

[b] Anticomplement immunofluorescence, stained with EBV-positive serum from a normal person

however, all FVNC and NC-37 cells were intensely positive for EBV-determined nuclear antigen (EBNA) (Osato et al., 1975b). FVNC cells were free of EBV-related early antigen (EA) immunofluorescence and murine type-C virus group-specific antigen (GSA) immunofluorescence;

FIG. 2. EPSTEIN-BARR VIRUS NUCLEAR ANTIGEN IN FVNC CELLS

All cells are intensely stained with Epstein-Barr virus-positive serum from a normal person. Anticomplement immunofluorescence x 620

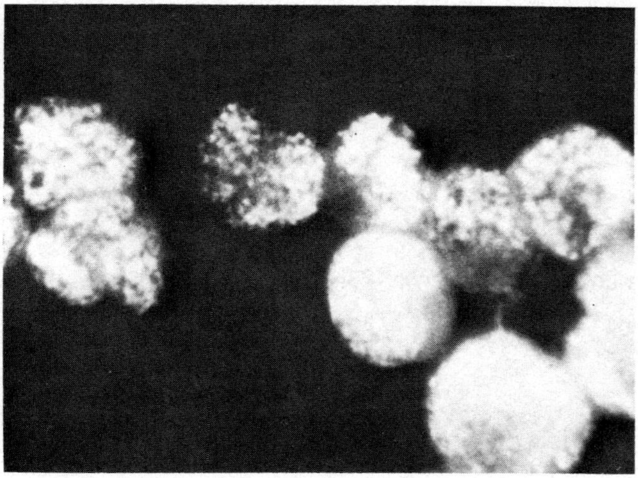

however, 5-iododeoxyuridine (IUDR) treatment resulted in both EA and GSA synthesis in all clones, indicating that each individual FVNC cell contains not only EBV but also type-C viral genome in a repressed form (Osato et al., 1975a).

SENSITIVITY OF FVNC CELLS TO SUPERINFECTION WITH EBV

As described above, FVNC cells contain very few EBV genomes, although as a result of type-C virus infection NC-37 cells from which they are derived contain a large number of EBV copies. Moreover, individual FVNC cells contains a repressed type-C viral genome, in addition to EBV. It was therefore considered to be of interest to examine the sensitivity of FVNC cells to EBV superinfection and to compare them with control NC-37 cells. When FVNC cells and NC-37 cells were exposed to EBV, three to four times more EA-positive cells were observed in infected FVNC, as observed by indirect immunofluorescence and stained with serum from a nasopharyngeal carcinoma patient (Table 2). This suggests that FVNC cells are much more sensitive than NC-37 cells in their response to EBV exposure (Osato et al., 1975b).

Table 2. Induction of Epstein-Barr virus early antigen (EA)-positivity in FVNC and NC-37 cells by superinfection with Epstein-Barr virus

Days after superinfection[a]	% EA-positive cells[b]	
	FVNC	NC-37
2	28.9	9.1
4	35.5	11.2
7	25.8	6.3
10	10.9	3.9

[a] EBV inoculum was obtained from P3HR-1 cells.

[b] Indirect immunofluorescence, stained with serum from a patient with nasopharyngeal carcinoma

TYPE-C VIRAL INDUCTION IN FVNC CELLS FOLLOWING EBV SUPERINFECTION

It was considered of further interest to see whether or not the repressed type-C viral genome in FVNC cells could be activated by exposure to EBV. The results are shown in Table 3, in which induction of murine GSA immunofluorescence as revealed by murine P30 antiserum, is evident (Osato et al., 1975b).

Table 3. Induction of type-C virus, as demonstrated by group-specific antigen (GSA) immunofluorescence, in FVNC and NC-37 cells by superinfection with Epstein-Barr virus

Days after superinfection[a]	% GSA-positive cells[b]	
	FVNC	NC-37
2	16.5	0
4	17.9	0
7	8.6	0

[a] EBV inoculum was obtained from P3HR-1 cells.

[b] Indirect immunofluorescence, stained with Rauscher leukaemia virus P30 antiserum

EBV INDUCTION IN FVNC CELLS BY EXPOSURE TO TYPE-C VIRUS

Although no significant GSA synthesis was evident in non-producer FVNC cells, we have recently isolated a clone that spontaneously produces type-C virus, as shown by P30 immunofluorescence and reverse transcriptase assay. Figures 3a and 3b illustrate EBNA and GSA immunofluorescence, stained differentially with rhodamine and fluorescein, respectively, in the same microscopic field. When FVNC cells

FIG. 3. CLONED FVNC CELLS THAT SPONTANEOUSLY PRODUCE TYPE-C VIRUS, POSITIVE FOR BOTH EPSTEIN-BARR VIRUS NUCLEAR ANTIGEN (EBNA) AND GROUP-SPECIFIC ANTIGEN (GSA)

(a) EBNA, stained with EBV-positive serum from a normal person, followed by tetramethyl-rhodamine isothiocyanate-labelled antibody x 620

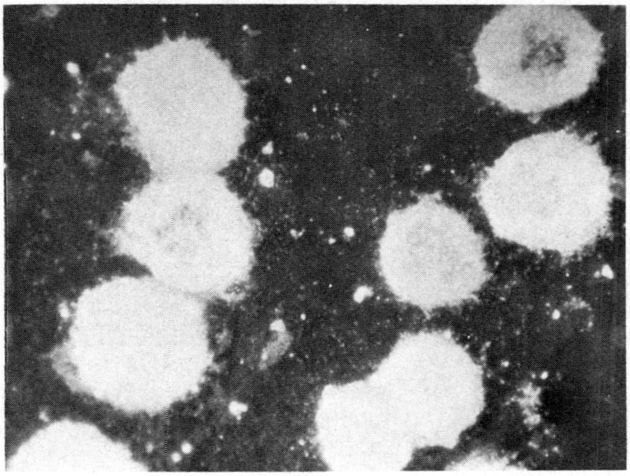

(b) GSA, stained with Rauscher type-C murine leukaemia virus P30 antiserum, followed by fluorescein isothiocyanate-labelled antibody x 620

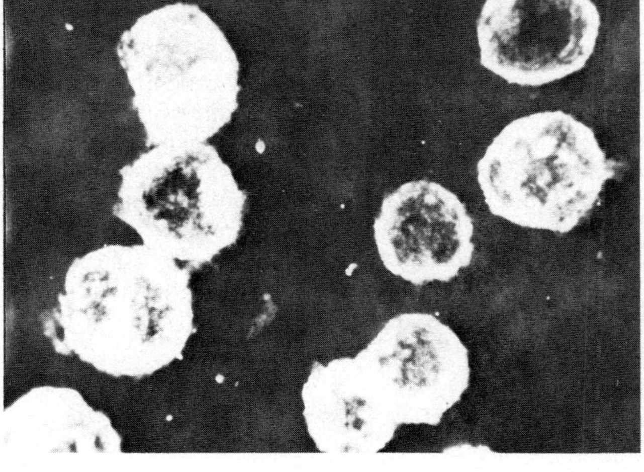

were exposed to type-C virus grown in the producer clone, a high frequency of induction of EBV-related early nuclear antigen, which we call ENA (Sugawara & Osato, 1973), was evident (Fig. 4), as detected by indirect immunofluorescence. ENA induction was also seen in control NC-37 cells, but at a much lower frequency.

FIG. 4. HIGH-FREQUENCY INDUCTION OF EPSTEIN-BARR VIRUS-RELATED EARLY NUCLEAR ANTIGEN IN FVNC CELLS BY EXPOSURE TO TYPE-C VIRUS

Stained with Epstein-Barr virus-positive serum from a normal person; indirect immunofluorescence x 300

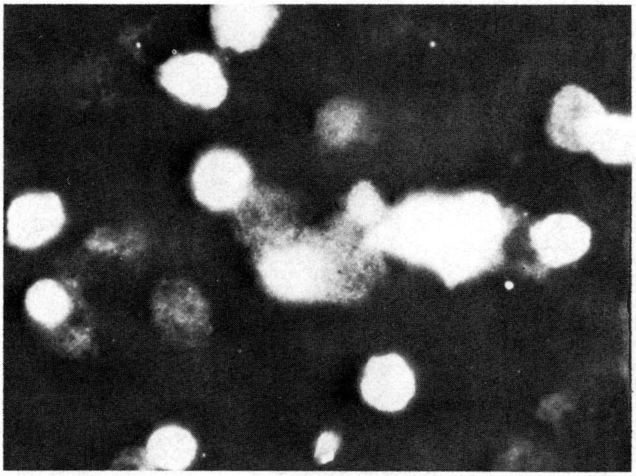

DIFFERENTIAL ASSOCIATION OF EBV AND TYPE-C VIRAL GENOMES WITH FVNC CELL CHROMOSOMES

In view of the responsiveness of FVNC cells to exposure to these viruses, we thought it worthwhile to investigate the association of EBV and type-C viral genomes with FVNC cell chromosomes. We used the method of human-mouse somatic-cell hybridization, in which a preferential and random loss of human chromosomes generally occurs. After hybrids between FV5 (clonal line of FVNC cells) and MCB-2 (clonal line of mouse MCB fibroblasts[1]) had been established, a number of clones that still retained a small number of various human chromosomes were isolated, and immunofluorescence investigations were carried out. The results showed that 15 of 19 hybrid clones were positive for both EBV and GSA immunofluorescence, two clones were EBNA- but not GSA-positive; and the remaining two were EBNA-negative but positive for GSA. No GSA immunofluorescence was detected in control sets, such as in IUDR-treated mouse MCB-2 cells and in IUDR-treated hybrid NC-37/MCB-2 cells. These data suggest

[1] Yamamoto et al., unpublished data

that the repressed EBV and type-C viral genomes may be associated with different chromosomes in FVNC human lymphoid cells.

DISCUSSION

The present findings confirm our previous results (Osato et al., 1975a, b), which showed that human lymphoid FVNC cells containing both repressed EBV and type-C viral genomes are remarkably sensitive to EBV superinfection, and that EBV exposure results in an obvious induction of type-C viral expression in such human cells. Similar investigations have been carried out recently, in which herpes simplex virus was used to activate endogenous murine type-C virus (Hampar et al., 1976).

Very recently, the resident EBV genome was found to be significantly activated by exposure to type-C virus grown for several years in human lymphoid FVNC cells; this is most probably a xenotropic murine type-C virus. Such EBV induction by 'human cell-adapted' type-C virus may be important, although these results are still preliminary. The high frequency of EBV induction in FVNC cells, as compared with NC-37 cells, may reflect an altered EBV-human lymphoid cell interaction due to their coexistence with type-C viral genomes; this would be compatible with the high sensitivity of FVNC cells to superinfection by EBV.

Our findings thus suggest that the high responsiveness of FVNC cells to exposure either to EBV or to type-C virus can probably be attributed to certain unstable conditions in the FVNC cells, in which two different oncogenic virus genomes are present in a repressed form (Osato et al., 1975b). In this respect, the differential association of EBV and type-C viral genomes with FVNC cell chromosomes may be of interest. Further investigations are in progress to clarify the interaction between EBV and type-C viruses in individual human lymphoid cells.

SUMMARY

The interaction between EBV and type-C viruses was studied in our FVNC experimental system, in which EBV and type-C viral genomes are contained in each cell. The data indicate that the human lymphoid FVNC cells are sensitive to both EBV and type-C virus exposure, showing high frequencies of induction of both repressed viral genomes. The two different viral genomes may be associated with different chromosomes in individual cells.

ACKNOWLEDGEMENTS

We thank Dr Y. Ikawa of the Cancer Institute, Tokyo, Japan, and Dr G.R. Pearson of the Mayo Clinic/Foundation, Rochester, Minn., USA, for supplying P30 antiserum, and Drs K. Fujinaga and Y. Yamazaki, Sapporo Medical College, for the reverse transcriptase assay. We also thank Miss J. Kusajima and Miss T. Izumi for assistance. This work was supported in part by grants from the Japanese Ministry of Education, Science and Culture, the Japanese Ministry of Health and Welfare, the Princess Takamatsu Cancer Research Fund and the Japanese Medical Association.

REFERENCES

Hampar, B., Aaronson, S.A., Derge, J.G., Chakrabarty, M., Showalter, S. D. & Dunn, C.Y. (1976) Activation of an endogenous mouse type-C virus by ultraviolet-irradiated herpes simplex virus types 1 and 2. *Proc. nat. Acad. Sci. (Wash.)*, *73*, 646-650

Miller, G. (1974) The oncogenicity of Epstein-Barr virus. *J. infect. Dis.*, *130*, 187-205

Osato, T., Yamamoto, K., Mizuno, F., Sugawara, K., Aya, T. & Sonta, S. (1975a) *Dual persistence of Epstein-Barr viral and type-C viral genomes in nonproducer human lymphoblastoid cells*. In: Ito, Y. & Dutcher, R.M., eds, *Comparative Leukemia Research 1973*, Tokyo, University of Tokyo Press, pp. 585-588

Osato, T., Mizuno, F., Yamamoto, K. & Nonoyama, M. (1975b) *Alteration in Epstein-Barr virus-human lymphoid cell interactions caused by the presence of type-C viral genome*. In: de-Thé, G., Epstein, M.A. & zur Hausen, H., eds, *Oncogenesis and Herpesviruses II, Part 2 (IARC Scientific Publications No. 11)*, Lyon, pp. 27-35

Sugawara, K. & Osato, T. (1973) Immunofluorescence antigen associated with Epstein-Barr virus induced by 5-iododeoxyuridine. *Nature (New Biol.)*, *246*, 72-73

DISCUSSION SUMMARY

W. HENLE

The Joseph Stokes, Jr Research Institute
at The Children's Hospital of Philadelphia
and Medical School,
University of Pennsylvania
Philadelphia, Pa., USA

Discussion centred on three areas:

(1) Since infectious mononucleosis is virtually unknown in regions of the world where primary Epstein-Barr virus infections occur in the population at an early age, it has been assumed that such childhood infections mostly remain silent. It was pointed out, however, that this might be an erroneous conclusion, since illnesses induced by Epstein-Barr virus at an early age might be lost among the numerous illnesses of the upper respiratory tract that children suffer annually; these could be detected only if Epstein-Barr virus-specific serodiagnostic and heterophil antibody tests were performed. Pertinent studies should be pursued.

(2) It was claimed that Caucasian nasopharyngeal carcinoma patients cannot be differentiated by Epstein-Barr virus-specific serology from patients with carcinomas elsewhere in the head and neck region. These remarks unleashed a prolonged discussion. Firstly, the need for uniform histopathological classification of the tumours was further stressed, since the association with Epstein-Barr virus seems largely to be limited to undifferentiated carcinomas of the nasopharynx. Secondly, Caucasian nasopharyngeal carcinoma patients seen at the Mayo Clinic showed serological patterns comparable with those seen in Chinese and African cases. It was pointed out further that it is essential to distinguish between antibodies to the two components of the early antigen complex: the dominant antibody in nasopharyngeal carcinoma is anti-D, which often reaches high titres, whereas antibodies to

the early antigen complex in other carcinomas are mostly of low titres and are usually directed against R. Finally, it was emphasized that differentiations must be made between nasopharyngeal carcinoma patients before and after treatment, between the stages of the disease at the time of serum collection, the period that has elapsed since initiation of therapy and the presence in long-term survivors of residual or recurrent tumour activity or of disease. This is important because untreated patients in stage I of the disease or treated patients who have shown no evidence of disease for several years may have spectra and titres of antibodies to Epstein-Barr virus-related antigens that are not readily distinguishable from those seen in healthy donors who had primary infections long before. If nasopharyngeal carcinoma patients are not subgrouped according to the above criteria, the distinct serological features of advanced cases of nasopharyngeal carcinoma become obscured. It must also be realized that the persistent viral carrier state which regularly follows primary Epstein-Barr virus infections can be activated by immunosuppressive diseases or by therapy, leading to enhanced anti-viral capsid antigen titres and often also to re-emergence of anti-early antigen. It has long been known, therefore, that Epstein-Barr virus-related serology alone is insufficient to establish an association of Epstein-Barr virus with a given malignancy and that additional evidence is required.

The demonstration of Epstein-Barr virus DNA, which provides such additional evidence, has been limited thus far to cases of Burkitt's lymphoma and nasopharyngeal carcinoma. Several reported exceptions were subsequently found to be due to mixing up of specimens. The limitation has been confirmed in a large series of biopsies, reported here, and by another extensive study carried out by Ho, in which a search was made for Epstein-Barr nuclear antigen-positive carcinoma cells in touch preparations from numerous biopsies of head-and-neck tumours. Such cells were found only in cases of undifferentiated nasopharyngeal carcinoma and carcinomas of the nasal fossa and not in moderately well-differentiated carcinomas of the nasopharynx nor in other carcinomas of the head and neck region.

(3) Several reports clearly indicate that undifferentiated carcinoma cells from nasopharyngeal carcinoma biopsies contain complete viral genomes. Cultured Epstein-Barr nuclear antigen-positive nasopharyngeal carcinoma cells can be maintained in culture for only a

few weeks during this period; some of them can be induced, by exposure to IdU, to synthesize early antigen, viral capsid antigen and virus particles. It is most important now to establish permanent lines of nasopharyngeal carcinoma cells, as well as cultures of the normal epithelial progenitors of the carcinoma cells, so as to study in detail the biological and molecular events involved in the transformation of the epithelial cells by Epstein-Barr virus, the role of the viral genome in the maintenance of the malignant state and the properties of virus rescued from nasopharyngeal carcinoma cells.

ETIOLOGY OF NASOPHARYNGEAL CARCINOMA – IMMUNOLOGICAL FACTORS

EPSTEIN-BARR VIRUS-RELATED SEROLOGY IN NASOPHARYNGEAL CARCINOMA AND CONTROLS

W. HENLE & G. HENLE

Division of Virology,
The Joseph Stokes, Jr Research Institute
at The Children's Hospital of Philadelphia
and Medical School,
University of Pennsylvania,
Philadelphia, Pa 19174, USA

J.H.C. HO

The Institute of Radiology,
Queen Elizabeth Hospital,
Kowloon, Hong Kong

INTRODUCTION

The first clue that suggested an association of Epstein-Barr virus (EBV) with anaplastic or poorly differentiated nasopharyngeal carcinoma (NPC) was provided by Old et al. (1966, 1968), who observed that sera from NPC patients often yielded one or more lines of precipitation in immunodiffusion tests with concentrated extracts of Burkitt's lymphoma cells from EBV-producing cultures. This observation was rapidly substantiated, using the indirect immunofluorescence technique for detection and titration of antibodies to EB viral capsid antigen (VCA) (Henle & Henle, 1966; Henle et al., 1966). Sera from NPC patients in various parts of the world were consistently found to contain antibodies to VCA at titres which, as a rule, substantially exceeded those observed in healthy control groups or in patients with malignant tumours of the head and neck region other than NPC (de Schryver et al., 1969, 1972; de-Thé et al., 1973, 1975; Henle & Henle, 1968; Henle et al., 1968, 1970a, 1973; Kawamura et al., 1970; Lin et al., 1972, 1973; Lynn et al., 1973a, b). While the majority of patients with malignant tumours of the postnasal space other than NPC or carcinomas elsewhere in the head and neck region had anti-VCA titres within the range observed in healthy controls, slightly more high anti-VCA titres were noted among such patients as compared to controls. NPC patients differed from these two control groups also by an increased incidence and concentration of antibodies to EBV-determined cell membrane antigens (MA) (de Schryver et al., 1969, 1972).

Since the initial studies, two groups of EBV-coded antigens, in addition to VCA and MA, have been identified by immunofluorescence techniques, i.e., (1) EBV-induced early antigens (EA) (Henle et al., 1970b; Hinuma et al., 1971), which are subdivided into D (diffuse) and R (restricted) components on the basis of immunofluorescence patterns and their resistance to methanol fixation (Henle et al., 1971); and (2) the EBV-associated nuclear antigen (EBNA), which is detectable only by the sensitive anticomplement immunofluorescence technique (Reedman & Klein, 1973). In turn, methods for detection and titration of the corresponding antibodies have been developed (see Henle et al., 1974). Furthermore, differentiation of VCA- or EA-specific IgG, IgM or IgA antibodies in indirect immunofluorescence tests with fluorescein isothiocyanate-conjugated antibodies to the appropriate human immune globulin classes has provided additional parameters for the study of EBV-associated diseases.

ANTIBODIES TO EBV-RELATED ANTIGENS IN NPC PATIENTS AND CONTROLS

Application of the whole series of EBV-related antibody tests has revealed a number of remarkable serological features of NPC patients as compared to healthy controls, patients with other EBV-associated diseases (infectious mononucleosis, Burkitt's lymphoma) or patients with various malignant or non-malignant diseases that are not considered to be EBV-associated but that due to their immunosuppressive effects may lead to activation of persistent viral infections and, concomitantly, to an over-representation of high anti-VCA titres and of anti-EA reactions as compared to controls (Henle & Henle, 1973). The last group of diseases includes Hodgkin's disease and other malignant lymphomas, chronic lymphocytic and other leukaemias, other types of cancers, as well as systemic lupus erythematosis, sarcoidosis and several other conditions.

Results obtained with the various EBV-related serological procedures in NPC patients and pertinent controls were as follows:

VCA-specific IgG antibodies

The titres of IgG antibodies to VCA of as yet untreated NPC patients are to a large extent related to the total tumour burden (Henle et al., 1970a, 1973; Lynn et al., 1973a). The geometric mean titre (GMT) in stage I is only slightly higher than the GMT of healthy controls; however, it increases stepwise as the disease advances from stage I to stage V, being ultimately about eight-fold higher than in stage I and about ten-fold higher than in healthy controls. Patients with other malignant tumours of the postnasal space or carcinomas elsewhere in the head and neck region may show an increased incidence of high anti-VCA titres as compared to controls, which is far less striking, however, than the increased incidence seen in NPC patients. Correspondingly, the GMT of anti-VCA in patients with various malignant tumours other than NPC is only about two to three times that of healthy controls (de Schryver et al., 1969, 1972; Henle et al., 1970a).

EA-specific IgG antibodies

The majority of NPC patients have antibodies to the EA complex that are directed against the D component, whereas in those with Burkitt's lymphoma anti-R predominates (Henle et al., 1971). The incidence and titres of anti-D increase with the total tumour burden: in stage I, only about 30% of patients have anti-D, mostly at low titres, but by stage III nearly all patients have antibodies to D, in part at substantial titres (Henle et al., 1973). Accordingly, the GMT of anti-D is low in stage I but increases stepwise to a six- to eight-fold higher level in stages III-V. A few patients in stage I or II of the disease may show low titres of anti-R as the sole or dominant antibody to the EA complex. As the anti-D titres increase with advance of the disease, anti-R is no longer measurable because R staining cannot be discerned in the presence of brilliant D immunofluorescence. Antibodies to EA components are found at only a low frequency and titres in healthy controls (Henle & Henle, 1973; Henle et al., 1970b, 1971). They are directed mostly against the R component and are observed only among those donors who maintain relatively high anti-VCA titres. Patients with carcinomas of the head and neck region other than NPC show, as mentioned above, a somewhat higher incidence of elevated anti-VCA titres than controls and, correspondingly, a slightly increased incidence of antibodies to R, although mostly at low titres; they rarely show anti-D, i.e., patterns that are comparable to those seen in NPC patients (Henle[1]).

Antibodies to EBNA

Anti-EBNA, like anti-VCA (IgG), is uniformly detectable in sera from NPC patients, often at elevated titres as compared to controls (de-Thé et al., 1973; Henle et al.[1]). The GMT of anti-EBNA in Chinese patients from Hong Kong tends to increase with the stage of the disease, although less strikingly than do the IgG GMTs of anti-VCA or anti-D. Since totally distinct antigens are involved, the ratios between the titres of anti-VCA and anti-EBNA in individual sera, whether from patients with NPC or from controls, can vary from well over 4 to less than 0.25; however, the GMTs of both antibodies are similar, and thus the ratios between the GMTs of anti-VCA and anti-EBNA are only slightly above unity in healthy controls and in NPC patients in stage I or II. This ratio increases gradually to about 4 with advance of NPC to stages III-V. These findings denote that anti-EBNA titres tend to increase in parallel with anti-VCA titres in the early stages of NPC and that in later stages only the anti-VCA titres show further substantial increases.

[1] Unpublished data

In East African NPC cases, anti-EBNA, but not anti-VCA, titres tend to be lower than in Chinese patients. Since information concerning stage of the disease has not been available for the African patients, only the total groups can be compared. The ratio between the GMTs of anti-VCA and anti-EBNA in the African cases turned out to be about 9, or four to five times higher than in Chinese NPC patients and six times higher than in African controls. African patients with carcinomas other than NPC showed ratios about half-way between those for the NPC and control groups. The relatively low anti-EBNA levels in African patients are unexplained but suggest that unknown, possibly immunosuppressive, conditions reduce the production of antibodies to EBNA but not to VCA.

EBV-related IgA antibodies

The report that NPC patients have increased serum IgA levels (Wara et al., 1975) suggested that this might be due to increased levels of EBV-specific IgA antibodies; and, indeed, high frequencies of VCA- and D-specific IgA antibodies are readily detectable in sera from NPC patients (Henle & Henle, 1976a, b; Ho et al., 1976). Before initiation of therapy, nearly all patients show IgA antibodies to VCA, and many also to D, at titres that occasionally match those of the corresponding IgG antibodies. The incidence and GMTs of the IgA antibodies increase with the total tumour burden like those of the other antibodies described. In contrast, IgA antibodies to VCA are rarely detectable in healthy donors (< 2%) and then at only low titres among those individuals who maintain relatively high VCA-specific IgG levels; IgA antibodies to EA components have thus far not been found. Patients with carcinomas other than NPC only occasionally (about 2%) show low VCA-specific IgA antibody titres.

The incidence and titres of serum IgA antibodies to herpes simplex virus are low in NPC patients and are not elevated when compared to those in control groups. VCA-specific serum IgA antibodies are observed in Burkitt's lymphoma patients and, transiently, in those with infectious mononucleosis in no more than 30-40% of the patients, generally at only low titres. Thus, the high frequency and, often, high titres of EBV-related serum IgA antibodies appear to be a unique but presently unexplained feature of NPC. Preliminary data indicate that the serum IgA antibodies are dominantly, if not entirely, of the systemic (7S) and not of the secretory (11S) type.

VCA-specific IgM antibodies

The detection of high titres of VCA-specific IgM antibodies provides the most important criterion for identifying a current primary EBV infection, whether or not it is accompanied by signs of infectious mononucleosis (see Henle et al., 1974). Following primary EBV infections, a persistent, latent viral carrier state is consistently established in the lymphoreticular system and is responsible for the life-long maintenance of nearly constant titres of VCA-specific IgG, neutralizing and EBNA-specific antibodies. The apparent equilibrium between the persistent viral carrier state and the immune responses of the host can, however, be upset by various immunosuppressive malignant or non-malignant diseases, as mentioned earlier. It is conceivable that reactivation of the latent infection leads to a transitory reemergence of VCA-specific IgM antibodies; this phenomenon has, in fact, been noted now in a small proportion of patients with Hodgkin's disease or other lymphomas, as well as in a few NPC patients (Henle[1]).

LONG-TERM SEROLOGICAL FOLLOW-UP STUDY OF NPC PATIENTS

The foregoing observations have shown that antibodies to a number of EBV-coded antigens increase in titre with an advance of NPC from stage I to stage V, i.e., with the total tumour burden. Exceptions are provided by cases in which the tumour rapidly invades the central nervous system without expanding to draining lymph nodes (see below). Correspondingly, one would expect declines in the titres of the various antibodies following reduction or elimination of the tumour burden by therapeutic measures. Support for this suggestion has been derived from a comparison of the VCA- and D-specific IgG antibody titres in two groups of patients, one composed of as yet untreated patients and the other of patients who had survived for five or more years (Henle et al., 1973). While the GMTs of anti-VCA and anti-D in the untreated patients showed the stepwise increases from stage I to stage IV or V of the disease, the GMTs of the long-term survivors no longer conformed to those of the stages recorded at commencement of therapy. Many of these patients showed no anti-D, the incidence of low anti-R titres was increased in the absence of interfering anti-D reactions, and the GMTs of anti-VCA and anti-D were distinctly lower than those in the untreated group. A significantly lower GMT of VCA-specific IgG antibodies in long-term survivors as compared to untreated patients has also been observed by Lynn et al. (1973b), and declines in anti-VCA titres during two years following therapy have been noted by de-Thé et al. (1973). In addition, when long-term survivors showed anti-VCA and anti-D titres comparable to those seen in untreated patients, they were known to have residual or recurrent tumours or had relapses subsequently (Henle et al., 1973).

These results indicated that EBV-related serology might serve to monitor the effectiveness of therapy and, thus, to provide information regarding the prognosis of patients. To verify this suggestion, a longitudinal serological follow-up study of over 100 NPC patients was initiated over five years ago, and is now nearing completion. Plotting of serological data from individual patients has revealed several different patterns.

At one end of the range are patients who responded well to therapy, with at most one or two minor, relatively early relapses at the primary site or in lymph nodes. Patients initially in stage I or II predominate in this group, although patients in stage III or IV at

[1] Unpublished data

commencement of therapy are also represented. The titres of VCA- and D-specific IgG and IgA antibodies showed a steady, gradual downward trend; and, depending upon the initial titres, those of the D-specific IgA and IgG and the VCA-specific IgA antibodies declined to non-detectable or low levels within one to several years, whereas those of the VCA-specific IgG antibodies merely decreased to levels within the range observed in healthy donors. In contrast, the anti-EBNA titres in this and the other groups of patients showed mostly minor changes.

At the other end of the range are patients who responded only transiently to therapy and who soon developed recurrences at the primary site or in lymph nodes, followed ultimately by wide-spread metastases. Patients initially in stage I or II showed remarkable increases in titres of IgA and IgG antibodies to VCA and D; those in stage III or IV also showed increments in various antibody titres, or maintained continuously high titres. In a few patients, transient peaks or persistent levels of IgM antibodies to VCA were also observed. Of special significance is the fact that in some patients significant rises in antibody titres were noted months in advance of the detection of major relapses or widespread metastases.

A third, small group of patients succumbed to NPC due to rapid invasion of the cranial cavity by the tumour, without significant involvement of cervical glands. These patients initially showed moderate or low VCA-specific IgG or IgA antibody titres, respectively, and no anti-D; these patterns are comparable to those seen in many stage I and a few stage II patients at admission. There were no major changes in the spectrum or titres of antibodies that would have warned of the invasion of the central nervous system prior to recognition of the clinical reality.

The remaining two groups had patterns intermediary between the first two discussed. Patients in both groups responded well to therapy and remained free of detectable disease for several years. In both groups, antibody titres declined initially. Then, in the first of these groups, the titres levelled off, so that IgA antibodies to VCA and D and IgG antibodies to D and, sometimes, to R remained detectable at low to moderate levels during the remainder of the observation period. Since most of these cases were initially in stage III and thus started with high antibody levels, this decline in titres might represent all that can be observed during four- to five-year intervals in patients without evidence of disease. However, in the second group of patients, the downward trend in various antibody titres changed to an upward trend, although some of these patients remained thus far free of detectable tumours. In a few, the increases in titres preceded the recognition of late relapses, which were again successfully treated. Such patients obviously require continued surveillance.

These results indicate that EBV-related serology may indeed serve to monitor the success of therapy in NPC. While the detection of a downward trend in antibody titres over several years of observation indicates a favourable prognosis, it must not be taken as cause for relaxation of intensive periodic check-ups of the patients. Reversals from the downward to an upward trend in antibody titres may be observed after several years, and this may occur months in advance of the recognition of recurrent tumours or metastases. This, in fact, may be the most significant observation derived from this longitudinal serological study. Close serological monitoring of NPC patients at frequent intervals might alert to an imminent recurrence of the tumour or to the development of metastases, and, thus, to the need for intensified examination of the patients and, if indicated, reinstitution of therapy.

CONCLUDING REMARKS

The foregoing presentation has demonstrated some unique features of EBV-related serology in NPC. For the studies reported it was of prime importance to include only well-documented cases of the disease, such as in the patients in Hong Kong. In these, the tumours were classified by uniform histopathological examinations, the patients were staged according to a standard procedure, and information on the clinical status before and for years after treatment was readily available. It is evident that untreated patients in stage I do not, as a rule, show the characteristic EBV-related serological pattern of NPC; similarly, years after effective therapy, the serological pattern may also no longer be characteristic of NPC. A serological analysis of NPC patients for whom stage of disease or clinical status at given times after treatment have not been specified or for whom dependable histopathological classification of the carcinoma by experienced pathologists has not been made might lead to confusing results. NPC is relatively rare in Europe and the United States, and classification of the limited numbers of patients according to the various criteria has often resulted in too small numbers of cases in given categories for valid statistical analyses to be made. While EBV-related serological patterns comparable to those seen in Chinese and East African patients were observed in some Caucasian patients, others had patterns which were not characteristic of NPC; this observation has led, perhaps prematurely, to the suggestion that NPC in Caucasian patients might differ somewhat from NPC in other races (de Schryver et al., 1974; Henderson et al., 1974; Henle[1]).

For these and other reasons, it has long been evident that an intimate association of EBV with human malignancies cannot be established by serology alone but requires additional evidence, such as a demonstration of EBV DNA- or EBNA-positive tumour cells in biopsies. Indeed, EBV DNA- and/or EBNA-positive carcinoma cells have been demonstrated in nearly all biopsies from Chinese and East African NPC patients,

[1] Unpublished data

as discussed by Epstein[1]. EBV DNA- and/or EBNA-positive cells have been detected thus far only in biopsies from NPC that were classified as anaplastic, undifferentiated or poorly differentiated carcinomas (Andersson-Anvret et al.[2]; Ho et al.[3]). Moderately to well-differentiated carcinomas of the postnasal space were devoid of EBV-DNA- or EBNA-positive cells, and the patients in whom they occurred had EBV-related serological patterns comparable to those seen in healthy donors. Biopsies from carcinomas arising elsewhere in the head and neck region, ranging from undifferentiated to well-differentiated, have thus far uniformly failed to reveal the presence of EBV genomes, with the exception of undifferentiated carcinomas of the nasal fossa. Since carcinomas of the nasal fossa and NPC arise in anatomically close proximity, they may well have similar origins. Corresponding studies of biopsies from Caucasian patients with carcinomas in the postnasal regions are needed to determine to what extent these are or are not associated with EBV.

---

[1] See p. 333

[2] See p. 347

[3] Unpublished data

ACKNOWLEDGEMENTS

Studies by the authors were supported by research grant CA-04568 and contract N01-CP-33272 from the National Cancer Institute, US Public Health Service. W. Henle is the recipient of Career Award 5-K6-AI-22683, National Institutes of Health, US Public Health Service.

REFERENCES

de Schryver, A., Friberg, S., Jr, Klein, G., Henle, W., Henle, G., de-Thé, G., Clifford, P. & Ho, H.C. (1969) Epstein-Barr virus (EBV)-associated antibody patterns in carcinoma of the postnasal space. *Clin. exp. Immunol.*, *5*, 443-459

de Schryver, A., Klein, G., Henle, G., Henle, W., Cameron, H., Santesson, L. & Clifford, P. (1972) EB-virus associated serology in malignant disease: antibody levels to viral capsid antigens (VCA), membrane antigens (MA) and early antigens (EA) in patients with various neoplastic conditions. *Int. J. Cancer*, *9*, 353-364

de Schryver, A., Klein, G., Henle, W. & Henle, G. (1974) EB virus-associated antibodies in Caucasian patients with carcinoma of the nasopharynx and in long-term survivors after treatment. *Int. J. Cancer*, *13*, 319-325

de-Thé, G., Sohier, R., Ho, J.H.C. & Freund, R.J. (1973) Nasopharyngeal carcinoma. IV. Evolution of complement-fixing antibodies during the course of the disease. *Int. J. Cancer*, *12*, 368-377

de-Thé, G., Ho, J.H.C., Ablashi, D.V., Day, N.E., Macario, A.J.L., Martin-Berthelson, M.C., Pearson, G. & Sohier, R. (1975) Nasopharyngeal carcinoma. IX. Antibodies to EBNA and correlation with response to other EBV antigens in Chinese patients. *Int. J. Cancer*, *16*, 713-721

Henderson, B.E., Louie, E., Bogdanoff, E., Henle, W., Alena, B. & Henle, G. (1974) Antibodies to herpes group viruses in patients with nasopharyngeal and other head and neck cancers. *Cancer Res.*, *34*, 1207-1210

Henle, G. & Henle, W. (1966) Immunofluorescence in cells derived from Burkitt's lymphoma. *J. Bact.*, *91*, 1248-1256

Henle, G. & Henle, W. (1976a) Epstein-Barr virus-specific IgA serum antibodies in nasopharyngeal carcinoma. *Bibl. haematol.*, *43*, 322-325

Henle, G. & Henle, W. (1976b) Epstein-Barr virus-specific IgA serum antibodies as an outstanding feature of nasopharyngeal carcinoma. *Int. J. Cancer*, *17*, 1-7

Henle, G., Henle, W. & Diehl, V. (1968) Relation of Burkitt tumor associated herpes-type virus to infectious mononucleosis. *Proc. nat. Acad. Sci. (Wash.)*, *59*, 94-101

Henle, G., Henle, W. & Klein, G. (1971) Demonstration of two distinct components in the early antigen complex of Epstein-Barr virus infected cells. *Int. J. Cancer*, *8*, 272-282

Henle, W. & Henle, G. (1968) Present status of the herpes-group virus associated with cultures of the hematopoietic system. *Persp. Virol.*, *6*, 105-117

Henle, W. & Henle, G. (1973) Epstein-Barr virus (EBV)-related serology in Hodgkin's disease. *Nat. Cancer Inst. Monogr.*, *36*, 79-84

Henle, W., Hummeler, K. & Henle, G. (1966) Antibody coating and agglutination of virus particles separated from the EB3 line of Burkitt lymphoma cells. *J. Bact.*, *92*, 269-271

Henle, W., Henle, G., Ho, H.C., Burtin, P., Cachin, Y., Clifford, P., de Schryver, A., de-Thé, G., Diehl, V. & Klein, G. (1970a) Antibodies to EB virus in nasopharyngeal carcinoma, other head and neck neoplasms and control groups. *J. nat. Cancer Inst.*, *44*, 225-231

Henle, W., Henle, G., Zajac, B., Pearson, G., Waubke, R. & Scriba, M. (1970b) Differential reactivity of human sera with EBV-induced 'early antigens'. *Science*, *169*, 188-190

Henle, W., Ho, H.C., Henle, G. & Kwan, H.C. (1973) Antibodies to Epstein-Barr virus-related antigens in nasopharyngeal carcinoma. Comparison of active cases and long term survivors. *J. nat. Cancer Inst.*, *51*, 361-369

Henle, W., Henle, G. & Horwitz, C.A. (1974) Epstein-Barr virus-specific diagnostic tests in infectious mononucleosis. *Human Path.*, *5*, 551-565

Hinuma, Y., Sairenji, T., Sekizawa, T. & Ida, S. (1971) A new antigen induced by the Epstein-Barr virus and its reactivity with sera from patients with malignant tumors. In: Nakahara, W., Nishioka, K., Hirayama, T. & Ito, Y., eds, *Recent Advances in Human Tumor Virology and Immunology*, Tokyo, University of Tokyo Press, pp. 351-359

Ho, H.C., Ng, M.H., Kwan, H.C. & Chau, J.C.W. (1976) Epstein-Barr virus-specific IgA and IgG serum antibodies in nasopharyngeal carcinoma. *Brit. J. Cancer*, *34*, 655-660

Kawamura, A.J., Takata, M. & Gotoh, A. (1970) Seroepidemiological studies on nasopharyngeal carcinoma by fluorescent antibody techniques with cultured Burkitt lymphoma cells. *Gann*, *61*, 55-71

Lin, T.M., Yang, C.S., Ho, S.W., Chiou, T.F., Liu, C.H., Tu, S.M., Chen, K.P., Ito, Y., Kawamura, A. & Hirayama, T. (1972) Antibodies to herpes-type virus in nasopharyngeal carcinoma and control groups. *Cancer*, *29*, 603-609

Lin, T.M., Yang, C.S., Chiou, J.F., Tu, S.S., Lin, C.C., Liu, C.H., Chen, K.P., Ito, Y., Kawamura, A. & Hirayama, T. (1973) Seroepidemiological studies on carcinoma of the nasopharynx *Cancer Res.*, *33*, 2603-2608

Lynn, T.C., Tu, S.M., Hirayama, T. & Kawamura, A.J. (1973a) Nasopharyngeal carcinoma and Epstein-Barr virus. I. Factors related to the anti-VCA antibody. *Jap. J. exp. Med.*, *43*, 121-133

Lynn, T.C., Tu, S.M., Hirayama, T. & Kawamura, A.J. (1973b) Nasopharyngeal carcinoma and Epstein-Barr virus. II. Clinical course and the anti-VCA antibody. *Jap. J. exp. Med.*, *43*, 135-144

Old, L.J., Boyse, E.A., Oettgen, H.F., Harven, E., Geering, G., Williamson, B. & Clifford, P. (1966) Precipitating antibody in human serum to an antigen present in cultured Burkitt's lymphoma cells. *Proc. nat. Acad. Sci. (Wash.)*, *56*, 1699-1704

Old, L.J., Boyse, E.A., Geering, G. & Oettgen, H.F. (1968) Serologic approaches to the study of cancer in animals and in man. *Cancer Res.*, *28*, 1288-1299

Reedman, B.M. & Klein, G. (1973) Cellular localization of an Epstein-Barr virus (EBV)-associated complement-fixing antigen in producer and non-producer lymphoblastoid cell lines. *Int. J. Cancer*, *11*, 499-520

Wara, W.M., Wara, D.W., Phillips, T.L. & Ammann, A.J. (1975) Elevated IgA in carcinoma of the nasopharynx. *Cancer*, *35*, 1313-1315

CLINICAL EVALUATION OF EBV SEROLOGY IN AMERICAN PATIENTS WITH NASOPHARYNGEAL CARCINOMA

G.R. PEARSON, H.L. COATES & H.B. NEEL, III

Departments of Microbiology and Otorhinolaryngology,
Mayo Clinic/Foundation,
Rochester, Minn. 55901, USA

P. LEVINE, D. ABLASHI & J. EASTON

National Cancer Institute,
National Institutes of Health,
Bethesda, Md. 20014, USA

INTRODUCTION

There is now extensive immunological, biological and biochemical evidence to support an etiological relationship between Epstein-Barr virus (EBV) and nasopharyngeal carcinoma (NPC) in patients from different geographical locations (Klein, 1973). Besides providing information on the question of etiology, the results from immunological investigations suggest that antibodies to some of the EBV-associated antigens might be of clinical importance in the diagnosis and prognosis of NPC. Levels of antibodies to the EBV-induced early antigen complex (EA) tend to increase with stage of disease (de-Thé et al., 1975; Henle et al., 1973); this is particularly true of the antibody response to the D component of this complex (Henle et al., 1973). Antibodies to other EBV-associated antigens also vary with stage of disease, but these differences are not as striking as those noted with EA, particularly when comparisons are made with control populations in which EA levels tend to be low or absent (de-Thé et al., 1975). Certain evidence suggests that antibody levels to EA might also be of prognostic significance in treated patients, since lower levels of antibodies to this group of antigens were detected in sera from long-term survivors than in sera collected from NPC patients before treatment (de Schryver et al., 1974; Henle et al., 1973). However, longitudinal studies on individual patients are needed before this association can be confirmed.

Recently, Henle & Henle (1976) reported on another immunological parameter that appeared to be relatively specific for NPC patients in comparison with patients with other types of head and neck cancers: this was the frequent presence of antibodies to EBV-associated antigens in the IgA immunoglobulin fraction. It had previously been reported that this immunoglobulin fraction was elevated in NPC patients (Wara et al., 1975). Approximately 93% of NPC patients had anti-EBV antibodies in the IgA serum fraction, as opposed to less than 10% of the control populations. Furthermore, high levels of antibodies were frequently detected in untreated patients but tended to decrease and occur less frequently in patients who had no clinical evidence of recurrent disease. These findings indicated that the presence and levels of antibodies to EBV antigens in the IgA immunoglobulin fraction might be a clinical parameter useful in the diagnosis and follow-up of patients with NPC.

The goals of the programme reported here were to confirm and extend these findings using American patients and control groups, to determine the potential clinical application of EBV serology to this patient population.

MATERIALS AND METHODS

Sera

Sera of patients with NPC were obtained from those examined at the Mayo Clinic or from those whose physicians had requested serological evaluation at the National Institutes of Health. The majority of the serum donors were Caucasian. Control sera were obtained from patients examined at the Mayo Clinic. Histopathological confirmation was obtained for all patients with NPC as well as for those with other cancers who were used as controls. For comparison, sera from Chinese and Tunisian patients with NPC were also examined in this study. All sera were heat-inactivated at 56°C for 30 min before testing.

Immunological assays

Sera were titrated for antibodies to VCA on acetone-fixed smears of the P3HR-1 cell line, as described previously (Henle et al., 1970; Pearson et al., 1971). These cultures contained 5-10% VCA-positive cells. Anti-EA serum titrations were performed on acetone-fixed smears of EBV-infected Raji cultures, containing approximately 20% EA-positive cells and less than 0.1% VCA-positive cells, as determined from standard control sera. Four-fold dilutions of sera in phosphate-buffered saline were prepared for the titrations; the last dilution that produced definitive fluorescence in a percentage of cells comparable to that in a control serum was taken as the serum titre. Anti-VCA serum titres were determined using fluorescein-conjugated goat anti-IgG or anti-IgA reagent (Hyland Laboratories, Los Angeles, Ca, USA). All preparations were examined under a vertical fluorescence microscope.

RESULTS

VCA and EA titres in American NPC patients and controls

Initial studies with American NPC patients were made to determine whether the patients examined had the same EBV serology profiles as have been observed in Chinese, African and European NPC patients. For this purpose, sera from 69 NPC patients, 85 patients with other head and neck cancers, 80 with lymphomas of various types, including Hodgkin's disease, and from 47 clinically normal individuals were titrated for antibodies to VCA and EA. The group of NPC patients included both untreated patients and individuals who had no further clinical evidence of disease following therapy. Results are shown in Table 1. All NPC patients were positive for antibodies to VCA, as opposed to 76-90% in the control groups. Geometric mean titres (GMT) of VCA were approximately 4-10-fold higher in NPC patients than in the different control groups. Ninety-seven percent of the NPC

Table 1. Serological findings on anti Epstein-Barr virus antibodies [viral capsid antigen (VCA) and early antigen (EA)] in sera of American patients with nasopharyngeal carcinoma (NPC) and other cancers and in normal controls

Serum donor	VCA		EA	
	No. positive/no. tested (%)	GMT	No. positive/no. tested (%)	GMT
NPC patients (NIH)	34/34(100)	376.7	33/33(100)	86.2
NPC patients (Mayo)	35/35(100)	261.2	33/35(94)	61.3
All NPC patients	69/69(100)	311.9	66/68(97)	77.6
Patients with other head & neck cancers	77/85(90)	81.2	38/85(44)	3.1
Lymphoma patients	70/80(88)	68.0	47/80(59)	7.0
Normal controls	36/47(76)	35.9	17/47(36)	2.7

GMT - geometric mean titre

patients were positive for antibodies to EA, as opposed to 44% of patients with other head and neck cancers, 59% of lymphoma patients and 36% of normal controls. The GMTs were substantially higher

(10-30 fold) in NPC patients. The antibodies to EA in the NPC group were primarily 'D' (diffuse), confirming the findings of Henle et al. (1973).

Although anti-VCA and EA titres in the sera from these American patients were significantly higher than those seen in the control groups, anti-EBV titres were substantially lower than those in Chinese and Tunisian NPC patients, as shown in Figure 1. Mean VCA titres were approximately 4-fold higher in these two groups than in American patients, while EA titres were similar in American and Tunisian patients but about 3-fold lower than the mean titre in Chinese.

FIG. 1. COMPARISON OF VIRAL CAPSID ANTIGEN (VCA) AND EARLY ANTIGEN (EA) TITRES BETWEEN AMERICAN, CHINESE AND TUNISIAN NASOPHARYNGEAL CARCINOMA PATIENTS

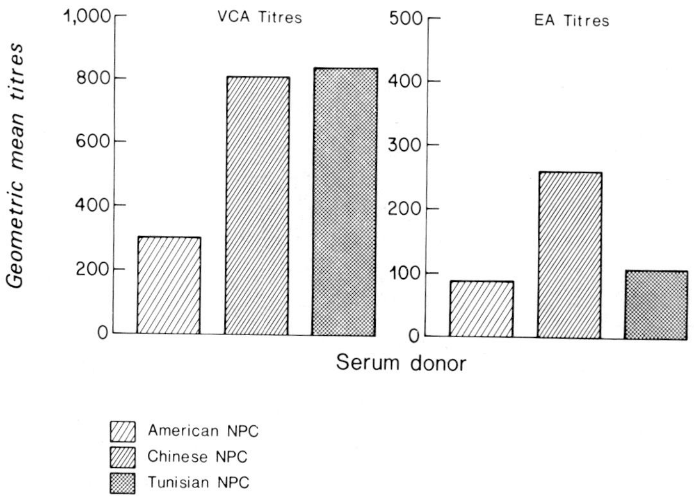

Interestingly, five sera from American-Chinese NPC patients had VCA and EA titres similar to those in the Chinese patients (Ablashi et al., 1977). Similar differences between American, Chinese and Tunisian NPC patients were also noted in levels of antibodies to Epstein-Barr nuclear antigen (EBNA) and 'S' antigen.

Occurrence of antibody to EBV-associated antigens in the IgA immunoglobulin fraction

Sera from the groups examined at the Mayo Clinic were also tested for antibodies to EBV in the IgA fraction. They were tested only for antibody to VCA, although similar results were obtained with some sera that were also tested against EA and membrane antigen (MA). Results from these investigations are presented in Table 2. Seventy-seven percent of the NPC sera were positive for IgA antibodies to VCA, with titres ranging from less than 5 to greater than 80. All of the negative sera in this group came from treated patients who had no clinical evidence of disease. Only 6-10% of the sera from the three control groups were positive in these tests, and most at a titre of less than 5. The most obvious exception was a serum from the lymphoma group that had a titre of 40; interestingly, the histological diagnosis of this patient's disease was poorly differentiated lymphocytic lymphoma of the right tonsil.

Table 2. Serum antibodies to Epstein-Barr virus-induced viral capsid antigen (VCA) in IgA immunoglobulin fraction of American patients with nasopharyngeal carcinoma (NPC) and other cancers and in normal controls

Serum donor	No. positive/no. tested (%)	No. with VCA titres[a]						
		≤ 5	5	10	20	40	80	>80
NPC patients	27/35(77)	8	4	8	3	3	5	3
Patients with other head & neck cancers	9/85(10)	76	5	2	2[b]			
Lymphoma patients	8/80(10)	72	5	2		1[c]		
Normal controls	3/47(6)	44	3					

[a] Serum from one NPC patient was not titrated.

[b] From patients with basal-cell carcinoma of the neck and carcinoma of the floor of the mouth

[c] Donor had a diagnosis of poorly differentiated lymphocytic lymphoma in the right tonsil.

Anti-EBV titres in untreated patients versus *those in remission*

To determine whether these antibody parameters vary with disease course, GMTs for VCA, EA and IgA-VCA were assessed in untreated patients and in those with recurrent disease and were compared with those in patients with no clinical evidence of disease. The results are shown in Figure 2. VCA GMTs were approximately 4-fold lower in patients in remission; however, there was a substantial difference in titres of EA and IgA-VCA between these two groups. These findings provide further evidence that these two parameters might be of prognostic value in patients undergoing treatment.

FIG. 2. COMPARISON OF VIRAL CAPSID ANTIGEN (VCA), EARLY ANTIGEN (EA) AND IgA (VCA) ANTIBODY TITRES IN AMERICAN NASOPHARYNGEAL PATIENTS IN UNTREATED AND RECURRENT DISEASE *VERSUS* IN REMISSION

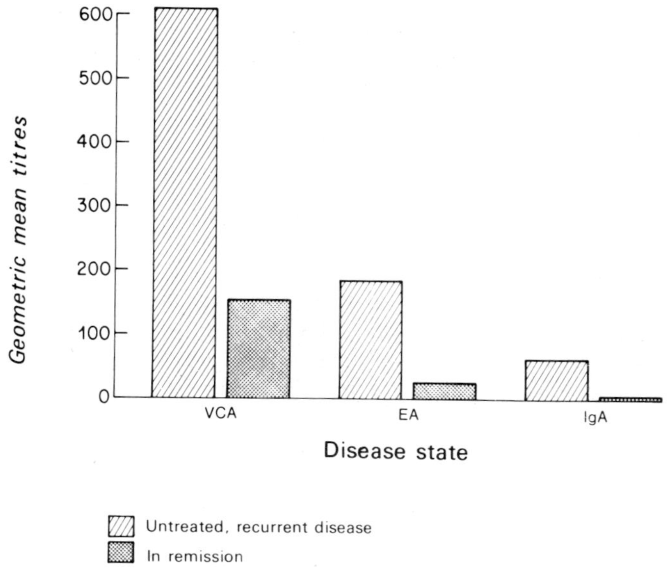

DISCUSSION

Most studies on EBV and NPC have been directed towards proving an etiological association between the two. In the course of such investigations, however, a number of viral parameters have been identified, which could have clinical application. The most important of these parameters from a clinical point of view would appear to be the patterns of antibody response to EBV-associated antigens.
A number of laboratories have now reported that NPC patients have elevated antibody titres to EBV antigens and that antibodies to some of these antigens increase with stage of disease (de-Thé et al., 1975; Henle et al., 1973). These observations suggest that identification of antibodies to these antigens, both quantitatively and qualitatively, might aid in the diagnosis of this disease. This is particularly

important in those situations in which absolute diagnosis of NPC on a pathological basis is uncertain. Other studies have indicated that antibody titres to EBV antigens vary with the course of the disease and may, therefore, be of prognostic importance. Should these parameters be true indicators of early recurrence, they would be very useful in new clinical studies directed towards the treatment of recurrent disease. However, for both of these applications, the specificity of these anti-viral parameters must be determined in different high- and low-incidence populations, and the potential clinical application determined in a prospective fashion. The main purpose of the experiments reported in this paper was to establish baseline parameters with respect to the specificity of the anti-EBV responses in American NPC patients, so that such studies could be initiated.

Our findings confirm and extend those of other studies on NPC in the US (Henderson et al., 1974), which showed that, as in other populations, antibody titres to EBV-associated antigens are generally elevated in NPC patients in comparison with those in control populations, including patients with other cancers of the head and neck.

Anti-EA antibodies appear to be the most reliable discriminating factor, particularly in a comparison of GMTs. However, occasional individual patients with other malignancies also showed high anti-EA titres: 7 of 85 sera from patients with other head and neck cancers had anti-EA titres between 40 and 100; 17 of 80 lymphoma patients had titres that ranged from 40 to 640.

The most specific immunological parameter appeared to be the presence of antibodies to EBV antigens in the IgA immunoglobulin fraction, as reported by Henle & Henle (1976). This again, however, was not absolute, since high titres were also noted occasionally in other cancer patients. In our studies, one patient with a poorly differentiated lymphoma of the right tonsil had a high IgA antibody titre (greater than 10), and two patients with head and neck cancers other than NPC had elevated titres. Although these discrepancies were rare, they are a point of concern when considering the use of EBV serology as a potential aid to pathology in the diagnosis of NPC.

The results reported here also confirm published findings which showed that antibody titres to EBV-associated antigens were generally lower in patients without clinically active disease than in untreated patients, suggesting that these parameters might be of prognostic value (de Schryver et al., 1974; Henle & Henle, 1976; Henle et al., 1973). This is particularly apparent with the anti-EA and IgA titres. In our early studies at the Mayo Clinic, we were thus able to identify two patients who subsequently developed clinical evidence of recurrence; however, we are still following one patient who has elevated anti-EA and IgA titres but who has no clinical evidence of recurrent disease. It will be important to follow such patients prospectively over an extended period of time before it can be determined whether some of the anti-EBV immunological parameters might indeed be early indicators of residual or recurrent disease. If indeed this is the case, such parameters would be invaluable in therapy programmes directed at the development of new therapeutic approaches to NPC.

It should also be mentioned that in the limited number of American patients studied to date EBV serology has not consistently correlated with pathology. This is somewhat of a paradox, since the EBV genome has so far been detected only in the epithelial cells of the anaplastic or poorly differentiated form of NPC (or lymphoepithelioma) (Desgranges et al., 1975; Huang et al., 1974; Klein et al., 1974; Wolf et al., 1973). Further studies should be made not only to determine the potential clinical application of EBV serology to NPC but also to clarify the relationship of these serological parameters to the pathological type of disease.

One other serological test now being applied in relation to the clinical course of NPC is the antibody-dependent lymphocyte cytotoxicity (ADLC) assay, which is a sensitive test for measuring antibodies to EBV-induced MA (Pearson & Orr, 1976). Antibody response to these antigens in an animal herpesvirus system followed a disease-related pattern when measured by the ADLC assay but not when measured by the standard membrane immunofluorescence test (Prevost et al., 1975, 1976). Similar studies are now underway with the EBV system to determine whether antibody levels to MA vary with disease course. Although the preliminary findings are encouraging, further studies are needed before any conclusions can be drawn concerning the potential clinical value of this assay.

SUMMARY

There is now extensive immunological, biological and biochemical evidence to support a possible etiological relationship between EBV and NPC in patients from different geographical locations. Besides providing information on the question of etiology, the results from immunological investigations suggest that antibodies to some of the EBV-associated antigens might also be of clinical importance in the diagnosis and prognosis of NPC. To determine the possible clinical application of EBV serology to American NPC, sera from patients seen at the Mayo Clinic and the National Institutes of Health were examined for antibodies to EBV-associated antigens in an effort to identify those parameters which most reliably distinguish NPC from other types of cancer. The results show that high antibody titres to EBV-induced EA and the presence of antibody to EBV antigens in the IgA immunoglobulin fraction were the two most specific discriminating parameters, although neither was infallible. These findings are discussed in relation to future studies that are needed in order to determine the potential clinical value of EBV serology to the diagnosis and prognosis of NPC.

ACKNOWLEDGEMENT

This work was supported in part by Comprehensive Cancer Center Grant No. 15083 awarded to the Mayo Foundation.

REFERENCES

Ablashi, D.V., Easton, J.M., Levine, P.H., Krueger, G.R.K. & Connally, R. (1977) *Immunological comparison of nasopharyngeal carcinoma and Burkitt's lymphoma from relatively high and low risk populations.* In: Severi, L., ed., *Proceedings of the 6th Perugia Quadrennial International Conference on Cancer: Tumours of Early Life in Man and Animals, Perugia, Italy,* Perugia, University of Perugia (in press)

de Schryver, A., Klein, G., Henle, W. & Henle, G. (1974) EB virus-associated antibodies in Caucasian patients with carcinoma of the nasopharynx and in long-term survivors after treatment. *Int. J. Cancer, 13*, 319-325

Desgranges, C., Wolf, H., de-Thé, G., Shanmugaratnam, K., Cammoun, N., Ellouz, R., Klein, G., Lennert, K., Muñoz, N. & zur Hausen, H. (1975) Nasopharyngeal carcinoma. 10. Presence of Epstein-Barr genomes in separated epithelial cells of tumors in patients from Singapore, Tunisia and Kenya. *Int. J. Cancer, 16*, 7-15

de-Thé, G., Ho, J.H.C., Ablashi, D.V., Day, N.E., Macario, A.J.L., Martin-Berthelon, M.C., Pearson, G. & Sohier, R. (1975) Nasopharyngeal carcinoma. 9. Antibodies to EBNA and correlation with response to other EBV antigens in Chinese patients. *Int. J. Cancer, 16*, 713-721

Henderson, B.E., Louie, E., Bogdanoff, E., Henle, W., Alena, B. & Henle, G. (1974) Antibodies to herpes group viruses in patients with nasopharyngeal and other head and neck cancers. *Cancer Res., 34*, 1207-1210

Henle, G. & Henle, W. (1976) Epstein-Barr virus-specific IgA serum antibodies as an outstanding feature of nasopharyngeal carcinoma. *Int. J. Cancer, 17*, 1-7

Henle, W., Henle, G., Zajac, B.A., Pearson, G., Waubke, R. & Scriba, M. (1970) Differential reactivity of human sera with early antigens induced by Epstein-Barr virus. *Science, 169*, 188-190

Henle, W., Ho, J.H.C., Henle, G. & Kwan, H.C. (1973) Antibodies to Epstein-Barr virus-related antigens in nasopharyngeal carcinoma: comparison of active cases with long-term survivors. *J. nat. Cancer Inst., 51*, 361-369

Huang, D., Ho, J.H.C., Henle, W. & Henle, G. (1974) Demonstration of Epstein-Barr virus-associated nuclear antigen in nasopharyngeal carcinoma cells from fresh biopsies. *Int. J. Cancer, 14*, 580-588

Klein, G. (1973) *The Epstein-Barr virus*. In: Kaplan, A.S., ed., *The Herpesviruses*, New York, Academic Press, pp. 521-555

Klein, G., Giovanella, B., Lindahl, J., Fialkow, P.J., Singh, S. & Stehlin, J. (1974) Direct evidence for the presence of Epstein-Barr virus DNA and nuclear antigen in malignant epithelial cells from patients with anaplastic carcinoma of the nasopharynx. *Proc. nat. Acad. Sci. (Wash.), 71*, 4737-4741

Pearson, G.R. & Orr, T.W. (1976) Antibody dependent lymphocyte cytotoxicity against cells expressing Epstein-Barr virus antigens. *J. nat. Cancer Inst., 56*, 485-488

Pearson, G.R., Henle, G. & Henle, W. (1971) Production of antigens associated with Epstein-Barr virus in experimentally infected lymphoblastoid cell lines. *J. nat. Cancer Inst., 46*, 1243-1250

Prevost, J.M., Orr, T.W. & Pearson, G.R. (1975) Augmentation of lymphocyte cytotoxicity by antibodies to *Herpesvirus saimiri* associated antigens. *Proc. nat. Acad. Sci. (Wash.), 72*, 1671-1675

Prevost, J.M., Pearson, G.R., Wallen, W.C., Rabin, H. & Qualtiere, L.F. (1976) Antibody responses to membrane antigens in monkeys infected with *Herpesvirus saimiri*. *Int. J. Cancer, 18*, 679-686

Wara, W.M., Wara, D.W., Phillips, T.L. & Ammann, A.J. (1975) Elevated IgA in carcinoma of the nasopharynx. *Cancer, 35*, 1313-1315

Wolf, H., zur Hausen, H. & Becker, V. (1973) EB viral genomes in epithelial nasopharyngeal carcinoma cells. *Nature (New Biol.), 244*, 245-247

THE GENETIC AND ANTIGENIC BASIS FOR THE IgA ANTIBODY RESPONSE TO EPSTEIN-BARR VIRAL CAPSID ANTIGEN

M.H. NG

Department of Microbiology,
University of Hong Kong,
Hong Kong

H.C. HO & H.C. KWAN

Medical and Health Department
Institute of Radiology and Oncology,
Queen Elizabeth Hospital,
Kowloon, Hong Kong

INTRODUCTION

Over 90% of nasopharyngeal carcinoma (NPC) patients, and none of a group of healthy subjects, have been shown to have detectable levels of IgA antibody to the viral capsid antigen (VCA) of Epstein-Barr virus (EBV) at a serum dilution of 1:10, although all had serum levels of IgG antibody to VCA (Ho et al., 1976). Henle & Henle (1976) reported that levels of serum IgA antibodies to EBV-determined antigens in patients with Burkitt's lymphoma or infectious mononucleosis were substantially lower than those sustained by NPC patients, although all three groups of patients had comparable levels of IgG antibodies. IgA antibody to VCA was also detected in concentrated saliva obtained from the majority of NPC patients; in all except one sample, these antibodies lacked the secretory factors that may be expected to be found in secretory IgA molecules (Tomasi et al., 1970). The antibody was not detected in saliva from any of the control subjects, including patients with other cancers of the head and neck and healthy subjects, under similar conditions. These results suggest that the IgA antibody response to EBV antigens may be a unique feature of NPC (Henle & Henle, 1976; Ho et al., 1976, 1977a).

EBV is a ubiquitous virus that causes inapparent infections in a substantial proportion of the local Chinese population of Hong Kong (Ho et al., 1976). This is evident from the presence of IgG antibodies to VCA in all control subjects, including healthy ones and patients with other cancers. EBV is also associated with Burkitt's lymphoma (see Miller, 1976) and may be causally related to infectious mononucleosis (Henle et al., 1968). The association between IgA antibody response to EBV antigens and NPC therefore suggests that the state of infection with this virus as it exists in NPC patients may be different, albeit subtly, from that which occurs in the inapparent infection of healthy subjects and patients with other cancers. It may also be different from that which exists in patients with other EBV-related diseases. Consistent with this contention is the now well-established fact that EBV persists in NPC tumour cells, which are epithelial in origin (Desgranges et al., 1975; Glaser et al., 1976; Huang et al., 1974, 1977; Klein et al., 1974; Trumper et al., 1976). As this constitutes the only known exception to the otherwise lymphotropic properties of EBV (see Klein, 1973), it seems reasonable to suppose that the antigenic stimulation for the IgA antibody response may be derived from NPC tumour cells (Ho et al., 1977b). The familial aggregation of individuals showing the IgA response, on the other hand, suggests that this antibody response might be determined, in part at least, by a recessive genetic trait that is prevalent among NPC patients and their family members (Ho, 1972). To test these possibilities, we studied and report here on levels of IgA antibody to VCA in sera obtained from NPC patients before and after radiation therapy, from their family members and from relapse-free survivors after radiation therapy.

MATERIALS AND METHODS

Sera were obtained from 126 NPC patients before radiation therapy, 10 patients at varying periods after therapy, 47 relapse-free survivors at up to 12 years after therapy and 57 healthy subjects. Plasma was obtained from 133 apparently healthy members of 60 families of NPC patients. All sera and plasma specimens were stored at -70°C without thawing until use. Unless otherwise stated, sera or plasma were diluted 1:10 in phosphate-buffered saline and tested for IgA antibody to VCA, as described previously (Ho et al., 1976).

RESULTS

A strong association was noted between levels of IgA antibody to VCA and NPC. The apparently healthy family members constituted an intermediate association group, showing a frequency of detection of

21.05%; none of the 57 healthy subjects showed detectable levels of IgA antibody to VCA (Table 1).

Table 1. IgA antibodies to Epstein-Barr viral capsid antigen (VCA) in sera obtained from nasopharyngeal carcinoma (NPC) patients before radiation therapy, from their non-NPC family members and from controls

Subjects	Mean age (yrs)	No. with IgA-anti-VCA ≥1:10	< 1:10	Total	% with IgA-anti-VCA ≥1:10	Relative disease risk[a]
NPC patients						
Stages I & II[c]	42 ± 11	34	4	38		
Stages III & IV	46 ± 15	87	1	88		
Total	45 ± 14	121	5	126	96.03	1
Non-NPC family members of NPC patients	35 ± 18	28	105	133	21.05	0.22
Controls[b]	32 ± 14	0	57	57	0	0

[a] Ratio of % of non-NPC groups with IgA-anti-VCA ≥1:10 to that of NPC patients

[b] 18 non-NPC traumatic ward patients due for discharge and 39 healthy blood donors

[c] Staging system of Ho (1970)

Ho (1972) reported that family members of NPC patients have a higher risk for NPC as compared with family members of patients with other cancers. These results suggest that the risk for the disease might be associated with the frequency of detection of IgA antibody to VCA. If the relative disease risk, i.e., the ratio of the percentage frequency of non-NPC groups with IgA-anti-VCA to that of NPC patients, assigned to NPC patients is 1, that for their family members can be calculated to be 0.22; the relative disease risk for healthy subjects was 0 (Table 1). These results indicate that individuals who show the IgA antibody response tend to aggregate in families and that such individuals are rarely observed among the healthy subjects. This suggests that the IgA antibody response to VCA might be genetically determined. It was interesting to note that as in the incidence of NPC, there was a preponderance of males in the sex distribution of individuals who showed this seroreactivity.

The distribution of individuals with IgA antibody to VCA among siblings from sibships of different sizes was analysed by the method of complete ascertainment (Table 2). In this analysis, the size of the sibships was taken as the number of siblings available for study, which, in some instances, did not represent the actual sizes of the sibships since other members were sometimes not available for various reasons. The table shows that the observed frequencies of occurrence of individuals with IgA-anti-VCA correlated with the expected frequencies, as if the IgA antibody response were determined by an autosomal recessive gene (see Thompson & Thompson, 1966). This also holds true

Table 2. Observed and expected distribution of nasopharyngeal carcinoma (NPC) patients and individuals showing the IgA-anti-VCA response in sibships of NPC patients

Size of sibship	Number of sibships	Number of siblings	Expected no.[a]	Observed no. with NPC	Observed no. with IgA-anti-VCA ≥1:10
2	15	30	17.14	19	24
3	8	24	10.38	10	12
4	6	24	8.78	7	9
5	4	20	6.56	5	7
6	1	6	1.82	3	5
8	2	16	4.44	2	5
				χ^2 = 3.05 (P <0.7)	8.66 (P <0.2)
			Correlation coefficient =	0.97	0.96

[a] Those with autosomal recessive trait, calculated by the method of complete ascertainment

for the distribution of NPC patients among these sibships.

IgA antibody to VCA was similarly tested in sera obtained from NPC patients with various stages of the disease and from survivors who had shown no clinical relapse for periods of one to twelve years after radiation therapy (Table 3). The frequency of detection of this seroreactivity was found to be slightly higher in NPC patients with regional disease than in those with local disease or in survivors who had had regional disease before therapy. The difference in either instance was not, however, significant. The frequency of detection was similar in NPC patients with local disease and in survivors who had been in the same disease stage before radiation therapy and in survivors who had had local or regional disease before therapy.

Sera were also obtained from 10 NPC patients before radiation therapy and at intervals for periods of up to 48 months afterwards. IgA antibody to VCA was found to persist in all of these patients, despite the fact that five had at least one episode of relapse. There was thus no apparent association between this seroreactivity and clinical evolution.

During our study, we encountered a family member who had no clinical symptoms of NPC but whose serum gave a positive result at a dilution of 1:10. Nine months later she developed symptoms that were diagnosed as NPC, and there was a concomitant and substantial rise in the titre of IgA antibody to VCA. The tumour disappeared after radiation therapy, and there was no clinical evidence of relapse for up to eight months afterwards. The patient sustained a high level of IgA antibody to VCA during this time. The level of IgG antibody to VCA was initially high and remained so throughout the entire period of observation (Fig. 1).

Table 3. Serum IgA antibody levels in nasopharyngeal carcinoma patients with local and regional tumours before radiation therapy and in relapse-free survivors after radiation therapy

Subjects	No. with IgA > 1:10	IgA < 1:10	χ^2	P
Patients with localized disease	34	4		
Survivors of localized disease	19	3		
	53	7	0.13	0.99
Patients with regional disease	87	1		
Survivors of regional disease	22	3		
	109	4	6.79	<0.1
Patients with localized disease	34	4		
Patients with regional disease	87	1		
	121	5	6.13	<0.2
Survivors of localized disease	19	3		
Survivors of regional disease	22	3		
	41	6	0.03	>0.99

DISCUSSION

There is a tendency for individuals who show detectable serum levels of IgA antibodies to VCA to aggregate in families. This, coupled with the rare occurrence of these individuals among healthy subjects and patients with other cancers, makes it likely that IgA antibody to VCA may be determined, in part at least, by a recessive genetic trait. The observed frequencies of siblings who show the IgA antibody response correlate with those expected for sibships of different sizes, as though this response were determined by an autosomal recessive gene (see Thompson & Thompson, 1966)

Ho (1972) observed that family members of NPC patients have a higher risk for NPC than do the family members of patients with other cancers.

FIG. 1. EVOLUTION OF ANTIBODY TITRES
IN A NASOPHARYNGEAL CARCINOMA PATIENT

Titres of IgA (●) and IgG (■) antibody to Epstein-Barr viral capsid antigen (VCA) in a nasopharyngeal carcinoma (NPC) patient with no evidence of disease (NED), with NPC and after radiation therapy (RT)

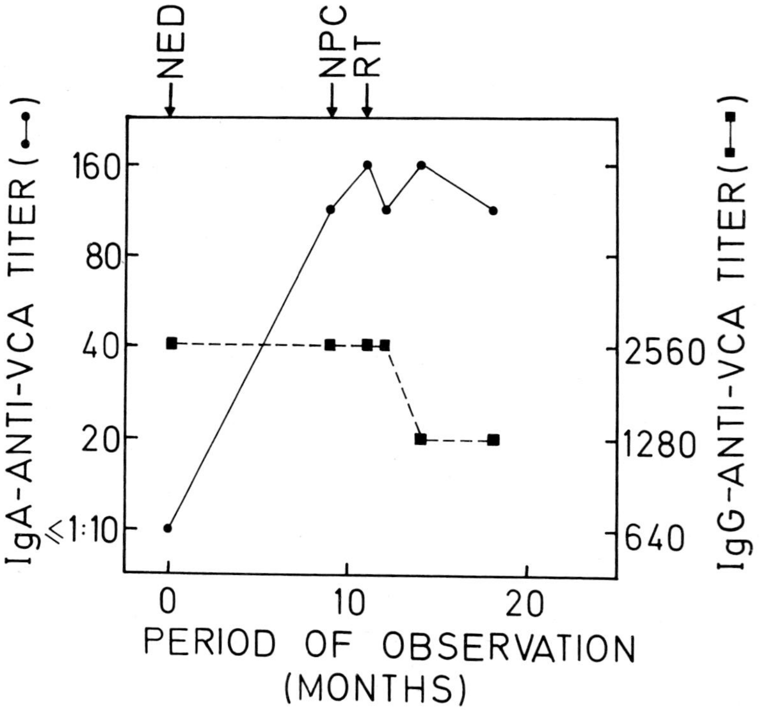

That the risk for NPC might be genetically determined was also suggested by the results of his pedigree study (Ho, 1972). On the basis of these results and of those of immunogenetic studies, Simons et al. (1974) postulated the existence of a disease susceptibility gene for NPC. The present results clearly demonstrate a close association between NPC and the frequency of detection of IgA antibody to VCA. From the genetic viewpoint, such an association may imply linkage between the hypothetical disease susceptibility gene and the gene that influences the IgA antibody response. Five of the NPC patients of the 126 studied showed no detectable IgA antibody to VCA; of these, four had local tumours, and the failure to detect IgA antibody in these patients might be due to insufficient antigenic stimulation. One of the patients, however, had a regional tumour, and the negative test results might be due to segregation of the two hypothetical genes. Unfortunately, family members of this patient were not available for immunogenetic studies.

In one patient we observed a substantial rise in titre of antibody to VCA concomitantly with the development of NPC, indicating that this antibody response is related to NPC. Consistent with this contention, slightly more NPC patients with regional tumours showed a positive test result as compared with those with local disease or with relapse-free survivors who had a regional tumour before radiation therapy, although the differences were not significant by chi square analysis. The finding that over 90% of NPC patients show detectable levels of IgA antibody to VCA and that they sustain substantially higher titres of this seroreactivity than do patients with Burkitt's lymphoma or infectious mononucleosis (Henle & Henle, 1976; Ho et al., 1976) provides further support for the above contention.

It is possible that the IgA antibody response to VCA is under dual control, i.e., due to stimulation with antigens originating from the NPC cells and to an autosomal recessive gene prevalent among NPC patients and their family members. The autosomal recessive gene may determine the capacity of an individual to mount the IgA antibody response, the increased capacity for this antibody response being evident in NPC patients by the elevated mean serum IgA concentration as compared with that in controls. This elevated IgA level may also reflect the intensity of antigenic stimulation (Ho et al., 1976; Wara et al., 1975).

Even though the IgA antibody response is increased, it is still limited relative to that of the IgG immune system: the serum IgG concentration was about four times that of IgA, probably implying that the IgA antibody response is more easily saturated by the antigenic load. The apparent lack of association between the frequency of detection of IgA antibody to VCA and clinical evolution of disease or disease staging might be attributed in part to the limited capacity of the IgA immune response system.

The detection of IgA antibody to VCA in presymptom serum obtained from one patient and in the sera from the majority of relapse-free survivors after radiation therapy suggests that the IgA response can be elicited by occult and subclinical residual tumours. The detection of this reactivity in apparently healthy family members of NPC patients might, therefore, indicate the presence of occult tumours. The importance of regular examination of these individuals cannot be overemphasized.

SUMMARY

There is a strong association between the frequency of detection of IgA antibody to VCA and NPC. Over 90% of NPC patients and none of 57 healthy subjects showed this reactivity. The healthy family members of NPC patients constitute an intermediate association group, showing a frequency of detection of 21.05%; this pattern of familial aggregation suggests that the IgA antibody response to VCA might be genetically determined. The observed frequencies of siblings who showed this seroreactivity correlated with the expected frequencies for sibships of different sizes, as though this response were determined by an autosomal recessive gene.

The association with NPC suggests that the IgA antibody response to VCA might depend on tumour burden. A substantial rise in IgA antibody titre was observed concomitantly with the appearance of clinical NPC in one patient. The limited capacity for mounting the IgA response, as compared with the IgG immune system, may account for the poor correlation between the frequency of detection of IgA antibody to VCA and tumour load or clinical evolution of disease.

This assay system appears to be highly sensitive for NPC and may provide an indication of the existence of occult and subclinical residual tumours.

ACKNOWLEDGEMENTS

This study was supported in part by a research contract with the International Agency for Research on Cancer, Lyon, France, and by the Hong Kong Anti-Cancer Society.

REFERENCES

Desgranges, G., Wolf, H., de-Thé, G., Shanmugaratnam, K., Cammoun, N., Ellouz, R., Klein, G., Lennert, K., Muñoz, N. & zur Hausen, H. (1975) Nasopharyngeal carcinoma. X. Presence of Epstein-Barr genomes in separated epithelial cells of tumors in patients from Singapore, Tunisia and Kenya. *Int. J. Cancer, 16*, 7-15

Glaser, R., de-Thé, G., Lenoir, G. & Ho, J.H.C. (1976) Superinfection of epithelial nasopharyngeal carcinoma cells with Epstein-Barr virus. *Proc. nat. Acad. Sci. (Wash.), 73*, 960-963

Henle, G. & Henle, W. (1976) Epstein-Barr virus specific IgA serum antibodies as an outstanding feature of nasopharyngeal carcinoma. *Int. J. Cancer, 17*, 1-7

Henle, G., Henle, W. & Diehl, V. (1968) Relation of Burkitt's tumor-associated herpes-type virus to infectious mononucleosis. *Proc. nat. Acad. Sci. (Wash.), 59*, 94-101

Ho, J.H.C. (1970) Head and neck tumors. *Oncology, 4*, 1-14

Ho, J.H.C. (1972) Nasopharyngeal carcinoma (NPC). *Advanc. Cancer Res., 15*, 57-92

Ho, H.C., Ng, M.H., Kwan, H.C. & Chan, J.C.W. (1976) Epstein-Barr virus specific IgA and IgG serum antibodies in nasopharyngeal carcinoma patients and controls. *Brit. J. Cancer, 34*, 655-660

Ho, H.C., Kwan, H.C. & Ng, M.H. (1977a) Detection of salivary IgA antibodies to Epstein-Barr virus capsid antigen in NPC patients and control subjects. *Brit. J. Cancer* (in press)

Ho, H.C., Ng, M.H. & Kwan, H.C. (1977b) Studies of the IgA antibody response to the Epstein-Barr virus capsid antigen in nasopharyngeal carcinoma patients before and after radiation therapy and controls. *Brit. J. Cancer* (in press)

Huang, D., Ho, J.H.C., Henle, W. & Henle, G. (1974) Demonstration of Epstein-Barr virus-associated nuclear antigen in nasopharyngeal carcinoma cells from fresh biopsies. *Int. J. Cancer, 14*, 580-588

Huang, D.P., Ho, H.C., Ng, M.H. & Liu, M. (1977) Possible transformation of nasopharyngeal epithelial cells in culture with Epstein-Barr virus derived from B95-8 cells. *Brit. J. Cancer* (in press)

Klein, G. (1973) *The Epstein-Barr virus.* In: Kaplan, A., ed., *The Herpesviruses*, New York, Academic Press, pp. 521-555

Klein, G., Giovanella, B., Lindahl, T., Fialkow, P.J., Singh, S. & Stehlin, J. (1974) Direct evidence for the presence of Epstein-Barr virus DNA and nuclear antigen in malignant epithelial cells from patients with anaplastic carcinoma of the nasopharynx. *Proc. nat. Acad. Sci (Wash.), 71*, 4737-4741

Miller, G. (1976) *Epidemiology of Burkitt's lymphoma.* In: Evans, A.S., ed., *Viral Infection of Humans*, New York and London, Plenum, pp. 481-499

Simons, M.J., Wee, G.B., Day, N.E., Morris, P.J., Shanmugaratnam, K. & de-Thé, G. (1974) Immunogenetic aspects of nasopharyngeal carcinoma. I. Differences in HL-A antigen profiles between patients and control groups. *Int. J. Cancer, 13*, 122-134

Thompson, J.S. & Thompson, M.W. (1966) *Genetics in Medicine*, Philadelphia, Saunders

Tomasi, T.B., Bull, D., Tourville, D. & Yurechak, A. (1969) *Concept of local immunity and the secretory system.* In: Dayton, D.H., Jr, et al., eds, *Symposium of the Secretory Immunologic System, Verobeach, Florida*, Washington, D.C., U.S. Government Printing office

Trumper, P.A., Epstein, M.A. & Giovanella, P.C. (1976) Activation *in vitro* by BUdR of a productive Epstein-Barr virus infection in the epithelial cells of nasopharyngeal carcinoma. *Int. J. Cancer, 17*, 578-587

Wara, W.M., Wara, D.W., Philips, T.L. & Amanann, A.J. (1975) Elevated IgA in carcinoma of the nasopharynx. *Cancer, 35*, 1313-1315

PRESENCE OF EPSTEIN-BARR VIRUS SPECIFIC IgA IN SALIVA OF NASOPHARYNGEAL CARCINOMA PATIENTS: THEIR ACTIVITY, ORIGIN AND POSSIBLE CLINICAL VALUE

C. DESGRANGES & G. DE-THE

Unit of Biological Carcinogenesis,
International Agency for Research on Cancer,
Lyon, France

INTRODUCTION

Recent studies have demonstrated the presence of Epstein-Barr (EBV)-specific IgA serum antibodies in nasopharyngeal carcinoma (NPC) patients (Henle & Henle, 1976; Ho et al., 1976). The high IgA antibody response to EBV antigens [viral capsid antigen (VCA) and early antigen (EA)] in serum seems to be a unique feature of NPC patients (Desgranges et al., 1977; Henle & Henle, 1976) when compared with Burkitt's lymphoma (BL) or infectious mononucleosis (IM) patients.

EBV-neutralizing IgA antibodies to VCA (VCA/IgA) were detected in the throat-washings of NPC patients but never in saliva from BL or IM patients. In this paper we report on the secretory nature of these IgA and on their origin in the tumour tissue.

MATERIALS AND METHODS

Saliva and sera

As already reported (Desgranges et al., 1977), salivas were collected from 10 NPC patients in Tunisia (Institut Salah Azaiz, Tunis) and from 13 NPC patients in Hong Kong (Medical and Health Department, Queen Elizabeth Hospital, Kowloon), from 21 BL patients in Arua, East Africa, from 18 IM patients in Lyon and from healthy controls in each country. The samples were frozen immediately and sent to Lyon. Salivas were used without any concentration after centrifugation at 1 500 rpm for 10 min at 4°C and filtration through a 0.8 μ mesh. Sera were collected from NPC patients and controls in Tunisia, Hong Kong and Singapore. These were frozen at $-70^{o}C$ before testing.

EBV-specific immunofluorescence (IF) tests

IgA reactivity to VCA in saliva was detected using acetone-fixed Jijoye cell smears, as described previously (Desgranges et al., 1977), but for the present study the smears were stained with fluorescein-conjugated anti-human IgA specific for alpha chains (FITC-anti-α) (Hyland, Los Angeles, USA) and anti-human secretory piece of IgA (FITC-anti-SP) (Dakopatts, Copenhagen, Denmark). The specificity of the IgA-α conjugates was tested with smears of human myeloma cells and for secretory piece (SP) with sera positive for IgG, IgA(α) and for IgM.

Detection of IgA(α) and SP in situ

Detection of IgA(α) and SP of IgA was carried out using fluorescein-conjugated rabbit antisera to human IgA(α) and SP (Dakopatts, Copenhagen, Denmark). Horse-radish peroxidase-conjugated antibodies to IgA(α) and SP (Dakopatts, Copenhagen, Denmark) were used in parallel by either direct or indirect testing.

In order to study the specificity of IgA present in NPC tumours, the biopsies were ground in phosphate-buffered saline, centrifuged at 2 000 rpm for 15 min and the supernatant tested for IgA/EBV-specific activity. Similar extracts were prepared from inflamed tonsils, adenoids and normal nasopharyngeal mucosal biopsies. These were tested on Jijoye smears using anti-human IgA(α) and anti-human SP antisera as above.

Leucocyte transformation test

Leucocytes from heparinized umbilical cord blood were separated using the technique previously described by Yata et al. (1975): 2×10^6 leucocytes suspended in 1 ml of RPMI 1640 supplemented with 20% foetal calf serum were mixed with 1 ml of the throat-washing filtrate and incubated at $37^{o}C$ in an atmosphere of 5% carbon dioxide for eight weeks, half of the medium being changed weekly. Each throat-washing was tested in triplicate on three different cord bloods. For positive and negative controls, each leucocyte suspension was inoculated with the transforming virus, B95.8 (Miller & Lipman, 1973), and with culture medium. Some cultures contained only throat-washing fluids in RPMI medium.

Gel filtration chromatographic analysis of EBV IgA antibodies in NPC salivas

A 1 ml sample of saliva positive for both IgA(α) and SP (HK976) was applied to columns of 6B sepharose in 0.01M hydrochloric acid-Tris buffer at pH 7.2. Fractions (3.5 ml) were collected, analysed for absorbance at 280 nm, grouped by three, lyophilized and resuspended in 0.5 ml distilled water. Each fraction was assayed by immunofluorescence on fixed Jijoye cells for their content of EBV IgA(α), IgA(SP), IgG and IgM.

RESULTS

Presence of neutralizing EBV-specific IgA in NPC saliva

Table 1 shows that 14 NPC salivas out of 23 were positive for EBV-specific IgA(α). We were never able to obtain the transformation of cord blood leucocytes with positive EBV-IgA salivas, whereas one EBV-IgG-positive saliva (HK975) contained transforming EBV.

Table 1. Presence of IgA and IgG antibodies to viral capsid antigen (VCA) and to early antigen (EA) in throat-washings from nasopharyngeal carcinoma patients

Registry number	IgA		IgG		Transformation
	VCA	EA	VCA	EA	
HK 604	+	-	++	-	-
HK 744	-	-	-	-	S[a]
HK 796	++++	+	+	+	-
HK 917	-	-	++	±	-
HK 918	+	-	++++	+++	-
HK 920	-	-	+++	++	-
HK 923	-	-	-	-	S[a]
HK 924	-	-	+++	-	-
HK 932	++	-	++++	+++	-
HK 971	+	-	++++	+++	-
HK 973	-	-	-	-	-
HK 975	-	-	++	-	+
HK 976	+++	+	++++	++++	-
Tu 12	+++	++	+++	++	-
Tu 17	+	-	+++	+++	-
Tu 19	+	-	+	+	-
Tu 21	++	+	+++	+	-
Tu 201	++	++	++++	++	-
Tu 238	+	++	+++	++	-
Tu 333	-	-	-	-	+
Tu 336	+	-	+	-	-
Tu 354	+	++	+++	+++	-
Tu 394	-	-	-	-	-

- undetectable; + undiluted; ++ $\frac{1}{8}$; +++ $\frac{1}{16}$; ++++ $>\frac{1}{16}$

[a] Stimulation of the culture for two months but no establishment of a lymphoblastoid line

The transforming activity of B95.8 virus (2 x 10^3 ID 50/ml) was neutralized by three IgA positive and non-transforming throat-washings (HK976, HK932 and HK796); the neutralizing end-point was 1/200 for both HK976 and HK796 and 1/20 for HK932.

Three different IgA-negative non-transforming salivas (HK A, HK C and HK F = Chinese control group) failed to neutralize B95.8 virus.

Secretory nature of EBV-specific IgA in saliva of NPC patients

Table 2 shows that of 12 NPC salivas positive for EBV-IgA(α), nine were also positive for the SP. Salivas negative for EBV-IgA(α) were also negative for the SP.

Table 2. Presence of IgA(α) and secretory piece (SP) in salivas of nasopharyngeal carcinoma patients[a]

Registry number	IgA(α)	SP
HK 604	+	+
HK 744	-	-
HK 917	-	-
HK 918	+	+
HK 920	-	-
HK 923	-	-
HK 924	-	-
HK 932	++	-
HK 971	+	+
HK 973	-	-
HK 975	-	-
HK 976	+++	+++
Tu 12	+++	++
Tu 17	+	-
Tu 19	+	+
Tu 21	++	++
Tu 32	+	-
Tu 238	+	+
Tu 333	-	-
Tu 354	+	+
Tu 394	-	-

[a] Determined by immunofluorescence using a fluorescein-labelled specific antihuman IgA or anti-SP

Figure 1 shows the profile obtained after chromatography on a 6B sepharose column with the positive HK976 saliva [IgA(α) and SP]. The IgA(α) and IgG activities were found in 7s fractions, whereas IgA-SP activities were localized in 11s fractions. No EBV IgM activity was detected in any of the fractions.

FIG. 1. GEL FILTRATION CHROMATOGRAPHIC ANALYSIS ON 6B SEPHAROSE OF SALIVA FROM NASOPHARYNGEAL CARCINOMA PATIENTS

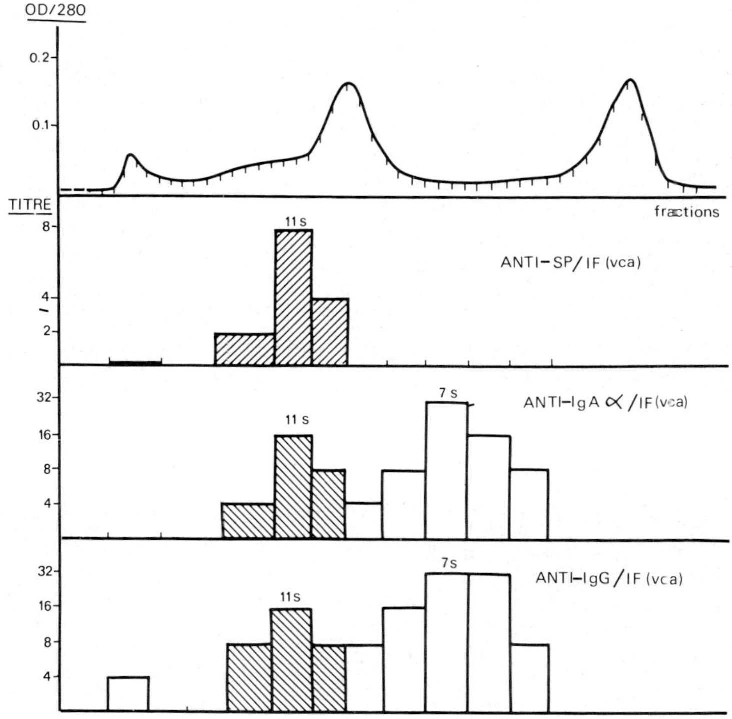

Origin of EBV-specific IgA in NPC patients

IgA(α) and SP were detected by IF in NPC biopsies in frozen as well as in Bouin-fixed sections. As seen in Figure 2, the plasmocytes with an exentric nucleus contained IgA(α) activity. IgA(SP) activity was found in cytoplasm and in the lumen of the glandular acini as well as on the surface of the epithelial tumour cells (Fig. 3).

The EBV specificities of the IgA(α) and SP in the NPCs were demonstrated in extracts of tumours tested on Jijoye cells

FIG. 2. IgA(α) IN PLASMOCYTES SURROUNDING EPITHELIAL TUMOUR CELLS x 300

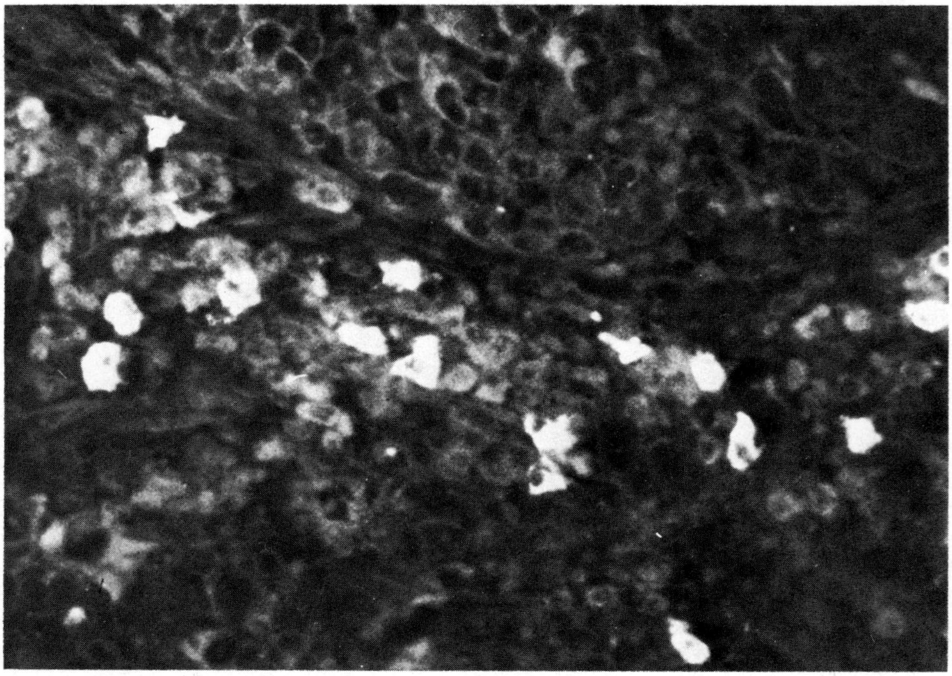

FIG. 3. IgA(SP) IN THE GLANDULAR ACINI AND ON THE SURFACE OF EPITHELIAL TUMOUR CELLS x 300

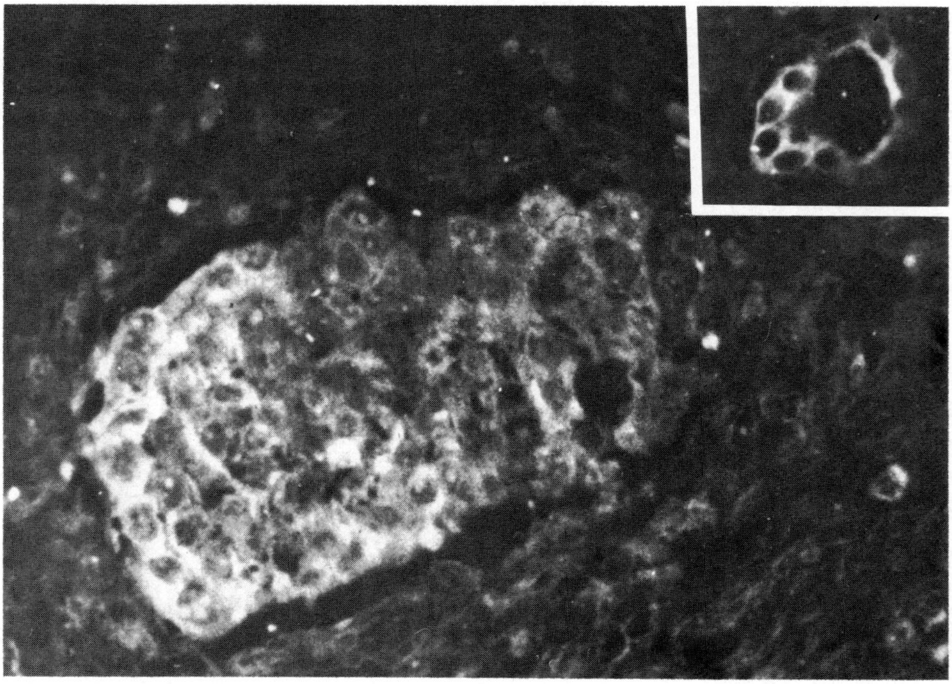

(Tu 12 - Tu 21). Tissue from adenoid, normal tonsil or normal nasopharyngeal mucosa that were positive for IgA was negative for EBV specificity when tested as above.

Clinical value of presence of EBV-IgA in salivas

As shown in Figure 4, throat-washings from NPC patients contained IgA directed to VCA and EA (54% and 27%, respectively) and IgG directed to VCA and EA (73% and 54%, respectively). In contrast, throat-washings from patients with BL, IM or other tumours of the head and neck and healthy controls were devoid of detectable IgA antibodies although positive for IgG in variable proportions.

FIG. 4. EPSTEIN-BARR VIRUS SPECIFIC IgA and IgG IN THROAT WASHINGS

Percentages of throat washings with Epstein-Barr virus-specific IgA and IgG in normal individuals and in patients with other tumours of the head and neck, infectious mononucleosis (IM), Burkitt's lymphoma (BL) and nasopharyngeal carcinoma (NPC). vca - viral capsid antigen; ea - early antigen

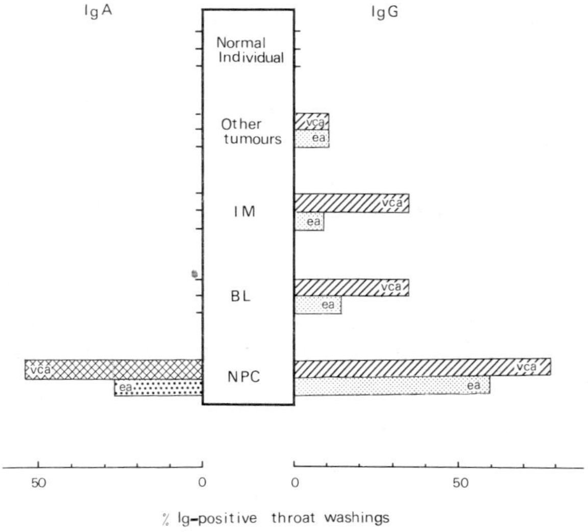

IgA and IgG in sera corresponding to throat-washings from patients with NPC and other tumours

Figure 5 shows the correlation between IgA and IgG antibodies to VCA and EA in sera corresponding to the throat washings described above. Sera from patients with BL and other cancers of the head and neck showed

FIG. 5. CORRELATION BETWEEN IgG AND IgA ANTIBODY TITRES TO VIRAL CAPSID ANTIGEN (VCA) AND EARLY ANTIGEN (EA)

Correlation between IgG and IgA antibody titres to VCA (left) and EA (right) in sera from patients with nasopharyngeal carcinoma, Burkitt's lymphoma and other tumours of head and neck

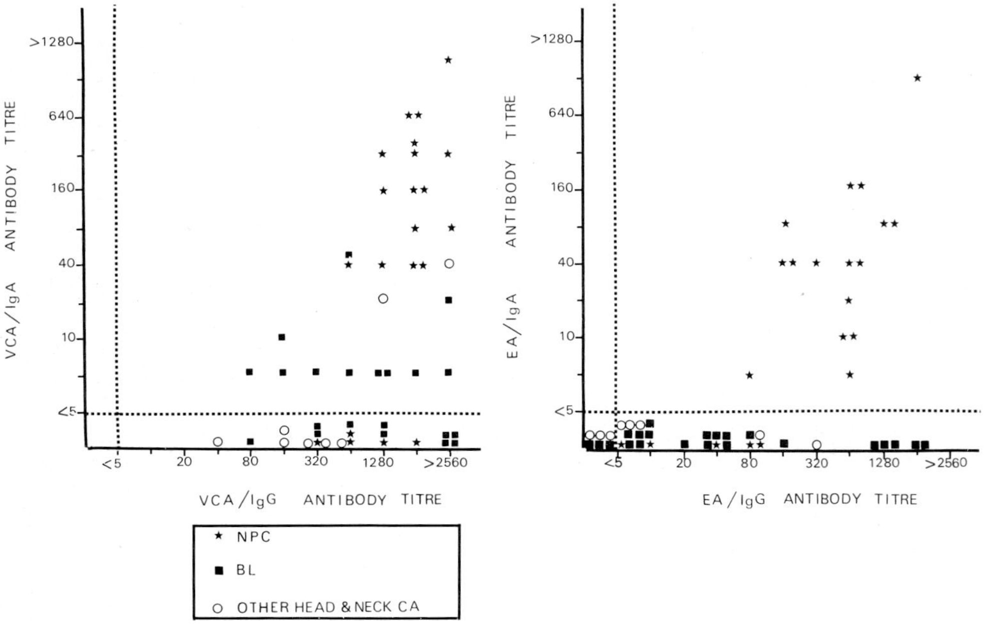

the presence of IgA-VCA at titres ranging from 1/10 to 1/40, while 76% of sera from patients with NPC showed high titres (1/40 to <1280). No group other than those with NPC had any significant levels of IgA-EA.

Table 3 shows the geometric mean titres (GMT) of IgA-VCA and EA in sera from Chinese NPC patients at different clinical stages of the disease. Stage III sera showed higher titres for IgA and IgG directed against both VCA and EA; decreases were noted in sera from patients in the last two stages of the disease.

Table 4 gives the percentages of sera positive for EBV/IgA in NPC patients, in NPC family members and in the normal population. NPC family members from Tunis, but not those from Hong Kong and Singapore, were more often positive for IgA-VCA than the general population. The reason for this difference among areas is unknown but is possibly due to the fact that only a small number of persons were tested in Hong Kong and Singapore.

Table 3. Epstein-Barr viral capsid antigen (VCA) and early antigen (EA)/IgG and IgA geometric mean titres (GMT) in sera from Chinese nasopharyngeal carcinoma (NPC) patients in different stages of the disease, in patients with other tumours and in controls.

Subjects	VCA/IgA		EA/IgA		VCA/IgG		EA/IgG	
	GMT	SE	GMT	SE	GMT	SE	GMT	SE
NPC Stage I	44.4	0.6	10.	0.5	512.	0.4	48.5	0.7
NPC Stage II	69.6	0.5	12.3	0.6	803.4	0.4	54.9	0.4
NPC Stage III	85.7	0.6	23.	0.6	1097.5	0.3	97.	0.6
NPC Stage IV	56.6	0.6	20.	0.6	630.4	0.4	84.4	0.7
NPC Stage V	52.8	0.9	16.8	0.9	724.1	0.5	101.6	0.5
Other tumours	3.3	0.1	2.5	0.0	279.2	0.3	3.3	0.3
Normal individuals	2.8	0.1	2.5	0.0	92.1	0.3	2.2	0.1

Table 4. Presence of Epstein-Barr virus/IgA in sera from nasopharyngeal carcinoma (NPC) patients, family members and normal population

	VCA	%	GMT/VCA	EA	%
HONG KONG					
NPC patients	58/62	93.6	70	49/62	79.1
NPC family members	3/20	15	2.77	0/31	0
Normal population	13/61	21.3	3.03	0/78	0
SINGAPORE					
NPC patients	24/31	70.9	33.45	15/31	48.4
NPC family members	25/125	20	3.07	1/124	0.8
Normal population	7/37	19	2.96	0/37	0
TUNIS					
NPC patients	45/52	86.6	95	42/52	80.8
NPC family members	60/133	45.1	3.81	1/134	0.8
Normal population	73/424	17.3	2.90	0/424	0

VCA - viral capsid antigen

GMT - geometric mean titre

EA - early antigen

DISCUSSION

Secretory IgA specific for EBV was detected in throat-washings from NPC patients but not in those with other conditions (such as BL or IM); the origin of this IgA was the tumour tissue itself. In a discussion of the origin of the EBV-specific IgA in NPC sera, Henle & Henle (1976) stressed that the tumour was localized in the area of Waldeyer's ring, the site of secretion of IgA. It is therefore of interest to have localized the synthesis of EBV/IgA in the tumour itself. The question that then arises is whether the synthesis of EBV/IgA precedes or follows tumour development. A longitudinal follow-up study of a high-risk population prior to tumour development would answer the question.

The local activity of this IgA found within the tumour is a matter of speculation; however, one may suggest that EBV-specific IgA on the surface of epithelial tumour cells could act as a blocking antibody against sensitive lymphocytes.

The presence of EBV/IgA in the sera of NPC patients in Stage I of the disease is pathognomonic for NPC as compared with other tumours and normal individuals. Detection of VCA and EA IgA should become an early diagnostic tool for NPC and could be used for detection of NPC in high-risk areas where this carcinoma represents the most frequent tumour in males.

A genetic control of EBV-specific IgA synthesis is suggested by the finding of a higher proportion of IgA-positive sera in NPC family members, as compared with the general population. Ng discusses this point elsewhere in this publication[1].

REFERENCES

Desgranges, C., de-Thé, G., Ho, J.H.C. & Ellouz, R. (1977) Neutralizing EBV specific IgA in throat-washings of nasopharyngeal carcinoma (NPC) patients. *Int. J. Cancer, 19*, 627-633

Henle, G. & Henle, W. (1976) Epstein-Barr virus-specific IgA serum antibodies as an outstanding feature of nasopharyngeal carcinoma. *Int. J. Cancer, 17*, 1-7

Ho, H.C., Ng, M.H., Kwan, H.C. & Chau, J.C.W. (1976) Epstein-Barr virus-specific IgA and IgG serum antibodies in nasopharyngeal carcinoma patients and controls. *Brit. J. Cancer, 34*, 655-660

---

[1] See p. 449

Miller, G. & Lipman, M. (1973) Release of infectious Epstein-Barr virus by transformed marmoset leukocytes. *Proc. nat. Acad. Sci. (Wash.)*, *70*, 190-194

Yata, J., Desgranges, C., Nakagawa, T., Favre, M.C. & de-Thé, G. (1975) Lymphoblastoid transformation and kinetics of appearance of viral nuclear antigen (EBNA) in cordblood lymphocytes infected by Epstein-Barr virus (EBV). *Int. J. Cancer*, *15*, 377-384

DIFFERENCES IN EBV ANTIBODY TITRES OF PATIENTS WITH NASOPHARYNGEAL CARCINOMA ORIGINATING FROM HIGH, INTERMEDIATE AND LOW INCIDENCE AREAS

G. DE THE, M.F. LAVOUE & L. MUENZ[1]

Units of Biological Carcinogenesis and Epidemiology,
International Agency for Research on Cancer,
Lyon, France

In collaboration with N. Cammoun and R. Ellouz, from the Institut Salah Azaiz, Tunis; J.H.C. Ho and H.C. Kwan, from the Institute of Radiology, Queen Elizabeth Hospital, Kowloon, Hong Kong; K. Shanmugaratnam, M.J. Simons[2] and S.H. Chan, from the Department of Pathology and the WHO Immunology Research and Training Centre, University of Singapore, Singapore; Y. Cachin, J. Brugère[3] and G. Schwaab from the Institut Gustave Roussy, Villejuif, France; G. Jausseran and G. Meyer, Institut Paoli, Marseille, France; B.E. Henderson and M.B. Gardner, University of Southern California School of Medicine, Los Angeles, Calif., USA; G. Klein, Tumor Biology, Karolinska Institutet, Stockholm, Sweden

---

[1] On secondment from the National Cancer Institute/National Institutes of Health, Bethesda, Md., USA

[2] New address: Immunodiagnostic Centre, Melbourne, Australia

[3] New address: Curie Foundation, rue d'Ulm, 75005 Paris, France

INTRODUCTION

The association between the Epstein-Barr virus (EBV) and nasopharyngeal carcinoma (NPC) rests upon two types of data. Patients with NPC have been shown to have high humoral (and sometimes cell-mediated) immune responses to a series of EBV-determined antigens, including structural antigens (viral capsid antigen, VCA), early antigens (EA) and nuclear antigens (EBNA) (de Schryver et al., 1974; de-Thé et al., 1975a; Henle et al., 1970a; Levine et al., 1976). Viral markers (EBV/DNA and EBNA) are also consistently present in poorly-differentiated tumour cells (Desgranges et al., 1975; de-Thé et al., 1973; Huang et al., 1974; Klein et al., 1974; Nonoyama & Pagano, 1973; Wolf et al., 1973; zur Hausen et al., 1970).

In order to compare the association between EBV and NPC in different geographical areas, we studied patients with NPC originating from areas with a high incidence of this tumour, such as Hong Kong and Singapore, with an intermediate incidence, such as North and East Africa, and with a low incidence, such as Europe and the USA. We first investigated the presence of EBV/DNA by separating epithelial tumour cells from lymphoid cells and found that EBV genomes were concentrated in tumour cells from all of the geographical area from which they came (Desgranges et al., 1975). We then carried out a comparative evaluation of the serological profiles of sera originating from NPC patients from the three NPC incidence areas and tested them 'blind', using standardized antigen batches for all sera. The recent challenge of Henderson et al. (1976) that questioned the serological association of EBV with this tumour, on the basis of differences observed among NPC patients of different racial groups in Los Angeles, prompted us to discuss these results here.

MATERIALS AND METHODS

Sera from 288 patients with nasopharyngeal carcinoma were selected for place of origin: 50 from Hong Kong Chinese, 50 from Singapore Chinese, 65 from Tunisia, 20 from Nairobi (through the courtesy of Dr G. Klein), 40 from Los Angeles (originating from 8 Chinese, 6 Blacks, 17 Whites and 9 varied), 35 from Paris (11 Arab migrant workers from Algeria, 3 from Tunisia, 3 from Morocco and 12 Caucasians from France, 6 from the South of Italy, Malta and Portugal), 16 from Marseilles (all born around the Mediterranean) and 13 Swedish cases from Stockholm.

The cases were also selected to correspond, as far as possible, to clinical stages III and IV, according to Ho (1970). We did not succeed everywhere, and half of the serum samples from Los Angeles and from Paris were from patients with early stage disease, I or II.

Of the samples from patients in Hong Kong, Singapore and Tunisia, 75% were from Stages III and IV combined and about 20% were Stage V and 5% Stage II. For sera from Nairobi, Sweden and Marseille there was insufficient clinical information to assess the stage of the disease.

The histological type of NPC was available for most cases, and the majority consisted of undifferentiated or poorly differentiated carcinomas (44/49 from Hong, 20/40 from Los Angeles, 49/55 from Tunis, 28/35 from Paris, 4/16 from Marseille); the diagnosis of differentiated squamous-cell carcinoma was given for only 29 cases (2 from Hong Kong, 13 from Los Angeles, 1 from Tunis, 5 from Paris, 8 from Marseille). The term 'lymphoepithelioma' was given to 8 cases from Los Angeles, 6 from Paris and 3 from Marseille but for none of those from the Far East. These data are given to indicate the variability in the histopathological diagnosis and to stress the necessity of standardizing the pathological classification of tumours arising in the nasopharynx.

In order to compare NPC cases with patients with other tumours and with normal individuals from the same geographical areas, we selected a further 39 sera from Hong Kong, 65 from Tunis and 37 from Paris, from patients with ear, nose and throat tumours other than NPC, and 45, 65 and 40 sera from normal individuals of the same age group as the patients (45-60 years) in Hong Kong, Tunis and Paris, respectively.

Antibodies to EBV-determined antigens were titrated by indirect immunofluorescent tests, using Jijoye cells for VCA (Henle & Henle, 1966). For EA antibodies (to both restricted and diffuse components), RAJI cells superimprinted with EBV were prepared (Henle et al., 1970b). Fluorescein-conjugated antisera to either human IgG or human IgA were used (Huntingdon Research Centre for NCI, Hyland). To titrate EBNA antibodies, RAJI cells (and for controls, MOLT-4 cells) were used in the anticomplement immunofluorescence test (Reedman & Klein, 1973). To improve readability, counterstaining with 0.006% Evans blue was used routinely. Complement fixation tests were carried out after checking for anticomplementary activity of the sera, using 2 units of EBV soluble antigen (CF/s) prepared from RAJI cell extracts (Sohier & de-Thé, 1972).

To avoid variability in titres resulting from either differences in antigen batches or the mode of reading, the same person carried out all of the tests, using one antigen batch for each of the serological reactivities. All of the sera were coded, and sera of different origins were included for each testing.

RESULTS

Table 1 gives the geometric mean titres (GMT) and the 95% confidence intervals of the four EBV reactivities (VCA, EA, EBNA and CF/s) of sera from NPC patients from different groups around the world.

Table 1. Geometric mean titres and 95% confidence intervals of EBV reactivities in different groups of nasopharyngeal carcinoma patients around the world

	HONG KONG	SINGAPORE	LOS ANGELES			
	Chinese	Chinese	Chinese	White	Varied[a]	Black
VCA (Jijoye)	1316 (957–1810)	1927 (1609–2307)	761 (318–1823)	416 (211–821)	527 (226–2456)	453 (179–1146)
No. of sera	50	50	8	17	9	6
EA (Raji)	182 (117–284)	277 (182–419)	129 (43–386)	29 (14–60)	61 (19–193)	42 (7–260)
No. of sera	50	50	8	17	9	6
CF (Raji)	88 (59–129)	185 (136–251)	74 (28–192)	30 (16–58)	83 (29–239)	101 (27–375)
No. of sera	43	43	8	17	9	6
EBNA (Raji)	776 (440–1370)	1643 (1025–2632)	614 (223–1689)	341 (168–691)	549 (220–1372)	1018 (225–4614)
No. of sera	48	50	8	17	9	6

	NAIROBI	TUNIS	PARIS		MARSEILLE	STOCKHOLM
	Black	Arabs	North Africans[b]	Caucasians[c]	Mediterraneans[d]	Caucasians
VCA (Jijoye)	1450 (905–2323)	1677 (1306–2153)	710 (397–1271)	978 (534–1790)	1337 (734–2435)	833 (411–1689)
No. of sera	20	65	17	18	16	13
EA (Raji)	343 (128–918)	119 (74–190)	111 (44–277)	194 (66–571)	167 (57–491)	52 (15–176)
No. of sera	20	65	17	18	16	13
CF (Raji)	113 (57–226)	75 (55–103)	31 (18–54)	32 (18–57)	236 (131–428)	66 (27–162)
No. of sera	16	58	17	18	16	9
EBNA (Raji)	1280 (695–4711)	593 (402–874)	85 (48–150)	118 (66–209)	Not done	281 (108–730)
No. of sera	20	65	17	18		13

[a] Filipino, Japanese, Mexican
[b] 11 Algerians, 3 Tunisians, 3 Moroccans
[c] 12 French, 3 Italians, 3 from Malta, Cayenne and Portugal
[d] These sera were received later and tested separately, with antigenic batches different from those usec for the other groups.

Each of the four reactivities varied up to three-fold between the highest and lowest ranking groups. There was overall agreement between VCA and EA reactivities in the different groups concerned, but less with regard to EBNA antibodies. If, for convenience, the GMTs of each reactivity are divided into three levels: high, intermediate and low, as in Table 2, it can be seen that there is a general downward trend of the GMT with increasing socio-economic level. Levels of antibodies to VCA and EA were highest in NPC sera from the Far East, North and East Africa, intermediate in the European cases, and lowest in Los Angeles (it must also be remembered that half of the cases from Los Angeles were stages I and II). Levels of antibodies to EBNA differed somewhat from the previous two (Table 2): Chinese tended to have intermediate levels, and Blacks from both East Africa and Los Angeles exhibited high GMTs.

In order to explore further the relative importance of environment *versus* 'racial' or 'genetic' background in the EBV profile of NPC patients, an 'income rank' was given to each group, from 1 to 10, according to the 1963 *UN Statistical Year Book*, as follows:

1. Nairobi Africans
2. Tunis Arabs
3. Arabs migrants in Paris
4. Hong Kong Chinese
5. Singapore Chinese
6. Paris Caucasians
7. Los Angeles Blacks
8. Los Angeles Chinese
9. Stockholm Caucasians
10. Los Angeles Caucasians

Table 2. Ranking of EBV GMT reactivities in NPC sera from various parts of the world

Geographical area	Ethnic group	VCA GMT			EA GMT			EBNA GMT		
		High > 1400	Intermediate 1399-700	Low <700	High > 175	Intermediate 174-85	Low <85	High > 1000	Intermediate 999-500	Low <500
Hong Kong	Chinese	X			X				X	
Singapore	Chinese	X			X			X		
Los Angeles	Chinese		X			X			X	
	White			X			X			X
	Black			X			X	X		
Nairobi	African	X			X			X		
Tunis	Arab	X				X			X	
Paris	Arab		X			X			X	
	Caucasian		X		X					X
Stockholm	Caucasian		X				X			X
Marseille	Mediterranean		X			X		X		

It was found that the income factor significantly influences the VCA GMTs ($P = 0.008$, or $P = 0.002$ if only two income groups, high and low, are considered), influences to a much lesser extent the EA antibody level ($P = 0.002$, or $P = 0.025$ if 10 or two income groups are considered), and has no effect on the humoral response either to EBNA ($P = 0.95$ or 0.18) or to soluble antigen, as tested by complement fixation tests (CF/s) ($P = 0.84$ or 0.32).

Unexpectedly, genetic or racial factors seemed to influence the GMTs of antibodies directed against EBNA ($P = 0.0001$, or $P = 0.001$ for 10 or two income groups) and of those against CF/s ($P = 0.0001$, or $P = 0.001$ for 10 or two income groups).

A comparison of EBV antibody titres in NPC patients with those in patients with other tumours and with those in normal individuals is shown in Table 3. Whereas VCA GMTs were increased in patients with tumours other than NPC, when compared to normal individuals, the GMTs of antibody to EA were identical in both control groups, but were

Table 3. EBV serological reactivities in NPC patients, patients with other tumours and normal individuals originating from three geographical areas

Group and EBV reactivities		NPC patients		Patients with other tumours		Normal individuals	
		GMT	No. of sera	GMT	No. of sera	GMT	No. of sera
Hong Kong	VCA	1316		376		119	
Chinese	EA	182		8		9	
	CF	88		18		21	
	EBNA	776		86		ND	
			49		39		45
Tunis	VCA	1677		190		114	
Arabs	EA	119		8		7	
	CF	75		ND		24	
	EBNA	593		142		ND	
			65		65		65
Paris	VCA	978		166		91	
Caucasians	EA	194		6		7	
	CF	32		10		10	
	EBNA	118		ND		ND	
			18		37		40

ND - Not done

raised by a factor of 20-fold in all NPC groups, regardless of their geographical origin, showing active EBV infection in these patients.

Further to the results of Desgranges & de Thé[1] IgA antibodies to both VCA and EA were titred in 20 NPC sera and in the sera from 20 patients with ear, nose and throat tumours other than NPC from four different geographical areas (Hong Kong, Nairobi, Tunis, Marseille). Table 4 shows that although IgA antibodies to VCA were present in a number of controls, the GMTs of IgA to VCA in NPC patients were 15- to 20-fold higher than those of controls. IgA to EA was detected only in about two-thirds of NPC cases, i.e., in those with high titres of IgA to VCA. Surprisingly, the Black African NPC patients exhibited lower IgA reactivities (both to VCA and EBNA) than did other NPC groups.

---

[1] See p. 459

Table 4. Titration of IgA to VCA and to EA in sera from NPC patients and controls from different geographical areas

	NPC patients				Patients with other tumours			Normal controls
	Hong Kong Chinese	Nairobi Africans	Tunis Arabs	Marseille Caucasians	Hong Kong Chinese	Tunis Arabs	Marseille Caucasians	Hong Kong Chinese
IgA to VCA No. positive	(20/20)	(14/18)	(17/20)	(18/20)	(6/20)	(11/20)	(10/18)	(2/20)
GMT	70	50	95	89	3.3	4.5	5.8	2.8
IgA to EA No. positive	(18/20)	(12/18)	(14/20)	(12/20)	(0/20)	(1/20)	(1/18)	(0/20)
GMT	21	13	27	22	-	-	-	-

DISCUSSION

Important variations (up to 3-fold) in the GMTs of IgG antibodies directed against EBV-determined antigens (VCA, EA, EBNA) were observed in sera from patients with NPC originating from different geographical areas. Although in some cases, the stage of the disease (not standardized for all areas) probably played a role, the main cause of these variations appeared to lie in the socio-economic environment of the patients. Socio-economic level is known to affect the age at primary infection by EBV (Henle et al., 1969). Would then the age at primary infection significantly influence the long-lasting titres of antibody response to VCA, as well as the level of the secondary response at the time of the EBV reactivation which appears to accompany NPC development? Results from sero-epidemiological surveys carried out under other circumstances (de-Thé et al., 1975b) would indicate that EBV infection very early in life, as in Uganda, could result in a very high antibody response to both VCA and EA. Antibodies to EA are known to decrease rapidly, over a few months or a year, whereas antibody titres to VCA are much more stable and decrease slowly over many years (de-Thé & Lenoir, 1977). Thus, the significant variations in EBV reactivities among NPC patients of different origins might reflect age at primary infection, associated with socio-economic environment, and, possibly, different levels of reinfection by this virus during life.

Of interest was the unexpected correlation between antibody titres to EBNA and racial/genetic background. In this context, the high VCA and EA reactivities in the Los Angeles Chinese NPC cases (as compared with the titres in Black and White NPC patients from the same area) were not related to income ranking nor to clinical staging. An analysis of individual EBV reactivities and HLA profiles in NPC patients and their family members in Singapore (Day, personal communication) did not, however, exhibit any particular pattern.

Is the strength of the association between EBV and NPC affected by the variations observed in the serology of NPC patients originating from different geographical areas? If one considers the results shwon in Tables 1 and 3, it is clear that, regardless of geographical origin, NPC is consistently associated with an *active* infection by EBV, as indicated by the presence of high titres of antibody to early antigens (EA). Since EA titres decrease rapidly after primary infection, rising titres later in life, as with NPC, would reflect either a reactivation of a latent infection (the favoured alternative) or a reinfection by EBV (no evidence exists that this could occur). Other reactivities also show large and significant differences among cases of NPC and of other tumours taken from the same area (Henle et al., 1970a). Finally, viral markers (EBV/DNA and EBNA) have been found consistently in NPC tumour cells originating from different geographical areas (Desgranges et al., 1975; zur Hausen et al., 1970), further strengthening the association between EBV and NPC.

Do the present results help to answer the critical question of whether EBV is a causal factor or a passenger host that is reactivated by the growth of a tumour in its natural nest, i.e., the nasopharynx? Henderson et al. (1976, 1977) tend to favour the latter hypothesis and base their arguments on the fact that a number of other tumours arising in the pharynx are associated with elevated VCA antibody titres. This is not, however, the experience of other authors (de-Thé et al., 1975a; Henle et al., 1970a), and a systematic study should be carried out to clarify this important point. A prospective study, of the type implemented in Uganda for Burkitt's lymphoma could supply critical data for the resolution of this problem by establishing the pre-tumour EBV profile. If 'candidates for NPC' were found to differ significantly in EBV profile from the general population, this would not only strengthen the causal association with EBV but would also permit characterization of individuals at highest risk for the tumour. This would allow further etiological studies and permit early detection of this cancer in countries where it is endemic and a public health problem, such as in the People's Republic of China and other areas of South-East Asia.

SUMMARY

In order to assess the differences in serological reactivities of NPC patients from high, intermediate and low incidence areas, 288 NPC sera from Hong Kong, Singapore, Tunis, East Africa, Paris and Los Angeles, together with sera from patients with ear, nose and throat tumours other than NPC and with those from normal individuals from the same areas, were tested 'blind' with the same batches of antigen. Important differences (up to 3-fold) in the GMTs of antibodies directed against VCA, EA and EBNA were observed between different ethnic groups. Although the stages of the disease varied somewhat between groups, the main cause of the variations appeared to lie in the socio-economic environment of the patients. Apart from these variations, and regardless of geographical or ethnic origins, NPC was consistently found to be associated with an *active* infection (or reactivation) by Epstein-Barr virus, which was not the case for patients with other tumours or for normal individuals from the same areas or of the same ethnic groups.

ACKNOWLEDGEMENT

This study was supported by Contract No. NO1 CP 43296 between the National Cancer Institute, Bethesda, Md., USA, and the International Agency for Research on Cancer, Lyon, France.

REFERENCES

de-Schryver, A., Klein, G., Henle, W. & Henle, G. (1974) EB virus-associated antibodies in Caucasian patients with carcinoma of the nasopharynx and in long-term survivors after treatment. *Int. J. Cancer*, *13*, 319-325

Desgranges, C., Wolf, H., de-Thé, G., Shanmugaratnam, K., Ellouz, R., Cammoun, N., Klein, G. & zur Hausen, H. (1975) Nasopharyngeal carcinoma. X. Presence of Epstein-Barr genomes in epithelial cells of tumours from high and medium risk areas. *Int. J. Cancer*, *16*, 7-15 de-Thé, G. & Lenoir, G. (1977) *Comparative diagnosis of Epstein-Barr virus related diseases: infectious mononucleosis, Burkitt's lymphoma and nasopharyngeal carcinoma.* In: Kurstak, E., ed., *Comparative Diagnosis of Viral Diseases*, New York, Academic Press, pp. 195-240

de-Thé, G., Ablashi, D.V., Liabeuf, A. & Mourali, N. (1973) Nasopharyngeal carcinoma. VI. Presence of an EBV specific nuclear antigen in fresh tumor biopsies. Preliminary results. *Biomedicine, 19*, 349-352

de-Thé, G., Ho, H.C., Ablashi, D.V., Day, N.E., Macario, A.J.L., Martin-Berthelon, M.C., Pearson, G. & Sohier, R. (1975a) Nasopharyngeal carcinoma. IX. Antibodies to EBNA and correlation with response to other EBV antigens in Chinese patients. *Int. J. Cancer, 16*, 713-721

de-Thé, G., Day, N.E., Geser, A., Lavoué, M.F., Ho, J.H.C., Simons, M.J., Sohier, R., Tukei, P., Vonka, V. & Zavadova, H. (1975b) *Sero-epidemiology of the Epstein-Barr virus. Preliminary analysis of an international study.* In: de-Thé, G., Epstein, M.A. & zur Hausen, H., eds, *Oncogenesis and Herpesviruses II*, vol. 2, Lyon, International Agency for Research on Cancer (*IARC Scientific Publications No. 11*), pp. 3-16

Henderson, B.E., Louie, E., Jing, J.S.H., Buell, P. & Gardner, M.B. (1976) Risk factors associated with nasopharyngeal carcinoma. *New Engl. J. Med., 295*, 1101-1106

Henderson, B.E., Louie, E.W., Jing, J.S. & Alena, B. (1977) Epstein-Barr virus and nasopharyngeal carcinoma. Is there an etiologic relationship? *J. nat. Cancer Inst., 59*, 1395-1398

Henle, G. & Henle, W. (1966) Immunofluorescence in cells derived from Burkitt's lymphoma. *J. Bacteriol., 91*, 1248-1256

Henle, G., Henle, W., Clifford, P., Diehl, V., Kafuko, G.W., Kirya, B. G., Klein, G., Morrow, R.H., Munube, G.M.R., Pike, M.C., Tukei, P. M. & Ziegler, J.L. (1969) Antibodies to Epstein-Barr virus in Burkitt's lymphoma and control groups. *J. nat. Cancer Inst., 43*, 1147-1157

Henle, W., Henle, G., Ho, J.H.C., Burtin, P., Cachin, Y., Clifford, P., de-Schryver, A., de-Thé, G., Diehl, V. & Klein, G. (1970a) Antibodies to Epstein-Barr virus in nasopharyngeal carcinoma other head and neck neoplasms and control groups. *J. nat. Cancer Inst., 44*, 225-231

Henle, W., Henle, G., Zajac, B., Pearson, G., Waubke, R. & Scriba, M. (1970b) Differential reactivity of human serums with early antigen induced by Epstein-Barr virus. *Science, 169*, 188-190

Ho, H.C. (1970) *The natural history and treatment of nasopharyngeal carcinoma.* In: Lee Clark, R., Cumley, R.W., McCay, J.E. & Murray, M., eds, *Oncology, Proceedings of the X International Cancer Congress*, Vol. 4, Chicago, Year Book Medical Publishers, pp. 1-14

Huang, D.P., Ho, H.C., Henle, W. & Henle, G. (1974) Demonstration of Epstein-Barr virus associated nuclear antigen in nasopharyngeal carcinoma cells from fresh biopsies. *Int. J. Cancer, 14*, 580-588

Klein, G., Giovanella, B.C., Lindahl, T., Fialkow, P.J., Singh, S. & Stehlin, J. (1974) Direct evidence for the presence of Epstein-Barr virus DNA and nuclear antigen in malignant epithelial cells from patients with poorly differentiated carcinoma of the nasopharynx. *Proc. nat. Acad. Sci. (Wash.), 71*, 4737-4741

Levine, P.H., de-Thé, G., Brugère, J., Schwaab, G., Mourali, N., Herberman, R.B., Ambrosioni, J.C. & Revol, P. (1976) Immunity to antigens associated with a cell line derived from nasopharyngeal carcinoma (NPC) in non-Chinese NPC patients. *Int. J. Cancer, 17*, 155-160

Nonoyama, M. & Pagano, J.S. (1973) Homology between Epstein-Barr virus DNA and viral DNA from Burkitt's lymphoma and nasopharyngeal carcinoma determined by DNA-DNA reassociation kinetics. *Nature (Lond.), 242*, 44-47

Reedman, B. & Klein, G. (1973) Cellular localization of an Epstein-Barr virus (EBV)-associated complement-fixing antigen in producer and non-producer lymphoblastoid cell lines. *Int. J. Cancer, 11*, 499-520

Sohier, R. & de-Thé, G. (1972) Evolution of complement-fixing antibody titres with the development of Burkitt's lymphoma. *Int. J. Cancer, 9*, 524-528

Wolf, H., zur Hausen, H. & Becker, V. (1973) EB viral genomes in epithelial nasopharyngeal carcinoma cells. *Nature New Biol., 244*, 245-257

zur Hausen, H., Schulte-Holthausen, H., Klein, G., Henle, W., Henle, G., Clifford, P. & Santesson, L. (1970) EBV-DNA in biopsies of Burkitt tumours and anaplastic carcinomas of the nasopharynx. *Nature (Lond.), 228*, 1056-1058

CELL-MEDIATED IMMUNITY, EPSTEIN-BARR VIRUS AND NASOPHARYNGEAL CARCINOMA

P.H. LEVINE

National Cancer Institute,
National Institutes of Health,
Bethesda, Md 20014, USA

J.-P. LAMELIN

Unit of Biological Carcinogenesis,
International Agency for Research on Cancer,
Lyon, France

D.A. STEVENS

Division of Infectious Diseases,
Department of Medicine,
Santa Clara Valley Medical Center
and Stanford University,
San Jose, Ca 95128, USA

This paper presents a review of cell-mediated immunity (CMI) to Epstein-Barr virus (EBV) and its relation to nasopharyngeal carcinoma (NPC). We describe our studies, which attempt to validate different techniques for the study of specific commitment of immune cells against EBV, and evaluate their usefulness.

The possible etiological relationship of EBV to NPC has been discussed extensively at this symposium. It should also not be necessary to reiterate the evidence for the importance of CMI in the control of cancer spread, which has been widely demonstrated in animal models. CMI to tumour antigens has also been demonstrated in man, and its probable importance in the control of cancer is suggested by recent experience with immunotherapy.

It is worthwhile to review briefly the evidence for the central role played by CMI in host defenses against human herpesviruses (Stevens, 1973), as suggested by clinical observations and defined by experimental models. The first such observation, for example, concerned herpes zoster and Hodgkin's disease; this disease is widely associated with CMI deficiencies, as documented with a variety of antigens. Further clinical associations were found subsequently, such as those of cytomegalovirus infections with acute leukaemia and renal and cardiac transplantation. Three human herpesviruses, cytomegalovirus, herpes simplex and varicella zoster, pose an overwhelming preponderance of the virological problems associated with human cancer and the immunosuppressed state. The other human herpesvirus, EBV, a major subject of our deliberations at this symposium, also appears to be activated following chemical immunosuppression (Staruch et al., 1974).

That the enhanced herpes infection is associated with defective CMI is also indicated by observations made in congenital immunodeficiencies, where pure humoral defects do not appear to be associated with enhanced viral infections. Congenital infections of the normal newborn, particularly those herpes simplex and cytomegalovirus infections that occur in the presence of passively transferred maternal antibodies, may also be due to depressed CMI. Stevens and coworkers (Stevens & Merigan, 1972; Stevens et al., 1975) have suggested that CMI plays a critical role in recovery from zoster infections, and several studies (Rasmussen et al., 1974; Wilton et al., 1972) have suggested that subtle, specific defects in CMI (i.e., defects demonstrable *in vitro* in some CMI parameters but not in others) can explain the different incidences of recurrent simplex infections amongst individuals with identical humoral immunity profiles. Such specific defects are likely to be most relevant to studies with ubiquitous and possibly oncogenic herpesviruses such as EBV.

The association between CMI deficiency and enhanced herpes infections is particularly clear in experiments with animal models, in which pure types of immunosuppression can be achieved and selective passive transfer experiments can be performed. Examples of such studies are those in mice with herpes simplex and antilymphocyte serum.

There is much less data with regard to oncogenic herpesviruses in lower animals. *Herpesvirus saimiri* is of special interest. In infection with this virus, the target cell is apparently the T lymphocyte (Wallen et al., 1974); circulating suppressor lymphocytes are found after the development of this simian malignancy (Wallen et al., 1975). In Marek's disease, the fact that passively transferred antibody can protect against it would argue against a central role for CMI (Biggs, 1975). However, in experiments in birds that have intact CMI, challenge virus neutralized with circulating passive antibody may be a potent stimulus to host CMI, and this could be important in protection. Passive antibody transfer into the embryonated egg does not modify the enhanced susceptibility of young birds.

It has, moreover, been shown that protection can be induced by vaccination in birds that lack an antibody-producing system (Else, 1974).

The potential importance of CMI in the control of EBV infection has led a number of investigators to the use of *in vitro* assays. In the primary infection, the best-defined target cell is the B lymphocyte, which possesses receptors for the virus. The infection presumably results in an antigenic alteration in the cells. When the primary infection is manifested as infectious mononucleosis (IM), there is an associated increase in T cells (Mangi et al., 1974), which incorporate thymidine (Virolainen et al., 1973). This increase in T cells, which are not infected by EBV, follows the increase in B cells and presumably represents a reaction against the infected cells. In IM, there is a concomitant depression in CMI to other antigens (as cited in Mangi et al., 1974).

Royston and coworkers (1975) showed that lymphoproliferation occurred in lymphocytes from IM patients in response to an EBV-infected cell line. This reactivity occurred concomitantly with depression of mixed leucocyte culture reactivity and response to mitogens. It was further shown that cytotoxicity in response to an EBV-infected B-cell line was increased in IM patients, in contrast to activity directed against an uninfected control line (which was not, however, a B-cell line). This activity reverted to the levels of normal controls in late stages of the disease. Hutt et al. (1975) showed that B-cell lines, whether infected with EBV or not, were more susceptible to lysis by leucocytes from IM patients than from controls (seropositive or seronegative). This activity subsided over the course of the disease.

The clue that perhaps explains the nonspecificity shown in these studies arises from the work of Svedmyr & Jondal (1975), who found that removal of the complement-bearing lymphocytes from mononuclear cell populations removes the cytotoxicity from normal individuals, and that, in IM patients, the resultant cytotoxic activity is directed only against genome-positive cell lines.

Attempts have been made to define the antigens involved in EBV-directed CMI reactions, to depart from the use of the whole cell as an antigenic stimulus. Gerber & Lucas (1972) demonstrated lymphocyte blastogenesis in seropositive individuals in response to inactivated virus from culture supernatants. Other *in vitro* CMI techniques have been applied to the problem. Fimmel et al. (1974) showed inhibition of leucocyte migration in seropositive individuals in response to P3HR-1-cell line extracts. Culture supernatants were, however, weak stimuli. These workers (Lai et al., 1975), using frozen-thawed P3HR-1-cell line antigen (which contained virus), later demonstrated EBV-specific inhibition of leucocyte migration and of migration inhibitory factor (MIF) production. Chan et al. (1977), using leucocyte adherence inhibition (LAI) and soluble (S) and ultra-violet (UV)-inactivated viral antigens, demonstrated enhanced activity in IM patients as compared with normal seropositive controls. Activity directed against viral antigens preceded activity against S antigens, the latter activity increasing with time. No such changes were seen with control simplex antigens.

We have omitted reference to the technique of antibody-dependent cellular cytotoxicity, discussed by Pearson elsewhere in this symposium[1]. Although this is a CMI-related assay and may be an important phenomenon *in vivo*, it does not require specifically committed lymphocytes.

Nikoskelainen & Stevens[2] have studied lymphocyte blastogenesis and production of the lymphokine, lymphotoxin, in IM patients, seropositive and seronegative controls and patients with other viral infections (It should be noted that the time periods discussed in the studies by these workers were calculated from the time of the first symptom of disease. They cannot be compared directly with the time periods studied by Chan et al. (1977), as cited above, since the latter group measured intervals from a later event, the time of diagnosis of disease. Thus, although reactivity in the LAI assay appears to occur earlier than reactivity in blastogenesis, a recalculation on the basis of time of diagnosis results in greater concordance with regard to onset of reactivity in the two assays than would appear on superficial comparison). Purified mononuclear cells from an autologous and EBV-seronegative blood group AB serum were tested with phytohemagglutinin (PHA) and a variety of antigens, including p3HR-1 culture supernatant, concentrated P3HR-1 and B95-8 viruses and P3HR-1 S antigen. Controls included a genome-negative cell line. Heterophile and immunofluorescence-sensitive antibodies to EBV capsid antigen (VCA) and to EBV nuclear antigen (EBNA) were assayed; IgG, IgM and IgA antibody to VCA were tested independently. These tests were correlated with clinical parameters (fever, pharyngitis, adenopathy, hepatitis, atypical and total mononucleosis).

In this study, EBV VCA- and S antigen-induced blastogenesis were significantly greater in seropositive donors, in contrast to PHA. These results conflict with those of Chang et al. (1976), who reported significant blastogenesis in seronegative donors. In IM patients, both PHA-induced and spontaneous transformation were depressed; such transformation, particularly the spontaneous type, was significantly increased by autologous serum but had returned to normal nine weeks after onset. Antigen-specific blastogenesis in IM patients was initially lower than that in seropositive donors ($P < 0.001$), and these patients showed low responses during the acute phase of the illness when clinical symptoms were present and antibody titres maximal. Specific blastogenesis rose to a peak at $3\frac{1}{2}$-9 weeks, when the patients had recovered, most laboratory findings had returned to normal and the antibody levels had declined. At its peak, specific blastogenesis in IM patients exceeded that of seropositive donors but later declined

---

1 See p. 439

2 Unpublished data

to the same level. Lymphotoxin production was also correlated with blastogenesis: notably, spontaneous production was augmented initially in IM. These results demonstrate specific CMI to EBV and show that these indices of CMI develop slowly in IM patients, in contrast to the evolution of the clinical events and humoral immunity. This provides additional evidence that CMI could be the mechanism by which lymphoproliferation is terminated in IM, especially in view of the close correlation of time sequences. IM patients have a transient serum factor that blocks transformation. In addition, this study demonstrates the importance of making serial studies in patients: the differences between IM patients and seropositive donors, for example, could not have been detected by random samplings of single blood specimens.

CMI studies in NPC patients, in contrast to the series of studies summarized above which provide a basis for further exploration, are in a more preliminary stage. The status of studies of non-specific CMI will be reviewed first.

Chan and co-workers have reported elsewhere in this symposium[1] an increased incidence of non-stimulation by PHA and of negative Mantoux tests in NPC patients; and they have correlated these findings with a poor prognosis and with a specific HLA type, A2 Sin 2. Goh and co-workers have also reported here[2] on the *in vitro* and *in vivo* restoration of these deficiencies by levamisole.

Further, Lamelin et al. (1977) have demonstrated depressed blastogenesis of peripheral blood lymphocytes in response to PHA and concanavalin A in NPC patients (similar findings have been observed in other forms of cancer) but no change in the blastogenic response to antilymphocytic globulins. This depression occurred concomitantly with a depression in the percentage of T lymphocytes. After radiotherapy these defects were more pronounced and included hyporesponsiveness to antilymphocytic globulins. A few long-term survivors were normal in their responses.

Levine and co-workers (1976) performed skin tests on NPC patients with extracts from lymphoblastoid cell lines. They noted a significant increase in positive responses in NPC patients treated with the NPC-derived cell line, HKLY 28 as compared with responses to extracts from cell lines derived from normal subjects and lymphoma patients. Most recent results (Table 1), from studies with 114 NPC patients from Hong Kong, France, USA and Tunisia, show that reactivity to the NPC line was 55% and that to other antigens 10% or less. It is also clear from this table that NPC patients are significantly more reactive to the antigen prepared from HKLY 28 than are patients with leukaemia, lymphoma or other solid tumours.

---

[1] See p. 495

[2] See p. 503

Table 1. Reactivities of cancer patients to skin testing with lymphoblastoid cell lines and other antigens, by type of cancer and country

	Total no. of patients tested	No. of patients positive (%)[a]											
		Raji		HKLY 28		F265		NC37		Molt		Recall[b]	
LYMPHOMA	84	40/69	(58)	3/16	(19)	6/73	(8)	0/10	(0)	...		70/83	(84)
Hodgkin's disease	11	2/5		1/5		0/5		0/4		...		7/11	(64)
France	4	0/3		0/4		0/3		0/4		...		2/4	
USA	7	2/2		1/1		0/2		...		...		5/7	
Non-Hodgkin's lymphoma	30	6/21	(29)	2/11	(18)	4/26	(15)	0/6		...		26/30	(87)
France	9	1/9		0/7		0/8		0/6		...		7/9	
USA	21	5/12	(42)	2/4		4/18	(22)	...		...		19/21	(90)
Burkitt's lymphoma (Ghana)	43	32/43	(74)	...		2/42	(5)	...		...		37/42	(88)
NASOPHARYNGEAL CARCINOMA	114	10/101	(10)	57/104	(55)	3/88	(3)	4/88	(5)	1/65	(2)	73/89	(82)
Hong Kong	78	1/78	(1)	41/78	(53)	0/63	(0)	1/65	(2)	1/65	(2)	55/65	(85)
France	17	2/16	(13)	9/17	(53)	2/17	(12)	1/17	(6)	...		13/17	(76)
USA	1	1/1		1/1		...		1/1		...		1/1	
Tunisia	18	6/6		6/8		1/18	(13)	1/5		...		4/6	
OTHER SOLID TUMOURS	206	46/161	(29)	24/114	(21)	3/87	(3)	14/130	(11)	0/10	(0)	162/191	(85)
Hong Kong	21	0/2		2/6		0/2		...		0/10	(0)	21/21	(100)
France	43	0/43	(0)	9/43	(21)	1/35	(3)	5/43	(12)	...		29/37	(78)
Tunisia[c]	126	46/109	(42)	12/61	(20)	2/44	(5)	9/87	(10)	...		105/126	(83)
USA	16	0/7		1/4		0/16	(0)	...		...		7/7	
ACUTE LYMPHOCYTIC LEUKAEMIA	65	26/65	(40)	...		1/54	(2)	...		6/17	(35)	...	
TOTAL	469	154/439	(35)	84/234	(36)	15/344	(4)	18/228	(8)	7/92	(8)	342/405	(84)

[a] Percentages were omitted for groups of < 10.

[b] Positive to at least one standard recall antigen

[c] All of these patients had carcinomas of the breast.

This reactivity was compared with stage of disease. Ho et al., elsewhere in this symposium[1], found depressed reactivity to an HKLY line in patients with disseminated disease (stage V in their classification).

The problems presented by the present results include lack of tumour specificity, since approximately 20% of non-NPC patients also showed positive reactions; and more highly purified preparations are needed: Levine et al. have, indeed, noted some lot to lot variations. On the other hand, this method of assay is particularly useful in that sophisticated laboratory equipment is not needed. Side effects are minimal, as noted by Levine et al.[2] in studies with over 400 patients with a variety of diseases; some patients have been monitored for over five years with no evidence of long-term side effects. The same antigens are now being utilized by this group in longitudinal studies, which have already suggested a correlation with tumour burden.

[1] See p. 545

[2] Unpublished data

Ng and co-workers[1] have studied MIF production from lymphocytes stimulated with Raji cell line extracts (using two methods of extraction: tris(hydroxymethyl)aminomethane (Tris)-glycerol and Tris-glycerol-ethylenediaminetetraacetic acid-sodium chloride and with extracts of pooled NPC biopsies (prepared by extraction with 2M potassium chloride followed by centrifugation at two different speeds). No differences in MIF production in response to purified protein derivative were noted between NPC patients and controls with other tumours; this result is in contrast to those of Chan et al. in NPC patients, cited above. Increased MIF production in response to Raji and pooled biopsy extracts was, however, significantly more common in NPC patients. These contrasting results obtained with different Raji extracts in *in vivo* and *in vitro* testing should be noted. In further studies with these antigens, Ng et al.[2] have found that lymphocyte blastogenesis in NPC patients is also enhanced over that in controls. This effect was especially pronounced when the pooled biopsy material was used in patients with stages III and IV of the disease. Current studies indicate an even sharper separation of NPC patients from their controls when the results of the two assays are considered together.

Stevens & Lamelin[1] have performed a pilot study with the LAI technique and the antigens used by Chan et al., referred to above. This study included 13 NPC patients from Tunis and Paris (all of the patients treated in France were of North African origin), another NPC patient who was analysed separately from the others because he alone had an EBNA-negative biopsy, and six controls with other head and neck tumours. Results from three of the NPC patients had to be discarded due to technical deficiencies. The antigens studied included Raji S antigen in four dilutions from 1:64 - 1:4096, Ly38 cell line S antigen in five dilutions (1:16 - 1:4096) and UV-inactivated viruses (B958 and P3HR-1 in three dilutions, 10^5 - 10^7; herpes simplex type I in 10^5 and 10^6; and herpes simplex type II in 10^6 and 10^7 particles/ml). The results are summarized in Table 2, in which a positive reaction is considered (by the common LAI test convention) to be $>$ 25% inhibition with any of the dilutions used. As the table indicates, results obtained using this technique do not at present suggest disease specificity. Out of interest, the same data were analysed by an opposite criterion, that is, $>$ 25% enhancement of leucocyte adherence with any dilution. The results were similar.

A smaller, preliminary study was performed by the same workers with a subgroup of the above population, measuring lymphocyte blastogenesis in response to four antigens: P3HR-1 and Raji supernatants, B958 virus, as utilized in the IM studies cited earlier, and a preparation of early antigen (EA) of EBV prepared by Lenoir et al. (1976).

[1] Unpublished data

Table 2. Leucocyte adherence inhibition in patients with nasopharyngeal carcinoma (NPC), including one Epstein-Barr-virus-nuclear-antigen (EBNA)-negative patient, and in patients with other cancers of the head and neck (controls). Results are presented as number positive (> 25% inhibition of adherence to at least 1 dilution) / number tested

	Subject category		
	NPC	NPC (EBNA-negative)	Controls
Antigen			
Raji S	5/10	1/1	2/6
B958 virus	6/10	0/1	2/6
P3HR-1 virus	8/10	1/1	4/6
HSV-1 virus	6/8	1/1	2/4
HSV-II virus	4/7	1/1	2/4
LY38 S	9/10	1/1	4/6

The results are presented in Table 3. Membrane extracts of the HKLY 38 cell line, extracted with various concentrations of sodium chloride from 0.9-0.1125%, were also examined in a pilot study with five NPC patients and four control patients with other cancers. Concentrations

Table 3. Lymphocyte stimulation in patients with nasopharyngeal carcinoma (NPC), including one Epstein-Barr-virus-nuclear-antigen (EBNA)-negative patient, and in patients with other cancers of the head and neck (controls). Results are presented as number positive/number tested; fractions to left of line in each column are based on criterion of transformation being > 1.5 times and those to right of line being > 3 times those of cultures without antigen.

	Subject category					
	NPC		NPC (EBNA-negative)		Controls	
Antigen[a]	> 1.5	> 3	> 1.5	> 3	> 1.5	> 3
EA	1/4	1/4	1/1	1/1	1/2	1/2
P3HR-1	2/4	1/4	-	-	1/2	0/2
Raji	1/4	0/4	-	-	0/2	0/2
B958	2/4	2/4	-	-	0/2	0/2

[a] EA - early antigen; P3HR-1 - culture supernatant; Raji - culture supernatant; B958 - concentrated inactivated virus from B958 cell line

of 0.1 to 250 mcg/ml were studied. PHA responses were positive, as expected, but all patients failed to respond to the extracts.

With regard to a possible role of CMI *in vivo*, as opposed to laboratory studies of the component parts such as as just detailed, the report of Chu et al. (1967) concerning cytotoxicity to autochthonous tumour in NPC patients should be noted. Klein has presented elsewhere[1] studies from his group that indicate the presence of EBV-specific killer T cells in NPC tumours and in the lymph nodes that drain them.

Obviously, considerably more information is needed on the role of CMI in NPC. Positive results reported from a single laboratory require confirmation elsewhere. There are, however, problems in the further pursuit of these studies. There is limited availability of purified antigens: the fact that EBV is cell-associated makes the preparation of viral antigens difficult; and S antigens, while available in adequate quantities, have not been completely purified. The soluble tumour extracts have also not been characterized. The present LAI technique incorporates the difficulties inherent in a visual assay, in particular, tediousness and subjectivity (the latter problem also occurs with the leucocyte migration inhibition and MIF techniques); however, the development of a ^{51}Cr method for LAI testing represents an advance. This test has a number of advantages: only small amounts of blood are required, allowing the use of numerous controls; and it is readily transportable, requiring a minimum amount of equipment, and can even be set up in one place and completed and read in another.

There are also significant problems in patient selection. A prime requirement is general agreement on the classification of the disease: the therapeutic status of the patients reported must be clear. This is also a factor to be considered in selection of appropriate controls, which is a particularly complex problem, given the variables of any disease and its treatment.

We believe that it is important to pursue these studies. It is essential to identify the relevant antigens with respect to CMI if there is to be a vaccine against EBV, as discussed recently (Epstein, 1976). It is also necessary to define these antigens if we are to study the effects of antibodies on host defenses against EBV-related tumours and if we are to study the possible relationship between altered immunity and the development of cancer after EBV infections. Such studies are critical if immunotherapy is ever to become a reality in this disease. All this information must be collected if prognostic patterns are to be revealed by CMI profiles, as has been done for humoral immunity. Finally, if CMI to EBV is unusual in comparison with other CMI parameters in NPC patients, EBV's etiological role in NPC will be further established.

---

[1] See p. 538

SUMMARY

Cellular immunity is apparently important in host defenses against cancer. A growing body of information on CMI to EBV is here reviewed, providing a strong basis for studies of such reactivity in NPC. Present work suggests that CMI responses to virus- and tumour-associated antigens may have implications for etiology, diagnosis and treatment.

ACKNOWLEDGEMENTS

We especially thank Dr G. B. de-Thé, Director, Unit of Biological Carcinogenesis, International Agency for Research on Cancer, for his numerous contributions to and sponsorship of many of the studies cited. Not mentioned in the text but contributors to parts of the studies were Dr G. Schwaab, Institut Gustave-Roussy, Paris, France, Dr R. Ellouz, Institut Salah Azaiz, Tunis, Tunisia and Dr M. Jean Brochier, Hôpital Edouard Herriot, Lyon, France.

REFERENCES

Biggs, P.M. (1975) *Vaccination against oncogenic herpesviruses: a review.* In: de-Thé, G., Epstein, M.A. & zur Hausen, H., eds, *Oncogenesis and Herpesviruses II, Part 2 (IARC Scientific Publications No. 11)*, Lyon, pp. 317-327

Chan, S.H., Wallen, W.C., Levine, P.H., Periman, P. & Perlin, E. (1977) Lymphocyte responses to EBV-associated antigens in infectious mononucleosis, Hodgkin's and non-Hodgkin's lymphoma patients using the leukocyte adherence inhibition assay. *Int. J. Cancer, 19*, 356-363

Chang, R.S. & Spina, C.A. (1976) *In vitro* stimulation of lymphocytes of donors seronegative for Epstein-Barr virus by preparation of inactivated Epstein-Barr virus. *J. infect. Dis., 133*, 676-680

Chu, E.H.Y., Stjernsward, J., Clifford, P. & Klein, G. (1967) Reactivity of human lymphocytes against autochthonous and allogeneic normal and tumor cells *in vitro*. *J. nat. Cancer Inst., 39*, 595-612

Else, R.W. (1974) Vaccinal immunity to Marek's disease in bursectomised chickens. *Vet. Rec.*, *95*, 182-187

Epstein, M.A. (1976) Epstein-Barr virus - is it time to develop a vaccine? *J. nat. Cancer Inst.*, *56*, 697-700

Fimmel, P.J., Lai, P.K., Keast, D., Alpers, M.P. & Mackay-Scollay, E.M. (1974) *In vitro* cellular immunity to Epstein-Barr virus in normal human subjects. *Int. J. Cancer*, *13*, 599-605

Gerber, P. & Lucas, S.J. (1972) *In vitro* stimulation of human lymphocytes by Epstein-Barr virus. *Cell. Immunol.*, *5*, 318-324

Hutt, L.M., Huang, Y.T., Dascomb, H.E. & Pagano, J.S. (1975) Enhanced destruction of lymphoid cell lines by peripheral blood leukocytes taken from patients with acute infectious mononucleosis. *J. Immunol.*, *115*, 243-248

Lai, P.K., Alpers, M.P. & Mackay-Scollay, E.M. (1975) *In vitro* evaluation of cell-mediated immunity to Epstein-Barr herpesvirus by cell migration inhibition tests. *J. nat. Cancer Inst.*, *55*, 1319-1322

Lamelin, J.-P., Ellouz, R., de-Thé, G. & Revillard, J.-P. (1977) Lymphocyte subpopulations and mitogenic responses in nasopharyngeal carcinoma, prior to and after radiotherapy. *Int. J. Cancer* (in press)

Lenoir, G., Berthelon, M.-C., Favre, M.-C. & de-Thé, G. (1975) Characterization of Epstein-Barr Virus (EBV) antigens: II. Detection of early antigen (S) using anticomplement immunofluorescence (ACIF) and complement fixation (CF) tests. *Biomedicine*, *23*, 461-464

Levine, P.H., de-Thé, G.B., Brugère, J., Schwaab, G., Mourali, N., Herberman, R.B., Ambrosioni, J.C. & Revol, P. (1976) Immunity to antigens associated with a cell line derived from nasopharyngeal cancer (NPC) in non-Chinese NPC patients. *Int. J. Cancer*, *17*, 155-160

Mangi, R.J., Niederman, J.C., Kelleher, J.E., Dwyer, J.M., Evans, A.S. & Kantor, F.S. (1974) Depression of cell-mediated immunity during acute infectious mononucleosis. *New Engl. J. Med.*, *291*, 1149-1153

Rasmussen, L.E., Jordan, G.W., Stevens, D.A. & Merigan, T.C. (1974) Lymphocyte interferon production and transformation after herpes simplex infections in humans. *J. Immunol.*, *112*, 728-736

Royston, I., Sullivan, J.L., Periman, P.O. & Perlin, E. (1975) Cell-mediated immunity to Epstein-Barr virus-transformed lymphoblastoid cells in acute infectious mononucleosis. *New Engl. J. Med.*, *293*, 1159-1163

Staruch, B., Andrews, L., Siegel, N. & Miller, G. (1974) Oropharyngeal excretion of Epstein-Barr virus by renal transplant recipients and other patients treated with immunosuppressive drugs. *Lancet*, *i*, 234-237

Stevens, D.A. (1973) Immunosuppression and virus infections. *Transplant Proc.*, *5*, 1259-1262

Stevens, D.A. & Merigan, T.C. (1972) Interferon, antibody and other host factors in herpes zoster. *J. clin. Invest.*, *51*, 1170-1178

Stevens, D.A., Ferrington, R.A., Jordan, G.W. & Merigan, T.C. (1975) Cellular events in zoster vesicles: relation to clinical course and immune parameters. *J. infect. Dis.*, *131*, 509-515

Svedmyr, E. & Jondal, M. (1975) Cytotoxic effector cells specific for B cell lines transformed by Epstein-Barr virus are present in patients with infectious mononucleosis. *Proc. nat. Acad. Sci. (Wash.)*, *72*, 1622-1626

Virolainen, M., Andersson, L.C., Lalla, M. & Von Essen, R. (1973) T-Lymphocyte proliferation in mononucleosis. *Clin. Immunol. Immunopath.*, *2*, 114-120

Wallen, W.C., Neubauer, R.H. & Rabin, H. (1974) *In vitro* immunological characteristics of lymphoid cells derived from owl monkeys infected with *Herpesvirus saimiri*. *J. med. Primat*, *3*, 41-53

Wallen, W.C., Neubauer, R.H. & Rabin, H. (1975) Evidence for suppressor cell activity associated with induction of *Herpesvirus saimiri*-induced lymphoma. *Clin. exp. Immunol.*, *22*, 468-472

Wilton, J.M.A., Ivanyi, L. & Lehner, T. (1972) Cell-mediated immunity in *Herpesvirus hominis* infections. *Brit. med. J.*, *i*, 723-726

GENERAL IMMUNOLOGICAL STATUS OF NASOPHARYNGEAL CARCINOMA PATIENTS IN SINGAPORE

S.H. CHAN

Department of Microbiology,
University of Singapore,
Singapore

E.H. GOH

Ear, Nose & Throat Unit,
Singapore General Hospital,
Singapore

T.H. KHOR

Radiotherapy Department,
Singapore General Hospital,
Singapore

T.S. CHEW

Department of Pathology,
Ministry of Health,
Singapore

INTRODUCTION

As part of an immunological programme for the study of nasopharyngeal carcinoma (NPC) patients in Singapore, general T-lymphocyte cell function was assessed in newly diagnosed NPC patients to see whether any of the tests were of prognostic value for predicting recurrence and survival.

Patients in whom NPC was suspected clinically were tested just prior to the taking of a postnasal biopsy and were classified as NPC-positive or -negative on the basis of the biopsy; those that were negative served as controls. NPC and control patients were of similar ethnic group (Chinese), male:female ratio and mean age. The study also included NPC-positive patients who had received radiotherapy nine months to nine years previously and who had no clinical evidence of the disease at the time of the study (treated 'remission' patients) and 42 normal Chinese blood donors.

GENERAL CELL-MEDIATED IMMUNE FUNCTION

General cell-mediated immune (CMI) function was assessed *in vivo* from the Mantoux response and *in vitro* from lymphocyte response to phytohaemagglutinin (PHA) (Chan et al., 1976a). When both tests were carried out on the same subject, they were performed on the same day. Thirty-eight (50%) of 76 untreated NPC-positive patients were found to be hyporesponsive ($\leqslant$ 5 mm of induration) in the Mantoux test (1 IU purified protein derivative intradermally, read at 72 hr), compared with 27 (25%) of 110 NPC-negative patients ($\chi^2 = 12.8$, $P < 0.001$). There was no difference in the frequency of Mantoux hyporesponsiveness between newly diagnosed and treated remission patients.

Forty-three (65.2%) of 66 untreated NPC-positive patients also showed lymphocyte hyporesponsiveness to PHA (responses > 2 SD below the mean response of 42 normal blood donors), compared with 15 (15.5%) of 97 NPC-negative patients ($\chi^2 = 42.3$, $P < 0.0001$). Total white cell and lymphocyte counts and the proportion of E rosette-forming cells were determined in 20 NPC and 28 control patients. Total white cell and lymphocyte counts were lower in NPC patients (6050 ± 2500 and 2800 ± 1800 per mm^3, respectively) than in control patients (8100 ± 3200 and 3800 ± 1000 per mm^3, respectively). However, the proportions of E rosette-forming cells were of a similar order in NPC patients (mean, 48%; range, 15-70%) and control patients (mean, 52%; range, 23-72%). As with the Mantoux test, treated remission NPC patients did not differ from untreated patients in the PHA assay.

In the early part of the study, 12 control patients were found to be PHA hyporesponsive; eight of these were found to have cancer at a subsequent biopsy (six had NPC, and two, carcinomas of the thyroid).

The four cancer-free, PHA hyporesponsive control patients and another 11 comprise the 15 control patients with PHA hyporesponsiveness reported here.

The Mantoux and PHA response tests were carried out on the same day on 83 NPC-positive and 61 NPC-negative patients. Thirty-five (42.2%) of 83 NPC-positive patients were hyporesponsive to both tests, compared with only two (3.3%) of 61 NPC-negative patients. There was no obvious correlation between the two tests (concordance, 56%); the PHA assay appears to be more discriminating than the Mantoux assay.

The newly diagnosed NPC patients were subdivided into early (tumour confined to nasopharynx) and late (clinical evidence of tumour spread) stages of disease. There was a trend towards a higher frequency of Mantoux hyporesponsiveness among those in the late disease stage than those in the early disease stage, but this difference was not significant. There was no difference in the frequency of PHA hyporesponsiveness between the two groups.

These results indicate that newly diagnosed NPC patients have impaired general CMI function, which occurs early in the course of the disease, and that treated remission patients fail to recover from these impairments.

PHA RESPONSIVENESS AND HLA PROFILE

It has been shown that the HLA profiles of A2 Sin 2 and Blank BW17 are associated with NPC in Chinese patients (Simons et al.[1]). We were able to correlate PHA responses with HLA profile in 49 newly diagnosed NPC patients: 10 (71%) of 14 patients with the HLA profile of A2 Sin 2 were hyporesponsive to PHA, compared with 16 (46%) of 35 patients with other HLA profiles. However, this difference was not statistically significant.

PHA RESPONSIVENESS AND EBV SEROLOGY

NPC patients also have high antibody titres to Epstein-Barr virus (EBV)-related antigens (de-Thé et al.[2]). We were able to correlate PHA responsiveness with EBV serology in 13 newly diagnosed NPC patients, and it was found that high EBV titres are associated with PHA hyporesponsiveness (Table 1). This association was most marked in the early antigen titres: 5 (83%) of 6 patients with PHA hyporesponsiveness had high early antigen titres ($\geqslant 320$), compared with 2 (29%) of 7 patients with normal PHA responses. However, this difference was not statistically significant.

---

[1] See p. 271

[2] See p. 471

Table 1. Phytohaemagglutinin (PHA) responsiveness and Epstein-Barr virus antibody titres

	No. patients positive/no. tested (%)		
PHA responsiveness	EA ⩾ 320	VCA ⩾ 640	EBNA ⩾ 640
Normal	2/7 (29)	5/7 (71)	4/7 (57)
Low	5/6 (83)	6/6 (100)	6/6 (100)

EA - early antigen
VCA - viral capsid antigen
EBNA - Epstein-Barr nuclear antigen

RESPONSES TO MANTOUX AND PHA TESTS AND SURVIVAL

NPC-positive patients, tested immunologically at the time of diagnosis, have now been followed up for over 3.5 years. All patients included in the study had completed a course of radiotherapy started within a month of diagnosis. Correlations between survival and responses to the Mantoux and PHA tests are shown in Figures 1 and 2.

FIG. 1. MANTOUX RESPONSE

Relationship between Mantoux response at time of diagnosis of nasopharyngeal carcinoma and survival of patients; ● ⩽5 mm ; ○ > 5 mm

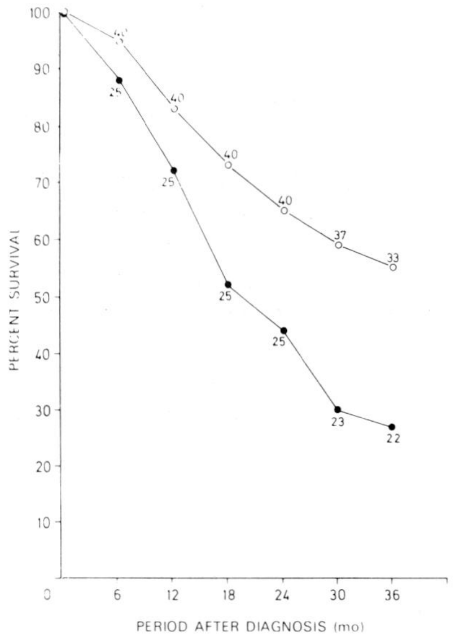

FIG. 2. PHYTOHAEMAGGLUTININ RESPONSE

Relationship between phytohaemagglutinin response at time of diagnosis of nasopharyngeal carcinoma and survival of patients; ● normal (mean ± 2 SD); ○ poor (2-4 SD below mean); ▲ very poor (> 4 SD below mean)

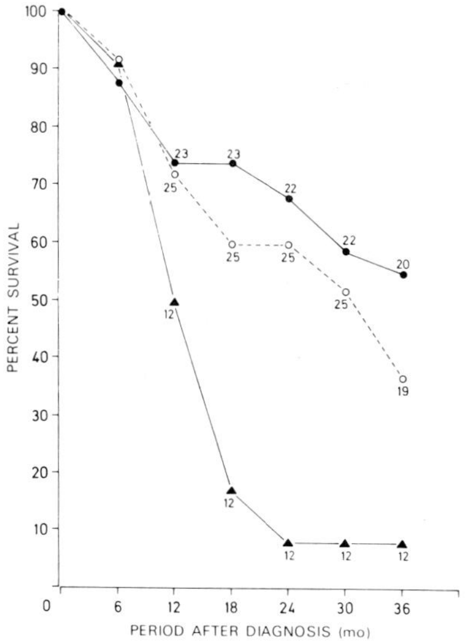

It can be seen that those with good responses in these tests survived longer than those with poorer responses. Twenty-two (59%) of 37 patients with a Mantoux response of >5 mm were still alive after 30 months, compared with 7 (30%) of 23 patients with a response of ⩽5 mm ($P < 0.05$). We divided the PHA response into three groups, normal, poor (2-4 SD below mean of normal response) and very poor (>4 SD below mean). Those with normal responses survived the longest, and those with very poor responses survived the least long. At 18 months after diagnosis, 17 (74%) of 23 normal, 15 (60%) of 25 poor and only 2 (17%) of 12 very poorly responsive patients were still alive. These results indicate that Mantoux and PHA responses at the time of diagnosis are of prognostic value in predicting survival.

AUGMENTATION OF PHA RESPONSES BY *IN VITRO* TREATMENT WITH LEVAMISOLE

The responses of PHA hyporesponsive lymphocytes can be partially or totally restored by their *in vitro* treatment with levamisole (Chan et al., 1976b). Similar effects were seen with PHA hyporesponsive lymphocytes from treated remission NPC patients.

In our study the PHA responses of 16 (36%) of 44 NPC patients were augmented by *in vitro* treatment with levamisole; no such effect was seen in 21 controls ($P < 0.005$). This effect was related to the PHA responsive states of the untreated lymphocytes, being most marked in those showing PHA hyporesponsiveness (3-5 SD below mean of normal response). The Mantoux and PHA responses could also be augmented by a short oral course of levamisole (Goh et al.[1]). Since the correlation between the augmentation of PHA responsiveness by *in vitro* and by *in vivo* administration of levamisole was good (88% concordance) (Table 2), the *in vitro* assay promises to be of value in predicting which NPC patients will benefit from levamisole treatment *in vivo*.

Table 2. Correlation between *in vivo* and *in vitro* augmentative effects of levamisole on phytohaemagglutinin responses in nasopharyngeal carcinoma patients

		In vivo augmentation		
		+	-	
In vitro augmentation	+	8	1	No. of
	-	2	13	patients
				24

Concordance, 88%
Cross product, 52

SUMMARY

Newly diagnosed NPC patients were found to have impaired general T-cell functions, as determined *in vivo* by the Mantoux test and *in vitro* by the PHA response assay. Treated remission patients were as hyporesponsiveness as newly diagnosed patients. PHA hyporesponsiveness was associated with the HLA profile of A2-B Sin 2 and with high antibody titres to EBV-related antigens, in particular to the early antigen. Impaired responses in the Mantoux or PHA tests were associated with poor survival. The impaired response could be partially or totally restored by *in vitro* treatment of the hyporesponsive lymphocytes with levamisole.

[1] See p. 503

ACKNOWLEDGEMENT

This work was supported in part by a collaborative research agreement between the Unit of Biological Carcinogenesis, IARC, Lyon, France and the IARC Research Centre, Department of Pathology, University of Singapore, under Contract No. N01-CP-43296 within the Virus Cancer Program of the National Cancer Institute, USA.

REFERENCES

Chan, S.H., Chew, T.S., Goh, E.H., Simons, M.J. & Shanmugaratnam, K. (1976a) Impaired general cell mediated immune function *in vivo* and *in vitro* in patients with NPC. *Int. J. Cancer, 18*, 138-144

Chan, S.H., Lee, S.K. & Simons, M.J. (1976b) Levamisole augmentation of lymphocyte hyporesponsiveness to phytohaemagglutinin in patients with pulmonary tuberculosis. *Proc. Soc. exp. Biol. Med. (N.Y.), 151*, 716-719

EFFECT OF LEVAMISOLE ON CELL-MEDIATED IMMUNE RESPONSES IN PATIENTS WITH NASOPHARYNGEAL CARCINOMA

E.H. GOH

Ear, Nose & Throat Unit,
Singapore General Hospital,
Outram Road,
Singapore

S.H. CHAN

Department of Microbiology,
University of Singapore,
Singapore

M.J. SIMONS

Immuno-diagnostic Centre,
Melbourne, Victoria, Australia

INTRODUCTION

Tetramisole, a broad-spectrum antihelminthic, has been used clinically for many years and has proven to be safe and effective. Recently, in both experimental animals and in man, tetramisole and its laevorotatory enantiomore, levamisole, have been shown to augment or improve cell-mediated immune (CMI) functions against previously sensitized antigens. The CMI functions include responses to skin tests (Tripodi et al., 1973), lymphocyte transformation (Chan et al., 1976a) and macrophage activity (Symoens, 1975). In laboratory animals, levamisole has no effect on primary invasion by virulent organisms or by tumour cells but increases resistance when the host has been previously sensitized.

Levamisole appears to improve CMI functions in patients in whom they are already impaired but does not affect normal subjects. Of particular interest to clinicians is the recent finding that levamisole increases CMI functions in patients with malignancies (Tripodi et al., 1973), in whom these functions are often impaired (Herberman, 1974). Clinical trials have been initiated in many centres. In a double-blind control trial on patients with bronchogenic carcinoma it was found that administration of levamisole resulted in a lower frequency of tumour recurrence and a higher survival rate (Study Group for Bronchogenic Carcinoma, 1976); similar findings have been observed in patients with breast cancer (Symoens, 1975). With regard to non-malignant diseases, levamisole was found to be effective in treating recurrent aphthous stomatitis, recurrent herpes labialis and genitalis, recurrent respiratory infection, chronic mucocutaneous candidiasis and recurrent warts (Symoens, 1975).

Patients with nasopharyngeal carcinoma (NPC) have been shown to have impaired CMI functions, as detected *in vivo* by the Mantoux test and *in vitro* by the phytohaemagglutinin (PHA) test (Chan et al., 1976b; Chan et al.[1]). This impairment was seen not only in newly diagnosed, untreated patients but also in patients treated nine months to nine years previously. The objective of the present study was to assess whether levamisole could augment CMI functions in a group of treated NPC patients.

MATERIALS AND METHODS

Patients

The study comprised 32 NPC patients who had been treated with radiotherapy nine months to nine years previously and who had no clinical signs of the disease at the time of study. All of the patients, with one exception, were Chinese; they had no unusual clinical manifestations. All patients received levamisole orally for four consecutive days; they were divided into three groups: group 1 (7 patients) received 150 mg thrice daily (total, 1800 mg), group 2 (10 patients) received 150 mg twice daily (total, 1200 mg), and group 3 (15 patients) received 50 mg thrice daily (total, 600 mg). Taking of peripheral blood for the PHA test and carrying out of the Mantoux test were done just before and at the end of the drug course.

Mantoux test

One IU tuberculin (in 0.1 ml; RT23, with Tween 80; Statens Serum Institute, Copenhagen, Denmark) was injected intradermally into the ventral aspect of the forearm, and skin induration was measured in two diameters at right angles to each other after 72 hr. The average of the two diameters was taken as a measure of the response

[1] See p. 495

to purified protein derivative (PPD): an average diameter of 5 mm or less was taken to indicate hyporesponsiveness (Chan et al., 1976b), and a difference of 5 mm or more in Mantoux readings before and after oral administration of levamisole was arbitrarily considered to be an effect of the drug.

Lymphocyte separation and culture

Peripheral blood leucocytes were separated by a Ficoll-isopaque density method (Boyum, 1968). Mononuclear cells comprised 85-95% of the cell population, and this preparation was considered to be a lymphocyte suspension.

Lymphocyte activation by PHA ('purified'; Burroughs Wellcome, UK) was quantitated on the basis of net percent incorporation of γ-emitting ^{75}Se-methionine (^{75}SeMe, Radio Chemicals, Amersham, UK), as a measure of *de novo* protein synthesis (Chan et al., 1976a, b). Briefly, 0.4 x 10^6 lymphocytes in 1 ml methionine-free Eagle's medium (Commonwealth Serum Laboratories, Melbourne, Australia), supplemented with 10% fetal calf serum and 0.05 μg/ml unlabelled methionine, were cultured in round-bottom glass tubes for 72 hr at 37°C in a humidified atmosphere of continuously flowing 5% CO_2/95% air. PHA (0.025-250 μg) and ^{75}SeMe (0.02-0.03 μCi; 10,000-15,000 cpm) were added at the beginning of incubation. At harvest, the cultures were centrifuged in a MSE minor centrifuge (2 000 rpm/15 min), and the supernatant was taken off. The cell pellet was washed twice with 1.5 ml phosphate-buffered saline, pH 7.3, and the washings were added to the separated supernatant. The cell pellet and the supernatant were then treated separately with 1% perchloric acid (PCA), and the sedimented precipitates were washed twice with 1% PCA and counted in a gamma spectrometer (Packard TRICARB model 3002).

The results were expressed as percentage incorporation of ^{75}SeMe, after correcting for the amount of radioactivity precipitated by PCA in control tubes containing medium alone. The percentages of ^{75}SeMe incorporated into the cell and supernatant compartments were added to give total percentage incorporation. The response of lymphocytes to PHA was expressed as net percent ^{75}SeMe incorporation (that in stimulated minus that in unstimulated cultures).

In a study of 42 blood donors, responses to PHA stimulation fell within a narrow range (Chan et al., 1976b): the mean net percentage ^{75}SeMe incorporation was 48.3 ± 8.4. Therefore, lymphocyte hyporesponsiveness to PHA was defined as a response more than 2 SD below the mean normal response, i.e., $< 31.5\%$ ^{75}SeMe incorporation.

Day-to-day variations in PHA responsiveness in individual normal subjects have been found to be small (Chan et al., 1976b); thus, a difference of 5% or more in ^{75}SeMe incorporation before and after oral administration of levamisole was considered to be an effect of the drug.

RESULTS

In vivo effect of levamisole

Table 1 shows the effects of the three dosages of levamisole on responses in the Mantoux and PHA tests. The immune response was augmented most in patients receiving the highest dosage: 3 (43%) of 7 patients showed an increased Mantoux response, and 5 (83%) of 6 showed an increased PHA response. Both responses were increased less frequently in patients receiving lower dosages. The frequency of augmentation of the PHA response appeared to be dose-dependent: 83%, 50% and 23% in the high, mid and low dosage groups, respectively.

Table 1. Effects of levamisole on Mantoux and phytohaemagglutinin (PHA) responses in nasopharyngeal carcinoma patients

Patients	Number of patients			
	Mantoux response		PHA response	
	No. tested	No. increased (%)	No. tested	No. increased (%)
Group 1 (1800 mg)	7	3 (43%)	6	5 (83%)
Group 2 (1200 mg)	10	1 (10%)	8	4 (50%)
Group 3 (600 mg)	15	2 (13%)	15	3 (20%)
Total	32	6 (19%)	29	12 (41%)

Side effects of the drug seen in some patients included nausea, diarrhoea, skin rashes and dizziness, starting generally on the second or third day and subsiding on cessation of administration of the drug. The frequency with which they occurred was also dose-dependent: 34.3%, 20% and 0% in groups 1, 2 and 3, respectively.

Comparisons of the augmentation of responses in the Mantoux and PHA tests were carried out for 29 patients (Table 2): 19 (66%) of 29 sets of results were concordant (+/+, -/-). Similar frequencies of concordance were seen for all three dosage groups: group 1, 67%; group 2, 63%; group 3, 67%. The frequency of augmentation of both Mantoux and PHA responses was dose-related; in addition, the frequency of augmentation of either the Mantoux or the PHA response was also dose-dependent: 83% in group 1, 50% in group 2 and 33% in group 3.

Table 2. Comparison of augmented Mantoux and phytohaemagglutinin (PHA) responses in groups of nasopharyngeal carcinoma patients given various dosages of levamisole

Patients	Number of patients Mantoux / PHA tests					
	No. tested	+/+	+/-	-/+	-/-	Either Mantoux or PHA test positive (%)
Group 1 (1800 mg)	6	3	0	2	1	5 (83%)
Group 2 (1200 mg)	8	1	0	3	4	4 (50%)
Group 3 (600 mg)	15	0	2	3	10	5 (33%)
Total	29	4	2	8	15	14 (58%)

Longitudinal study

The CMI functions of five NPC patients (four in group 1 and one in group 3) given a single course of levamisole were assessed longitudinally for up to one year (Table 3). The augmentative effect of the dosage could still be detected in at least some NPC patients over the entire period.

DISCUSSION

The present findings indicate that levamisole can augment responses in both the Mantoux and PHA tests in patients with NPC, in a dose-dependent manner. In patients who received a total of 1800 mg levamisole, augmentation of Mantoux responses was seen in 3 (43%) of 7 and augmentation of PHA responses in 5 (83%) of 6; there was a correlation between augmentation of Mantoux and PHA responses at all three dosage levels. The frequency of side effects of the drug, nausea, diarrhoea, skin rashes and dizziness, was also dosage dependent; these effects were transient.

Three patients in the present study developed clinical recurrences of their tumours within three months of receiving the drug course. In two, the recurrence was indicated by histopathological evidence, and the third patient had enlarged, mobile lymph nodes and was given radiotherapy. All three patients were in group 3 (600 mg levamisole) and had shown evidence of impairment of CMI functions before the

Table 3. Longitudinal immunological study of nasopharyngeal carcinoma patients given a single course of levamisole

Patient	Date in relation to treatment		Mantoux response (mm)	Phytohaemagglutinin response[a]
LKC (Group 1)	9.2.74	Pre-levamisole	0	9.9
	26.2.74	Post-levamisole	0	30.3
	5.3.74	Follow-up	0	21.9
	28.1.75	Follow-up	0	26.3
LSC (Group 1)	19.2.74	Pre-levamisole	16	12.7
	26.2.74	Post-levamisole	19	27.4
	21.1.75	Follow-up	14	23.4
NKS (Group 1)	26.2.74	Pre-levamisole	1	22.7
	5.3.74	Post-levamisole	7	41.8
	25.2.74	Follow-up	4	36.5
	25.3.74	Follow-up	4	49.2
TPL (Group 1)	26.2.74	Pre-levamisole	2	41.2
	5.3.74	Post-levamisole	18	50.8
	21.1.75	Follow-up	12	21.2
TKS (Group 3)	7.5.74	Pre-levamisole	15	11.4
	14.5.74	Post-levamisole	20	16.2
	21.1.75	Follow-up	19	19.3

[a] For units, see 'Materials and Methods'

course of levamisole; in none of the three had levamisole augmented responses in the Mantoux or PHA tests. At present it is uncertain whether the recurrences were associated with the dose level of levamisole received or whether microscopic recurrences were already present in these patients before the course of the drug.

Recently, we have found an association between CMI status (Mantoux and PHA responses) at the time of diagnosis and three-year survival rates in NPC patients (Chan et al.[1]): those patients who had higher

[1] See p. 495

responses in the Mantoux or PHA tests survived longer than those showing poor responses. Since levamisole can augment CMI functions in NPC patients, therefore, it may prolong survival. We have also recently developed an *in vitro* assay to measure augmentation of CMI functions by levamisole (Chan et al., 1976a; Chan et al.[1]): preliminary data show a strong correlation between the ability of levamisole to augment CMI functions *in vitro* and *in vivo*. We hope to use this *in vitro* assay to select patients who will respond to an oral course of the drug.

SUMMARY

CMI functions, as monitored by responses in the Mantoux and PHA tests, can be augmented by a short oral course of levamisole. The augmentation is dosage dependent and, in some patients, of long duration.

REFERENCES

Boyum, A. (1968) Separation of leukocytes from blood and bone marrow. *Scand. J. clin. lab. Invest., 21*, Suppl. 97

Chan, S.H., Lee, S.K. & Simons, M.J. (1976a) Levamisole augmentation of lymphocyte hyporesponsiveness to phytohaemagglutinin in patients with pulmonary tuberculosis. *Proc. Soc. exp. Biol. Med., 151*, 716-719

Chan, S.H., Chew, T.S., Goh, E.H., Simons, M.J. & Shanmugaratnam, K. (1976b) Impaired general cell-mediated immune functions *in vivo* and *in vitro* in patients with nasopharyngeal carcinoma. *Int. J. Cancer, 18*, 139-144

Herberman, R. (1974) Cell-mediated immunity to tumour cells. *Advanc. Cancer Res., 19*, 207-263

Study Group for Bronchogenic Carcinoma (1976) Immunopotentiation in resectable bronchogenic carcinoma: a double-blind placebo control trial. *Brit. med. J.* (in press)

Symoens, J. (1975) *The effects of levamisole on host defence mechanisms.* In: Chirigos, M.A., ed., *Modulation of Host Immune Resistance in the Prevention or Treatment of Induced Neoplasias*, New York, Academic Press, Fogarty Int. Centre Proceedings

Tripodi, D., Parks, L.C. & Brugmans, J. (1973) Drug-induced restoration of cutaneous delayed hypersensitivity in anergic patients with cancer. *New Engl. J. Med.*, *289*, 354-357

CHANGES IN T-CELL SUBSETS AND THEIR CLINICAL SIGNIFICANCE IN CANCER PATIENTS

J. YATA

Departments of Pediatrics and Immunology,
Toho University,
Omorinishi, Otaku,
Tokyo, Japan

T. SHIMBO

Department of Immunology,
Toho University,
Omorinishi, Otaku,
Tokyo, Japan

S. SAWAKI

Department of Otorhinolaryngology,
Yokohama City University,
Yokohama, Japan

INTRODUCTION

Immunological events are carried out with the participation of various types of lymphocytes. Killer T cells have been shown to play the most important role in cancer immunity, their generation being mediated by amplifier (or helper) T cells and their suppression by suppressor T cells (Cerottini & Brunner, 1974).

Antibodies may have an antitumour effect by inducing complement-mediated cytolysis or antibody-dependent cell-mediated cytotoxicity, or they may suppress antitumour immunity by forming blocking substances (Hellström & Hellström, 1974). Antibody formation is also controlled by helper and suppressor T cells.

It was considered, therefore, that a study of T-cell subsets in cancer patients might provide important information for assessing their antitumour immune status.

We report in this paper on changes in the proportion of T cells that have a receptor for the Fc portion of IgG immunoglobulin molecules, one of the T-cell subsets that corresponds either to part of the killers or to the suppressors, in the functioning of T-cell helpers in immunoglobulin production and in the blastogenic response of lymphocytes to mitogenic substances; these changes were related to the clinical status of the patients.

MATERIALS AND METHODS

Demonstration of T cells with receptors for the Fc portion of IgG (IgG-Fc R^+ T cells)

Mononuclear cells were isolated from heparinized peripheral blood in a Hypaque-Ficoll density gradient. Then, 2 x 10^5 cells were suspended in 0.1 ml phosphate-buffered saline and mixed with 0.1 ml of a solution containing 1 x 10^7/ml chicken erythrocytes sensitized with 7S antibody (CkEA). The cells were reacted for 18 hours at 4-10°C. The supernatant was then removed, and 2 x 10^6 sheep erythrocytes (ShE) suspended in 0.2 ml heat-inactivated fetal calf serum were added to the pellet and mixed gently. The cells were centrifuged at 400 *g* for 5 min and cooled in iced water for 18 hours; they were then resuspended and observed under a microscope. Those cells that contain IgG-Fc receptors form rosettes with CkEA, and T cells form rosettes with ShE; thus, the proportion of cells that formed double rosettes with CkEA and ShE was scored.

Estimation of helper effect of T cells on in vitro *immunoglobulin production*

The mononuclear cells obtained as above from peripheral blood were separated into T cells and non-T cells (B cells and monocytes) by sedimentation of rosettes formed with ShE, as described previously (Yata et al., 1973). The following cell populations were prepared:

Bn: 2 x 10^5 non-T cells from a healthy donor

BnTn: 2 x 10^5 non-T cells and 8 x 10^5 T cells from a healthy donor

BnTp: 2 x 10^5 non-T cells from a healthy donor and 8 x 10^5 T cells from a patient

Tn: 8 x 10^5 T cells from a healthy donor

Tp: 8 x 10^5 T cells from a patient

Each cell population was suspended in 1 ml RPMI 1640 medium supplemented with 20% fetal calf serum, to which were added 10 μg pokeweed mitogen, and incubated under 5% CO_2 at 37°C for seven days. The cells were counted, smeared on glass slides and reacted with fluorescein-labelled antihuman immunoglobulin antibody; the immunoglobulin-producing (Ig) cells detected as cytoplasmic fluorescence-positive cells under an ultraviolet microscope were scored.

The helper effect of the T cells was calculated from:

$$\frac{\text{Ig cells from BnTp} - \text{Ig cells from Bn}}{\text{Ig cells from BnTn} - \text{Ig cells from Bn}} \times 100$$

An almost negligible number of T cells were Ig-producing, and only a few Ig cells were formed from non-T cells alone.

Estimation of the blastogenic response of lymphocytes to mitogenic substances

Peripheral blood lymphocytes (1×10^6) were suspended in 1 ml RPMI 1640 medium supplemented with 20% fetal calf serum, and 10 μg phytohaemagglutinin (PHA) or 10 μg concanavalin A (Con A) were added to the culture. After incubation under 5% CO_2 for 72 hr at 37°C, 1 μCi of ^{3}H-thymidine was added; the cells were collected after 2 hours and washed with phosphate-buffered saline and trichloracetic acid. The radioactivity incorporated into the cells was estimated in a liquid scintillation counter. The stimulation index (SI), the ratio of the radioactivity incorporated into cells stimulated with mitogen to that in untreated cells, was used to evaluate the responsiveness of the lymphocytes.

RESULTS

Increases in the percentage of IgG-Fc R^+ T cells in cancer patients

The proportion of IgG-Fc R^+ cells among circulating T cells in normal individuals was less than 10%; this percentage was markedly increased in certain cancer patients (Fig. 1).

Relationship between percentage of IgG-Fc R^+ T cells and progress of tumour

The percentages of IgG-Fc R^+ T cells, estimated before surgical operation, were compared in stomach cancer patients whose tumour could be completely removed and in those whose tumour had progressed too far for resection. The percentage of IgG-Fc R^+ T cells was found to be higher in the latter group (Fig. 2).

Effect of removal of tumour on percentage of IgG-Fc R^+ T cells

The proportion of IgG-Fc R^+ T cells was estimated serially before and after surgical operation in patients with stomach cancer. The percentage fell from a high pre-operative level to within the normal range one to two weeks after complete removal of the tumour (Fig. 3).

FIG. 1. PERCENTAGES OF IgG-Fc R^+ T CELLS IN VARIOUS CANCER PATIENTS

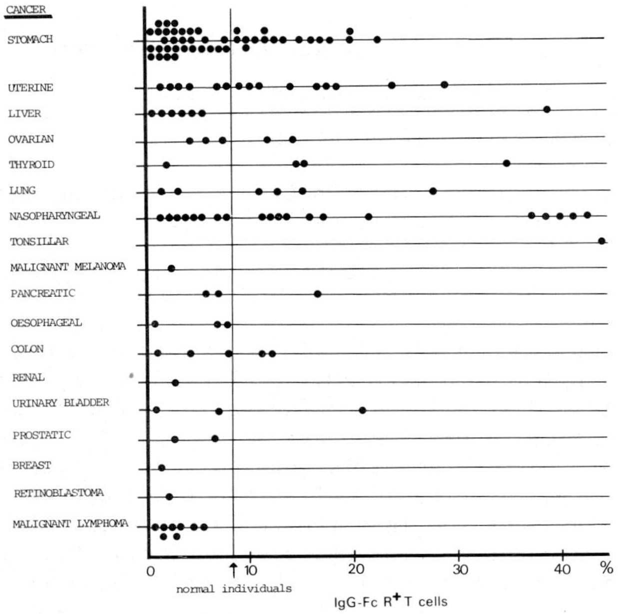

FIG. 2. PERCENTAGES OF IgG-Fc R^+ T CELLS IN PATIENTS WITH INOPERABLE AND OPERABLE TUMOURS

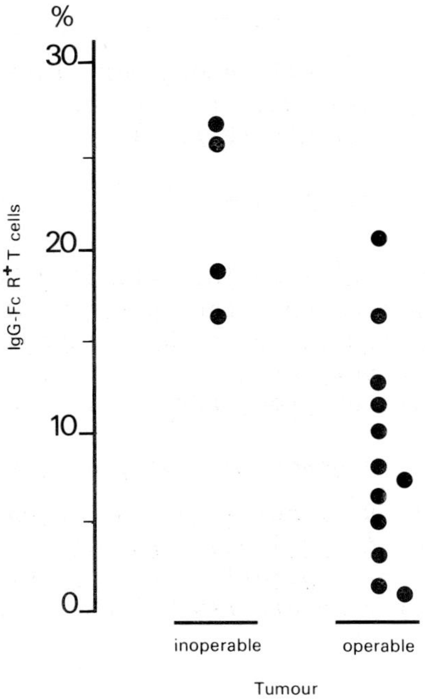

FIG. 3. EFFECT OF TUMOUR REMOVAL ON PERCENTAGE OF IgG-Fc R^+ T CELLS

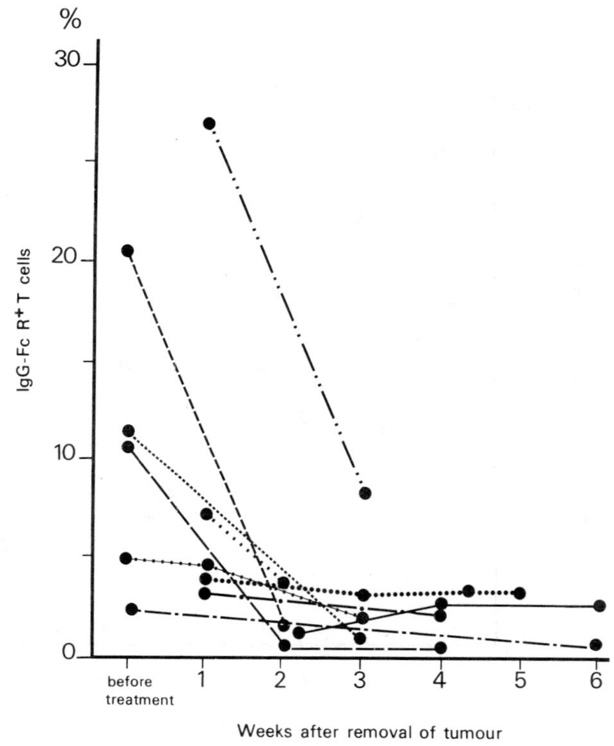

Relationship of changes in percentages of IgG-Fc R^+ T cells to the blastogenic response of lymphocytes to mitogenic substances

Lymphocyte populations with a normal proportion of IgG-Fc R^+ T cells usually showed a good response to PHA, while those with a high percentage showed decreased responsiveness (Fig. 4). In contrast, even lymphocyte populations with a high proportion of IgG-Fc R^+ T cells responded well to Con A. Thus, the ratio of the SI of Con A to that of PHA increased with increasing percentages of IgG-Fc R^+ T cells (Fig. 5).

Helper function of T cells in immunoglobulin production in relation to percentage of IgG-Fc R^+ T cells

Patients with tumours in advanced stages had increased proportions of IgG-Fc R^+ T cells and lowered helper function, while those who had been successfully treated had normal numbers of IgG-Fc R^+ T cells and normal helper function. A reverse relationship was thus observed between these two parameters (Fig. 6).

FIG. 4. RELATIONSHIP BETWEEN PERCENTAGE OF IgG-Fc R^+ T CELLS AND PHYTOHAEMAGGLUTININ (PHA) RESPONSIVENESS OF LYMPHOCYTES

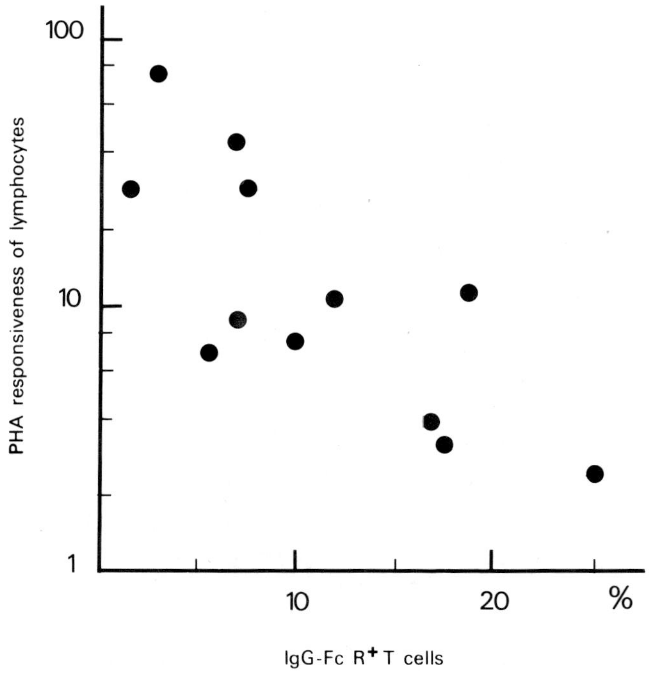

Changes in percentages of IgG-Fc R^+ T cells with stage of nasopharyngeal carcinoma

Patients were divided into three groups according to their clinical status. Percentages of IgG-Fc R^+ T cells were usually high in patients with advanced, relapsed or metastasizing tumours; most patients with early tumours had normal values; and slight increases were observed in patients who had been treated by radiation and had been free of all signs of their tumour for more than six months (Fig. 7).

DISCUSSION

T cells are divided into subsets according to their functions; they consist of helpers and suppressors of antibody production, killer T cells, amplifiers and suppressors of the killers and delayed hypersensitivity initiator T cells. Histocompatibility alloantigens have been used to identify these subsets in mice.

FIG. 5. RELATIONSHIP BETWEEN PERCENTAGE OF IgG-Fc R^+ T CELLS AND RATIO OF RESPONSIVENESS TO CONCANAVALIN A (Con A) AND PHYTOHAEMAGGLUTININ (PHA)

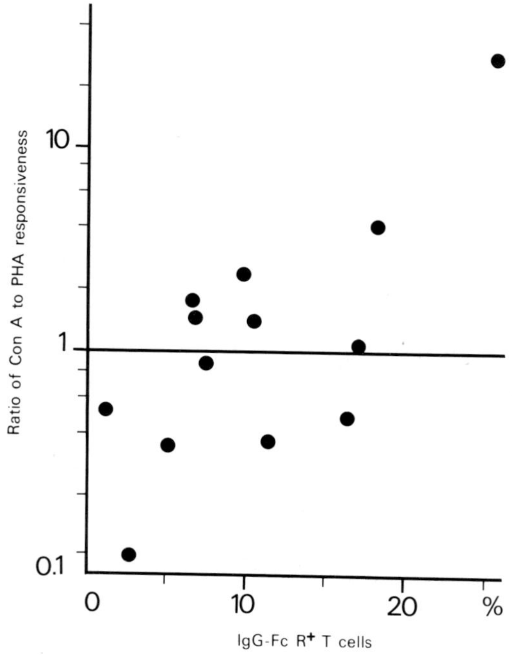

Cantor & Boyse (1975) have suggested that Ly 1 is present on helper T cells and that Ly 23 is expressed on killer and suppressor T cells. Stout & Herzenberg (1975) have reported that the presence or absence of the receptor for the Fc portion of the IgG molecule is also related to the T-cell subsets and appears to be expressed on a portion of the killer cells. Cooper et al. (1976) have proposed that human T cells that have receptors for IgM-Fc are probably helper T cells, while those that have receptors for IgG-Fc are suppressor T cells.

Our data, showing that the response of lymphocytes to PHA and the functioning of T cell helpers in immunoglobulin production are decreased when the lymphocytes comprise more IgG-Fc R^+ T cells, indicate that an increase in the proportion of this T-cell subset may be related to a reduction in T-cell function. Suppressor T cells appear to respond well to Con A and only poorly to PHA. Therefore, our finding that lymphocyte populations with a higher percentage of IgG-Fc R^+ T cells respond in this way might indicate that IgG-Fc R^+ T cells are suppressor T cells.

FIG. 6. RELATIONSHIP BETWEEN HELPER FUNCTION OF T CELLS IN IMMUNOGLOBULIN PRODUCTION AND PERCENTAGE OF IgG-Fc R^+ T CELLS

○ before treatment and ● after removal of tumour

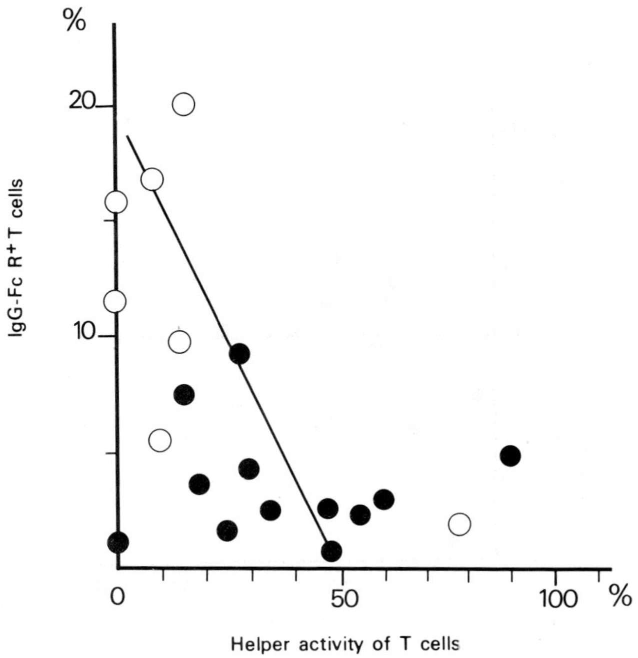

Increased numbers of suppressor T cells have been reported in tumour-bearing hosts by Fujimoto et al. (1976) and other authors. If the increased percentages of IgG-Fc R^+ T cells seen by us in cancer patients are related to a potentiation of the number of suppressors, these may be acting to diminish antitumour immunity and thus permit the progress of tumour growth. An alternative explanation is that IgG-Fc R^+ T cells are actually killer T cells, and an increase in the proportion of this subset is in some indirect way related to a reduction of other lymphocyte functions, such as response to PHA or immunoglobulin production. Greater numbers of these killer T cells would then appear in the circulatory system as growth of the tumour progressed.

Whatever the explanation, the fact that the increase in percentage of IgG-Fc R^+ T cells was greater in patients with advanced tumours and that it fell within the normal range after complete removal of the tumour indicates that these changes are related

FIG. 7. CHANGES IN PERCENTAGES OF IgG-Fc R^+ T CELLS WITH STAGE OF NASOPHARYNGEAL CARCINOMA

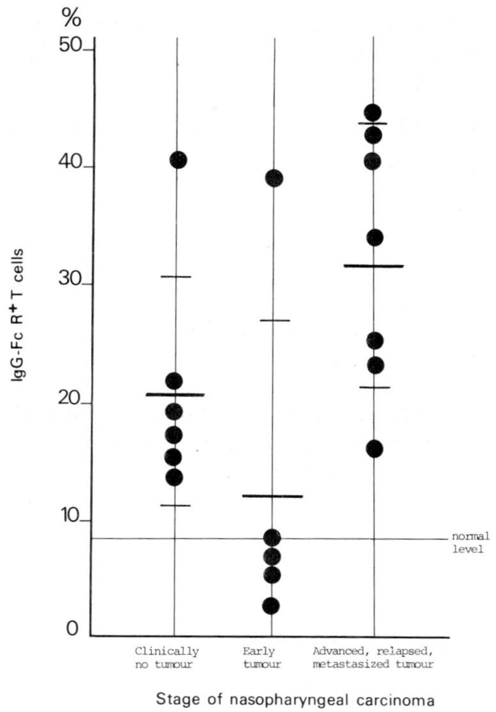

to the presence of the tumour and reflect the status of host-tumour interactions.

SUMMARY

The proportion of T cells that have receptors for IgG-Fc (Fc R^+ T cells), the functioning of T cell helpers in immunoglobulin production and the blastogenic response of lymphocytes to PHA and Con A were measured in cancer patients.

Increases in the percentage of IgG-Fc R^+ T cells were observed in most patients; these were greater in patients with advanced tumours and fell within the normal range after complete surgical removal of the tumour.

The functioning of T cell helpers in immunoglobulin production and response of lymphocytes to PHA were poor in those patients in whom IgG-Fc R^+ T cell percentages were increased. The lymphocytes of such patients responded well to Con A.

These changes in T-cell subsets appear to be related to the presence and progress of tumours.

ACKNOWLEDGEMENT

This work was supported by a cancer research subsidy awarded by the Japanese Ministry of Welfare.

REFERENCES

Cantor, H. & Boyse, E.A. (1975) Functional subclasses of T lymphocytes bearing different Ly antigens. II. Cooperation between subclasses of Ly^+ cells in the generation of killer activity. *J. exp. Med.*, *141*, 1390-1399

Cerottini, J.-C. & Brunner, K.T. (1974) Cell-mediated cytotoxicity allograft rejection, and tumor immunity. *Advanc. Immunol.*, *18*, 67-132

Cooper, M.D., Moretta, L., Webb, S.R., Pearl, E.R., Okos, A.J. & Lawton, A.R. (1976) *Analysis of defects in human B-cell differentiation and in development of two T-cell subpopulations*. In: Kobayashi, N., ed., *Immunodeficiency, Its Nature and Etiological Significance in Human Diseases*, Tokyo, University of Tokyo Press

Fujimoto, S., Greene, M.I. & Sehon, A.H. (1976) Regulation of immune response to tumor antigens. I. Immunosuppressor cells in tumor-bearing hosts. *J. Immunol.*, *116*, 791-799

Hellström, K.E. & Hellström, I. (1974) Lymphocyte mediated cytotoxicity and blocking serum activity to tumor antigens. *Advanc. Immunol.*, *18*, 209-217

Stout, R.D. & Herzenberg, L.A. (1975) The Fc receptor on thymus derived lymphocytes. II. Mitogen responsiveness of lymphocytes bearing the Fc receptor. *J. exp. Med.*, *142*, 1041-1051

Yata, J., Desgranges, C., Tachibana, T. & de-Thé, G. (1973) Separation of human lymphocytes forming spontaneous rosettes with sheep erythrocytes. *Biomedicine*, *19*, 475-478

AUTOANTIBODIES (COLD LYMPHOCYTOTOXINS, ANTIACTIN ANTIBODIES AND ANTINUCLEAR FACTORS) IN NASOPHARYNGEAL CARCINOMA PATIENTS

J.-P. LAMELIN & G. DE-THE

Unit of Biological Carcinogenesis,
International Agency for Research on Cancer,
Lyon, France

J.P. REVILLARD

Immunology Laboratory,
National Institute for Health and Medical Research (INSERM),
Hôpital Edouard Herriot,
Lyon, France

G. GABBIANI

Department of Pathology,
University of Geneva,
Geneva, Switzerland

INTRODUCTION

Cold lymphocytotoxic (Mottironi & Terasaki, 1970), smooth muscle (Andersen, 1975; Holborow et al., 1973) and nuclear antibodies (Kaplan & Tan, 1968) are byproducts of primary Epstein-Barr virus (EBV) infection. Whether these autoantibodies also occur in other EBV-associated diseases (in which the EBV infection is not primary), and what relationship may exist between them, was investigated in patients with nasopharyngeal carcinoma (NPC).

Sera from patients with acute viral infections such as rubella, measles and infectious mononucleosis were found by Mottironi & Terasaki (1970) to have cytotoxic activity against a panel of normal human lymphocytes; this cytotoxicity was complement-dependent and optimal at +15°C. 'Cold' lymphocytotoxic antibody (LTA) was later found to occur in various pathological conditions such as systemic lupus erythematosus (Mittal et al., 1970; Ooi et al., 1974; Terasaki et al., 1970; Winchester et al., 1974), in which the presence of LTA was found to correlate with that of anti-native DNA and of anti-single-stranded RNA antibodies (DeHoratius et al., 1975).

Antibodies that react in indirect immunofluorescence with smooth muscle (Johnson et al., 1965) and a variety of other tissues (Biberfeld et al., 1974; Fagraeus et al., 1973, 1974, 1975; Farrow et al., 1971; Gabbiani et al., 1973) were initially described in patients with chronic active hepatitis. Since staining was no longer observed in these tissues after absorption of the sera with a smooth-muscle extract, these antibodies were referred to as anti-smooth-muscle antibodies (SMA). It was later shown that these antibodies were specific for actin (Gabbiani et al., 1973; Lidman et al., 1976). Anti-SMA reactivity has been found not only in patients with chronic active hepatitis but also in sera from patients with other diseases, including infectious mononucleosis (Andersen, 1975; Holborow et al., 1973), malignant diseases (Whitehouse & Holborow, 1971) and various types of leukaemias and lymphomas (Andersen et al., 1976). Antinuclear antibodies (ANA), a major feature of systemic lupus erythematosus have also been found in various malignant conditions (Yoshida, 1974), including NPC (Yoshida, 1971; Yoshida et al., 1975).

The full results of our investigations, on which partial reports have already been published (Lamelin et al., 1977b, c) are presented below.

MATERIALS AND METHODS

Tests and control sera

Ninety-eight sera from patients with NPC diagnosed in Hong Kong (43 cases), Tunis (42 cases) and Paris (13 cases), selected so that the various stages of the disease (Ho, 1970) were statistically equally distributed among the three groups, were assayed for LTA. Control groups in each study consisted of age-matched, normal individuals. The SMA study was limited to 30 of the Tunisian patients and had an additional control group made up of 72 family relatives of these NPC cases. Sera from the same families (29 NPC cases and 119 relatives) were also assayed for ANA.

Assay for LTA

Preparation of lymphocytes. Pre-warmed (37°C), heparinized blood from normal Caucasian donors was passed through a nylon fibre column (Rhodiaceta TD3, Roger Bellon, Neuilly, France; 5 g/ml of blood) at a rate of 2-4 ml/min. The eluate was mixed thoroughly with dextran (6 x 10^5 mol. wt.; 0.5% final) and left at room temperature for 20 min. The lymphocyte-rich upper fraction was cleared of contaminating erythrocytes by treatment with 0.85% ammonium chloride, centrifuged, washed once at 4°C and resuspended in RPMI 1640. This selected population, 90-95% T lymphocytes, was 98-99% viable. The final suspension was adjusted to 2 x 10^6 cells/ml.

Complement. A pool of rabbit sera, selected for its lack of cytotoxicity toward human lymphocytes and kept frozen at -60°C, was used as the source of complement.

Cytotoxicity assay. The cytotoxicity of each test serum was evaluated against a panel of normal lymphocyte populations under oil in Terasaki microplates, as described by Mottironi & Terasaki (1970), with minor modifications. In brief, 1 µl portions of the test sera (serially diluted up to 1:16) were mixed with 1 µl cell suspension (i.e., 2000 cells). After 30 min at 4°C, 4 µl rabbit serum were added and the mixture left for 3.5 hr at 15°C. After the addition of 2 µl 5% eosin and 5 µl 40% formaldehyde (pH 7.2), the percentage of dead cells was scored, as follows: 0-20% = negative; 20-40% = +; 40-60% = ++; 60-80% = +++; 80-100% = ++++. Controls included negative and positive sera.

For each test serum, three additional assays were run in parallel: one at 37°C and two others at 15°C and 37°C in the presence (v/v) of 0.01M dithiotreitol (DTT), a reducing agent known to abrogate IgM, but not IgG, antibody activity. Sera containing anti-HLA activity were cytotoxic at 37°C, resistant to DTT treatment and usually active against only a small number of cell suspensions from the panel. In contrast, LTA-containing sera were cytotoxic at 15°C, but not at 37°C, sensitive to DTT treatment and killed all or most cell suspensions.

Expression of results. A serum was considered to be positive when there were >20% dead cells in at least two lymphocyte suspensions of the panel. With most of the positive sera, this activity could be titrated by dilution. Since these dilutions were different for the various suspensions of the panel, the geometric mean titre (GMT) of the last dilutions that gave 20% or more dead cells was calculated and taken as the LTA titre of the serum.

Assay for SMA

Cryostat sections of rat small intestine were fixed on glass slides for 5 min in acetone. Test sera, diluted 1:10 (or higher, if required for determining titres) in phosphate-buffered saline (PBS), were layered on a series of these sections. After 15 min at room temperature, the slides were washed in PBS and stained for 15 min with fluorescein-conjugated IgG fraction of goat antiserum to human IgG (Miles Seravac, Lausanne, Switzerland). After rewashing with PBS and mounting in glycerol:PBS (9:1), the level of fluorescence of smooth muscle was compared with that of preparations treated with human sera selected for their negativity or positivity (at a known dilution) with regard to SMA activity.

Assay for ANA

This assay was kindly performed by Dr T.O. Yoshida, as previously described (Yoshida et al., 1975).

EBV serology

Antibodies against viral capsid antigen (VCA) and early antigen (EA) were titrated by the indirect immunofluorescence technique described by Henle et al. (Henle & Henle, 1966; Henle et al., 1970). The anticomplement immunofluorescence test of Reedman & Klein (1973) was used to determine activity against Epstein-Barr nuclear antigen (EBNA).

Statistical analyses

The percentages of individuals with LTA were compared among various groups by the χ^2 test. The GMTs of positive sera within each group were determined and compared by Student's *t-test*.

RESULTS

(1) *The frequency of LTA-positive sera and their GMTs were higher among NPC patients than among their matched controls* in both Chinese (84% *vs.* 28.6% and 3.2 *vs.* 1.2, respectively) and Caucasians (62% *vs.* 17% and 1.7 *vs.* 1.1, respectively). The frequency of LTA-positive sera was identical (64%) in Tunisian NPC cases and in controls, although the GMT was higher in the NPC than in the control group (2.4 *vs.* 1.3; $P < 0.01$) (Table 1).

Table 1. Percentages and geometric mean titres (GMTs) of cold lymphocytotoxic antibody-positive sera in nasopharyngeal carcinoma (NPC) and control groups from geographical areas with different risks for the disease

Subjects	Percentage (no. positive/no. tested)			GMT (TSE)		
	NPC	Controls	P	NPC	Controls	P
Chinese	84 (36/43)	28 (8/29)	<0.0005	3.2 (1.17)	1.2 (1.12)	<0.01
Tunisian	64 (27/42)	64 (9/14)	NS	2.4 (1.17)	1.3 (1.10)	<0.01
Caucasian	62 (8/13)	17 (10/60)	<0.001	1.7 (1.19)	1.1 (1.09)	<0.05

TSE - transformed standard error

NS - not significant

In all positive sera the cytotoxic activity was shown to be complement-dependent and, in accordance with the postulated IgM nature of the antibodies (Chalopin et al., 1975), DTT-sensitive. The absorption of a few highly positive sera with platelets, polymorphonuclear cells and EBV-positive B lymphoblastoid cells (line 4091) had no effect on cytotoxicity, in contrast to the loss of cytotoxicity observed after absorption with T lymphocytes.

(2) *The GMTs of LTA-positive NPC sera from different geographical areas increased with the risk for NPC in the corresponding population (Table 1).*

The GMTs were 1.7 for Caucasians (low risk), 2.4 for Tunisians (intermediate risk) and 3.2 for Chinese (high risk); the difference between Caucasians and Chinese was significant ($P < 0.01$).

(3) *The GMTs of LTA-positive sera from patients with different stages of the disease increased with its spread (Table 2).*

In the homogeneous Chinese group, although the frequency of LTA-positive sera was similar in the three groups (I + II, III and IV), a steady increase in their GMTs was found with stage of disease (2.0, 3.0 and 4.9).

Table 2. Percentages and geometric mean titres (GMTs) of cold lymphocytotoxic antibody-positive sera in nasopharyngeal carcinoma patients from Hong Kong with different stages of the disease

Subjects	Percentage (no. positive/no. tested)	P[a]	GMT (TSE)	P
Controls	28 (8/29)		1.19 (1.37)	
Stages I + II	71 (10/14)	<0.01	2.0 (1.30)	NS
Stage III	93 (13/14)	<0.001	3.03 (1.30)	<0.05
Stage IV	87 (13/15)	<0.001	4.92 (1.28)	<0.01

[a] Level of significance of the difference between each stage and the control group

TSE - transformed standard error

NS - not significant

The last two values were significantly higher ($P < 0.05$ and $P < 0.01$, respectively) than the GMT of the positive control sera.

When data from all geographical areas were pooled, the difference between the GMTs of early and late stages (I + II *vs.* IV) was still significant (data not shown), despite the greater heterogeneity introduced into the sampling.

(4) *There was a correlation between the level of LTA activity and the anti-EBV antibody titres of NPC sera (Table 3).*

Positive correlations between titres of LTA and anti-VCA antibodies were found in the Chinese [correlation coefficient (r) = 0.31; $P < 0.05$] and in the Tunisian ($r = 0.33$; $P < 0.05$) groups. In addition, 27 NPC sera from Tunis were tested for the presence of anti-EBNA antibodies: a strong positive correlation ($r = 0.53$; $P < 0.01$) was again found between EBNA titres and LTA. In contrast, no correlation was found between LTA and anti-EA titres in the group of 26 NPC cases examined.

Table 3. Correlation coefficients (r) and levels of significance (P) of the association between cold lymphocytotoxic antibody and Epstein-Barr virus titres [anti-viral capsid antigen (VCA), anti-nuclear antigen (EBNA) and anti-early antigen (EA)]

		Chinese		Tunisian		Caucasian	
anti-VCA	r P	0.31 <0.05	(43)[a]	0.33 <0.05	(38)	0.50 NS	(13)
anti-EBNA	r P	ND		0.53 <0.01	(27)	ND	
anti-EA	r P	ND		-0.085 NS	(26)	0.411 NS	(13)

[a] Number of NPC cases is given in parentheses.

ND - not determined

NS - not significant

(5) *SMA were found at a higher frequency in sera from NPC patients than in sera from controls.*

Seven of 30 patients from Tunis were found to have SMA, as compared with none among 17 unrelated controls ($P < 0.05$) and five among 72 NPC family members ($P < 0.05$). When these controls were pooled, the significance of this difference reached a P value of < 0.001.

Six sera chosen from those that were SMA-positive were shown, by immunodiffusion, to give a strong precipitation line against purified actin (Fig. 1), confirming the presence of antiactin antibodies in immunofluorescence reactive sera.

FIG. 1. IMMUNODIFFUSION OF SMOOTH-MUSCLE ANTIBODY-POSITIVE SERUM (CENTRAL WELL) FROM A NASOPHARYNGEAL CARCINOMA PATIENT AGAINST PURIFIED ACTIN

(1.2 mg/ml in the upper well, and, clockwise, 1:2 serial dilutions)

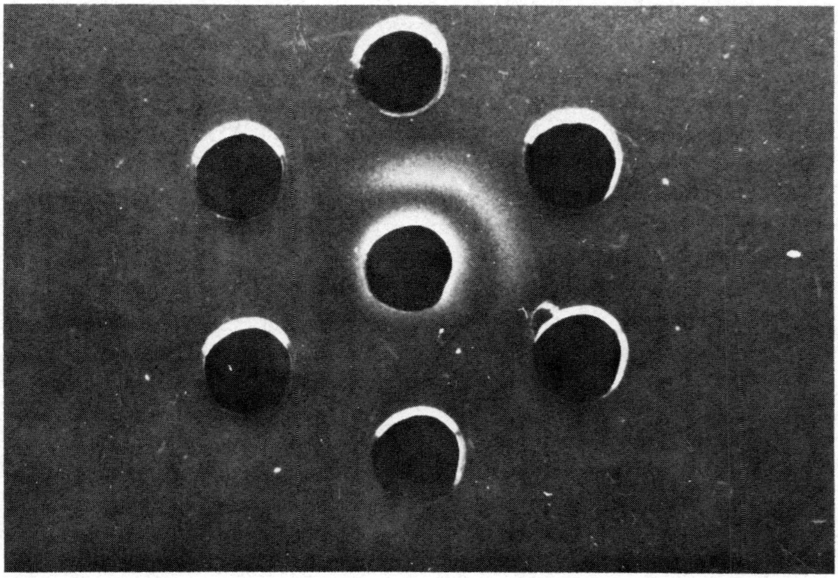

(6) *There was no correlation between the level of SMA and titres of anti-VCA, anti-EA or anti-EBNA antibodies (data not shown).*

(7) *LTA and SMA occurred independently in individual sera from NPC patients and controls (Table 4).*

Table 4. Distribution of smooth-muscle antibody (SMA)- and cold lymphocytotoxic antibody (LTA)-positive and -negative sera among pooled nasopharyngeal carcinoma patients and controls from Tunis

		SMA	
		-	+
LTA	-	40	3
	+	34	5

($\chi^2 = 0.79$; $P > 0.30$)

(8) *ANA were found at a higher frequency among NPC patients (11/29) than among their relatives (17/119).*

The difference between the frequency of positive sera within the two groups was statistically significant ($P < 0.01$). In individual sera from NPC patients, ANA was found independently of LTA and SMA (Fig. 2).

FIG. 2. SEROLOGY OF NASOPHARYNGEAL CARCINOMA PATIENTS

Lack of correlation between antinuclear antibody (ANA) (ordinate) and lymphocytotoxic antibody (LTA) (left abscissa) or smooth-muscle antibody (SMA) (right abscissa) titres in individual sera from nasopharyngeal carcinoma patients

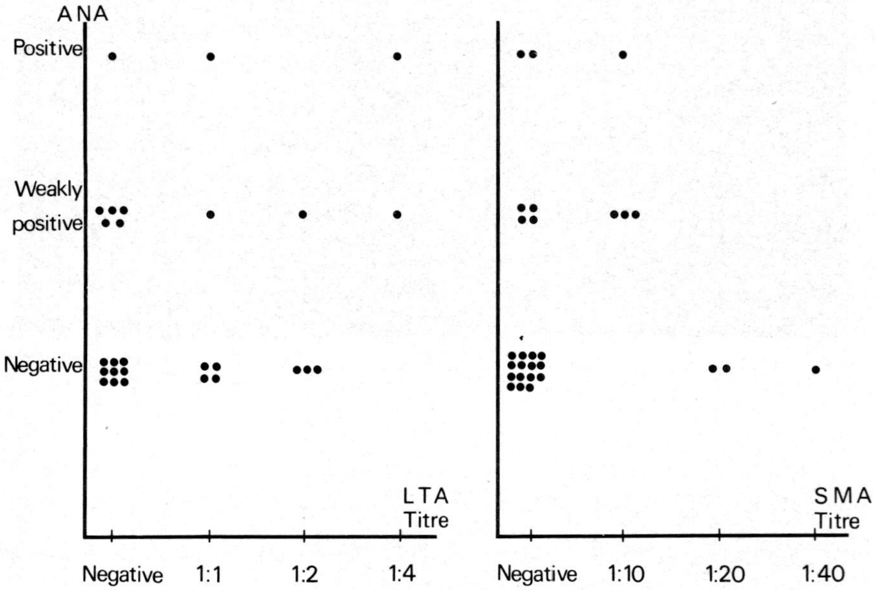

DISCUSSION

Antibodies specific for lymphocyte membrane-borne determinants, for actin and for nuclear antigen were found at a higher frequency in sera from NPC patients than in sera from matched controls. As noted above, these antibodies are commonly observed in sera from patients with infectious mononucleosis and with various other diseases in which the role of viruses is either established or postulated. The list is not exhaustive, and they even occur in some of the 'healthy' individuals chosen as controls.

The differentiation of B lymphocytes into cells that produce antibodies with these specificities and the biological significance of those autoantibodies are poorly understood. With regard to NPC, two alternatives can be proposed:

(1) *Autologous structures, such as lymphocyte membrane-borne determinants and actin and nuclear antigens, that belong to normally tolerated 'self' components become immunogenic in NPC patients.*

LTA, which are known to be produced preferentially during the acute phase of various viral infections, might represent a nonspecific byproduct of the antibody response either against virus-modified cell membranes or against structures characteristic of cells from the clones of stimulated lymphocytes, thus reflecting the operating of some regulatory process.

How actin, a weak immunogen in experimental animals (Pollard & Weihing, 1974), can become immunogenic in humans is not known. One possible interpretation in viral-associated diseases is that actin, known to be present in the coats of some viruses (Wang et al., 1975), is presented under an immunogenic form. The suggestion that the modified membrane of malignant cells might contain immunizing actin-like determinants is an alternative but not a comprehensive hypothesis (Whitehouse & Holborow, 1971).

The possibility that an actin-like structure, present on the lymphocyte surface, might act as a target for at least part of the LTA, is contradicted both by the lack of correlation between SMA and LTA activities (Table 4) and by the failure to stain live lymphocytes in suspension with SMA by indirect fluorescence (Fagraeus et al., 1974). This last observation is in accordance with the electron microscopic evidence that the myosin-like structures visualized by immunoferritin techniques are restricted to the inner surface of the plasma membrane (Painter et al., 1975).

Finally, both viral and host nucleic acids can be expected to be released from tumour cells exposed to infiltrating cytotoxic T cells (Klein[1]) and are therefore potential immunogens in NPC patients.

(2) *Some regulatory mechanism fails to turn off antibody synthesis against self components,* resulting in production of autoantibodies with various specificities in NPC patients.

Because of the genetic link between genes that code for T-cell functions and the HLA major histocompatibility complex (NPC is an HLA-associated disease) (Simons et al., 1975), the possible involvement of T lymphocytes deserves consideration. One consequence of the still ill-defined T-cell defect observed in NPC patients (Chan et al., 1976; Lamelin et al., 1977a; Stjernswärd & Clifford, 1970) could indeed be a failure

[1] See p. 538

to exert the positive controls that normally restrain the synthesis of autoantibodies by B cells (Allison et al., 1971). All that would rest to be explained is how this defect could have selective effects: on LTA in one patient, SMA in another, ANA in a third. Finally, the hypothesis that LTA activity is the cause rather than the consequence of the dysregulation is very unlikely in view of the complete lack of correlation between LTA and either SMA (Table 4) or ANA (Fig. 2).

In addition to these two hypotheses to explain the mechanism of autoantibody production in NPC patients, two further observations are worth consideration:

The existence of a link, in a given geographical area, between the incidence of NPC and the proportion of NPC patients with high LTA titres indirectly supports the hypothesis that EBV plays a role in NPC. If, indeed, EBV 'reactivation' is one of the single events (or cofactors) that increases the probability with which NPC occurs and is, at the same time, responsible for LTA production, then a difference in the frequency of this 'reactivation' would be expected to result in parallel variations in both the incidence of NPC in the general population and the level of LTA in those patients.

Our finding of a positive correlation between titres of anti-VCA and anti-EBNA antibody and LTA supports the interpretation that LTA and active viral infections are closely related. The failure to find a correlation between anti-EA - a marker of EBV replication - and LTA titres may be only an apparent paradox. These are, indeed, the kinds of results expected when two parameters, linked by a feedback mechanism, are compared without taking into account the onset of the regulatory mechanism.

Nothing is known about the biological significance of the auto-antibodies. No correlation could be found between the presence of LTA and the performances of the T-cell populations, as determined by the percentage of E-rosette-forming cells and the response to T mitogens (Lamelin et al., 1977a). From a clinical viewpoint, only longitudinal studies could indicate whether assays of LTA and SMA might help in establishing prognosis. As to the mechanism of their production, its elucidation will probably have to wait until the general biological phenomenon of autoimmunity is understood.

SUMMARY

LTA, SMA and ANA were found at higher frequencies in sera from NPC patients than in those from matched controls. The frequency and GMTs of LTA-positive sera varied with the origin of the patient (Chinese > North African > Caucasian, thus paralleling the risk for NPC in each ethnic group) and the stage of the disease (stage IV > stage I). A positive correlation was found between LTA and anti-EBV titres with regard to anti-VCA and anti-EBNA antibodies.

SMA were specific for actin, and their titres did not correlate with anti-EBV (VCA, EBNA and EA) titres.

Although there was no evidence for an abnormal immunogenicity of the self components recognized by the three autoantibodies, their independent augmentations did not favour the alternative hypothesis of a common central mechanism for their production. The origin and the biological significance of these autoantibodies remains, therefore, to be explained.

ACKNOWLEDGEMENTS

This study was supported by contract no. NO 1 CP 43296 within the Virus Cancer Program of the National Cancer Institute, USA and grant no. 3.0330.73 from the Fonds National Suisse pour la Recherche Scientifique.

REFERENCES

Allison, A.C., Denman, A.M. & Barnes, R.D. (1971) Cooperating and controlling functions of thymus-derived lymphocytes in relation to autoimmunity. *Lancet, ii*, 135-140

Andersen, P. (1975) Smooth-muscle antibodies in sera with Paul-Bunnell heterophil antibodies. *Acta path. microbiol. scand., Sect. C., 83*, 19-27

Andersen, P., Molgaard, J., Andersen, I. & Andersen, H.K. (1976) Smooth-muscle antibodies and antibodies to cytomegalovirus and Epstein-Barr virus in leukemias and lymphomata. *Acta path. microbiol. scand., Sect. C., 84*, 86-92

Biberfeld, G., Fagraeus, A. & Brighton, W.D (1974) Reaction of human smooth muscle antibody with thyroid cells. *Clin. exp. Immunol., 18*, 371-377

Chalopin, J.M., Ekladios, E., Revillard, J.P., Bonnet, M.C., Bétuel, H. & Creyssel, R. (1975) Anticorps lymphocytotoxiques dans les gammapathies monoclonales idiopathiques ou réactionnelles. *Lyon Méd., 234*, 507-514

Chan, S.H., Chew, T.S., Goh, E.H., Simons, M.J. & Shanmugaratnam, K. (1976) Impaired general cell-mediated immune functions *in vivo* and *in vitro* in patients with nasopharyngeal carcinoma. *Int. J. Cancer, 18*, 139-144

DeHoratius, R.J., Pillarisetty, R., Messner, R.I.P. & Talal, N. (1975) Antinucleic acid antibodies in systemic lupus erythematosus patients and their families: incidence and correlation with lymphocytotoxic antibodies. *J. clin. Invest., 56*, 1149-1154

Fagraeus, A., The, H. & Biberfeld, G. (1973) Reaction of smooth muscle antibody with thymus medullary cells. *Nature (New Biol.), 246*, 113-115

Fagraeus, A., Lidman, K. & Biberfeld, G. (1974) Reaction of human smooth muscle antibodies with human blood lymphocytes and lymphoid cell lines. *Nature (Lond.), 252*, 246-247

Fagraeus, A., Lidman, K. & Norberg, R. (1975) Indirect immunofluorescence staining of contractile proteins in smeared cells by smooth muscle antibodies. *Clin. exp. Immunol., 20*, 469-477

Farrow, L.J., Holborow, E.J. & Brighton, W.D. (1971) Reaction of human smooth muscle antibody with liver cells. *Nature (New Biol.), 232*, 186-187

Gabbiani, G., Ryan, G.B., Lamelin, J.-P., Vassalli, P., Majno, G., Bouvier, C.A., Cruchaud, A. & Luscher, E.F. (1973) Human smooth muscle autoantibody: its identification as antiactin antibody and a study of its binding to 'nonmuscular' cells. *Amer. J. Path., 72*, 473-484

Henle, G. & Henle, W. (1966) Immunofluorescence in cells derived from Burkitt's lymphoma. *J. Bact., 91*, 1248-1256

Henle, W., Henle, G., Zajac, B.A., Pearson, G., Waubke, R. & Scriba, M. (1970) Differential reactivity of human serums with early antigens induced by Epstein-Barr virus. *Science, 169*, 188-190

Ho, H.C. (1970) *The natural history and treatment of nasopharyngeal carcinoma.* In: Clark, R.L., Cumley, R.W., McCay, J.E. & Copeland, M.M., eds, *Oncology, Proceedings of the X International Cancer Congress*, Vol. 4, Chicago, Year Book Medical Publishers, pp. 1-14

Holborow, E.J., Hemsted, E.H. & Mead, S.V. (1973) Smooth muscle autoantibodies in infectious mononucleosis. *Brit. med. J., iii*, 323-325

Johnson, G.D., Holborow, E.J. & Glynn, L.E. (1965) Antibody to smooth muscle in patient with liver disease. *Lancet, ii*, 878-879

Kaplan, M.E. & Tan, E.M. (1968) Antinuclear antibodies in infectious mononucleosis. *Lancet, i*, 561-563

Lamelin, J.-P., Ellouz, R., de-Thé, G. & Revillard, J.P. (1977a) Lymphocyte subpopulations and mitogenic responses in nasopharyngeal carcinoma, prior to and after radiotherapy. *Int. J. Cancer* (in press)

Lamelin, J.-P., Revillard, J.P., Chalopin, J.M., Ho, J.H.C., Souissi, T. & de-Thé, G. (1977b) Cold lymphocytotoxic antibodies in nasopharyngeal carcinoma. *Brit. J. Cancer, 35*, 426-432

Lamelin, J.-P., Williams, E.H., Souissi, T., de-Thé, G. & Gabbiani, G. (1977c) Smooth muscle antibody in Burkitt's lymphoma and in nasopharyngeal carcinoma. *Clin. exp. Immunol., 27*, 157-162

Lidman, K., Bibérfeld, G., Fagraeus, A., Norberg, R., Torstensson, R., Utter, G., Carlsson, L., Luca, J. & Lindberg, U. (1976) Anti-actin specificity of human smooth muscle antibodies in chronic active hepatitis. *Clin. exp. Immunol., 24*, 266-272

Mittal, K.K., Rossen, R.D., Sharp, J.T., Lidsky, R.D. & Butler, W.T. (1970) Lymphocyte cytotoxic antibodies in systemic lupus erythematosus. *Nature (Lond.), 225*, 1255-1256

Mottironi, V.D. & Terasaki, P.J. (1970) *Lymphocytotoxins in disease. I. Infectious mononucleosis, rubella and measles.* In: Terasaki, P.J., ed., *Histocompatibility Testing*, Copenhagen, Munksgaard, pp. 301-308

Ooi, B.S., Orlina, A.R., Pesce, A.J., Mendoza, N., Masaitis, L. & Pollak, V.E. (1974) Lymphocytotoxic antibodies in patients with systemic lupus erythematosus. *Clin. exp. Immunol., 17*, 237-244

Painter, R.G., Sheetz, M. & Singer, S.J. (1975) Detection and ultrastructural localization of human smooth muscle myosin-like molecules in human non-muscle cells by specific antibodies. *Proc. nat. Acad. Sci. (Wash.), 72*, 1359-1363

Pollard, T.D. & Weihing, R.R. (1974) Actin and myosin and cell movement. *Crit. Rev. Biochem., 2*, 1-65

Reedman, B.M. & Klein, G. (1973) Cellular localization of an Epstein-Barr virus (EBV)-associated complement-fixing antigen in producer and non-producer lymphoblastoid cell lines. *Int. J. Cancer, 11*, 499-520

Simons, M.J., Wee, G.B., Chan, S.H., Shanmugaratnam, K., Day, N.E. & de-Thé, G. (1975) *Immunogenetic aspects of nasopharyngeal carcinoma (NPC). III. HL-A type as a genetic marker of NPC predisposition to test the hypothesis that EBV is an etiological factor in NPC.* In: de-Thé, G., Epstein, M.A. & zur Hausen, H., eds, *Oncogenesis and Herpesviruses II, Part 2 (IARC Scientific Publications No. 11)*, Lyon, pp. 249-258

Stjernswärd, J. & Clifford, P. (1970) *Tumour-distinctive cellular immune reactions against autochthonous cancer.* In: Severi, L., ed., *Proceedings of the 4th Perugia Quadriennal International Conference on Cancer: Immunity and Tolerance in Oncogenesis, Perugia, Italy*, Perugia, University of Perugia, pp. 749-758

Terasaki, P.I., Mottironi, V.D. & Barnett, E.V. (1970) Cytotoxins in disease: autocytotoxins in lupus. *New Engl. J. Med., 283*, 724-728

Wang, E., Wolf, B.A., Lamb, R.A., Choppin, P.W. & Goldberg, A.R. (1975) The presence of actin in enveloped viruses. *J. cell. Biol., 67*, 445a

Whitehouse, J.M.A. & Holborow, E.J. (1971) Smooth muscle antibodies in malignant disease. *Brit. med. J., iv*, 511-513

Winchester, R.J., Winfield, G.B., Siegal, F., Wernet, P., Bentwich, Z. & Kunkel, M.G. (1974) Analyses of lymphocytes from patients with rheumatoid arthritis and systemic lupus erythematosus: occurrence of interfering cold reactive anti-lymphocyte antibodies. *J. clin. Invest., 54*, 1082-1092

Yoshida, T.O. (1971) *High incidence of antinuclear antibodies in the sera of nasopharyngeal cancer patients.* In: Nakahara, W., Nishioka, K., Hirayama, T. & Ito, Y., eds, *Recent Advances in Human Tumour Virology and Immunology*, Tokyo, University of Tokyo Press, pp. 443-460

Yoshida, T.O. (1974) Autoantibodies in the sera of various cancer patients. *Gann Monogr., 16*, 63-70

Yoshida, T.O., Yasuda -Yasaki, Y. & Utsumi, K.R. (1975) *Autoantibodies in the sera of patients with nasopharyngeal carcinoma.* In: de-Thé, G., Epstein, M.A. & zur Hausen, H., eds, *Oncogenesis and Herpesviruses II, Part 2 (IARC Scientific Publications No. 11)*, Lyon, pp. 259-273

DISCUSSION SUMMARY

T. TACHIBANA

*The Research Institute for Tuberculosis and Cancer,
Tohoku University,
Sendai, Japan*

It was pointed out that antibody titres in sera of nasopharyngeal carcinoma (NPC) patients could also be influenced by clinical immunosuppressive treatment as well as by tumour burden.

Antibodies to Epstein-Barr virus (EBV) are invariably demonstrated not only in EBV-carrying tumours such as NPC and Burkitt's lymphoma and in EBV-associated infections such as mononucleosis but also in non-EBV-carrying tumours such as Hodgkin's disease, chronic lymphocytic leukaemia and other carcinomas of the head and neck region, and even in healthy donors. It would therefore be of interest to know if there are any differences in antibody levels, immunoglobulin classes and specificities of antibodies between persons with EBV-associated and those with non-associated diseases.

In general, the viral capsid antigen-specific IgG level was highest in those with EBV-associated diseases, intermediate in those with tumours that did not carry EBV and lowest in healthy donors. The most striking finding was that the sera of patients with NPC had higher incidences and titres of EBV-specific IgA than did patients with other EBV-associated diseases (infectious mononucleosis and Burkitt's lymphoma); patients with other carcinomas of the head and neck and healthy donors also had a low or no EBV-specific IgA antibody response, although a few of these patients showed antibody patterns similar to those of NPC patients. Whether these tumours are truly associated with EBV can only be established by demonstrating EBV genomes and/or Epstein-Barr nuclear antigen-positive malignant cells in biopsies.

Viral capsid antigen-specific IgM antibody should be induced by reactivation of a persistent EBV infection; however, in NPC patients, the EBV-specific IgM response has been seen to endure, albeit at a lower level and infrequently.

Although EBV-specific IgA of the secretory type was found in saliva of NPC patients, the IgA antibody found in sera was of the systemic 7S type. It remains to be clarified why and how this type of IgA is produced in patients with NPC but not in those with Burkitt's lymphoma or infectious mononucleosis.

Ng reported results on IgA in the saliva of NPC patients in Hong Kong. Twenty-four of 30 patients studied had EBV-specific IgA, as demonstrated by the presence of anti-α conjugate; however, only one of these positive salivas contained the secretory type of IgA, in contrast with the results obtained in Lyon. On the other hand, in Tunis, the frequency of IgA positivity in the sera of family members of NPC patients was similar to that seen in normal, healthy controls. The question was raised as to why there were discrepancies between the results from Hong Kong and those from Tunisia: it is not yet clear whether technical problems and/or ethnic differences are involved. In this connexion, it is noteworthy that there are differences in serological profile between different Caucasian ethnic groups: when examining French (except Arabs), Germans and Americans (except Chinese), the highest titre was detected in the French and the lowest in Germans.

The cell-mediated immunity test was designed by Ng to determine whether there is an NPC-associated immunity. Both the macrophage migration inhibition (MIF) test and lymphocyte blast transformation with purified protein derivative were done, using two antigen preparations from Raji cells and two from pooled NPC biopsies. Only lymphocytes from NPC patients responded to all four extracts; those from other cancer patients, tested as a control, exhibited no response to the four extracts. In contrast, there was no difference in the responses to purified protein derivative tested by either of the two assay methods, between the two groups of cancer patients.

Miller asked about the specificity of the killer T cells which are found in biopsies from NPC patients and about the target of these cells. Klein replied that T lymphocytes were separated in samples drawn from lymph nodes and the tumour site by rosetting with sheep red blood cells. The former was a much better source of the T cells. The lymphocytes were then exposed to ammonium chloride to remove the red blood cells and were recovered for cytotoxicity testing against EBV-positive and -negative cell lines. They showed specific cytotoxicity for EBV-positive cell lines and for biopsies from Burkitt's lymphomas. No HLA restriction was seen in this system.

In Singapore, there was evidence of a high-risk HLA haplotype in NPC patients and an association of this haplotype with a low response to phytohaemagglutinin. Chan added that NPC-negative patients that have the high-risk HLA haplotype, A2 and Sin 2, do not show hypo-responsiveness to phytohaemagglutinin; four normal family members of NPC patients also had the A2 and Sin 2 haplotype and showed hyporesponsiveness to phytohaemagglutinin, although they were not followed up.

The association of an HLA profile with NPC has been shown not only in Chinese living in Singapore, but also in Chinese from Malaysia, Hong Kong and the United States; this important problem should be studied in other ethnic groups.

Yata was asked what evidence he had that suppressor T cells carried the receptor for the Fc part of IgG (FcR). In rat and mouse lymphocytes sensitized to chemically induced tumours in a diffusion chamber, there is generation of T blast cells bearing FcR^+ which have killer activity. Yata replied that human FcR^+ T lymphocytes were separated by rosetting and this cell fraction was added to lymphocytes that were stimulated with phytohaemagglutinin; added FcR^+ T cells suppressed the response of the lymphocytes. There was also a correlation between decreased immunological function and increment of FcR^+ T cell population in patients with tumours, suggesting that FcR^+ T cells have a suppressive capacity.

de-Thé commented that atypically elevated responses to Epstein-Barr nuclear antigen and early antigen might relate to the occurrence of antibody to nuclear antigens, even if other factors were also involved.

It was noted that the presence of cold lymphocytotoxic antibodies is not an obligatory side effect of tumour development. In the follow-up of 75 Caucasian breast cancer patients, 17 (23%) were positive as compared to 8 out of 40 (20%) in the age-sex matched control population. These percentages remained stable during and following cobaltotherapy up to three months. It is also known that cold lymphocytotoxic antibodies occur patients with in systemic lupus erythematosus (SLE), Hodgkin's disease and Graves' disease and in normal pregnant women and to some extent in normal individuals. When normal people were tested recently for antibody activity, using B lymphocyte preparations, almost 25% had cold autoantibodies.

Miller stressed the necessity of major histocompatibility complex (MHC) identity between responding and stimulating cells for T cell activation. In mice, MHC identity was shown to be necessary for the generation of cytotoxic T cells and for the activation of cells involved in delayed type hypersensitivity (DTH). Therefore, in testing cell-mediated immunity in NPC or Burkitt's lymphoma patients *in vitro*, the target cells should have an HLA identical to that of the patient from whom the sensitized lymphocytes were taken. Even though there appears to be no allogeneic restriction in NPC for cell-mediated immunity testing at the present time, more detailed HLA groupings should be made in the future.

An interesting exception was the DTH response of mice to *Plasmodium berghei*-associated antigens, which showed no MHC restriction.

Concerning CMI to tumours, Stanley touched on the possible role of natural killer cells which are neither T cells nor B cells. These cells may be effector cells against endogenous C type RNA viruses. Stanley referred to an area which, with the exception of the brief report by Osato, had been virtually neglected at this meeting. He stated that all of us now recognize the excellence of the work on EBV - it has, perhaps more than work with any other virus, demonstrated the value of a concerted and integrated technical attack on its natural history, evolution and pathogenesis. At the same time as we acknowledge the constant association of EBV with NPC, we recognize the multifactorial etiology of this carcinoma, the obvious genetic predisposition to its occurrence, and the less obvious involvement of other cofactors.

He believes the time has now come when material from NPC (both human and laboratory-produced) should be processed for C-type RNA viruses, for the following reasons: (1) to eliminate or to involve them as a cofactor; (2) in view of the demonstration of Kotler et al. (1975) of primate C-type RNA virus in P3HR-1 and Raji lines of Burkitt's lymphoma grown in arginine-deficient media; (3) in view of the observation of Osato et al. (1975) of a possible synergism between herpesviruses and C-type RNA viruses; (4) due to improved techniques for demonstrating C-type RNA virus; and (5) in view of interactions between C-type RNA and herpesviruses in both Marek's disease and guineapig leukaemia.

Miller summarized his recent work on the immune response (Ir) genes in mice, which seem to act not at the level of the T lymphocyte itself, as was suggested sometime ago by Benacerraf and McDevitt, but at the level of stimulator cells.

The transfer of DTH by sensitized lymphocytes could be done successfully between two syngeneic strains but not between two congenic strains of mice, which differ at the I-A region of the MHC. DTH could also be transferred from both parental mice to the F_1 offspring, but not from one parent to the other. Conversely, when sensitized lymphocytes from F_1 offspring of two strains of mice that were congenic except for the I region were used, DTH could be transferred to both parents and to the syngeneic F_1 mice. Thus, it was shown that haplotype identity was required for successful transfer of DTH.

When F_1 mice were sensitized not by giving antigen but by giving antigen-pulsed macrophages derived from one of the parental strains, successful transfer of DTH occurred only with recipients that had a haplotype identical to that of the parental strain from which macrophages were derived. This suggests that F_1 mice have two subsets of T lymphocytes with respect to the specificity of their antigen-combining sites: one directed towards antigen and the I-region gene product of one parental strain, the other directed towards antigen and the I-region gene product of the other parental strain.

Moreover, when F_1 offspring of a responder and a non-responder strain were sensitized to an antigen under MHC-linked genetic control, DTH transfer could be made from sensitized F_1 lymphoid cells to both mice of the responder haplotype and to syngeneic F_1 mice, but not to mice of the non-responder haplotype strain. This suggests that the Ir gene is expressed at the level of the cells (macrophages) which present antigen to T lymphocytes, and it may be essential for an appropriate molecular interaction between the Ir gene product and the antigen. If the Ir gene in the non-responder is unable to produce such a stable molecular interaction, the antigen may come off the surface of the stimulator cells and be available as free antigen to stimulate suppressor T cells. It has been demonstrated that non-responders have specific suppressor T cells and no sensitized cells.

These experimental results on DTH transfer would indicate that cells from patients with a high-risk NPC haplotype could act as stronger stimulators in the cell-mediated immunity tests for lymphocytes sensitized to EBV specific antigens, as compared with the stimulating capacity of cells from patients which do not have the high-risk haplotype.

REFERENCES

Kotler, M., Balabanova, H., Weinberg, E., Friedmann, A. & Becker, Y. (1975) Oncornavirus-like particles released from arginine-deprived human lymphoblastoid cell lines. *Proc. nat. Acad. Sci. (Wash.)*, *72*, 4592-4596

Osato, T., Yamamoto, K., Mizuno, F., Sugawara, K., Aya, T. & Sonta, S. (1975) *Dual persistence of Epstein-Barr viral and type C viral genomes in non-producer human lymphoblastoid cells*. In: Yohey, I.K. & Dutcher, R.M., eds, *Comparative Leukemia Research*, Tokyo, University of Tokyo Press, pp. 585-588

PRESENT CONCEPTS ON TREATMENT AND CURRENT CLINICAL RESEARCH

IN VIVO CELL-MEDIATED IMMUNITY IN CHINESE PATIENTS WITH NASOPHARYNGEAL CARCINOMA

J.H.C. HO, J.C.W. CHAU & K.C. TSE

Medical and Health Department Institute of Radiology and Oncology,
Queen Elizabeth Hospital,
Kowloon, Hong Kong

M.H. NG

Department of Microbiology,
Pathology Building,
University of Hong Kong
Queen Mary Hospital Compound,
Hong Kong

P.H. LEVINE

Clinical Studies Unit,
Laboratory of Viral Carcinogenesis,
National Cancer Institute,
Bethesda, Md 20014, USA

INTRODUCTION

There is a close serological association between Epstein-Barr virus (EBV) and nasopharyngeal carcinoma (NPC), irrespective of geography, and EBV DNA and nuclear antigen (EBNA) have been demonstrated in some NPC cells (de-Thé et al., 1973; Huang et al., 1974; Klein et al., 1974; Wolf et al., 1973). However, the role played by EBV in NPC and the nature of the close serological association between the two are not known.

In order better to understand this association, the *in vivo* cell-mediated immunity (CMI) of untreated NPC patients to EBV-related and

EBV-unrelated antigens was studied horizontally, using patients with other cancers (OC) as controls, and longitudinally, at intervals after completion of radiation therapy, with parallel observation of the clinical evolution of the disease. The NPC patients were incidentally found to have significantly elevated antibody titres to the capsid antigen (VCA) and to other antigens associated with EBV, but these data are not included in this preliminary report.

MATERIALS AND METHODS

A total of 104 Chinese patients with NPC and 24 patients with other cancers (OC), registered at the Queen Elizabeth Hospital, were given skin tests, prior to any specific therapy, with a battery of crude membrane extracts from EBV-related (HKLY 28, Raji, F265 and NC37) and EBV-unrelated (Molt) T-lymphoid cell lines and some standard antigens (*Trichophyton, Candida albicans* and streptokinase/streptodornase). The cell extracts were prepared by Litton Bionetics, USA, by a modification of the method of Davies (Oren & Herberman, 1971), and adjusted to a protein concentration of 0.1 mg/0.1 ml, the dosage administered intradermally to each patient. Extracts from the same source were used by Herberman et al. (1975) and by Levine et al. (1976) in their studies on the CMI of non-Chinese NPC patients. Skin indurations at the site of injection less than 5 mm in diameter, measured 43-45 hr after injection, were considered to be negative delayed hypersensitivity reactions, 5-9 mm as one-plus and 10-24 as two-plus. None of the NPC patients had more than a two-plus reaction.

The 24 OC patients who agreed to participate in the study consisted of four with bronchial carcinomas, three with carcinomas of the nasal fossae, two with squamous carcinomas of the hypopharynx, four with squamous carcinomas of the larynx, two with carcinomas of the tongue, one with a carcinoma of the alveolar mucosa, one with a squamous carcinoma of the buccal mucosa, one with a squamous carcinoma of the oesophagus, one with a squamous carcinoma of the skin, one with a basal-cell carcinoma of the cheek, one with a sarcoma of the thigh, one with an adenocarcinoma of the parotid gland, one with a carcinoma of the urinary bladder and one with a carcinoma of testis.

In the longitudinal study, 73 NPC patients with stages I to IV (non-disseminated) of the disease (Ho, 1970) were given skin tests prior to and two and six months after the completion of radiation therapy and thereafter at six-monthly intervals until 24 months or death, default or migration, which ever occurred earlier.

RESULTS

The results of the skin tests given prior to specific therapy in NPC and OC patients without clinical evidence of distant spread of disease (non-disseminated) are given in Table 1, and results for those

Table 1. Frequencies of positive[a] skin tests in nasopharyngeal carcinoma (NPC) and other cancer (OC) patients without clinical evidence of distant spread of the disease

Antigen	NPC No. (%)	OC No. (%)	Comparison
HKLY 28	55/86 (63.2)	1/18 (5.6)	$\chi^2 = 19.92$; $P = 0.000008$
Molt	4/74 (5.4)	1/18 (5.6)	NS
Raji	4/87 (4.6)	0/18	NS
F265	1/53 (1.9)	0/18	NS
NC37	1/58 (1.7)		
Trichophyton	69/74 (93.2)	17/18 (94.4)	NS
Candida albicans	61/68 (89.7)	12/12 (100)	NS
Streptokinase/ streptodornase	8/12 (66.7)	9/16 (56.3)	NS

[a] A reaction of ⩾ 5 mm induration, measured 43-45 hr after injection of an antigen

NS - not significant

with disseminated disease are shown in Table 2. It is evident from Table 1 that NPC patients had a significantly higher frequency of positive skin reactions to HKLY 28 extract than OC patients; no significant differences in the frequencies of positive reactions to the other antigens were observed between the two groups of patients.

The frequency of positive skin reactions to HKLY 28 extract in NPC patients appeared to be related to the stage of the disease (Fig. 1), in that it was low in those with stage I, high in those with stages II, III and IV and very low in those with stage V. The sharp fall in frequency in those with stage V (disseminated disease) might be due to a depression of CMI that is specific to antigens associated with HKLY 28, since there was no concomitant sharp fall in the frequency of positive skin reactions to the standard antigens (Tables 1 and 2).

For the 73 NPC patients initially included in the longitudinal study, data on only 35 are analysed in this preliminary report. These include 33 who were followed for at least 12 months and two who were followed for only six months, at which time they developed recurrence of their primary tumours. Of the cases followed for at least 12 months, 15 were excluded from the analysis because they had a persistently negative skin reaction to HKLY 28; their reactions to

Table 2. Frequencies of positive[a] skin tests in nasopharyngeal carcinoma (NPC) and other cancer (OC) patients with clinical evidence of distant spread of the disease

Antigen	NPC No. (%)	OC No. (%)
HKLY 28	1/18 (5.6)	1/6 (16.7)
Molt	0/18	0/6
Raji	0/18	0/6
F265	0/15	0/6
NC37	0/10	-
Trichophyton	12/18 (66.7)	4/6 (66.7)
Candida albicans	11/15 (73.3)	3/4 (75.0)
Streptokinase/ streptodornase	3/6 (50.0)	0/3

[a] A reaction of $\geqslant$ 5 mm induration, measured 43-45 hr after injection of an antigen

the antigens associated with the extract were thus so weak that their inclusion would only have introduced confusion into the interpretation of the data from patients who had a known capacity to react to the test material. The clinical evolution of nine of these persistently negative reactors was favourable, i.e., they showed no evidence of the disease during the period of observation following radiation therapy; in the other six, the clinical evolution was unfavourable; there was thus a sort of random distribution. Two other patients were excluded because they were last tested with a batch of extract with poor potency, which elicited negative reactions, although up to that time they had shown positive reactions. The poor potency of the extract was discovered when it was used simultaneously with another extract of known potency. We have not been able to re-test the two patients with a more potent extract.

Table 3 summarizes the association between clinical evolution and skin reactivity to HKLY 28 extract in 35 NPC patients with stages I - IV of the disease who showed a capacity to respond detectably to the test at least once, before or following radiation therapy. The four skin response patterns identified were as follows:

FIG. 1. POSITIVE SKIN REACTIONS

Frequencies of untreated nasopharyngeal carcinoma patients with positive skin reactions to crude membrane extract from HKLY 28 cells by stage of disease (as described by Ho, 1970).

Comparisons: I vs II-IV - $\chi^2 = 3.93$; $P = 0.047$
V vs II-IV - $\chi^2 = 21.88$; $P = 0.000003$
V vs I -IV - $\chi^2 = 19.92$; $P = 0.000008$
I vs V - not significant

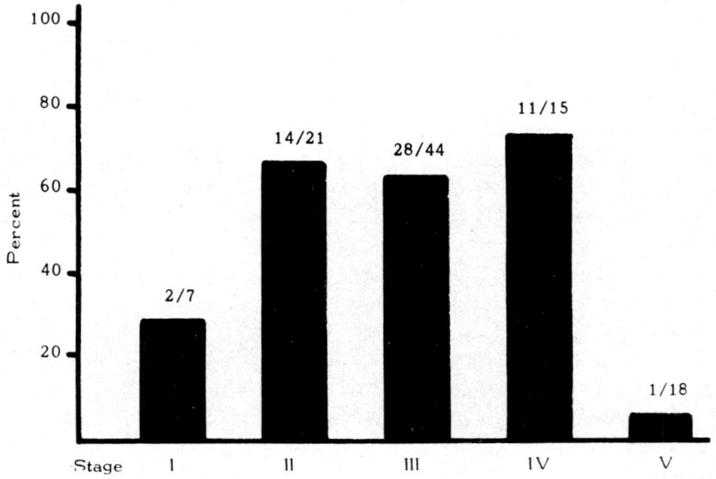

Table 3. Association between clinical evolution and skin reactivity to crude membrane extracts from HKLY 28 cells in patients with stages I-IV of nasopharyngeal carcinoma[a] before and following radiation therapy for 6-24 months

Reactivity	Clinical evolution (number of patients)		
	Favourable	Unfavourable	Total
(a) + becoming -	18	1	19
(b) persistently +	1	4	5
(c) + then fluctuated	2	3	5
(d) - then fluctuated	5	1	6
Total	26	9	35

[a] Ho, 1970

(a) positive becoming negative,
(b) persistently positive,
(c) positive with subsequent fluctuation, and
(d) negative with subsequent fluctuation.

Clinical evolution was found to have a significant association with all four skin response patterns ($P = 0.0016$); the association with patterns (a) and (b) was even more significant ($P = 0.00025$). Favourable clinical evolution was more frequently associated with (a) or (d) and unfavourable evolution with (b).

DISCUSSION

The present horizontal study was carried out in parallel with one by Levine et al. (1976) on 27 non-Chinese NPC patients, using the same antigens from the same source. All but one of the non-Chinese NPC patients studied by Levine et al. had received radiation therapy prior to, but none within one month of, skin testing, whereas the Chinese patients in the Hong Kong study were all tested before radiation therapy. However, the same percentage (63%) of patients in the two groups, both with apparently non-disseminated disease, showed positive skin reactions to the antigens derived from HKLY 28, a lymphoid cell line developed from a NPC biopsy obtained from a Hong Kong Chinese patient. The immediate effect of radiation therapy on skin reactivity to HKLY 28 is not known, but its immediate effect on CMI is one of depression; whatever its effect on the former, it appeared largely to have recovered within one month of the last treatment. The first post-radiation therapy skin testing was carried out in the Hong Kong patients at two months, to allow for CMI recovery and for the occurrence of major tumour regression.

Of the four EBV-associated cell lines used to prepare antigens for skin testing, HKLY 28 is the only one that is EBV-producing and the only one derived from an NPC biopsy. It is not clear, therefore, whether the much higher frequency of positive skin reactions to HKLY 28 extract, compared with the frequencies observed with the extracts from the other three cell lines, in NPC, and not in OC, patients is EBV- or NPC-associated or both. Further testing with extracts from non-EBV-producing cell lines derived from NPC and from EBV-producing cell lines from other sources, in place of Molt, F265 and NC37, is necessary for elucidation of this problem. It is also important that the reacting antigens in HKLY 28 be purified and characterized in order to determine their relationship to the skin reactions in NPC patients.

In the longitudinal study, four patterns of skin reactivity response to extracts from HKLY 28 were observed. Although clinical evolution of the disease was found to have a significant association with all four, and especially with three, of them, a significant number of patients showed a persistently negative response, from which no information with regard to prognosis could be obtained. As it stands, this test, using this particular HKLY 28 crude extract, appears to be of little practical value in monitoring the clinical evolution of NPC.

SUMMARY

Delayed hypersensitivity to antigens derived from four EBV-related (HKLY 28, Raji, F265 and NC37) and one EBV-unrelated (Molt) T-lymphoid cell lines and to standard antigens (*Trichophyton*, *Candida albicans* and streptokinase/streptodornase) was measured in 104 NPC patients and 24 patients with other cancers. Of the NPC patients with non-disseminated disease, 55/86 (63.2%) had a positive skin reaction to HKLY 28 extract, compared with only 1/18 (5.6%) OC patients with non-disseminated disease. The frequencies of these NPC patients with positive skin reactions to the other cell-line extracts were significantly lower (1.7-5.4%). From the preliminary results of a longitudinal study, skin testing with this particular crude membrane extract from HKLY 28 cells appears to be of little practical value in monitoring the clinical evolution of NPC, although a significant association between clinical evolution and certain patterns of skin reactivity response to the extract was found in about two-thirds of the cases analysed.

ACKNOWLEDGEMENTS

This work was supported by IARC/CRA and financed by Contract No. N01 CP 43296 with the National Cancer Institute, USA. Thanks are given to Mr C.M. Lam for statistical calculations, Mr R. Abesser for the figure, Mrs P. Liu for typing the manuscript and Mr K.W. Leung for photographic assistance.

REFERENCES

de-Thé, G., Ablashi, D.V., Liabeuf, A. & Mourali, N. (1973) Nasopharyngeal carcinoma (NPC). VI. Presence of an EBV nuclear antigen in fresh tumour biopsies: preliminary results. *Biomedicine, 19*, 349-352

Herberman, R.B., Char, D., Oldham, R., Levine, P., Leventhal, B.G., McCoy, J.L., Ho, J.H.C. & Chau, J.C.W. (1975) *Cell-mediated immunity in human acute leukemia.* In: Ito, Y. & Dutcher, R.M., eds, *VI International Symposium on Comparative Leukaemia Research, 1973, Leukemogenesis*, Basel, Karger, pp. 649-656

Ho, J.H.C. (1970) *The natural history and treatment of nasopharyngeal carcinoma.* In: Lee-Clark, R., Cumley, R.W., McCay, J.E. & Copeland, M., eds, *Proceedings of the X International Cancer Congress*, Vol. 4, Chicago, Yearbook Medical Publishers, pp. 1-14

Huang, D.P., Ho, H.C., Henle, W. & Henle, G. (1974) Demonstration of Epstein-Barr virus-associated nuclear antigen in nasopharyngeal carcinoma cells from fresh biopsies. *Int. J. Cancer, 14*, 580-588

Klein, G., Giovanella, B.C., Lindale, T., Kiaklow, P.J., Singh, S. & Stehlin, J.S. (1974) Direct evidence for the presence of Epstein-Barr virus DNA and nuclear antigen in malignant epithelial cells from patients with poorly differentiated carcinoma of the nasopharynx. *Proc. nat. Acad. Sci. (Wash.), 71*, 4737-4741

Levine, P.H., de-Thé, G.B., Brugère, J., Schwaab, G., Mourali, N., Herberman, R.B., Ambrosioni, J.C. & Revol, P. (1976) Immunity to antigens associated with a cell line derived from nasopharyngeal cancer (NPC) in non-Chinese patients. *Int. J. Cancer, 17*, 155-160

Oren, M.E. & Herberman, R.B. (1971) Delayed cutaneous hypersensitivity reactions to membrane extracts of human tumor cells. *Clin. exp. Immunol., 9*, 45-56

Wolf, H., zur Hausen, H. & Becker, V. (1973) EB viral genomes in epithelial nasopharyngeal carcinoma cells. *Nature (New Biol.), 244*, 245-247

CLINICAL EVALUATION OF CYTOLOGICAL DIAGNOSIS OF NASOPHARYNGEAL MALIGNANCIES

R. MOLINARI, S. PILOTTI & F. RILKE

Istituto Nazionale Tumori,
Via Venezian 1,
20133 Milan, Italy

INTRODUCTION

Early diagnosis of malignant nasopharyngeal tumours is one of the most difficult problems in head and neck oncology; most of these tumours become evident from lymph-node metastases. Anatomical, physiological and histopathological difficulties work together to make problematic both the symptomatology and histopathological confirmation of the tumour.

Various diagnostic techniques designed to overcome these problems have not proved effective in all cases: sectional radiography can only detect lesions that exceed a certain size or that produce bone alterations; the various tools elaborated to obtain a more reliable clinical view of the nasopharynx (soft palate retractors, transnasal and transoral photography and motion shots) often upset the patient, so that difficulties are sometimes increased rather than reduced.

On the other hand, early diagnosis of nasopharyngeal tumours should be an almost mandatory goal in view of the negative influence on prognosis of both local and regional progression of the lesion, as well as the marked radiosensitivity of most of these cancers.

In Europe, this problem is of relatively small dimensions, whereas it rises to a sociological level in some Asian regions in which nasopharyngeal cancers are the most frequent malignant tumours. Consequently, we decided to investigate simpler, quicker and at the same time more reliable techniques for early diagnosis and undertook a reevaluation of cytology in this respect.

In a previous paper, Rilke & Pilotti (1973) examined the histopathological aspect of the problem and described our first cumulative findings.

The present paper deals with a more accurate analysis of the results, mainly with regard to the reliability of cytology from the clinical point of view; finally, the results of combined cyto- and histological examinations are reported.

MATERIALS AND METHODS

Collecting method

Although the nasopharynx is accessible to the collection of material for cytological examination, few attempts have been made in the past to assess the usefulness of cytology in diagnosis (Djojopranoto, 1960; Hopp, 1958; Liang et al., 1962; Ma & Chen, 1958; Morrison et al., 1949); Ali & Shanmugaratnam (1967) concluded that cytology was of little interest in the diagnosis of nasopharyngeal cancer, in view of only 44% concordance between cytological and histopathological results. Nevertheless, an exhaustive analysis of the literature reveals discrepancies among the collecting methods used by different investigators.

Most introduced soft cotton flocks through the nose or, in some cases, obtained mucus by blowing the nose of the patient. Material obtained in this way contains a large amount of mucus and only a few cells, which, besides, do not derive from nasopharynx. Furthermore, cells withdrawn on a cotton flock introduced through the nose are derived from only a limited area of the nasopharyngeal walls.

We decided to use a more direct and extended approach to the nasopharynx, by introducing *via* the mouth an angled forceps holding a small rough pad of compressed gauze and by collecting throughout the entire cavity. The object of this method was to involve the whole mucosal surface and to execute, at least theoretically, a sort of squeezing of the intracryptic neoplastic cells.

The forceps are introduced under the soft palate directly into the nasopharynx, and the gauze is rubbed relatively energetically on the surface two or three times. The procedure is simple and easy, a little disturbing but almost painless for most patients; it takes only a few seconds, so that, after the first few attempts, we performed it without anaesthesia. A little bleeding frequently occurs but is never extensive; we considered the presence of some blood on the gauze mandatory for good collection.

Biopsy is performed immediately afterwards, using the same forceps without a pad, with the aid of an angled mirror when possible; in most cases the sample is taken in a blind fashion, on the basis of visual memory of prior posterior rhinoscopy.

Material for cytological examination is laid on two slides by multiple stipplings and fixed immediately with a spray fixative. More recently, the material has not been fixed but is stained by Papanicolaou's method and examined.

Case material

Between 1971 and the end of 1975, a consecutive series of 225 pairs of cytological and histological samples were taken, by the procedure described above, from the nasopharynxes of 216 patients. In 207 cases, the two samples were taken once; in nine patients (seven with carcinomas and two with lymphomas), biopsy or cytological examination or both were repeated in order to confirm or definitively exclude the presence of a nasopharyngeal tumour. In 16 patients, a lymph-node biopsy had previously been performed elsewhere, and consultation of the slides indicated a tumour of the nasopharynx. The other 200 patients were selected for combined examination according to the following criteria:

patients with macroscopically visible growths in the nasopharynx;

patients with clinical signs of nasal obstruction of a suspicious nature; and

patients with cervical adenopathies located in lymphatic regions of the neck related to the nasopharynx.

Subsequently, all of the patients were followed until a definitive diagnosis was established on the basis of various examinations, a cervical lymph-node biopsy or the clinical course of their illness. In particular, all of the patients with histology negative for the tumour were followed up for at least two years. The final diagnoses are summarized in Table 1.

Table 1. Definitive diagnoses of tumours in 216 patients seen at the Istituto Nazionale dei Tumori, 1971-1976

Diagnosis	No. of patients
Definite nasopharyngeal carcinoma	90
Definite nasopharyngeal lymphoma	24
Lymphoma in head or neck	12
Lymphoma at other sites	12
Nasopharyngeal tumours definitely excluded	78
Total	216

Among the 78 cases in which a nasopharyngeal tumour was excluded, six patients were considered theoretically capable of having one, since lymph-node metastases of squamous-cell cancer had previously been removed from the neck, although no primary tumour had been found in the head and neck area. None showed clinical signs of nasopharyngeal cancer, and both cytological and histological examinations were negative. Three of them underwent radical neck dissection: two are alive and well at present (after four and three years); the third died from recurrence of the neck malignancy. The remaining three patients were irradiated and died either from evolution of their neck malignancies or from distant metastases with no primary tumour having been detected. These patients were considered not to have nasopharyngeal malignancies.

In two additional cases, of malignant melanoma and adenoid cystic carcinoma, cytological and histological examinations were positive; however, these were not considered in the present study.

RESULTS

As far as technical problems are concerned, no complications occurred in the 216 patients; in particular, the bleeding observed at no time required tamponade or similar procedures. In three patients, very abnormal anatomical conditions made collection difficult; in two of these, both histological and cytological examinations were negative, and they were counted as failures of the method.

In the group of 78 patients in which a nasopharyngeal tumour was definitively excluded, all cytological examinations were negative; thus, no false-positive findings occurred.

Among malignant tumours, three main histological categories could be distinguished: lymphoma, squamous-cell carcinoma and undifferentiated carcinoma of the nasopharyngeal type. Table 2 shows the positive cytological and histological findings obtained for these three categories of tumours.

Table 2. Accuracy of cytological and histological diagnoses of nasopharyngeal tumours in 114 patients showing positive results, by histological type of tumour

Histological type	No. of cases	No. with positive cytology	(%)	No. with positive histology	(%)
Lymphoma	24	16	(66.6)	22	(91.7)
Squamous-cell carcinoma	15	11	(73.3)	13	(86.6)
Undifferentiated carcinoma	75	60	(80.0)	65	(86.6)
	114	87	(76.3)	100	(87.7)

As mentioned above, cytological or histological examinations or both were repeated in nine patients who showed negative responses. In four cases in which there was disagreement between cytological and histological findings, only the initially negative examination was repeated; the new findings were all positive. In five cases, both first results were negative; in two of them (one definitely cancer and one lymphoma), both cytological and histological findings were again negative, whereas in the remaining three patients the new samples showed positive results. The results presented in Table 1 and in this analysis, however, are taken only from the first pairs of examinations.

Lymphomas

Within the lymphoma group, only those cases with positive biopsies or cytological findings could be analysed. As shown in Table 1, in 24 cases a nasopharyngeal localization was indisputable; however, since lymphoma is a potentially diffuse illness which can involve all of the lymphoreticular tissues, another 24 cases (12 of the head and neck area other than the nasopharynx and 12 of other locations in the body) could theoretically have had microscopic nasopharyngeal involvement, in spite of negative clinical, histological and cytological findings.

Despite these limitations, the results presented in Table 3 should still be valid. In this table the results of cytological and histological examinations are correlated with the degree of suspicion at clinical examination by rhinoscopy and X-ray study. Cytological findings were positive in 66.6% and histological findings in 91.7%; however, because of the above-mentioned reasons, analysis should be limited to the suspicious or obvious cases, so that 75% (15/20) of positivity can be considered to be a more reliable value for cytological findings.

Table 3. Correlation of suspicion of lymphoma at clinical examination with positivity of cytological and histological findings in 24 cases of confirmed nasopharyngeal lymphoma

Clinical suspicion	No. of cases	No. with positive cytology	(%)	No. with positive histology	(%)
Negative	1	1	(25)	1	(100)
Doubtful	3	0		3	
Suspicious	6	4	(66.6)	5	(83.3)
Definite	14	11	(78.6)	13	(93.0)
Total	24	16	(66.6)	22	(91.7)

Carcinomas

Among the 90 patients with confirmed nasopharyngeal carcinomas (Table 4), cytological findings were positive in 70 cases (78%) and histological findings positive in 78 (86.6%); a combination of both

Table 4. Correlation of suspicion of carcinoma at clinical examination with positivity of cytological and histological findings in 90 cases of confirmed nasopharyngeal carcinoma

Clinical suspicion	No. of cases	No. with positive cytology	(%)	No. with positive histology	(%)	No. with positive combination	(%)
Negative	6	3	(50)	5	(83)	5	(83)
Doubtful	14	9	(64.3)	12	(85.7)	13	(93)
Suspicious	18	14	(77.8)	16	(88.9)	18	(100)
Definite	52	44	(84.6)	45	(86.5)	49	(94.2)
Total	90	70	(77.8)	78	(86.6)	85	(94.4)

methods allowed confirmation of the diagnosis in 85 of 90 patients (94.4%). Histological findings appeared to be independent of the size of the nasopharyngeal tumour, as evaluated by means of posterior rhinoscopy and X-ray study, while positivity of cytological results correlated with the degree of clinical suspicion, ranging from 50% to 84.6%.

As shown in Table 5, complete concordance between positive cytological and histological results was found in 70% of cases; false negative cytological findings occurred in 16.6%, but histological findings were also erroneously negative in 7.8% of patients. In only 5.5% of cases were both diagnostic procedures negative; in this small group we found three cases with evident, bulky tumours which had an important necrotic component.

Table 5. Correlation of cytological and histological findings in 90 confirmed cases of nasopharyngeal carcinoma with degree of clinical suspicion

Clinical suspicion	No. of cases	No. with cytology + histology +	(%)	No. with cytology + histology -	(%)	No. with cytology - histology +	(%)	No. with cytology - histology -	(%)
Negative	6	3	(50)	0	(0)	2	(33)	1	(16.5)
Doubtful	14	8	(57.1)	1	(7.1)	4	(28.3)	1	(7.1)
Suspicious	18	12	(66.6)	2	(11.1)	4	(22.2)	0	(0)
Definite	52	40	(76.9)	4	(7.7)	5	(9.6)	3	(5.8)
Total	90	63	(70)	7	(7.8)	15	(16.6)	5	(5.5)

Table 6 shows the correlation of positivity of cytological or histological findings, or a combination of both, in the group of undifferentiated carcinomas with clinical suspicion of the extent of the tumour. In comparison with the findings shown in Table 4, cytology appears to be a slightly more reliable diagnostic tool for this group of cancers than for the rest of the series. This fact is even more evident in Table 7, in which the three histological types of malignancies are compared.

Table 6. Correlation of cytological and histological findings in 75 confirmed cases of undifferentiated carcinoma with degree of clinical suspicion

Clinical suspicion	No. of patients	No. with positive cytology	(%)	No. with positive histology	(%)	No. with positive combination	(%)
Negative	5	3	(60)	5	(100)	5	(100)
Doubtful	12	8	(66.6)	10	(83.3)	11	(91.6)
Suspicious	16	13	(81.2)	14	(87.5)	16	(100)
Definite	42	36	(85.7)	36	(85.7)	40	(95.2)
Total	75	60	(78.7)	65	(86.6)	72	(96)

Table 7. Correlation of positivity of cytological findings in three histological types of nasopharyngeal tumour with degree of clinical suspicion

Clinical suspicion	Lymphoma		Squamous-cell carcinoma		Undifferentiated carcinoma	
	No. of cases (%)	No. with positive cytology (%)	No. of cases (%)	No. with positive cytology (%)	No. of cases (%)	No. with positive cytology (%)
Negative or doubtful	4 (16.6)	1 (25)	2 (13.3)	0 (0)	17 (22.6)	11 (64.7)
Suspicious or definite	20 (83.4)	15 (75)	13 (86.6)	11 (84.6)	58 (77.4)	49 (84.5)
Total	24	16 (66.6)	15	11 (73.3)	75	60 (80)

DISCUSSION

In spite of the findings reported in the literature, cytology appears to offer a consistent aid to the diagnosis of malignant nasopharyngeal tumours.

A first encouraging finding was the absence of false-positive results in the series of cases in which a malignancy was undoubtedly excluded. A certain number of tumours (25%) could not be detected by cytology, false-negative results varying according to histological type (1/3 lymphomas, 1/4 squamous-cell carcinomas and 1/5 undifferentiated carcinomas).

On the other hand, histology does not always provide positive correlation; accuracy was 87.7% (91% for lymphomas and 86.6% for carcinomas). Thus, instead of calculating the percentage of positivity of cytological findings on the basis of the whole series of cases, we think it more reasonable to do so only on the basis of cases with positive histological findings; this would give us a more correct measure of the usefulness of cytology in this respect. By doing this, many confounding factors, such as the actual incidence of lymphomas, the presence of abundant necrotic tissue on the surface of the tumour and patient-related conditions (anatomy, cooperation), could be taken into account for both procedures. When this is done, the values for correlation of cytology presented in Table 7 are modified as follows: 72.7% in lymphoma, 84.6% in squamous-cell carcinoma and 92.3% in undifferentiated carcinoma.

The latter type of tumour appears to show the highest and most significant values, probably because of its extensive vascularization and rich cell population.

Correctness of clinical diagnosis of the tumours in this series varied according to histological type. Clinically evident cases strongly predominate in the group of squamous-cell carcinomas (13/15); this is logical, since these tumours show a later spreading and a slower local growth and are consequently generally diagnosed on the basis of symptoms due more to the primary tumour than to neck metastases. Early diagnoses are thus very rare, and, with the most limited tumours, both cytological and histological findings are nearly always negative.

The composition of degree of clinical suspicion is quite different in the group of lymphomas, with 4.2% positive cytological findings for negative clinical diagnoses, 12.5% for doubtful, 25% for suspicious and 58.3% for definite.

For the group of undifferentiated carcinomas, the frequency of occurrence of more limited tumours is slightly greater than for the other two histological types (22.6% *versus* 16.6% and 13.3%, respectively). It is evident that a correct cytological diagnosis can be made more frequently for this last group of tumours (80%) and that such a diagnosis can be made at an early stage in a high percentage of cases (65%), as shown in Table 7.

As far as general clinical application of cytology is concerned, there are two main possibilities, its use:

(1) as a complementary examination with histology, in order to confirm microscopically the existence of a malignant tumour in the nasopharynx in patients with neoplastic symptoms such as a metastatic cervical lymph node: and

(2) as an early diagnostic means, to be used in mass screening of a general population.

In the first case, the absence of false-positive results makes combined cyto-histological findings of great value. Systematic use of this double diagnostic modality provides microscopic verification of 96% of undifferentiated carcinomas (with no wide variation, depending on the extent of the tumour), of 86.6% of squamous-cell carcinomas (with a high significance for extensive tumours but very rarely for limited ones) and of 95% of lymphomas (with the same frequency in the various stages of tumour spread, even considering the statistical limits due to preselection of cases).

A judgement of the use of cytology as a means of mass screening for nasopharyngeal cancers can be made on the basis of these findings: the frequency of positive diagnoses and the absence of false positive results seems to justify its use as an effective diagnostic tool in every stage (even the early ones) of undifferentiated carcinoma. For squamous-cell carcinomas, its use appears to be effective only for the most extensive tumours. The problem of its use, therefore, involves mainly the relative incidence of these two types of tumours in any population under consideration. A review of the literature shows a large variability in this connection, since, in the large number of reports published before the era when nasopharyngeal carcinoma was recognized as such, diagnoses such as 'epidermoid carcinoma' or 'squamous carcinoma' ranged from 15% to 80%. There is no evidence whether these depend on an actual variability in geographical distribution, and consequently on epidemiological factors, or on lack of agreement among pathologists about the criteria for classifying nasopharyngeal tumours.

In view of a study carried out at our institute, which shows that the various histological types have very different natural histories, agreement on the criteria for histological classification is highly desirable.

In our opinion the present collected findings justify a wider study of the effectiveness of cytology using a large population, such as in a mass screening. This is hardly possible in Europe, where nasopharyngeal cancer is rare; we therefore suggest that such an evaluation be organized in south-east Asian countries where these malignancies give shape to a true sociological problem.

SUMMARY

Between 1970 and 1975 cytological examination was applied to the diagnosis of nasopharyngeal malignancies in a series of 216 consecutive patients who had either a tumour in the nasopharynx or clinical signs of nasopharyngeal carcinoma, or who were locally asymptomatic but had enlarged cervical lymph nodes.

Smears were taken by introducing a small rough pad of compressed gauze through the mouth into the nasopharynx with an upward-angled forceps. In each case the cytological smear was taken immediately before biopsy; often, a lymph node was removed subsequently.

When morphological diagnoses were doubtful and histological findings were at variance with positive cytological findings, the patients were reexamined clinically, and diagnosis was postponed.

The case material was made up of 90 nasopharyngeal carcinomas, 24 lymphomas, one malignant melanoma, one adenoid cystic carcinoma and 100 patients without malignancies.

Cytological findings from the first smear were positive in 77.8% of nasopharyngeal carcinomas, in 66.6% of lymphomas and in the cases of melanoma and adenoid cystic carcinoma. There were no false-positive results. When the nasopharyngeal carcinomas were subdivided into undifferentiated carcinomas of the nasopharyngeal type and squamous-cell carcinomas, cytological findings were positive in 80% and 73%, respectively.

Positivity of histological findings was distributed as follows: 91.7% for malignant lymphomas, 86.6% for undifferentiated carcinomas and 86.6% for squamous-cell carcinomas.

With respect to clinical suspicion of malignancy, positive cytological findings were obtained in 50% of clinically occult cases and in 84.6% of patients with obvious malignancies; intermediate figures were found for clinically doubtful (64.3%) and for highly suspicious (77.8%) cases. Cyto-histological concordance was shown in 70% of cases; false-negative histological results were obtained in 7.8% and false-negative cytological results in 16.6% of cases.

Combined cyto-histological positive results allowed diagnostic accuracy from the first samples in 94.4% of cases. Undifferentiated carcinoma appeared to be the malignancy most accessible to cytological diagnosis, with positive results ranging from 65% in clinically negative or doubtful cases to 84.5% in those with obvious tumours.

Assessment of the cytology of the nasopharynx, using the new sampling method described herein, may be a useful diagnostic tool in nasopharyngeal malignancies.

REFERENCES

Ali, M.Y. & Shanmugaratnam, K. (1967) Cytodiagnosis of nasopharyngeal carcinoma. *Acta cytol., 11*, 54-60

Djojopranoto, M. (1960) [Incidence and pathology of nasopharyngeal tumors] *Doctoral thesis*, Airlangga Di Surabaja University, Java, Indonesia

Hopp, E.S. (1958) Cytologic diagnosis and prognosis in carcinoma of the mouth, pharynx and nasopharynx. *Laryngoscope, 68*, 1281-1287

Liang, P.-C., Ch'En, C.C., Chu, C.C., Hu, Y.F., Chu, H.M. & Tsung, Y.S. (1962) The histological classification, biological characteristics and histogenesis of nasopharyngeal carcinoma. *Chin. med. J., 81*, 629-658

Ma, S.S. & Chen, L.H. (1958) Cytology in diagnosis of nasopharyngeal carcinoma. *Mem. Coll. Med. nat. Taiwan Univ., 5*, 1-14

Morrison, L.F., Hopp, E.S. & Wu, R. (1949) Diagnosis of malignancies of the nasopharynx: cytological studies by the smear technic. *Ann. Otolaryngol., 58*, 18-32

Rilke, F. & Pilotti, S. (1973) Die zytologische Diagnose der Epipharynxkarzinome. *Verh. Dtsch. Ges. Path, 57*, 373-377

EUROPEAN ORGANIZATION FOR RESEARCH ON TREATMENT OF CANCER (E.O.R.T.C.) CONTROLLED TRIALS OF CHEMOTHERAPY AS AN ADJUVANT OR PALLIATIVE TREATMENT OF NASOPHARYNGEAL CARCINOMA

R. MOLINARI[1]

Istituto Nazionale Tumori,
Via Venezian 1,
20133 Milan, Italy

Nasopharyngeal carcinomas (NPC) are usually treated by radiotherapy at all stages, and, considering that they are localized in a hidden region, their local and regional extent at time of diagnosis and the depth of the anatomical site to be treated, the results of such treatment are unexpectedly good: overall survival after five years is 40-45% (70% in T1-2 NO cases) (Brugère et al., 1974; Zucali, 1974). This rate is much higher than that for tumours that are usually treated earlier and more easily, such as oral, oropharyngeal and hypopharyngeal cancers, and this is due to the fact that NPCs are more radiosensitive and progress more slowly.

Nevertheless, the frequency of distant metastasis, isolated or mediated by neck recurrences, is very high, approaching 44% in all cases (Table 1). In addition, it must be borne in mind that 55-60% of NPC patients die because radiotherapy cannot control local or distant progress of the illness.

We therefore decided to add another form of therapy to radiotherapy. The choice was between chemotherapy and immunotherapy or a combination of both; however, since results obtained in the latter field are still debatable, we decided to try chemotherapy and proposed a therapeutic trial to the Head and Neck Group of the E.O.R.T.C.

---

[1] President-in-charge, Head and Neck Cooperative Group of the EORTC - a collective proposal

Table 1. Cause of death in 159 patients with nasopharyngeal cancers

	At risk No.	Died from cancer No.	%	T, N or T + N No.	%	M No.	M + N + T No.	Total M No.	%
Squamous-cell carcinoma	21	18	85.7	16/18	88.9	0	2	2/18	11.1
Undifferentiated carcinoma	138	86	62.3	42/86	48.8	24	20	44/86	51.1
Total	159	104	65.4	58/104	55.8	24	22	46/104	44.2

T - tumour; N - lymph-node involvement; M - metastasis

The basis of the trial was a retrospective study carried out at the Istituto Nazionale Tumori, Milan. A series of drugs were tested in the treatment of advanced NPCs, and the results were evaluated in terms of frequency and extent of regressions achieved. The drugs shown to be most active in this study were adriamycin, cyclophosphamide, bleomycin and methotrexate, which produced 39%, 31%, 28% and 17% regression, respectively. Each drug was used alone; however, recently they have been administered in various combinations, although the results of these tests are not yet available. Radiotherapy modalities (fields and doses) for the trials were standardized at that time.

The most difficult problem arose from the fact that the pathologists did not agree initially with our proposed classification, based on the wide difference we had noted in survival between patients with undifferentiated carcinomas and those with squamous-cell cancers (Fig. 1). The Head and Neck Cooperative Group therefore appointed a Pathologists' Study Group to set up a histological classification, which was accepted by all participants.

A second problem arose from the fact that nasopharyngeal or cervical recurrences can sometimes be re-treated by radiotherapy or surgery. We had therefore to take into consideration not only whether or not to leave these patients in the trial after new local therapy, but also what type of treatment was to be used in case of relapse.

GENERAL AIM OF THE TRIAL

The general aim of the proposed trial is to evaluate the usefulness of chemotherapy in all stages of NPC.

Since there are not many patients with NPC in Europe, it was considered advisable to use the clinical material as rationally and exhaustively as possible, in order to evaluate at the time and in the

FIG. 1. ACTUARIAL SURVIVAL CURVES OF NASOPHARYNGEAL CANCER PATIENTS (according to histological type) ◆———◆ undifferentiated cancer (138 cases) ■———■ squamous cancer (21 cases)

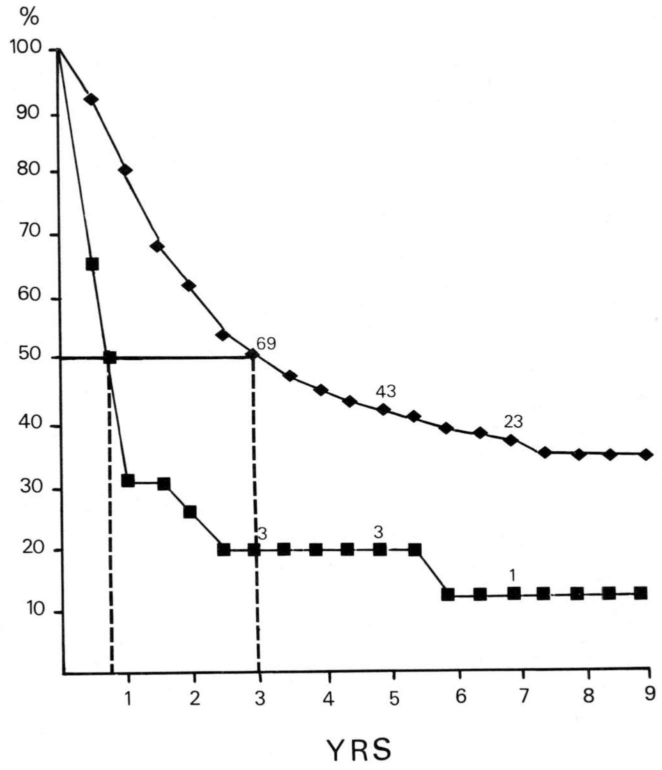

same series the effectiveness of long-term prophylactic chemotherapy after radiotherapy and also the palliative effects of aggressive chemotherapy on local or regional recurrences and on general diffusion of the illness. Consequently, two controlled trials are foreseen:

NPC 1 trial (long term chemotherapy): to evaluate in a randomized series the effectiveness of long-term chemotherapy (cyclophosphamide) in preventing or delaying general diffusion and local or regional recurrences after radiotherapy.

NPC 2 trial (aggressive chemotherapy): to test successive schemes of palliative chemotherapy in patients with advanced NPC (distant metastases or regional and/or local not otherwise treatable recurrences).

Different drugs and regimens will be compared, two by two, in order to select schemes of chemotherapy to be employed in long-term treatment, as alternatives to cyclophosphamide, in possible new trials after completion of NPC 1 trial.

GENERAL DESIGN OF THE TRIALS

Every patient with a malignant nasopharyngeal tumour observed at the cooperating centres is to be recorded on a special form. All of those with NPCs will be eligible for both trials; those with malignancies other than carcinomas are to be excluded. The general design is outlined in Scheme 1. Classification of tumours is based on the TNM system (UICC, 1974).

SCHEME 1. GENERAL DESIGN OF THE TRIALS

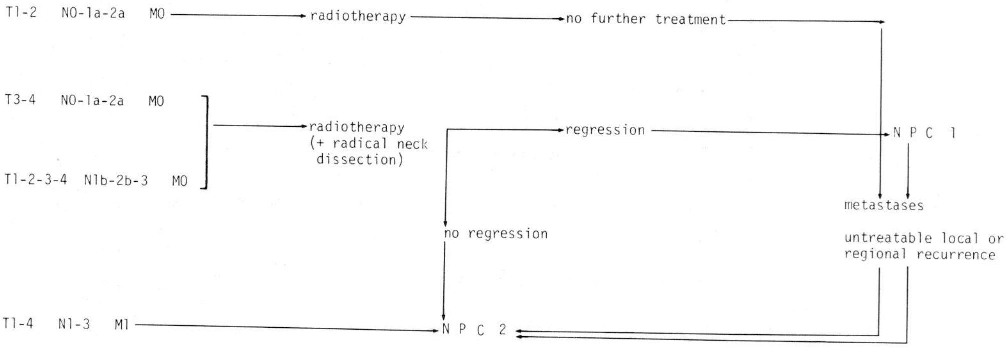

All cases classified as T1-2 NO-1a-2a MO are to be treated by radiotherapy alone. All patients classified as T3-4 NO MO and T1-2-3-4 N1b-2b-3 will be eligible for the NPC 1 trial. Those entering the NPC 2 trial will be: patients with distant metastases (M1) when first seen; patients presenting distant metastases or/and not otherwise treatable local or regional recurrences during the course of the NPC 1 trial; and patients classified as T1-2 NO-1a-2a MO (not included in NPC 1) presenting distant metastases and/or not otherwise treatable local or regional recurrences.

Number of patients required

On the basis of previous statistical evaluations, 50 patients must be entered into each arm of the NPC 1 trial in order to detect a significant difference between the two treatment groups. Since it is foreseen that 30 patients per year will enter this trial, the required duration of patient entry will be approximately 3.3 years.

For the NPC 2 trial, the inclusion of 50 patients in each arm of the trial, followed until death, will be sufficient to detect a ratio of 1.65:1 in the median (or mean) duration of survival (assumed exponential) for the two treatment groups.

Histopathological classification

The Pathologists' Study Group appointed by the Head and Neck Cooperative Group has proposed a classification that is correlated with the natural history of the different types of NPC, as follows:

- Carcinoma
  - undifferentiated carcinoma of the nasopharyngeal type
    - solid type
    - Schminke's type
    - Regaud's type
    - sclerosing type
  - squamous-cell carcinoma
    - well-differentiated
    - moderately-differentiated
    - poorly-differentiated
  - adenocarcinoma
    - adenoid cystic carcinoma
    - miscellaneous
  - malignant mucoepidermoid carcinoma
  - unclassifiable carcinoma
- Malignant lymphoma
- Other malignant tumour
- Unclassifiable malignant tumour
- Metastatic tumour

Since this classification is an unusual one, the study group decided to review all of the NPC slides, by circulating them after inclusion of the patients in the trials.

Initial radiation therapy

Radiotherapy must be delivered using high energy sources (Co^{60}, linear accelerator, etc.). Irradiation fields must include the nasopharynx, the base of the skull and bilateral cervical lymph nodes, including the mastoid, spinal and supraclavicular chains. The base of the skull must be irradiated even if radiological examination is negative for bone involvement.

Radiation to the primary tumour and clinically positive cervical nodes must reach a total dose of 6,000-7,000 rads. The following schedule is proposed: 7,000 rads over seven weeks; 6,500 rads over six weeks; and 6,000 rads over five weeks (in NSD equivalents), taking into account the R.E.T.

Clinically negative lymph nodes must receive a minimum of 5,000 rads, whereby the upper nodes will obviously receive approximately the same dose as the primary tumour.

NPC 1 TRIAL - LONG-TERM CHEMOTHERAPY

Cyclophosphamide is the drug of choice. It will be administered as a single dose of 1.2 g/m^2 intravenously every three weeks for 10 cycles. Chemotherapy will start six weeks after completion of radiation therapy, or, if radical neck dissection is planned, 15 days after this operation.

Design of the trial (Scheme 2)

All of the patients accepted for the NPC 1 trial will be examined six weeks after completion of radiotherapy, and the results will be evaluated. Patients with complete regression of T and N will be directly randomized with regard to adjuvant chemotherapy. Patients with complete regression of T and incomplete regression of N will be divided into two categories:

(1) If possible, radical neck dissection will be performed, and these patients will then be randomized for the NPC 1 trial.

(2) If further treatment of N is not feasible or is locally incomplete, they will be randomized for the NPC 2 trial.

Patients with no or incomplete regression of T and N will be randomized for the NPC 2 trial.

All of the patients assigned to the NPC 1 trial will be randomized, the choice being between chemotherapy, with cyclophosphamide given at the dose of 1.2 g/m^2 intravenously every three weeks for 10 cycles, and no further treatment.

Local/regional relapse and conditions for treatment

If a local recurrence of the primary tumour occurs during long-term chemotherapy or during follow-up, a new local treatment with

SCHEME 2. DESIGN OF NPC 1 TRIAL

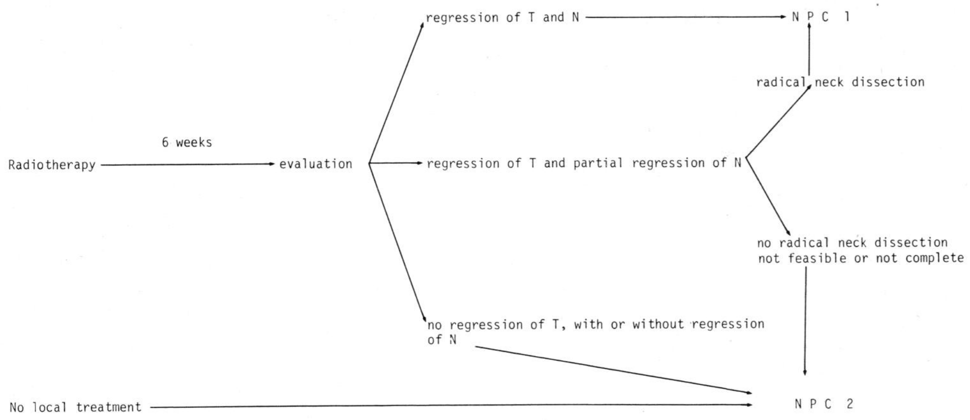

radiotherapy is to be considered, taking into account the initial dose of radiation and the interval between radiotherapy and recurrence. When possible, a new course of radiotherapy or a radical neck dissection will be performed with curative purpose and the patient left in the trial. If treatment is not feasible or is unsuccessful, the patient will be included in the NPC 2 trial.

Criteria for evaluation and end-point of the trial (Scheme 3)

The main criterion for evaluation of therapy is the appearance of distant metastases. A second will be the interval between radiotherapy and relapse, and the five-year survival rate will constitute a final one.

NPC 2 TRIAL - TREATMENT MODALITY

A comparison will be made between the effects of monochemotherapy (adriamycin alone) and polychemotherapy (adriamycin + vinblastine + bleomycin). Patients will be randomized and will undergo two different types of treatment:

(1) Adriamycin, at a dose of 75 mg/m^2 intravenously every four weeks, or

SCHEME 3. DEVELOPMENT OF NPC 1 TRIAL

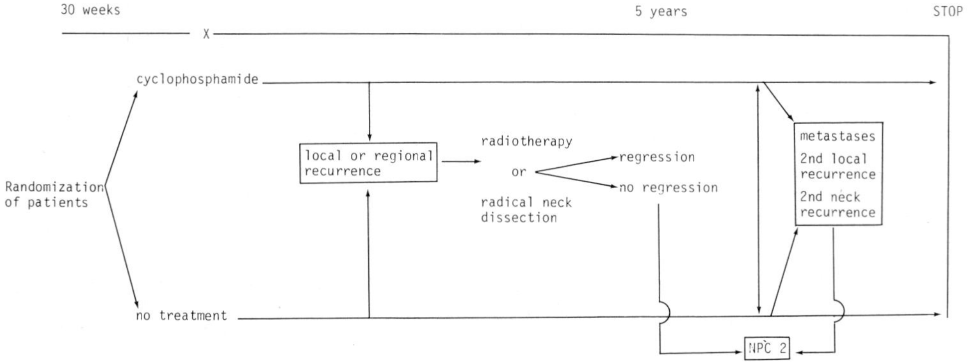

(2) Adriamycin, 30 mg/m^2, vinblastine, 6 mg/m^2 and bleomycin, 15 mg/m^2 intravenously every three weeks.

The total dose of adriamycin must not exceed 550 mg/m^2 and that of bleomycin, 250 mg/m^2. If initial signs of cardiac toxicity (adriamycin) or pulmonary fibrosis (bleomycin) occur, administration of the drug will be interrupted and the patient removed from the trial.

Collateral treatment may be needed. For instance, in the case of critical metastases in bones (vertebrae, mediastinum, etc.) or nodes, radiotherapy will be considered a valid treatment. In the case of a sole critical localization, the patient will not be included in the trial.

Design and development of the trial (Scheme 4)

All of the patients accepted for the trial will be divided into two categories (stratification): those previously entered into the NPC 1 trial and those not previously entered into the NPC 1 trial. After stratification, the patients will be randomized for the two regimens described above.

If the treatment achieves a positive response and is well tolerated, it will be continued until maximum prudent doses are achieved. At this point, chemotherapy will be interrupted and the patient followed until signs of progression appear.

SCHEME 4. DEVELOPMENT OF NPC 2 TRIAL

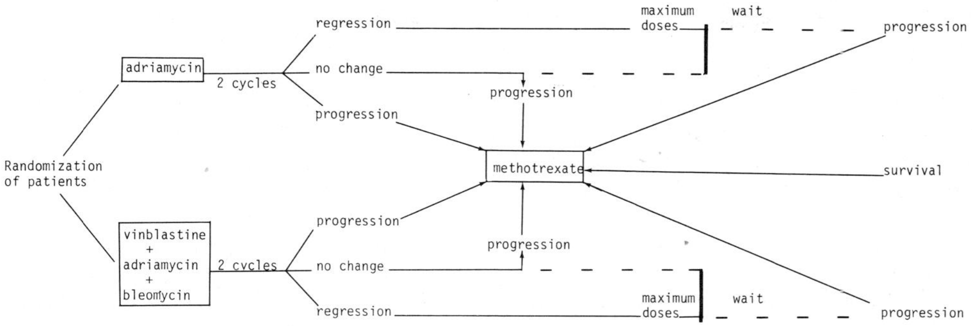

If progression occurs during the trial, treatment will be interrupted and the patient removed from the trial.

Criteria of evaluation and end-point of the trial

Regression of any measurable lesion and the duration of this regression are the main criteria for evaluating the trial; two cycles of chemotherapy are generally enough to judge the effectiveness of a treatment. Length of survival is another important criterion, provided that every patient receives the same treatment during follow-up after progression. Different responses can be expected with different localizations of relapse, and these can be considered to be collateral criteria for evaluation.

COMMENT

We expect to obtain a great deal of collateral information from this trial. Firstly, we plan to study the immunological status of the patient before and after chemotherapy. Secondly, forms have been designed to collect data regarding histological and clinical classification, taking into account histological variants of the primary tumour and number, size and level of enlarged lymph-nodes.

Finally, the trial will provide the opportunity of increasing knowledge about the epidemiology of NPC in Europe and, in cooperation with Dr de-Thé and the IARC, of studying particular immunological aspects, such as Epstein-Barr virus and specific tumour antigens.

SUMMARY

The E.O.R.T.C. Head and Neck Cooperative Group has designed a relatively complex international programme for a multidisciplinary approach to the treatment of NPC. The aim of the programme is to evaluate the usefulness of chemotherapy in preventing metastases and recurrences and, at the same time, to test other chemotherapeutic regimens and to compare them subsequently with the first one. Two contemporaneous controlled trials are foreseen: (1) long-term chemotherapy after radiotherapy for T3-4 N0 and T1-4 N1-3 M0 cases (NPC 1) and (2) aggressive chemotherapy for M1 cases and for patients who develop local or regional recurrences during the first trial (NPC 2). A search of the literature and a pilot study carried out at the Istituto Nazionale dei Tumori in Milan on advanced cases of NPC showed the following percentages of regression after various kinds of chemotherapy: cyclophosphamide, 38%; adriamycin, 39%; bleomycin, 28%; and methtrexate, 17%. On this basis, the following regimens were chosen:

NPC 1 trial: cyclophosphamide (1.2 g/m^2 every three weeks for 10 cycles) and a control group receiving no chemotherapy

NPC 2 trial: adriamycin alone *versus* a combination of vinblastine + bleomycin + adriamycin.

The programme was begun a short time ago, and no results are yet available.

REFERENCES

Brugère, J., Schlienger, M. & Cachin, Y. (1974) Les carcinomes du rhinopharynx de l'adulte: particularités cliniques et évolutives, traitement et résultats. *Cah. ORL*, *8*, 859-881

UICC (1974) *TNM Classification of Malignant Tumours*, 2nd ed., Geneva

Zucali, R. (1974) Histoire clinique, traitement et évolution des cancers du rhinopharynx. *Cah. ORL*, *8*, 839-848

USE OF IMMUNOLOGICAL STUDIES IN EVALUATING THE CLINICAL COURSE OF NASOPHARYNGEAL CARCINOMA

S. SAWAKI

Department of Otolaryngology,
Yokohama City University,
School of Medicine,
Yokohama 232, Japan

A. KAWAMURA, Jr

Department of Immunology,
Institute of Medical Science,
University of Tokyo,
Tokyo 108, Japan

T. TACHIBANA

Department of Immunology,
Research Institute for Tuberculosis, Leprosy and Cancer,
Tohoku University,
Sendai 980, Japan

INTRODUCTION

The prognosis of nasopharyngeal carcinoma (NPC) is very poor; therapeutic results vary, but the average five-year survival rate is about 30%. Cause of death is either distant metastasis or intracranial involvement.

At present, there is no absolute index which can project the result of treatment. Staging, as outlined in the TNM classification, has been regarded as an index of prognosis in that very advanced cases are considered to be incurable; and other factors, such as histological characteristics and anti-Epstein-Barr viral capsid antigen (VCA) antibody titres, have been advocated in this respect (Lynn et al., 1973a). It has been reported at this Symposium that the immune response of the peripheral lymphocytes has an influence on the clinical course of carcinoma cases (Chan et al.[1]).

The peripheral lymphocytes of 27 patients with NPC were examined from this point of view, and the results were compared with those using other indices.

MATERIALS AND METHODS

The case material consisted of 27 patients with NPC who had been treated at our clinic between 1973 and 1974. The age at first hospital visit varied between 12 and 78 years, but most were aged between 60 and 70 years. Twenty-one of the patients were males, and six, females.

All patients were treated with Linac X-ray irradiation, at differing doses. Generally, however, 7 000 rads were applied both to the region of the primary tumour and to metastases in the neck.

T cell and B cell peripheral lymphocytes were measured by Tachibana's plate method (Sawaki et al., 1975). Reduction of monocytes was not performed, however, and the two cell types were measured as erythrocyte rosette-forming cells (ERFC), corresponding to T cells, and complement receptor cells (CRC), corresponding to B cells. These were determined before, during and after radiation treatment.

RESULTS

The proportions of ERFC and CRC observed in a healthy control subject over a period of nearly a year were relatively constant (Fig. 1), indicating that our results are reliable.

Cases were divided into three types according to variations in the two subpopulations of peripheral lymphocytes. In type I cases, the CRC rate was constantly low throughout the course of the disease. The pattern was similar to that of the healthy control (Fig. 2).

In Type II cases, the level of CRC fluctuated with time (Fig. 3), and the clinical findings were complex. Although the primary tumour seemed to disappear with treatment, it recurred in lymph nodes or in distant organs. This metastatic growth can be controlled well by irradiation, but recurrences are frequent, and such patients always die as a result.

---

[1] See p. 495

FIG. 1. LEVELS OF ERYTHROCYTE ROSETTE-FORMING CELLS (ERFC) AND COMPLEMENT RECEPTOR CELLS (CRC) IN A HEALTHY CONTROL SUBJECT WITH TIME

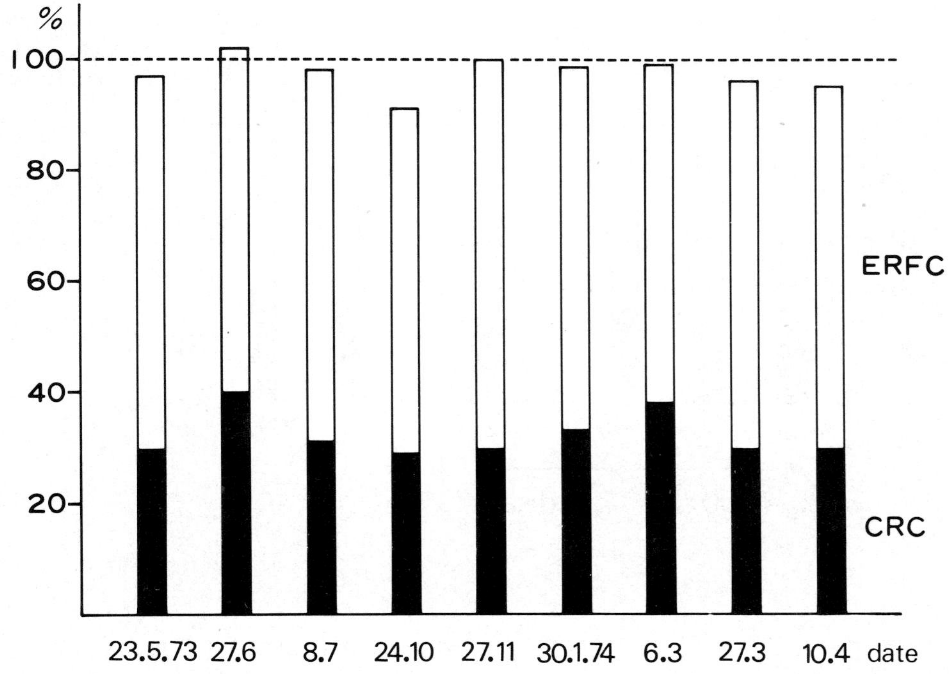

Inevitably, the clinical course of this type is long.

In Type III cases the CRC levels are constantly high, from the early stages of the disease (Fig. 4). The clinical course is unpredictable, and distant metastases appear suddenly: in the case shown in Figure 4, the tumour metastasized into the humerus only four months after initial treatment. The clinical course was thus extremely short, and the patient died from general weakness.

The prognoses of patients with the three types of immune responses are shown in Table 1. Those for patients with Type I responses were good, but those for the other two types were poor.

FIG. 2. LEVELS OF ERYTHROCYTE ROSETTE-FORMING CELLS (ERFC) AND COMPLEMENT RECEPTOR CELLS (CRC) WITH TIME IN A TYPE I CASE

A 78-year old female complaining of a 'full' sensation in the ear, found to have a T1 N1 M0 nasopharyngeal carcinoma in the superior position, diagnosed histologically as a squamous-cell carcinoma, alive and without a tumour in January 1977

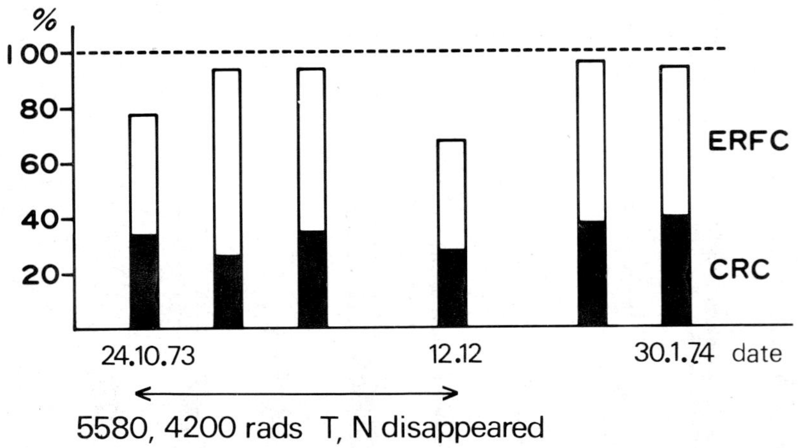

FIG. 3. LEVELS OF ERYTHROCYTE ROSETTE-FORMING CELLS (ERFC) AND COMPLEMENT RECEPTOR CELLS (CRC) WITH TIME IN A TYPE II CASE

A 12-year old male complaining of a neck swelling, found to have a T2 N2 M0 nasopharyngeal carcinoma in the superior position, diagnosed histologically as an undifferentiated squamous-cell carcinoma, died January 1977, five years after first visit

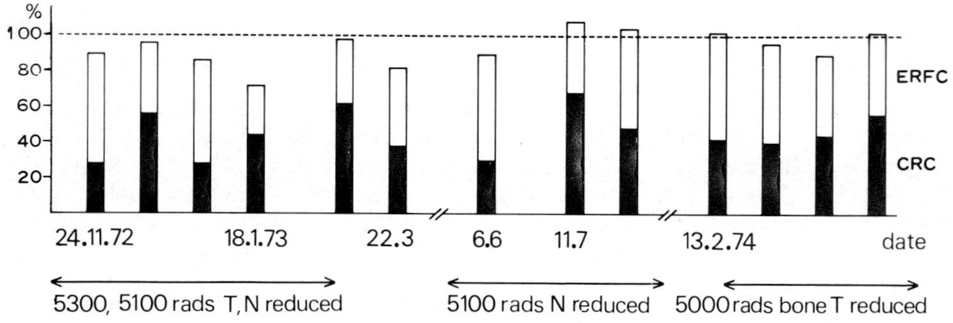

FIG. 4. LEVELS OF ERYTHROCYTE ROSETTE-FORMING CELLS (ERFC) AND COMPLEMENT RECEPTOR CELLS (CRC) WITH TIME IN A TYPE III CASE

A 22-year old male complaining of a neck swelling, found to have a T2 N2 M0 nasopharyngeal carcinoma in the inferior position, diagnosed histologically as a transitional-cell carcinoma, died 20 July 1973, nine months after first visit

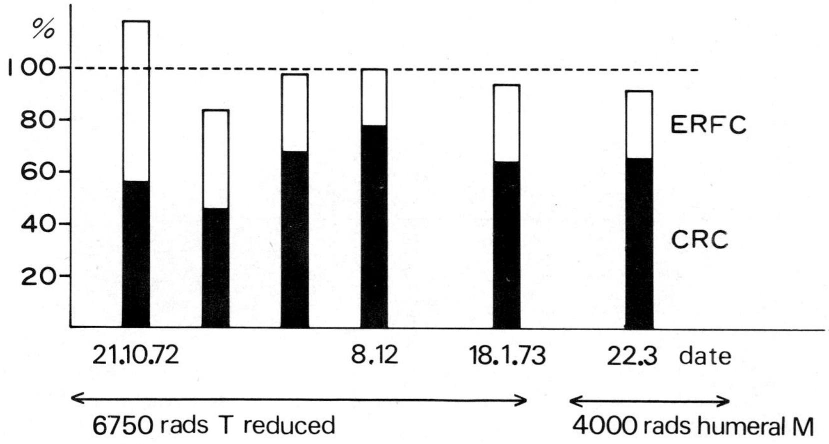

Table 1. Prognosis of nasopharyngeal carcinoma patients as indicated by type of immune response

Type	No. of patients		
	Alive	Dead	Total
I	5	6	11
II	1	8	9
III	0	7	7

The prognoses were then examined with regard to other indices. Survival rate according to clinical stage of disease is shown in Table 2. Most cases fell into stages III and IV, and no marked difference was observed between these two stage groups. Patients

Table 2. Prognosis of nasopharyngeal carcinoma patients as indicated by stage classification of disease

Stage grouping	No. of patients		
	Alive	Dead	Total
II	1	0	1
III	4	13	17
IV	1	8	9

were also analysed from the standpoint of histological classification (Table 3): the prognoses of those with transitional-cell carcinoma and lymphoepithelioma were extremely poor, and that of those with undifferentiated carcinoma was intermediate.

Table 3. Prognosis of nasopharyngeal carcinoma patients as indicated by histological classification of their tumour

Histological type	No. of patients		
	Alive	Dead	Total
Unclassified	1	1	2
Well-differentiated	1	0	1
Undifferentiated	4	9	13
Transitional-cell	0	6	6
Lymphoepithelioma	0	5	5

Finally, prognosis was examined with regard to anti-VCA-antibody titres. It was shown (Table 4), however, that this cannot serve as an index of prognosis for NPC patients.

Table 4. Prognosis of nasopharyngeal carcinoma patients as indicated by anti-Epstein-Barr viral capsid antigen (VCA) antibody titre

Anti-VCA antibody titre	No. of patients		
	Alive	Dead	Total
× 2560	1	8	9
× 640	4	6	10
× 160	0	5	5
⩽ × 40	1	2	3

The relationship between CRC population and anti-VCA-antibody titre was examined by means of a plot diagram (Fig. 5), using repeated measurements in the same patients. There may be some relation between an elevated CRC population and a high antibody titre, but no precise results were obtained.

FIG. 5. RELATION BETWEEN POPULATION OF COMPLEMENT RECEPTOR CELLS (CRC) AND ANTI-EPSTEIN-BARR VIRAL CAPSID ANTIGEN (VCA) ANTIBODY TITRE IN NASOPHARYNGEAL CARCINOMA PATIENTS WITH TYPE I (●), II (◎) AND III (○) IMMUNE RESPONSES AND IN A HEALTHY CONTROL (×)

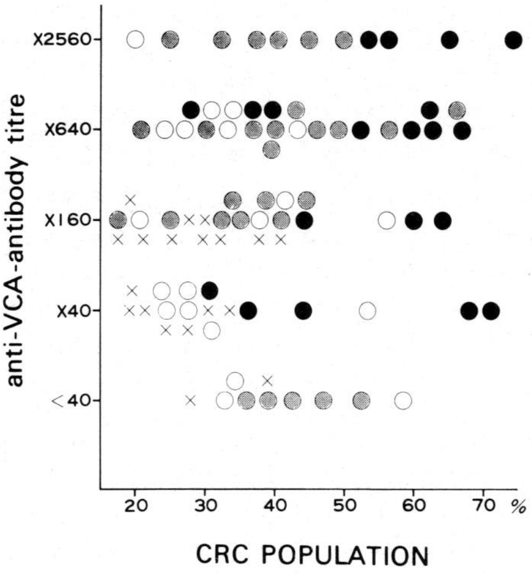

DISCUSSION

Usually, the prognosis of NPC patients is poor, and they die from general weakness due to distant metastases or from complications resulting from intracranial invasion. It is important to consider what steps should be taken in order to improve the therapeutic results in this disease. Many factors, such as clinical stage of the disease, histological characteristics of the tumour and anti-VCA-antibody titres, are considered to indicate the prognosis of NPC patients; and early diagnosis is essential.

Some patients die quickly, even if the cancer is detected at an early stage, and others may be cured, even if treatment is begun only at a later stage of the disease. Thus, the clinical stage at which treatment is begun is not always a reliable index of prognosis.

It is well known that, histologically, the vast majority of NPCs are undifferentiated squamous-cell carcinomas, including transitional-cell carcinomas and lymphoepitheliomas. This type of tumour is very sensitive to irradiation. It must be kept in mind, however, that radiosensitivity is not always synonymous with radiocurability; in fact, lymphoepitheliomas metastasize easily to distant organs, such as lung and bone. Histological characteristics, therefore, appear to be important indicators for prognosis.

NPC also has an intimate association with the Epstein-Barr virus, and it is a well-known fact that many NPC patients have high anti-VCA-antibody titres. Lynn (1973a,b) examined the relationship between anti-VCA-antibody titres and prognosis in 49 NPC cases and reported that the average titre of patients who died was significantly higher. It would appear, therefore, that anti-VCA-antibody titre indicates the prognosis of NPC cases.

Recently, tumour immunology has been advocated as an index of prognosis, and many studies have been reported (Burnet, 1970; Prehn, 1971). In particular, the immune response of the peripheral lymphocytes, i.e., the proportions of the T cell and B cell subpopulations, seems to reflect the general condition of NPC patients.

These four indices were investigated in 27 NPC patients in relation to their prognosis after an adequate lapse of time. It was concluded that the pattern of change of the proportions of the two subpopulations of peripheral lymphocytes over a period of time gave a fairly precise indication of prognosis. It is generally considered that the T cells are concerned with immunological surveillance of the tumour (Burnet, 1970; Prehn, 1971). On the other hand, cellular immunity is decreased by X-ray irradiation. Thus, the prognosis of a patient whose ERFC population is reduced and whose CRC population is increased is poor. In some cases, the ERFC population is abruptly decreased by irradiation. Theoretically, therefore, immune therapy, which would enforce the function of the T cells, could be expected to improve prognosis. Picabanil®, a lyophilized preparation of *Streptococcus pyogenes*, is considered to be one drug useful in such treatment.

The anti-VCA-antibody titres were high in many of the patients. If titres of dilutions of 640 or above are considered to be positive, the rate of positivity was 63%. There was, however, no intimate association between the type of immune response of the peripheral lymphocytes and anti-VCA-antibody titres (Table 5).

Table 5. Relationship between type of immune response of peripheral lymphocytes and anti-Epstein-Barr viral capsid antigen antibody titres in 27 nasopharyngeal carcinoma patients

Titre[a]	Type		
	I	II	III
× 2560	2	4	2
× 640	4	3	2
× 160	2	2	3
× 40	3	0	0

[a] ⩾ × 640 considered to be positive

The relationship between anti-VCA-antibody titres and histological type of tumour has been examined in 84 patients with NPC (Lynn, 1973b). The rates of positivity and geometric mean titres of anti-VCA-antibody were remarkably high in the group with lymphoepithelioma. The cellular immune response, on the other hand, does not correspond to histological classification.

The four indices described above were also compared in relation to the average survival time of those of the 27 NPC patients in this study who died. With regard to type of immune response, the average times were 33.8 months (type I), 36.9 months (type II) and 13.1 months (type III). It is evident that the life expectancy of those with type III responses is very short, indicating that the anti-tumour defense of persons with this type is very weak.

With regard to clinical course of disease, patients were divided into those in stages III and IV, and the average survival times were found to be 31.2 and 23.4 months, respectively. No significant difference was observed between the two. Neither was any difference found among the survival times of patients with three different histological types of tumours: undifferentiated squamous-cell carcinoma, 27.5 months; transitional-cell carcinoma, 21.3 months; and lymphoepithelioma, 28.4 months.

With respect to anti-VCA-antibody titres, the average survival time of patients with high titres was rather longer than in those with low titres, but no significant phenomenon was observed.

Thus, length of survival was not related to clinical stage of disease, histological type of tumour or anti-VCA-antibody titre. Only the type of immune response of the peripheral lymphocytes gave a good indication of the prognosis of the NPC patients.

SUMMARY

The prognosis of a NPC patient is influenced by many factors, including the therapeutic method used and the clinical stage and histological characteristics of the tumour. The immune response of the peripheral lymphocytes was examined in 27 patients with NPC, and it was concluded that this response accurately indicates the clinical course of the diseases as compared with clinical stage of disease, histological type of tumour and anti-VCA-antibody titre.

ACKNOWLEDGEMENT

These investigations were carried out in part with the support of a grant from the Ministry of Health and Welfare, the Government of Japan.

REFERENCES

Burnet, F.M. (1970) *Immunological Surveillance*, Oxford, Pergamon Press

Lynn, T.C., Tu, S.M., Hirayama, T. & Kawamura, A., Jr (1973a) Nasopharyngeal carcinoma and Epstein-Barr virus. I. Factors related to the anti-VCA-antibody. *Jap. J. exp. Med.*, *43*, 121-133

Lynn, T.C., Tu, S.M., Hirayama, T. & Kawamura, A., Jr (1973b) Nasopharyngeal carcinoma and Epstein-Barr virus. II. Clinical course and the anti-VCA antibody. *Jap. J. exp. Med.*, *43*, 135-144

Prehn, R.T. (1971) Immunosurveillance, regeneration and oncogenesis. *Progr. exp. Tumor Res.*, *14*, 1-24

Sawaki, S., Sugano, H., Hirayama, T., Kawamura, A., Jr & Tachibana, T. (1975) Histopathological and immunological studies of nasopharyngeal carcinoma. *Chin. J. Microbiol.*, *8*, 73-81

DISCUSSION SUMMARY

R.A. MANAKER

National Cancer Institute,
Laboratory of DNA Tumour Viruses,
Bethesda, Maryland, USA

It was pointed out that in Ho's study, the Epstein-Barr virus-producing HKLy-28 cells were injected into cancer patients. The potency of some antigen was determined by checking against a preparation of known potency in the same patient on the same day. It was commented that controls other than the Raji cell are needed, i.e., a B-cell line not containing Epstein-Barr virus.

The discrepancy between the report that T-cell functions are depressed even at an early stage of disease and the observations of Dr Ho was due to the fact that the former studies were made *in vitro*, and Ho was using an *in vivo* approach.

It was pointed out that purified protein derivative was used to show blast responses, and there was no real evidence of a general depression of cell-mediated immune response.

No statement could be made about a blocking effect since this was a preliminary report. The sera were sent to Dr P. Levine and are in storage.

There is uncertainty about the antigens involved. The Ly-28 line is lymphoid, so the responses are not to a tumour-specific antigen. The antigens involved are not known. Raji cells were used as a control, but the work was limited by the supply of antigen.

The objective of the Hong Kong study was not to seek subtle differences but to ascertain the pattern of changes with treatment which reduces the tumour load.

After Molinari's paper, Ho pointed out that the period selected for observation in the controlled trials was short, since these tumours grow slowly; sometimes six months elapse before tumour growth is observed. There is some question of whether chemotherapy would prove effective, since skeletal metastases are common, and these do not respond well.

These points had been discussed in planning the study, and it was decided to conduct the trial to determine whether some kind of treatment would prevent or delay the frequency of distant metastases.

Ho pointed out that in view of the poor prognosis even with such treatment, one may question whether the expensive maintenance therapy was warranted.

RECOMMENDATIONS

RECOMMENDATIONS

Participants were grouped by discipline to discuss questions which appeared to be most relevant to the etiology and control of nasopharyngeal carcinoma (NPC), to make recommendations and to suggest priorities for future studies.

HISTOPATHOLOGICAL CLASSIFICATION[1]

The variations in the terminology/classification/definitions of NPC found in the literature were exemplified in the papers presented at this conference.

Despite these variations, important biological differences have been recognized between differentiated squamous-cell carcinomas of the nasopharynx and undifferentiated tumours. In general, NPCs of the differentiated squamous-cell type (in contradistinction to undifferentiated carcinomas and 'lymphoepitheliomas') were found more commonly in older patients, comprised a greater proportion of cases in low-risk populations, were less radiosensitive and were associated with lower levels of antibodies against various Epstein-Barr virus (EBV)-related antigens. However, while these correlations were recognized, they were not regarded as absolute.

Recommendations

1. The uniform use of the proposed WHO classification/definitions of NPCs is strongly recommended, in order to promote comparability of international and interdisciplinary studies (See WHO Recommendations in Annex, p. 605)
2. A panel of pathologists with particular experience in this area should be set up to review problem cases and to ensure uniformity and comparability of data.
3. Pathological studies should be correlated with clinical, epidemiological (especially age and race), immunovirological and molecular biological variables.
4. The cytochemical, histochemical and electron microscopic features of difficult or debatable tumours should be investigated in greater detail.
5. The use of the abbreviation 'NPC' has led to some confusion, as it has been variously interpreted to mean 'nasopharyngeal carcinoma' (most commonly) and, occasionally 'nasopharyngeal cancer' (i.e., including malignant epithelial and non-epithelial tumours, lymphomas, etc.). Thus, it is important to investigate tumours of the nasopharynx other than nasopharyngeal carcinoma, and tumours occurring in other parts of the body (e.g., salivary gland, tonsil, thymus, small intestine) in which tumours of 'lympho-epitheliomatous structure' are known to occur.

---

[1] The subgroup comprised Dr Cammoun, Dr Kawamura, Dr Lennert, Dr Lin, Dr Micheau, Dr Saw, Dr Shanmugaratnam (*Moderator*), Dr Sugano and Dr Weiland.

CLINICAL STAGING[1]

To improve comparability between clinical and experimental studies, the following stage classification of NPC is recommended for general adoption, prospectively, for a trial period of five years:

Anatomical limits of the nasopharynx

Lower limit: posterior margin of the soft palate in the resting position

Anterior limit: stops short of the posterior margin of the nasal septum and the margin of the choanal orifices, both of which should be included in the nasal fossae

T. Primary tumour

UICC classification	Proposed classification (adapted from Ho's classification, 1970)	
	T 1S	Not included
T 0 T 1 T 2	T 1	Tumour confined to the nasopharyngeal mucosa, or no tumour visible, but biopsy positive
T 3	T 2	Tumour extended to the nasal fossa, oropharynx or adjacent muscles or nerves below the base of the skull
T 4	T 3	Tumour extended beyond T2 limits and subclassified as follows:
		T3a Bone involvement below the base of the skull (floor of the sphenoid sinus is included in this category)
		T3b Involvement of the base of skull
		T3c Involvement of cranial nerve(s)
		T3d Involvement of the orbit, laryngopharynx (hypopharynx) or infratemporal fossa

[1] The subgroup comprised Dr Brugère, Dr Cachin, Dr Chau, Dr Ellouz, Dr Goh, Dr Ho (*Moderator*), Dr Hsu, Dr Molinari, Dr Poon, Dr Prasad and Dr Sawaki.

N. Cervical lymph nodes

N0 None palpable (nodes thought to be benign excluded)

N1 Node(s) wholly in the upper cervical level bounded below by a line joining the upper margin of the sternal end of the clavicle on the opposite side to the apex of an angle between the lateral surface of the neck and the superior margin of the trapezius on the same side (see Fig. 1).

N2 Node(s) extending below the lower boundary line of N1

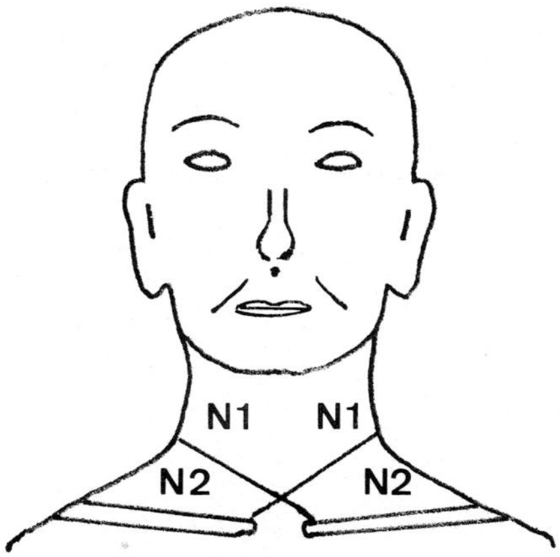

M. Haematogenous metastasis

and/or involvement of the skin or lymph node(s) extending below the clavicles

Stage grouping

To avoid confusion with any other stage grouping in present use, the stages will be designated A, B, C and D, as follows:

A : T1 N0

B : T1 N1, T2 N0, T2 N1, T3 N0 or T3 N1

C : N2 irrespective of T

D : M present

Primary tumour \ Node(s)	N 0	N 1	N 2
T 1	A	B	C
T 2	B	B	C
T 3	B	B	C
M	D	D	D

Comparison between the present recommended stage classification and that of Dr Ho[1]

	Recommended classification	Ho's classification
Stage	A	I
Stage	B	II
Stage	C	III and IV combined
Stage	D	V

The above proposed clinical staging may raise some difficulties, which were stressed by the European Group, since patients T2 N1 and T2 N0 are combined with T1 N1.

[1] Ho, H.C. (1970) *The natural history and treatment of nasopharyngeal carcinoma.* In: Lee Clark, R., Cumley, R.W., McCay, J.E. & Murray, M., eds, *Oncology, Proceedings of the X International Cancer Congress*, Vol. 4, Chicago, Year Book Medical Publishers, pp. 1-14

EPIDEMIOLOGY[1]

1. Is there really a double peak in the age-distribution of NPC? If there is, in what areas? Is the NPC seen in childhood and adolescence epidemiologically different (i.e., exposure to environmental agents) from NPC in adults?

   Recommendation:

   A multidisciplinary approach to young NPC patients and proper controls in selected areas are recommended.

2. How can we monitor time trends in NPC incidence and patterns in Chinese in the USA, Japan, Singapore and Hong Kong? In China? How can we explain the reported changes in trends (i.e., change in traditional life style and/or socio-economic status)?

   Recommendation:

   Set up morbidity and mortality monitoring programmes in these areas, utilizing existing cancer registries and vital statistics.

3. What is the natural history of NPC in relation to EBV infection and exposure to 'co-factors'? What is the EBV serological profile prior to the development of the disease? To what extent have we evidence that specific environmental chemicals that could explain the high incidence of NPC in Southern Chinese exist in their environment? To what extent is the HLA haplotype associated with the risk for NPC, particularly in older persons? Is the high incidence of NPC in Southern Chinese the result of a combined action of multiple risk factors?

   Recommendation:

   Carry out a multidisciplinary, longitudinal, cohort study in a high-risk population: e.g., five-year follow-up of 5 000 Cantonese males of 45-49 years of age.

---

[1] The subgroup comprised Dr de-Thé, Dr Geser and Dr Hirayama (*Moderator*).

4. What is the epidemiological significance of the presence of the EBV genome in different histopathological types?

Recommendation:

Study material from an agreed pathological classification of NPC. Close coordination with the pathology group is recommended.

GENETICS[1]

The main questions and recommendations were to:

1. Identify more precisely HLA profiles of NPC cases from populations with intermediate and low risks.

   This could be achieved by typing freshly diagnosed NPC cases with a satisfactorily matched control series from the following groups:

   a) Malays from Kuala Lumpur and Singapore
   b) Tunisians
   c) Japanese
   d) Caucasians
   e) American Indians (if sufficient cases are forthcoming)

   It is a strongly recommended that lymphocytes from the above groups be stored, so that if and when IA or locus D antigens of interest are identified, typing can be carried out immediately.

2. Identify the locus A blank in Chinese and Malays by:

   a) Use of a more specific anti-sera for the AW19 group of antigens, in particular AW33 and AW34 (Malay)
   b) Screening of sera
   c) Study of families to establish the activity as part of the HLA locus A series

3. Identify HLA-related genotypes related more specifically to NPC, in particular IA and locus D, by:

   a) Screening of sera from pregnant women to identify anti-IA activities specifically related to NPC
   b) Development of primed lymphocyte typing and its use for identification of a NPC-related locus D antigen.

4. Establish the relationship between immunological status and prognosis related to HLA type by:

   HLA typing and, preferably, genotyping of all patients entered into longitudinal studies of NPC patients (WSr HK).

5. Determine whether particular immune responses are linked to the HLA type associated with NPC, by:

---

[1] The subgroup comprised Dr Day, Dr Simons and Dr Terasaki (*Moderator*).

Studying immunological parameters in families (a single case sufficient, multiple cases preferred) with NPC, to study joint segregation with the NPC-related haplotypes. The parameters to be studied should be determined by the immunology subgroup but might include IgA and antibody activity.

6. Determine the full risk associated with the HLA region by:

   Studying the HLA relationship between related cases of NPC (multiple-case family studies). There is great difficulty in finding further multiple-case families in Singapore and Hong Kong. It is recommended that some approach be made to the relevant authorities in the People's Republic of China, where a study of this type would be feasible.

7. Follow up the fact that various components of complement are known to be coded by genes close to the HLA region. It is recommended that studies be made of complement allotypes in families of NPC cases. The close association between C3 and the Epstein-Barr virus receptor also calls for further investigation.

8. Study other genetic systems, Gu, Iuv, red-cell antigens and enzymes, and carry out genetic studies of susceptibility to the carcinogens found in salted fish. The priority for this proposal is low, until more is known of the relevant systems under genetic control.

VIROLOGY[1]

The following suggestions were felt to have high priority:

1. To characterize biologically, antigenically and biochemically EBV strains obtained from different diseases and geographical areas.

   This includes attempts to isolate the EBV from NPC tumour cells, studies on viral DNA from biopsy tissue culture and established lines, etc.

2. To conduct a correlative study of all types of cancers arising in the nasopharynx and at other sites in the head and neck, as to exact histology (using the WHO classification), presence or absence of EBV markers in tumour cells [viral DNA and Epstein-Barr nuclear antigen (EBNA)] and EBV serological reactivities in patients' sera.

   To determine whether the detection of EBV DNA (EBNA-positive tumour cells) is limited to one specific histological type of carcinoma in the nasopharynx or whether it extends to other histological types and other sites. To determine whether it would be helpful in the diagnosis of a distinct type of carcinoma, i.e., to differentiate between different histological diagnoses.

3. a) To attempt to culture the epithelial progenitors of NPC cells

   b) To transform epithelial elements from normal nasopharyngeal mucosa by EBV from various sources. This would allow study of the histological and biochemical events in the transformation.

   c) To study the local immunopathology and viral replication of EBV in the oropharynx of patients with infectious mononucleosis, Burkitt's lymphoma and NPC.

4. To conduct a prospective study in a Chinese population to characterize preclinical events with regard to EBV serology and to detect IgA in saliva prior to tumour development. This study is related to recommendation 2 of the epidemiology group. It is suggested that such studies be carried out in family members of NPC patients.

---

[1] The subgroup comprised Dr Ablashi, Dr Epstein, Dr zur Hausen, Dr Henle (*Moderator*), Dr G. Henle, Dr Hinuma, Dr Huang, Dr Lenoir, Dr Manaker, Dr Nonoyama, Dr Osato, Dr Stanley and Dr Yoshida.

5. To pursue longitudinal studies on NPC patients with regard to humoral antibody patterns and general and EBV-specific cell-mediated immune responses. The aim of these studies would be to see the prognostic implications of these immune markers, which could help in early detection and in monitoring therapy.

6. To search for new and to characterize known EBV-determined antigens, both from the biochemical viewpoint and for use in immunological studies (see below).

7. To develop an experimental model system in non-human primates in order better to understand the relationship and pathogenesis of the oncogenic potential of EBV in humans, specifically by the establishment of a breeding centre for cotton-top marmosets, since these animals are very difficult to obtain and appear to be most susceptible to EBV.

IMMUNOLOGY[1]

Three questions are highly relevant to NPC etiology and control:

- What antigens are relevant in the cellular immune response?
- What influence has cellular immunity on the course of the disease?
- Can susceptible groups be defined, i.e., in terms of HLA genotypes?

The following research projects are recommended:

1. *Purification and standardization of antigen preparations*

It is evident that, if meaningful studies of cellular immunity are to be carried out, uniformly pure, standard antigen preparations should be used. This we consider to be of high priority and suggest that more than one laboratory pursue such studies.

(a) Selection of antigens for purification

Epstein-Barr nuclear antigen (EBNA), early antigen-diffused (EA-D), early antigen-restricted (EA-R), viral capsid antigen (VCA), lymphocyte determined membrane antigen (LYDMA) and surface glycoproteins including membrane antigen (MA) were mentioned. One should bear in mind the possibility that NPC-specific antigens, not associated with EBV, may exist.

(b) Assays

Assays for the identification of antigen preparations would be the usual *in vitro* tests, i.e., lymphocyte transformation and proliferation, macrophage inhibition factor (MIF), etc. Lymphocytes from both seropositive and seronegative donors should be tested.

2. *Cellular immunity studies*

Both *in vivo* and *in vitro* studies should be carried out and should encompass both specific and non-specific cell-mediated immunity. The studies should be carefully correlated, not only with parallel investigations of humoral immunity, but also with the stages of the disease. It is strongly recommended that a uniform and standardized clinical staging of the disease should be available. In addition, there should be a uniform selection of standard types of control patients.

---

[1] The subgroup comprised Dr Chan, Dr Lamelin, Dr Miller (*Moderator*), Dr Ng, Dr Pearson, Dr Stevens, Dr Tachibana and Dr Yata.

For *in vitro* studies, the target cells should be defined precisely. Among the targets to be considered are autochthonous biopsy materials and lymphoblastoid cell lines.

It is also recommended that the HLA genotypes of both patients and targets be determined whenever possible. Thus, one should know whether there is HLA identity between the *in vivo* stimulator cells of the patient and the *in vitro* target cells. It would also be useful to know whether target cells that have the high-risk HLA haplotype are better or worse than target cells with other HLA types.

3. *Animals models*

A search for appropriate animal models must be instigated and facilities for breeding susceptible animals, i.e., cotton-top marmosets, be made available for all immuno-virological studies. Hence, the induction of carcinomas in the nasopharyngeal area of susceptible animals should be explored with a view to initiating well-defined and -controlled immunovirological investigations.

ANNEX

HISTOLOGICAL CLASSIFICATION OF TUMOURS OF THE NASOPHARYNX RECOMMENDED BY THE WORLD HEALTH ORGANIZATION[1]

EPITHELIAL TUMOURS

A. BENIGN

1. Squamous cell papilloma
2. Oxyphilic adenoma [oncocytoma]
3. Pleomorphic adenoma [mixed tumour]
4. Others

B. MALIGNANT

1. Nasopharyngeal carcinoma
   (*a*) Squamous cell carcinoma [keratinizing squamous cell carcinoma]
   (*b*) Non-keratinizing carcinoma
   (*c*) Undifferentiated carcinoma [undifferentiated carcinoma of nasopharyngeal type]
2. Adenocarcinoma
3. Adenoid cystic carcinoma
4. Others

[1] Shanmugaratnam, K. & Sobin, L.H. (1978) *Histological typing of upper respiratory tract tumours (International Histological Classification of Tumours*, No. 19), Geneva, World Health Organization

Nasopharyngeal carcinoma

A malignant tumour of the epithelium lining the surface and crypts of the nasopharynx.

On the basis of electron microscopic findings, all types of nasopharyngeal carcinoma may be regarded as variants of squamous cell carcinoma. These tumours may be classified into the following groups according to their predominant pattern on light microscopy.

(*a*) *Squamous cell carcinoma* [keratinizing squamous cell carcinoma]. A nasopharyngeal carcinoma showing definite evidence of squamous differentiation with the presence of intercellular bridges and/or keratinization over most of its extent. It may be graded as well, moderately, or poorly differentiated.

(*b*) *Nonkeratinizing carcinoma*. A nasopharyngeal carcinoma showing evidence of differentiation with a maturation sequence that results in cells in which squamous differentiation is not evident on light microscopy. The tumour cells have fairly well defined cell margins and show an arrangement that is stratified or pavemented and not syncytial. A plexiform pattern is common. Some tumours may exhibit a clear cell structure due to the presence of cytoplasmic glycogen. There is no evidence of mucin production or of glandular differentiation.

(*c*) *Undifferentiated carcinoma* [undifferentiated carcinoma of nasopharyngeal type]. The tumour cells have oval or round vesicular nuclei and prominent nucleoli. The cell margins are indistinct and the tumour exhibits a syncytial rather than pavemented appearance. Spindle-shaped tumour cells, some with hyperchromatic nuclei, may be present. The tumour cells are arranged in irregular and moderately well defined masses and/or in strands of loosely connected cells in a lymphoid stroma. The tumour cells do not produce mucin. These cytological and histological features are fairly characteristic and when present in metastatic tumours, which are particularly common in the upper cervical lymph nodes, may enable a presumptive diagnosis of nasopharyngeal carcinoma to be made.

The term 'lymphoepithelial carcinoma' [lymphoepithelioma] is used to describe nonkeratinizing and undifferentiated nasopharyngeal carcinomas in which numerous lymphocytes are found among the tumour cells. The lymphoid elements in such tumours are not neoplastic. Lymphoepithelial carcinomas, like other undifferentiated carcinomas of the nasopharynx, show ultrastructural evidence of squamous differentiation.

INDEX OF AUTHORS

INDEX OF AUTHORS

Ablashi, D.V., *85, 439*
Anderson, E.N., Jr., *231*
Anderson, M.L., *231*
Andersson-Anvret, M., *347*
Aya, T., *413*

Ball, G., *299*
Behi, J., *13, 115*
Ben Attia, R., *13, 115*
Betuel, H., *271*
Blake, N.M., *283*
Brugère, J., *241*

Cachin, Y., *131*
Cammoun, M., *13, 95, 115*
Chan, S.H., *271, 283, 495, 503*
Charnay, N., *213*
Chau, J.C.W., *271, 545*
Chen, H.C., *65*
Chew, T.S., *495*
Chia, K.B., *199*
Coates, H.L., *439*

Darmalingam, S., *271*
Day, N.E., *213, 271, 329*
Desgranges, C., *459*
De-Thé, G., *213, 271, 377, 459, 471, 523*

Easton, J.M., *85, 439*
Ellouz, R., *13, 115*
Epstein, M.A., *299, 333*

Finerty, S., *299*
Forsby, N., *347*
Fresen, K.-O., *391*
Fujinaga, K., *403*

Gabbiani, G., *523*
Geser, A., *213*
Giovanella, B.C., *299*
Glaser, R., *85, 397*
Goh, E.H., *199, 271, 495, 503*
Gough, T.A., *309*

Hamajima, K., *65*
Henderson, B.E., *251*
Henle, G., *427*
Henle, W., *347, 421, 427*
Hinuma, Y., *385*
Hirayama, T., *27, 147, 167*
Ho, J.H.C., *99, 213, 231, 271, 309, 315, 359, 427, 449, 545*
Huang, D.P., *309, 315, 359*

Jarvis, J.E., *299*

Kaiserling, E., *51*
Kawamura, A., Jr.,*65, 575*
Khor, T.H., *495*
Kirk, R.L., *283*
Klein, G., *347, 369*
Kwan, H.C., *449*

Lamelin, J.-P., *483, 523*
Lavoué, M.F., *471*
Lennert, K., *51*
Lenoir, G., *377*
Levine, P.H., *439, 483, 545*
Louie, E., *251*

Maeda, M., *385*
Manaker, R.A., *587*
Marandas, P., *131*

Matsuo, T., *413*
Mazzanti, T., *51*
Mickey, M.R., *263*
Mizuno, F., *413*
Molinari, R., *553, 565*
Muenz, L., *471*
Murata, M., *65*

Neel, H.B., III, *439*
Ng, M.H., *359, 449, 545*
Nonoyama, M., *397, 413*

Ojima, S., *403*
Osato, T., *413*
Osono, M., *65*

Pearson, G.R., *439*
Perdue, S.T., *263*
Pilotti, S., *553*
Point, D., *241*
Prasad, U., *271*

Revillard, J.P., *523*
Rilke, F., *553*

Sairenji, T., *385*
Sakamoto, G., *27*
Sancho-Garnier, H., *131, 241*
Saw, D., *315*
Sawada, Y., *403*
Sawaki, S., *27, 147, 511, 575*
Schwaab, G., *131, 241*
Serjeantson, S., *283*
Shanmugaratnam, K., *3, 191, 199, 271*
Shimbo, T., *511*
Simons, M.J., *271, 283, 503*
Stevens, D.A., *483*
Sugano, H., *27, 147*

Tachibana, T., *537, 575*
Tanaka, A., *397*
Teoh, T-B., *315*
Terasaki, P.I., *263*
Trumper, P.A., *299*
Tse, K.C., *545*
Tye, C.Y., *199*

Wee, G.B., *271*
Weiland, L.H., *41*

Yamamoto, K., *413*
Yano, S., *403*
Yata, J., *511*

zur Hausen, H., *391*

PUBLICATIONS OF THE INTERNATIONAL AGENCY FOR RESEARCH ON CANCER

SCIENTIFIC PUBLICATIONS SERIES

No. 1 LIVER CANCER (1971)
176 pages US$ 10.00; Sw. fr. 30.–

No. 2 ONCOGENESIS AND HERPESVIRUSES (1972)
Edited by P.N. Biggs, G. de Thé & L.N. Payne
515 pages US$ 25.00; Sw. fr. 100.–

No. 3 N-NITROSO COMPOUNDS – ANALYSIS AND FORMATION (1972)
Edited by P. Bogovski, R. Preussmann & E.A. Walker
140 pages US$ 6.25; Sw. fr. 25.–

No. 4 TRANSPLACENTAL CARCINOGENESIS (1973)
Edited by L. Tomatis & U. Mohr
181 pages US$ 12.00; Sw. fr. 40.–

No. 5 PATHOLOGY OF TUMOURS IN LABORATORY ANIMALS. VOLUME I TUMOURS OF THE RAT PART 1 (1973)
Editor-in-Chief V.S. Turusov
216 pages US$ 15.00; Sw. fr. 50.–

No. 6 PATHOLOGY OF TUMOURS IN LABORATORY ANIMALS. VOLUME I TUMOURS OF THE RAT PART 2 (1976)
Editor-in-Chief V.S. Turusov
315 pages US$ 35.00; Sw. fr. 90.–

No. 7 HOST ENVIRONMENT INTERACTIONS IN THE ETIOLOGY OF CANCER IN MAN (1973)
Edited by R. Doll & I. Vodopija
464 pages US$ 40.00; Sw. fr. 100.–

No. 8 BIOLOGICAL EFFECTS OF ASBESTOS (1973)
Edited by P. Bogovski, J.C. Gilson, V. Timbrell & J.C. Wagner
346 pages US$ 32.00; Sw. fr. 80.–

No. 9 N-NITROSO COMPOUNDS IN THE ENVIRONMENT (1974)
Edited by P. Bogovski & E.A. Walker
243 pages US$ 20.00; Sw. fr. 50.–

No. 10 CHEMICAL CARCINOGENESIS ESSAYS (1974)
Edited by R. Montesano & L. Tomatis
230 pages US$ 20.00; Sw. fr. 50.–

No. 11 ONCOGENESIS AND HERPESVIRUSES II (1975)
Edited by G. de Thé, M.A. Epstein & H. zur Hausen
Part 1, 511 pages, US$ 38.00; Sw. fr. 100.–
Part 2, 433 pages, US$ 30.00; Sw. fr. 80.–

No. 12 SCREENING TESTS IN CHEMICAL CARCINOGENESIS (1976)
Edited by R. Montesano, H. Bartsch & L. Tomatis
666 pages US$ 48.00; Sw. fr. 120.–

No. 13 ENVIRONMENTAL POLUTION AND CARCINOGENIC RISKS (1976)
Edited by C. Rosenfeld & W. Davis
454 pages US$ 20.00; Sw. fr. 50.–

No. 14 ENVIRONMENTAL N-NITROSO COMPOUNDS – ANALYSIS AND FORMATION (1976)
Edited by E.A. Walker, P. Bogovski & L. Griciute
512 pages US$ 45.00; Sw. fr. 110.–

No. 15 CANCER INCIDENCE IN FIVE CONTINENTS, VOL. III (1976)
Edited by C.S. Muir, J. Waterhouse, P. Correa & J. Powell
584 pages US$ 40.00; Sw. fr. 100.–

No. 16 AIR POLLUTION AND CANCER IN MAN (1977)
Edited by U. Mohr, D. Schmähl & L. Tomatis
331 pages US$ 35.00; Sw. fr. 90.–

No. 17 DIRECTORY OF ON-GOING RESEARCH IN CANCER EPIDEMIOLOGY (1977)
Edited by C.S. Muir & G. Wagner
599 pages US$ 10.00; Sw. fr. 25.–

No. 18 ENVIRONMENTAL CARCINOGENS SELECTED METHODS OF ANALYSIS (1978) Vol. 1-ANALYSIS OF VOLATILE NITROSAMINES IN FOOD
Edited by H. Egan, R. Preussmann, M. Castegnaro, E.A. Walker & E.A. Wassermann
218 pages US$ 45.00; Sw. fr. 90.–

No. 19 ENVIRONMENTAL ASPECTS OF *N*-NITROSO COMPOUNDS
Edited by E.A. Walker, M. Castegnaro, L. Griciute & R.E. Lyle
566 pages US$ 50.00; Sw. fr. 100.–

No. 20 NASOPHARYNGEAL CARCINOMA: ETIOLOGY AND CONTROL
Edited by G. de-Thé & Y. Ito
610 pages US$ 60.00; Sw. fr. 100.–

No. 21 CANCER REGISTRATION AND ITS TECHNIQUES
Edited by R. MacLennan, C.S. Muir, R. Steinitz & A. Winkler
235 pages US$ 25.00; Sw. fr. 40.–

No. 26 DIRECTORY OF ON-GOING RESEARCH IN CANCER EPIDEMIOLOGY 1978
Edited by C.S. Muir & G. Wagner
550 pages Sw. fr. 30.–

IARC MONOGRAPHS ON THE EVALUATION OF THE CARCINOGENIC RISK OF CHEMICALS TO MAN

Volume 1, 1972
Some inorganic substances, chlorinated hydrocarbons, aromatic amines, N-nitroso compounds, and natural products
184 pages US$ 4.20; Sw. fr. 12.–

Volume 2, 1973
Some inorganic and organometallic compounds
181 pages US$ 3.60; Sw. fr. 12.–

Volume 3, 1973
Certain polycyclic aromatic hydrocarbons and heterocyclic compounds
271 pages US$ 5.40; Sw. fr. 18.–

Volume 4, 1974
Some aromatic amines, hydrazine and related substances, N-nitroso compounds and miscellaneous alkylating agents
286 pages US$ 7.20; Sw. fr. 18.–

Volume 5, 1974
Some organochlorine pesticides
241 pages US$ 7.20; Sw. fr. 18.–

Volume 6, 1974
Sex hormones
243 pages US$ 7.20; Sw. fr. 18.–

Volume 7, 1974
Some anti-thyroid and related substances, nitrofurans and industrial chemicals
326 pages US$ 12.80; Sw. fr. 32.–

Volume 8, 1975
Some aromatic amines
357 pages US$ 14.40; Sw. fr. 36.–

Volume 9, 1975
Some aziridines, N-, S- and O-mustards and selenium
268 pages US$ 10.80; Sw. fr. 27.–

Volume 10, 1976
Some naturally occurring substances
353 pages US$ 15.00; Sw. fr. 38.–

Volume 11, 1976
Cadmium, nickel, some epoxides and miscellaneous industrial chemicals, and general considerations on volatile anaesthetics
306 pages US$ 14.00; Sw. fr. 34.–

Volume 12, 1976
Some carbamates, thiocarbamates and carbazides
282 pages US$ 14.00; Sw. fr. 34.–

Volume 13, 1977
Some miscellaneous pharmaceutical substances
255 pages US$ 12.00; Sw. fr. 30.–

Vol. 14, 1977
Asbestos
106 pages US$ 6.00; Sw. fr. 14.–

Volume 15, 1977
Some fumigants, the herbicides 2,4-D and 2,4,5-T, chlorinated dibenzodioxins and miscellaneous industrial chemicals
354 pages US$ 20.00; Sw. fr. 50.–

Volume 16, 1977
Some aromatic amines and related nitro compounds – Hair dyes, colouring agents and miscellaneous industrial chemicals
400 pages US$ 20.00; Sw. fr. 50.–

Volume 17, 1978
Some N-Nitroso compounds
365 pages US$ 20.00; Sw. fr. 50.–

Volume 18, 1978
Polychlorinated biphenyls and polybrominated biphenyls
140 pages US$ 13.00; Sw. fr. 20.–

Non-serial publication (in French only)
Alcool et Cancer
42 pages Fr. fr. 35.–; Sw. fr. 14.–

WHO/IARC publications may be obtained, direct or through booksellers, from:

ALGERIA: Société Nationale d'Edition et de Diffusion, 3 bd Zirout Youcef, ALGIERS

ARGENTINA: Carlos Hirsch SRL, Florida 165, Galerías Güemes, Escritorio 453/465, BUENOS AIRES

AUSTRALIA: *Mail Order Sales:* Australian Government Publishing Service Bookshops, P.O. Box 84, CANBERRA A.C.T. 2600; *or over the counter from* Australian Government Publications and Inquiry Centres *at:* 113–115 London Circuit, CANBERRA CITY A.C.T. 2600; Shop 42, The Valley Centre, BRISBANE, Queensland 4000; 347 Swanston Street, MELBOURNE VIC 3000; 309 Pitt Street, SYDNEY N.S.W. 2000; Mt Newman House, 200 St. George's Terrace, PERTH WA 6000; Industry House, 12 Pirie Street, ADELAIDE SA 5000; 156–162 Macquarie Street, HOBART TAS 7000 — Hunter Publications, 58A Gipps Street, COLLINGWOOD VIC 3066

AUSTRIA: Gerold & Co., Graben 31, 1011 VIENNA I

BANGLADESH: The WHO Programme Coordinator, G.P.O. Box 250, DACCA 5 — The Association of Voluntary Agencies, P.O. Box 5045, DACCA 5

BELGIUM: Office international de Librairie, 30 avenue Marnix, 1050 BRUSSELS — *Subscriptions to World Health only:* Jean de Lannoy, 202 avenue du Roi, 1060 BRUSSELS

BRAZIL: Biblioteca Regional de Medicina OMS/OPS, Unidade de Venda de Publicações, Caixa Postal 20.381, Vila Clementino, 04023 SÃO PAULO, S.P.

BURMA: *see* India, WHO Regional Office

CANADA: *Single and bulk copies of individual publications (not subscriptions):* Canadian Public Health Association, 1335 Carling Avenue, Suite 210, OTTAWA, Ont. K1Z 8N8. *Subscriptions: Subscription orders, accompanied by cheque made out to the* Royal Bank of Canada, OTTAWA, Account World Health Organization, *should be sent to the* World Health Organization, P.O. Box 1800, Postal Station B, OTTAWA, Ont. K1P 5R5. *Correspondence concerning subscriptions should be addressed to the* World Health Organization, Distribution and Sales, 1211 GENEVA 27, Switzerland

CHINA: China National Publications Import Corporation, P.O. Box 88, PEKING

COLOMBIA: Distrilibros Ltd, Pío Alfonso García, Carrera 4a, Nos 36–119, CARTAGENA

CZECHOSLOVAKIA: Artia, Ve Smeckach 30, 111 27 PRAGUE 1

DENMARK: Ejnar Munksgaard, Ltd, Nørregade 6, 1164 COPENHAGEN K

ECUADOR: Librería Científica S.A., P.O. Box 362, Luque 223, GUAYAQUIL

EGYPT: Nabaa El Fikr Bookshop, 55 Saad Zaghloul Street, ALEXANDRIA

EL SALVADOR: Librería Estudiantil, Edificio Comercial B No 3, Avenida Libertad, SAN SALVADOR

FIJI: The WHO Programme Coordinator, P.O. Box 113, SUVA

FINLAND: Akateeminen Kirjakauppa, Keskuskatu 2, 00101 HELSINKI 10

FRANCE: Librairie Arnette, 2 rue Casimir-Delavigne, 75006 PARIS

GERMAN DEMOCRATIC REPUBLIC: Buchhaus Leipzig, Postfach 140, 701 LEIPZIG

GERMANY, FEDERAL REPUBLIC OF: Govi-Verlag GmbH, Ginnheimerstrasse 20, Postfach 5360, 6236 ESCHBORN — W. E. Saarbach, Postfach 101610, Follerstrasse 2, 5 COLOGNE 1 — Alex. Horn, Spiegelgasse 9, Postfach 3340, 6200 WIESBADEN

GREECE: G. C. Eleftheroudakis S.A., Librairie internationale, rue Nikis 4, ATHENS (T. 126)

HAITI: Max Bouchereau, Librairie "A la Caravelle", Boîte postale 111-B, PORT-AU-PRINCE

HONG KONG: Hong Kong Government Information Services, Beaconsfield House, 6th Floor, Queen's Road, Central, VICTORIA

HUNGARY: Kultura, P.O.B. 149, BUDAPEST 62 — Akadémiai Könyvesbolt, Váci utca 22, BUDAPEST V

ICELAND: Snaebjørn Jonsson & Co., P.O. Box 1131, Hafnarstraeti 9, REYKJAVIK

INDIA: WHO Regional Office for South-East Asia, World Health House, Indraprastha Estate, Ring Road, NEW DELHI 110002 — Oxford Book & Stationery Co., Scindia House, NEW DELHI 110000; 17 Park Street, CALCUTTA 700016 (*Sub-Agent*)

INDONESIA: M/s Kalman Book Service Ltd, Jln. Cikini Raya No. 63, P.O. Box 3105/Jkt., JAKARTA

IRAN: Iranian Amalgamated Distribution Agency, 151 Khiaban Soraya, TEHERAN

IRAQ: Ministry of Information, National House for Publishing, Distributing and Advertising, BAGHDAD

IRELAND: The Stationery Office, DUBLIN 4

ISRAEL: Heiliger & Co., 3 Nathan Strauss Street, JERUSALEM

ITALY: Edizioni Minerva Medica, Corso Bramante 83–85, 10126 TURIN; Via Lamarmora 3, 20100 MILAN

JAPAN: Maruzen Co. Ltd, P.O. Box 5050, TOKYO International 100–31

KOREA, REPUBLIC OF: The WHO Programme Coordinator, Central P.O. Box 540, SEOUL

KUWAIT: The Kuwait Bookshops Co. Ltd, Thunayan Al-Ghanem Bldg, P.O. Box 2942, KUWAIT

LAO PEOPLE'S DEMOCRATIC REPUBLIC: The WHO Programme Coordinator, P.O. Box 343, VIENTIANE

LEBANON: The Levant Distributors Co. S.A.R.L., Box 1181, Makdassi Street, Hanna Bldg, BEIRUT

LUXEMBOURG: Librairie du Centre, 49 bd Royal, LUXEMBOURG

MALAYSIA: The WHO Programme Coordinator, Room 1004, Fitzpatrick Building, Jalan Raja Chulan, KUALA LUMPUR 05–02 — Jubilee (Book) Store Ltd, 97 Jalan Tuanku Abdul Rahman, P.O. Box 629, KUALA LUMPUR 01–08 — Parry's Book Center, K. L. Hilton Hotel, Jln. Treacher, P.O. Box 960, KUALA LUMPUR

MEXICO: La Prensa Médica Mexicana, Ediciones Científicas, Paseo de las Facultades 26, Apt. Postal 20–413, MEXICO CITY 20, D.F.

MONGOLIA: *see* India, WHO Regional Office

MOROCCO: Editions La Porte, 281 avenue Mohammed V, RABAT

MOZAMBIQUE: INLD, Caixa Postal 4030, MAPUTO

NEPAL: *see* India, WHO Regional Office

NETHERLANDS: N. V. Martinus Nijhoff's Boekhandel en Uitgevers Maatschappij, Lange Voorhout 9, THE HAGUE 2000

NEW ZEALAND: Government Printing Office, Mulgrave Street, Private Bag, WELLINGTON 1, *Government Bookshops at:* Rutland Street, P.O. Box 5344, AUCKLAND; 130 Oxford Terrace, P.O. Box 1721, CHRISTCHURCH; Alma Street, P.O. Box 857, HAMILTON; Princes Street, P.O. Box 1104, DUNEDIN — R. Hill & Son, Ltd, Ideal House, Cnr Gillies Avenue & Eden St., Newmarket, AUCKLAND 1

NIGERIA: University Bookshop Nigeria Ltd, University of Ibadan, IBADAN — G. O. Odatuwa Publishers & Booksellers Co., 9 Hausa Road, SAPELE, BENDEL STATE

NORWAY: Johan Grundt Tanum Bokhandel, Karl Johansgt. 43, 1010 OSLO 1

PAKISTAN: Mirza Book Agency, 65 Shahrah–E–Quaid–E–Azam, P.O. Box 729, LAHORE 3

PAPUA NEW GUINEA: WHO Programme Coordinator, P.O. Box 5896, BOROKO

PHILIPPINES: World Health Organization, Regional Office for the Western Pacific, P.O. Box 2932, MANILA — The Modern Book Company Inc., P.O. Box 632, 926 Rizal Avenue, MANILA

POLAND: Składnica Księgarska, ul Mazowiecka 9, 00052 WARSAW *(except periodicals)* — BKWZ Ruch, ul Wronia 23, 00840 WARSAW *(periodicals only)*

PORTUGAL: Livraria Rodrigues, 186 Rua do Ouro, LISBON 2

SIERRA LEONE: Njala University College Bookshop (University of Sierra Leone), Private Mail Bag, FREETOWN

SINGAPORE: The WHO Programme Coordinator, 144 Moulmein Road, G.P.O. Box 3457, SINGAPORE 1 — Select Books (Pte) Ltd, 215 Tanglin Shopping Centre, 2/F, 19 Tanglin Road, SINGAPORE 10

SOUTH AFRICA: Van Schaik's Bookstore (Pty) Ltd, P.O. Box 724, 268 Church Street, PRETORIA 0001

SPAIN: Comercial Atheneum S.A., Consejo de Ciento 130–136, BARCELONA 15; General Moscardó 29, MADRID 20 — Librería Díaz de Santos, Lagasca 95, MADRID 6; Balmes 417 y 419, BARCELONA 6

SRI LANKA: *see* India, WHO Regional Office

SWEDEN: Aktiebolaget C. E. Fritzes Kungl. Hovbokhandel, Regeringsgatan 12, 103 27 STOCKHOLM

SWITZERLAND: Medizinischer Verlag Hans Huber, Länggass Strasse 76, 3012 BERNE 9

SYRIAN ARAB REPUBLIC: M. Farras Kekhia, P.O. Box No. 5221, ALEPPO

THAILAND: *see* India, WHO Regional Office

TUNISIA: Société Tunisienne de Diffusion, 5 avenue de Carthage, TUNIS

TURKEY: Haset Kitapevi, 469 Istiklal Caddesi, Beyoglu, ISTANBUL

UNITED KINGDOM: H. M. Stationery Office: 49 High Holborn, LONDON WC1V 6HB; 13a Castle Street, EDINBURGH EH2 3AR; 41 The Hayes, CARDIFF CF1 1JW; 80 Chichester Street, BELFAST BT1 4JY; Brazennose Street, MANCHESTER M60 8AS; 258 Broad Street, BIRMINGHAM B1 2HE; Southey House, Wine Street, BRISTOL BS1 2BQ. *All mail orders should be sent to* P.O. Box 569, LONDON SE1 9NH

UNITED STATES OF AMERICA: *Single and bulk copies of individual publications (not subscriptions):* WHO Publications Centre USA, 49 Sheridan Avenue, ALBANY, NY 12210. *Subscriptions: Subscription orders, accompanied by check made out to the* Chemical Bank, New York, Account World Health Organization, *should be sent to the* World Health Organization, P.O. Box 5284, Church Street Station, NEW YORK, NY 10249. *Correspondence concerning subscriptions should be addressed to the* World Health Organization, Distribution and Sales, 1211 GENEVA 27, Switzerland. *Publications are also available from the* United Nations Bookshop, NEW YORK, NY 10017 *(retail only), and single and bulk copies of individual* International Agency for Research on Cancer *publications (not subscriptions) may also be ordered from the* Franklin Institute Press, Benjamin Franklin Parkway, Philadelphia, PA 19103

USSR: *For readers in the USSR requiring Russian editions:* Komsomolskij prospekt 18, Medicinskaja Kniga, MOSCOW — *For readers outside the USSR requiring Russian editions:* Kuzneckij most 18, Meždunarodnaja Kniga, MOSCOW G-200

VENEZUELA: Editorial Interamericana de Venezuela C.A., Apartado 50785, CARACAS 105 — Librería del Este, Apartado 60337, CARACAS 106

YUGOSLAVIA: Jugoslovenska Knjiga, Terazije 27/II, 11000 BELGRADE

ZAIRE: Librairie universitaire, avenue de la Paix N° 167, B.P. 1682, KINSHASA I

Special terms for developing countries are obtainable on application to the WHO Programme Coordinators or WHO Regional Offices listed above or to the World Health Organization, Distribution and Sales Service, 1211 Geneva 27, Switzerland. Orders from countries where sales agents have not yet been appointed may also be sent to the Geneva address, but must be paid for in pounds sterling, US dollars, or Swiss francs.

Price: Sw. fr. 100.— US $ 60.00 Prices are subject to change without notice.

IARC/2/78